Introduction to
Radiologic
& Imaging Sciences
& Patient Care

Introduction to

Radiologic
& Imaging Sciences
& Patient Care

SEVENTH EDITION

ARLENE M. ADLER
MEd, RT(R), FAEIRS
Professor Emerita
Radiologic Sciences Programs
Indiana University Northwest
Gary, Indiana

RICHARD R. CARLTON
MS, RT(R)(CV), FAEIRS
Former Chair and Associate Professor of Radiologic and Imaging Sciences
Grand Valley State University
Grand Rapids, Michigan

ELSEVIER

ELSEVIER

3251 Riverport Lane
St. Louis, Missouri 63043

INTRODUCTION TO RADIOLOGIC AND IMAGING SCIENCES AND
PATIENT CARE, 7th EDITION

ISBN: 978-0-323-56671-1

Notices

Knowledge and best practice in this field are constantly changing. As new research and experience broaden our understanding, changes in research methods, professional practices, or medical treatment may become necessary.

Practitioners and researchers must always rely on their own experience and knowledge in evaluating and using any information, methods, compounds, or experiments described herein. In using such information or methods they should be mindful of their own safety and the safety of others, including parties for whom they have a professional responsibility.

With respect to any drug or pharmaceutical products identified, readers are advised to check the most current information provided (i) on procedures featured or (ii) by the manufacturer of each product to be administered, to verify the recommended dose or formula, the method and duration of administration, and contraindications. It is the responsibility of practitioners, relying on their own experience and knowledge of their patients, to make diagnoses, to determine dosages and the best treatment for each individual patient, and to take all appropriate safety precautions.

To the fullest extent of the law, neither the Publisher nor the authors, contributors, or editors, assume any liability for any injury and/or damage to persons or property as a matter of products liability, negligence, or otherwise, or from any use or operation of any methods, products, instructions, or ideas contained in the material herein.

Library of Congress Preassigned Control Number: 2018953141

Content Strategist: Sonya Seigafuse
Senior Content Development Manager: Luke Held
Publishing Services Manager: Julie Eddy
Senior Project Manager: Cindy Thoms
Design Direction: Renee Duenow
Marketing Manager: Jennifer Rolwes

Printed in Canada

Last digit is the print number: 9 8 7 6 5 4 3 2 1

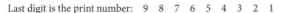

Working together to grow libraries in developing countries

www.elsevier.com • www.bookaid.org

To Don, Meredith, and Katie Adler and to D. Raleigh and Hazel Carlton

and

In memory of Ronald J. Berg, a wonderful patient model

CONTRIBUTORS

Arlene M. Adler, MEd, RT(R), FAEIRS
Professor Emerita
Radiologic Sciences Programs
Indiana University Northwest
Gary, Indiana

Angie Arnold, MEd, RT(R)
Department Chair and Program Director,
    Radiologic Technology
Sinclair Community College
Dayton, Ohio

Vesna Balac, MS, RT(R)(MR)
Program Director and Assistant Clinical Professor
Radiologic Sciences Programs
Indiana University Northwest
Gary, Indiana

Norman E. Bolus, MSPH, MPH, CNMT, FSNMMI-TS
Assistant Professor and Program Director
Nuclear Medicine Program
University of Alabama at Birmingham
Birmingham, Alabama

Jan Bruckner, PhD, PT, CLT-LANA
Physical Therapist
Physical Medicine and Rehabilitation
Aria Health-Jefferson
Philadelphia, Pennsylvania

Lynn Carlton, MSRS, RDMS, RT(R)(M)
Former Director and Assistant Professor of
    Diagnostic Medical Sonography
Grand Valley State University
Grand Rapids, Michigan

Richard R. Carlton, MS, RT(R)(CV), FAEIRS
Former Chair and Associate Professor of
    Radiologic Sciences
Grand Valley State University
Grand Rapids, Michigan

Elizabeth Cloyd, BS, RT(R)(CT)(MR)
Course Director
Nuclear Medicine Department
University of Alabama at Birmingham
Birmingham, Alabama

Melynie Durham, MS, RT(R)(MR)
Clinical Assistant Professor
Radiologic Sciences Programs
Indiana University Northwest
Gary, Indiana

Linda C. Galocy, MS, RHIA, FAHIMA
Program Director and Clinical Associate Professor
Health Information Management Programs
Indiana University Northwest
Gary, Indiana

Julie Gill, PhD, RT(R)(QM)
Department Chair and Professor, Allied Health
University of Cincinnati Blue Ash College
Cincinnati, Ohio

Joanne S. Greathouse, EdS, RT(R), FASRT, FAEIRS
Educational Consultant
Sun City, Arizona

Randy Griswold, MPA, RT(R)
Instructor, Northeast Wisconsin Technical College
Educational Consultant and Lecturer
Green Bay, Wisconsin

Kelli Welch Haynes, EdD, RT(R)
Program Director and Associate Professor
Northwestern State University
Shreveport, LA

Kenya Haugen, DM, MS, RT(R)
Clinical Assistant Professor, Radiologic Sciences
The University of North Carolina at Chapel Hill
Chapel Hill, North Carolina

Tracy Herrmann, PhD, RT(R)
Interim Associate Dean of Academic Affairs
Professor, Allied Health
University of Cincinnati Blue Ash College
Blue Ash, Ohio

James M. Ketchum, MSEd, DHA, RT(R)
Assistant Professor, Radiologic Sciences Program
University of Mississippi Medical Center
Jackson, Mississippi

Rebecca Lamberth, MJ, MS, RT(R)(MR), CRA, FAHRA
Director of Imaging Services
Saint David's South Austin Medical Center
Austin, Texas

Kristi Moore, PhD, RT(R)(CT)
Chair, Program Director and Associate Professor
Radiologic Sciences Program
University of Mississippi Medical Center
Jackson, Mississippi

Ann M. Obergfell, JD, RT(R)
Associate Vice Chancellor and Professor
Indiana University Fort Wayne
Fort Wayne, Indiana

Bettye G. Wilson, MAEd, RT(R)(CT), ARRT, RDMS, FASRT
Education Consultant and Associate Professor Emerita
School of Health Professions
University of Alabama at Birmingham
Birmingham, Alabama

REVIEWERS

Jerry Fox, MEd, RT(R)(N)
Director, Radiography Program
Kishwaukee College
Malta, Illinois

Ericka M. Lasley, MSRS, RT(R)
Program Manager/Director
Mary Washington Hospital School of Radiologic Technology
Fredericksburg, Virginia

Thomas G. Sandridge, MS, MEd, RT(R)
Program Director
Northwestern Memorial Hospital School of Radiography
Chicago, Illinois

It has now been over 25 years and 7 editions since we first published *Introduction to Radiologic and Imaging Sciences and Patient Care*. We continue to be pleased with the success of the book, because it was quickly adopted in radiologic and imaging science classrooms, and we continue to receive comments and suggestions from our colleagues as they make it part of their teaching. We have been delighted with the success of many of our contributing authors over the years, and we think you will find this new edition to be no exception in the quality and relevance of their coverage of the critical issues for beginning clinical practice in our field.

We are always pleased when we are contacted by a teacher and even more pleased when we are contacted by a student in regard to this book. We encourage you to email, phone, write, or simply come up and talk with us at professional meetings. We consider dialogue with you to be absolutely critical to improving our profession, and we do value each and every comment, suggestion, correction, or improvement that you can provide. As with all our new editions, there are numerous updates, clarifications, expanded coverage, and new topics that we added as a result of the commentary we received from students and faculty.

We remain committed to providing a reasonably priced but comprehensive introduction to our profession. We continue to strive to provide the breadth necessary to permit well-informed and properly oriented students their first real clinical practice. We attempt to sufficiently pry open the doors to technical areas so that students will respect not only what they know but how much they don't know as well. We have found that the most dangerous person in a school may well be the first-year student who has had an introduction to psychology but has not yet glimpsed the vast depth of knowledge in this field. He or she runs around trying to apply elementary concepts in interpersonal relationships just enough to thoroughly damage the friendships with anyone foolish enough to take their advice. The danger, of course, is not in what the student knows, but in the failure to appreciate what they do not know. We hope we have avoided setting anyone up for this error by treating our readers as serious new professionals, who are perfectly capable of deducing the potential dangers of the clinical environment while at the same time beginning to learn how to function competently in a manner that begins to make a contribution to our field.

The major changes you will find in the seventh edition include the following:

- Updates made consistent with the relevant Introduction and Patient Care sections of the ASRT curriculum
- Expansion and significant updates to Introduction to Clinical Education
- Additional ethical dilemma examples
- Updates on the current status of digital imaging instrumentation
- Ancillary support for teachers that includes an updated test bank and PowerPoint slides, as well as all artwork for cut and paste use by faculty members—this is available on the accompanying Evolve site online at https://evolve.elsevier.com.
- Patient care laboratories and review questions are included in the printed text and are also available to students on the accompanying Evolve website at http://evolve.clscvicr.com to provide evidence that students have met the necessary clinical prerequisite information before beginning clinical experience.

We continue to assume full responsibility for any errors, including those that may be construed as having arisen from quoting others out of context. We have made every effort to ensure the accuracy of the information. We ask that you remember that it is the responsibility of every practitioner to evaluate the appropriateness of a particular procedure in the context of an actual clinical situation. Consequently, neither the authors nor the publisher take responsibility or accept any liability for the actions of persons applying the information contained herein in an unprofessional manner.

We highly value your point of view. We have learned that the most precious commodity to an author is criticism. As the reader, your perceptions are very important to us and we always appreciate that you communicate with us regarding any aspect of the book you like, dislike, or would like to see changed. As in all our books, we point out that a book such as this is never finished but merely abandoned until the next edition.

Arlene M. Adler, Indiana University Northwest
aadler@iun.edu
Richard R. Carlton, Grand Valley State University
carltonr@gvsu.edu

ACKNOWLEDGMENTS

Students are always the best teachers, and we have had some of the very greatest at Indiana University Northwest in Gary, Indiana; Michael Reese Hospital in Chicago; Grand Valley State University in Grand Rapids, Michigan; Wilbur Wright College in Chicago; Lima Technical College in Lima, Ohio; City College of San Francisco; Mills-Peninsula School of Radiologic Technology, Burlingame, California; Memphis' Methodist School of Radiologic Technology; and Arkansas State University. We thank you all for listening and valuing what we have tried to teach you.

Rick offers many thanks for the constant and solid support of Lynn Carlton, MS, RDMS, RT(R)(M) at Grand Valley State University. Arlene would like to thank her professional colleagues: Robin Jones, MS, RT(R); Sharon Lakia, RDMS, MS, RT(R); Vesna Balac, MS, RT(R)(MR); Amanda Sorg, BS, RT(T); Sue Woods, AS, RT(R); Shannon Baimakovich, AS, RT(R) Angela Brite, AS, RT(R), Helen Campbell, RT(R); Char Gilpin, RT(R); Sue Janosky, BS, RT(R); Heather Govert, BS, RT(R), Patricia Lewis, RT(R); Sheri Stremplewski, BS, RT(R); Becky Wantland RT(R); Sue Wilson, AS, RT(R); and Laura Zlamal, RT(R), all with the Radiologic Sciences Programs at Indiana University Northwest.

Special thanks are owed to the Radiology Department at Methodist Hospital Southlake in Merrillville and Julie Aguayo, AS, RT(R), St. Rita's Medical Center in Lima, Ohio; Ronald and Rita Berg, Edyta Postolowicz, Dennis Stryker, Brian Nye, John Jacobs, Jill Steinbrenner; Sally Singer, Jeff Lloyd, and Kay Williams at Spectrum Health in Grand Rapids, Michigan. Appreciation is also extended to our photographers, John Geiger and Jenny Torbett, from the Biomedical Communications Department at The Ohio State University; the late George D. Greathouse of Phoenix, Arizona; and Curt Steele of Arkansas State University. Our early edition photographs were great because of the spectacular performance of the best pediatric model ever, Meredith Adler, who has now headed off to college and been replaced by the spectacular performances of Landon Parkison and Emma Speck.

Arlene M. Adler, MEd, RT(R), FAEIRS
Richard R. Carlton, MS, RT(R)(CV), FAEIRS

CONTENTS

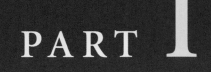

PART I

The Profession of Radiologic Technology

1

Introduction to Imaging and Radiologic Sciences

Arlene M. Adler, MEd, RT(R), FAEIRS,
Richard R. Carlton, MS, RT(R)(CV), FAEIRS

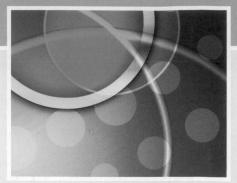

During World War I, the demand for x-ray technicians in military hospitals was so great that a shortage of technical workers became acute at home. The value of the well-trained technician was emphasized, and the radiologist was no longer satisfied with someone who knew only how to throw the switch and develop films.

Margaret Hoing, The First Lady of Radiologic Technology
A History of the American Society of X-Ray Technicians, 1952

OBJECTIVES

On completion of this chapter, the student will be able to:
- Explain the use of radiation in medicine.
- Provide an overview of the history of medicine.
- Describe the discovery of x-rays.
- Define terms related to radiologic technology.
- Explain the career opportunities within the profession of radiologic technology.
- Identify the various specialties within a radiology department.
- Describe the typical responsibilities of the members of the radiology team.
- Explain the career-ladder opportunities within a radiology department.
- Discuss the roles of other members of the health care team.

OUTLINE

KEY TERMS

Bone Densitometry (BD) Measurement of bone density using dual-energy x-ray absorptiometry (DEXA or DXA) to detect osteoporosis

Cardiovascular Interventional Technology (CVIT) Radiologic procedures for the diagnosis and treatment of diseases of the cardiovascular system

Computed Tomography (CT) Recording of a predetermined plane in the body using an x-ray beam that is measured, recorded, and then processed by a computer for display on a monitor

Diagnostic Medical Sonography Visualization of deep structures of the body by recording the reflections of pulses of ultrasonic waves directed into the tissue

Energy Capacity to operate or work

Ionization Any process by which a neutral atom gains or loses an electron, thus acquiring a net charge

Magnetic Resonance Imaging (MRI) Process of using a magnetic field and radiofrequencies to create sectional images of the body

Mammography Radiography of the breast

Nuclear Medicine Technology Branch of radiology that involves the introduction of radioactive substances into the body for both diagnostic and therapeutic purposes

Positron Emission Tomography (PET) The creation of sectional images of the body that demonstrate the physiologic function of various organs and systems

Radiation Energy transmitted by waves through space or through a medium

Radiation Therapy Branch of radiology involved in the treatment of disease by means of x-rays or radioactive substances

Radiography Making of records (radiographs) of internal structures of the body by passing x-rays or gamma rays through the body to act on specially sensitized film or an imaging plate or system

Radiologic Technologist (RT) General term applied to an individual who performs radiography, radiation therapy, or nuclear medicine technology

Radiologist Physician who specializes in the use of x-rays and other forms of both ionizing and nonionizing radiation in the diagnosis and treatment of disease

Radiologist Assistant (RA) An advanced-level radiographer who extends the capacity of the radiologist in the diagnostic imaging environment, thereby enhancing patient care

Radiology Branch of the health sciences dealing with radioactive substances and radiant energy and with the diagnosis and treatment of disease by means of both ionizing (e.g., roentgen rays) and nonionizing (e.g., ultrasound) radiation

Roentgen Ray Synonym for *x-ray*

X-ray Electromagnetic radiation of short wavelength that is produced when electrons moving at high velocity are suddenly stopped

MEDICAL RADIATION SCIENCES

When the term *radiation* is used, it generally evokes concern and a sense of danger. This circumstance is unfortunate because radiation not only is helpful but also is essential to life. **Radiation** is energy that is transmitted by waves through space or through a medium (matter); it has permeated the universe since the beginning of time and is a natural part of all of our lives. For example, the sun radiates light energy, and a stove radiates heat energy.

Energy is the capacity to operate or work. The many different forms of energy include mechanical, electrical, heat, nuclear, and electromagnetic energy. Many forms of energy are used in medicine to create images of anatomic structures or physiologic actions. These images are essential for the proper diagnosis of disease and treatment of the patient. All of these energy forms can be described as *radiation* because they can be, and in many instances must be, transmitted through matter.

Some higher energy forms, including x-rays, have the ability to ionize atoms in matter. **Ionization** is any process by which a neutral atom gains or loses an electron, thus acquiring a net charge. This process has the ability to disrupt the composition of the matter and, as a result, is capable of disrupting life processes. Special protection should be provided to prevent excessive exposure to ionizing radiation.

Sound is a form of mechanical energy. It is transmitted through matter, and images of the returning sound waves can be created. Diagnostic medical sonography is the field of study that creates anatomic images by recording reflected sound waves. Sound waves are a form of nonionizing radiation.

Electrocardiography and *electroencephalography* are methods of imaging the electrical activities of the heart and of the brain, respectively. The graphs they produce provide useful information about the physiologic activities of these organs.

The body's naturally emitted heat energy can also produce images for diagnostic purposes. These images are called *thermograms,* and they can be useful in demonstrating conditions such as changes in the body's circulation.

Nuclear energy is emitted by the nucleus of an atom. Nuclear medicine technology uses this type of energy to create images of both anatomic structures and physiologic actions. It involves the introduction of a radioactive substance into the body for diagnostic

and therapeutic purposes. These substances emit gamma radiation from their nuclei. *Gamma radiation* is a form of electromagnetic energy that has the ability to ionize atoms. As a result, proper radiation protection is important in the nuclear medicine department.

Electromagnetic energy has many forms (Fig. 1.1). Many of these forms are used in medicine to deliver high-quality patient care. For example, light is an essential energy form in many of the scopes used by physicians to view inside the body. In addition, x-rays are a human-made form of electromagnetic energy. They are created when electrons moving at high speed are suddenly stopped. X-rays, also called **roentgen rays**, named after their discoverer, Wilhelm Conrad Röntgen, allow physicians to visualize many of the anatomic structures that were once visible only at surgery.

Radiography is the making of records, known as *radiographs*, of internal structures of the body by passage of x-rays or gamma rays through the body to act on, historically, specially sensitized film or, most commonly, on a digital imaging plate or detector. In the diagnostic radiography department, images are created using x-rays that pass through the body (Fig. 1.2). In addition, very-high-energy x-rays are used in the radiation therapy department for the treatment of many forms of cancer. In both of these departments, proper radiation protection is essential.

Radio waves are another form of electromagnetic radiation. They are a nonionizing form of radiation and are important in **magnetic resonance imaging (MRI)** (Fig. 1.3).

Medical radiation science involves the study of the use of radiation throughout medicine. The fact that many forms of radiation are used in all branches of medicine should be apparent. Because many laypeople assume that the terms *radiation* and *ionizing radiation* are used interchangeably, the term *imaging sciences* has been preferred to the term *radiation* or *radiologic sciences* in areas that use a nonionizing form of radiation such as diagnostic medical sonography and MRI. Furthermore, because radiation therapy is primarily involved in treatment and not imaging, the term *imaging sciences* alone is not encompassing enough. As a result, many feel that our profession is best described by both terms, *imaging* and *radiation* or *radiologic sciences*. With regard to the profession, the term *radiologic technology* is used by the American Registry of Radiologic Technologists (ARRT) to encompass all of our individual disciplines.

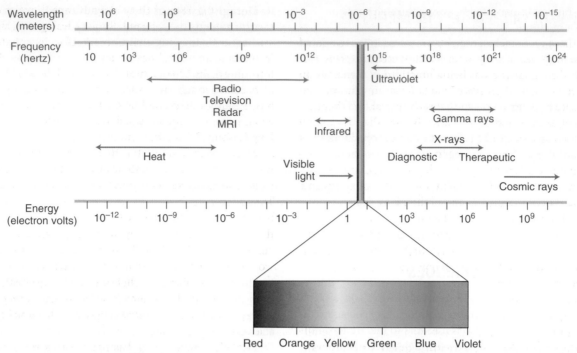

Wavelength (meters)

Frequency (hertz)

Radio
Television
Radar
MRI

Heat

Infrared

Visible light

Ultraviolet

Gamma rays

X-rays

Diagnostic   Therapeutic

Cosmic rays

Energy (electron volts)

Red   Orange   Yellow   Green   Blue   Violet

Fig. 1.1 The electromagnetic spectrum. *MRI,* Magnetic resonance imaging.

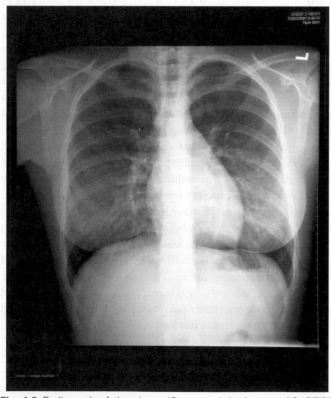

Fig. 1.2 Radiograph of the chest. (Courtesy Julie Aguayo, AS, RT[R], Methodist Hospital Southlake Campus, Merrillville, IN.)

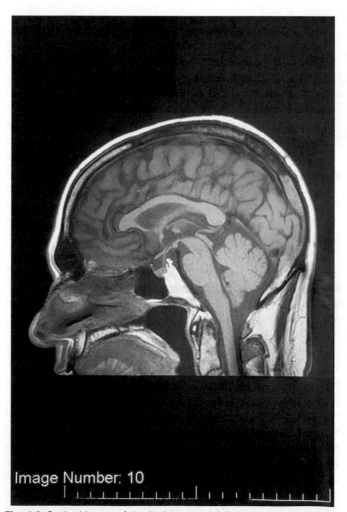

Image Number: 10

Fig. 1.3 Sagittal image of the brain created using magnetic resonance imaging. (Courtesy Julie Aguayo, AS, RT[R], Methodist Hospital South-lake Campus, Merrillville, IN.)

OVERVIEW OF THE HISTORY OF MEDICINE

Humankind's attempt to treat and cure diseases can be dated back almost 5000 years to Egypt and Mesopotamia, where evidence exists that medicine was being practiced in combination with religious beliefs. Prehistoric skulls found in Europe and South America also demonstrate that early humans deliberately removed bone from the skull successfully. Whether this action was performed as a surgical treatment or as a religious attempt to release evil spirits is unknown. In addition, evidence exists that many potent drugs still in use today, such as castor oil and opium, were used in ancient Egypt for medicinal purposes. However, the Egyptians demonstrated little knowledge of anatomy, despite their sophisticated embalming skills.

The understanding of human anatomy and physiology by the early Greek philosophers was of such high quality that it was not equaled for hundreds of years. Hippocrates (c. 460–370 BC) was a Greek physician who is considered the father of Western medicine. Little is really known about him, but the fact that he was a contemporary of Socrates and was one of the most famous physicians and teachers of medicine of his time is generally accepted. More than 60 medical treatises, called the *Hippocratic Corpus*, traditionally have been attributed to him; however, Hippocrates did not write most of them himself. The writings are similar in that they emphasize rational and natural explanations for the treatment of disease and reject sorcery and magic. Hippocrates emphasized the importance of carefully observing the patient. He believed in the powers of nature to heal over time and taught the prevention of disease through a regimen of diet and exercise. He is also attributed with developing a high standard of ethical conduct, as incorporated in the Hippocratic Oath, which provided guidelines for physician-patient relationships, for the rights of patients to privacy, and for the use of treatment for curative purposes only. The Hippocratic Oath still governs the ethical conduct of physicians today.

The Romans recognized the importance of proper sanitation for good public health, evidenced by their construction of aqueducts, baths, sewers, and hospitals. Unfortunately, during the Middle Ages the destruction or neglect of the Roman sanitary facilities resulted in many local epidemics that eventually led to the great plague, known as the *Black Death*, during the 14th century. Medicine was strongly controlled by religious groups during this period, and it was not until the early 1500s that a physician in England had to be licensed to practice.

By the 17th century, medicine began to develop an increasingly scientific experimental approach. William Harvey (1578–1657), an English physician, is considered by many scholars to have laid the foundation of modern medicine. Harvey was first to demonstrate the function of the heart and the circulation of the blood. This feat is especially remarkable because it was accomplished without the aid of a microscope. By the end of the 17th century, bacteria had been described by Anton Van Leeuwenhoek (1632–1723), a Dutch zoologist, who isolated the microorganism with a microscope he made. With the development of improved microscopes, the discovery of the capillary system of the blood helped complete Harvey's explanation of blood circulation.

During the 18th century a significant number of developments in medicine occurred. Surgery was becoming an experimental science, a large number of reforms were taking place in the area of mental health, and the heart drug digitalis was introduced. In 1796, Edward Jenner (1749–1823), an English physician, introduced a vaccine to prevent smallpox when he inoculated an 8-year-old boy, which proved that cowpox provided immunity against smallpox. This discovery served as the foundation for the field of immunology.

In the 19th century the theory that germs cause disease was established. Louis Pasteur (1822–1895), a French chemist, worked with bacteria to prove the germ theory of infection. Through his work, the process of pasteurization was developed. Robert Koch (1843–1910), a German bacteriologist, established the bacterial cause for many infections, such as anthrax, tuberculosis, and cholera. In 1905 Koch received a Nobel Prize for his work in developing tuberculin as a test for tuberculosis. During the mid-1800s Florence Nightingale (1820–1910), an English nurse, developed the foundations for modern nursing. In 1895, Wilhelm Röntgen discovered x-rays, and the radiologic imaging sciences had their start.

The 20th century saw development of the use of the scientific method throughout medicine. The early part of the century welcomed discovery of the first antibiotics. Sir Alexander Fleming (1881–1955), a Scottish bacteriologist, discovered penicillin in 1928. Further medical advances included the increased use of chemotherapy and a better understanding of the immune system, which resulted in the increased prophylactic use of vaccines such as the Salk vaccine, discovered by Jonas Salk (1914–1995), which helped to control and prevent poliomyelitis. Increased knowledge of the endocrine system has helped to treat diseases resulting from hormone imbalance, including the use of insulin to treat diabetes.

In 1953, at Cambridge University in England, Francis Crick (1916–2004), an English scientist, and James Watson (b. 1928), an American biologist, announced that they had discovered the *secret of life*. Through their work, they identified the molecular structure of deoxyribonucleic acid (DNA), a key to heredity and genetics. Currently, much research is being devoted to the field of genetics. Completed in 2003, the Human Genome Project (HGP) was a 13-year international scientific research project coordinated by the US Department of Energy and the National Institutes of Health. During the early years of the HGP, the Wellcome Trust (United Kingdom) became a major partner; additional partners came from Japan, France, Germany, China, and others. The project goals were to:

- *Identify* all of the approximately 20,000 to 25,000 genes in human DNA
- *Determine* the sequences of the 3 billion chemical base pairs that make up human DNA
- *Store* this information in databases
- *Improve* tools for data analysis
- *Transfer* related technologies to the private sector
- *Address* the ethical, legal, and social issues that may arise from the project

Although the HGP is finished, analyses of the data will continue for many years. The replacement of faulty genes through gene therapy offers promises of cures for a variety of hereditary diseases, and, through genetic engineering, important pharmaceuticals have been developed.

HISTORY OF RADIOLOGIC TECHNOLOGY

The field of radiologic technology began on November 8, 1895, when Wilhelm Röntgen, a German physicist, was working in his laboratory at the University of Wurzburg. Röntgen had been experimenting with cathode rays and was exploring their properties outside glass tubes. He had covered the glass tube to prevent any visible light from escaping. During this work, Röntgen observed that a screen that had been painted with barium platinocyanide was emitting light *(fluorescing)*. This effect had to be caused by invisible rays being emitted from the tube. During the next several weeks, Röntgen investigated these invisible rays. During his investigation, he saw the very first radiographic image—his own skeleton. Röntgen became the first radiographer when he produced a series of photographs of radiographic images, most notably the image of his wife's hand (Fig. 1.4). He termed these invisible rays *x-rays* because *x* is the symbol for an unknown variable.

Wilhelm Röntgen was born in Lennep, Germany, on March 27, 1845. In 1872, he married Anna Bertha Ludwig (1839–1919), and they had one adopted daughter. In 1888, Röntgen began working at the University of Wurzburg in the physics department. During the 1870s and 1880s, many physics departments were experimenting with cathode rays, electrons emanating from the negative (cathode) terminal of a tube. During his discovery, Röntgen worked with a Crookes tube. Sir William Crookes (1832–1919) used a large, partially evacuated glass tube that encompassed a cathode and an anode attached to an electrical supply. His tube was the early version of the modern fluorescent light. Crookes actually produced x-rays during his experimentation in the 1870s but failed to grasp the significance of his finding. He often found that photographic plates stored near his worktable were fogged. He even returned fogged photographic plates to the manufacturer, claiming they were defective. Many physicists created x-rays during the course of their work with cathode rays, but Röntgen was the first to appreciate the significance of the penetrating rays.

The actual day that the significance of Röntgen's finding became clear to him is the subject of much debate. However, Friday, November 8, 1895, is believed by historians to be the day that Röntgen created the famous image of his wife's hand (see Fig. 1.4). On Saturday, December 28, 1895, Röntgen submitted his first report, titled *On a New Kind of Rays,* to the Wurzburg Physico-Medical Society. Through his investigative methods, Röntgen identified the properties of x-rays. His methods were so thorough that no significant additions have been made to his work.

For his efforts, Röntgen was honored in 1901 with the first Nobel Prize in physics. He refused to patent any part of his discovery and rejected many commercial company offers. As a result, he saw little financial reward for his work. He died on February 10, 1923, of colon cancer.

Throughout the 20th century, the use of x-rays advanced significantly to include the imaging of almost all aspects of

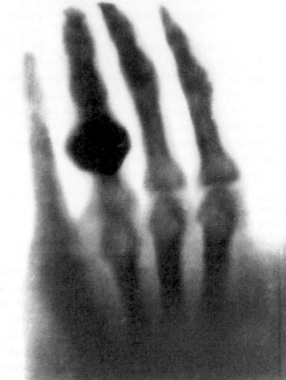

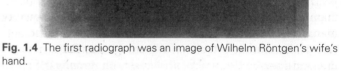

Fig. 1.4 The first radiograph was an image of Wilhelm Röntgen's wife's hand.

the human body and the treatment of diseases with radiation therapy. In addition, radioactive substances came into use for both imaging (nuclear medicine) and treatment. By the 1970s, imaging had further advanced to include diagnostic medical sonography, computed tomography (CT), and MRI. Today, through the use of hybrid scanners that combine nuclear medicine imaging with either CT or MRI, both anatomic and physiologic function can be assessed in a single examination.

OPPORTUNITIES IN RADIOLOGIC TECHNOLOGY

Radiologic technology is the technical science that deals with the use of x-rays or radioactive substances for diagnostic or therapeutic purposes in medicine. **Radiologic technologist (RT)** is a general term applied to persons qualified to use x-rays *(radiography)* or radioactive substances *(nuclear medicine)* to produce images of the internal parts of the body for interpretation by a physician known as a **radiologist.** Radiologic technology also involves the use of x-rays or radioactive substances in the treatment of disease *(radiation therapy)*.

In addition to using x-rays and radioactive substances, RTs are also involved in using high-frequency sound waves (diagnostic medical sonography) and magnetic fields and radio waves (MRI) to create images of the internal anatomy of the body.

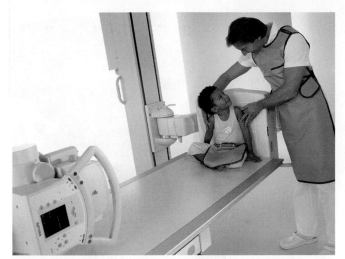

Fig. 1.5 A radiographer positions a patient for a radiographic examination. (Courtesy Philips Medical Systems.)

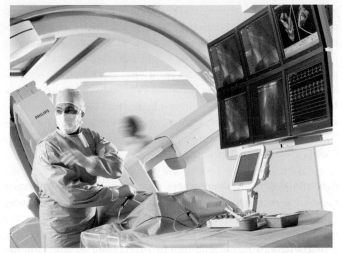

Fig. 1.6 A physician performs a cardiovascular interventional procedure in a vascular suite, which may be located in the cardiology, radiology, or surgery department. (Courtesy Philips Medical Systems.)

The ARRT is the credentialing organization for medical imaging, interventional procedures, and radiation therapy. The organization identifies the following disciplines that are included in the profession of radiologic technology: radiography (R), nuclear medicine technology (N), radiation therapy (T), magnetic resonance imaging (MR), sonography (S), cardiovascular-interventional radiography (CV), mammography (M), computed tomography (CT), quality management (QM), bone densitometry (BD), vascular sonography (VS), cardiac-interventional radiography (CI), vascular-interventional radiography (VI), breast sonography (BS), and radiologist assistants (RRA). From this list, one can see how all-encompassing the profession of radiologic technology truly is.

Radiography

An RT specializing in the use of x-rays to create images of the body is known as a *radiographer* (Fig. 1.5). Radiographers perform a wide variety of diagnostic x-ray procedures, including examinations of the skeletal system, the chest, and the abdomen. They administer contrast media to permit visualization of the gastrointestinal (GI) tract and the genitourinary system. They also assist the radiologist during more specialized contrast media procedures, such as those used to visualize the spinal cord *(myelography)* and the joint spaces *(arthrography)*.

To become a registered radiographer, one must complete an ARRT-recognized radiography program. Programs are most commonly sponsored by hospitals, community colleges, and universities. There are approximately 730 ARRT-recognized radiography programs, primarily in the United States. On successful completion of a recognized program, individuals are awarded a certificate, an associate degree, or a baccalaureate degree and are eligible to take the national examination in radiography offered by the ARRT. Effective January 1, 2015, all candidates must have earned an academic degree to qualify for this certification. A registered radiographer uses the initials *RT(R) (ARRT)* after his or her name. This abbreviation means *registered technologist (radiography)*.

Appendix A contains Clinical Practice Standards for Radiography, developed by the American Society of Radiologic Technologists. These practice standards help to define the role of the radiographer and establish criteria used to judge performance.

Cardiovascular Interventional Technology. Radiographers can specialize in performing radiologic examinations of the cardiovascular system, a discipline called cardiovascular interventional technology (CVIT) (Fig. 1.6). These procedures involve the injection of iodinated contrast media for diagnosing diseases of the heart and blood vessels. *Angiography* is the term for radiologic examination of the blood vessels after injection of a contrast medium. Most often, the contrast material is injected through a catheter, which can be directed to a variety of major arteries or veins for visualization of these structures. By way of a catheter, injecting contrast media into structures such as the carotid arteries leading to the brain, the renal arteries leading to the kidneys, the femoral artery of the leg, and many other sites is relatively easy.

Placing a catheter into one of the chambers of the heart is termed *cardiac catheterization.* This catheter then can be directed into one or both of the two main arteries that supply blood to the heart itself. These arteries are called the *coronary arteries.*

Coronary arteriography is an extremely valuable tool in diagnosing atherosclerosis, which can block the coronary arteries and cause a heart attack *(myocardial infarction)*. By way of a special catheter with a balloon tip, effective treatment of atherosclerosis is possible. This treatment of a blocked blood vessel is termed *angioplasty*. Angioplasty is used to treat patients without having to use invasive open heart surgery. In addition to angioplasty, blocked vessels are also treated by placing a stent in the vessel to physically keep it open.

CVIT involves the use of highly specialized equipment and complex procedures. This specialization of equipment and supplies has resulted in a need for radiographers to be specially prepared in this advanced technology. Most of this advanced education occurs through continuing education classes and on-the-job clinical experience. In 1991 the ARRT began offering a postprimary examination in CV. This examination is no longer offered but has been split into two separate examinations, one for cardiac interventional (CI) technology and another for vascular interventional (VI) technology. To qualify to take either examination, individuals must be ARRT certified in radiography and meet clinical requirements. An ARRT-certified individual uses the initials *RT(CI)(ARRT)* and/or *RT(VI) (ARRT)* after his or her name.

Mammography. Radiographers can specialize in performing radiologic examination of the breast, a procedure called **mammography**. Mammography is a valuable diagnostic tool for the early detection of breast disease, especially breast cancer. Current statistics indicate that one of every eight or nine women in the United States will develop breast cancer. Men are not excluded from this disease; approximately 1% of breast cancers are found in men. Early detection of breast cancer is important to successful treatment and cure. As a result, the American Cancer Society has recommended regular mammography screening for all women older than 40 years.

This emphasis on screening mammography has resulted in an increase in the number of mammographic examinations being performed across the country. Special breast imaging centers have been built to accommodate the demand for these procedures. Equipment and supplies, such as a specially designed x-ray tube and high-resolution digital imaging detectors, are used to create high-quality breast images. This specialization of equipment and supplies has resulted in a need for radiographers to be specially prepared in this advanced technology. Most of this advanced education occurs through continuing education classes and on-the-job clinical experience. In 1992 the ARRT began offering a postprimary examination in mammography. To qualify to take the examination, individuals must be ARRT certified in radiography and meet educational and clinical requirements. An ARRT-certified individual uses the initials *RT(M)(ARRT)* after his or her name.

Radiologist Assistant. A **radiologist assistant (RA)** is an advanced-level radiographer who extends the capacity of the radiologist in the diagnostic imaging environment, thereby enhancing patient care. The RRA is an ARRT-certified radiographer who has completed an advanced academic program encompassing a nationally recognized RRA curriculum and a radiologist-directed clinical preceptorship. RRAs perform a wide variety of patient care procedures under the direction of the radiologist. These procedures include fluoroscopic examinations such as GI studies, myelograms, arthrograms, and central venous line placements, along with contrast media and general medication administration. RAs also evaluate images for completeness and diagnostic quality and report clinical observations to the radiologist.

The concept of the RRA has moved in and out of popularity in the United States. Pilot programs at the University of Kentucky and Duke University were launched in the mid-1970s to educate technologists to carry out certain tasks traditionally

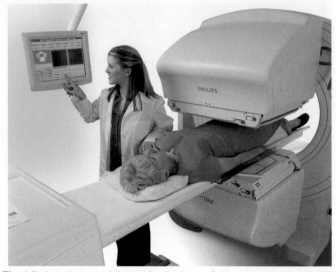

Fig. 1.7 A nuclear medicine technologist performs procedures requiring the use of radioactive substances. (Courtesy Philips Medical Systems.)

performed by radiologists. The programs produced a small number of graduates before they were forced to close when federal funding was cut in the late 1970s. The American College of Radiology was not in support of the concept, and the programs slowly died over the next 20 years. A new era of RRA programs began in 1995, when Weber State University in Utah started a 2-year educational program for registered RTs who had at least 5 years of experience and wanted to work in an advanced clinical role. Although this program has also been somewhat controversial, it was joined in 2003 by a Bachelor of Science program at Loma Linda University in California and in 2004 by several other undergraduate programs around the country. In 2005 the ARRT began offering a postprimary examination for RRAs. To qualify to take the examination, individuals must be ARRT certified in radiography, earn a bachelor's degree, have at least 1 year of acceptable clinical experience in radiography, complete an ARRT-approved RRA education program, and meet the educational, ethics, and examination standards established by the ARRT. Currently, eight ARRT-Recognized RRA Educational Programs are listed on the ARRT website at http://www.arrt. org. In addition to RRAs, there are RTs who have also completed a physician assistant program and who work with radiologists much as the RRA does. An ARRT-certified individual uses the initials *R.R.A. (ARRT)* after his or her name.

Nuclear Medicine

The branch of radiologic technology that involves procedures that require the use of radioactive materials for diagnostic or therapeutic purposes is **nuclear medicine technology** (Fig. 1.7). Nuclear medicine procedures usually involve the imaging of a patient's organs—such as the liver, heart, or brain—after the introduction of a radioactive material known as a *radiopharmaceutical*. Radiopharmaceuticals are usually administered intravenously but can be administered orally or by inhalation. Procedures can also be performed on specimens such as blood or urine. Samples from a patient can be combined with a radioactive substance to measure various constituents

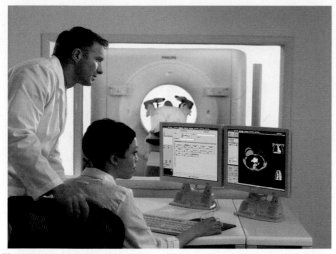

Fig. 1.8 A radiation therapist administers radiation treatments to patients with lesions. A radiation therapist is using a specialized oncology computed tomography unit to perform initial treatment-planning studies on a patient. (Courtesy Philips Medical Systems.)

in the sample. Radiopharmaceuticals are also used to perform **positron emission tomography (PET)** procedures. After the injection of a positron-emitting radioisotope, PET scans create sectional images of the body that demonstrate the physiologic function of various organs and systems. Today many PET scanners are combined with CT or MR to acquire both the functional images that PET can provide with the anatomic references that CT and MR accomplish. These hybrid imaging techniques have advantages over either system performed separately.

To become a registered nuclear medicine technologist, completing an accredited nuclear medicine technology program is necessary. There are approximately 115 ARRT-recognized programs, primarily in the United States. Most commonly sponsored by hospitals, community colleges, or universities, these programs vary in length from 1-year programs to 4-year baccalaureate programs. One-year programs are usually designed for persons who already hold credentials in radiography, medical technology, or nursing or who possess a baccalaureate degree in one of the basic sciences. Effective January 1, 2015, all candidates must have earned an academic degree to qualify for ARRT certification. Graduates of an accredited program are eligible to take the national examination in nuclear medicine technology offered by either the ARRT or the Nuclear Medicine Technology Certification Board (NMTCB). Successful completion of one of these two examinations is usually required for employment. An ARRT-certified person uses the initials *RT(N) (ARRT)* after his or her name, meaning *registered technologist (nuclear medicine technology).* An NMTCB-certified individual uses the initials *CNMT* after his or her name, signifying *certified nuclear medicine technologist.*

Radiation Therapy

A **radiation therapy** technologist, or *radiation therapist,* is a person who administers radiation treatments to patients according to the prescription and instructions of a physician, known as a *radiation oncologist* (Fig. 1.8). *Radiation oncology* involves the use of high-energy ionizing radiation to treat primarily malignant tumors *(cancer).* Therapists are responsible for administering

a planned course of prescribed radiation treatments using high-technology therapeutic equipment and accessories. They provide specialized patient care and observe the clinical progress of their patients. Radiation therapists can specialize in the area of medical dosimetry. *Medical dosimetrists* are involved in treatment planning and dose calculations. This specialized area usually requires advanced education and certification.

To become a registered radiation therapist, it is necessary to complete an ARRT-recognized radiation therapy program. There are approximately 110 educational programs, primarily in the United States. Programs are most commonly sponsored by hospitals, community colleges, or universities and vary in length from 1-year programs to 4-year baccalaureate programs. One-year programs are usually designed for persons who already have credentials in radiography or who can demonstrate competence in the areas identified in the essentials for a radiation therapy program. Effective January 1, 2015, all candidates must have earned an academic degree to qualify for certification. Graduates of an ARRT-recognized program are eligible to take the national examination in radiation therapy offered by the ARRT. An ARRT-certified individual uses the initials *RT(T) (ARRT)* after his or her name. This abbreviation means *registered technologist (radiation therapy).*

Bone Densitometry — → checking bone/calcium levels

Bone densitometry (BD) is most often used to diagnose osteoporosis, a condition that is often recognized in menopausal women but can also occur in men. Osteoporosis involves a gradual loss of calcium, causing the bones to become thin, fragile, and prone to fractures. Routine x-ray examinations can diagnose bone fractures but are not the best way to assess bone density. To detect osteoporosis accurately, dual-energy x-ray absorptiometry (DEXA or DXA) is used. DEXA BD is the current standard for measuring bone mineral density. Measurement of the lower spine and hips is most often performed. The International Society for Clinical Densitometry has offered the Certified Bone Densitometry Technologist credential since 1993. In 2001 the ARRT began offering a postprimary examination in BD. To qualify to take the examination, individuals must be ARRT certified in radiography, nuclear medicine technology (or NMTCB certified), or radiation therapy and meet clinical requirements. An ARRT-certified individual uses the initials *RT(BD)(ARRT)* after his or her name.

Computed Tomography — → higher levels of radiation than x-ray

Computed tomography (CT) is the recording of a predetermined plane in the body using an x-ray beam that is measured, recorded, and then processed by a computer for display on a monitor (Fig. 1.9). This technology allows physicians to visualize patient anatomy in various sectional planes.

CT involves the use of highly specialized equipment and complex procedures, which has resulted in a need for radiographers to be specially prepared in this advanced technology. Most of this advanced education occurs through continuing education courses and on-the-job clinical experience. In 1995 the ARRT began offering a postprimary examination in CT. To qualify to take the examination, individuals must be ARRT

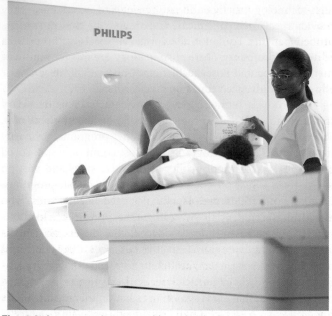

Fig. 1.9 A computed tomographic technologist uses a computerized x-ray system to produce sectional anatomic images of the body. (Courtesy Philips Medical Systems.)

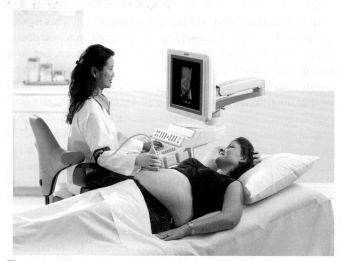

Fig. 1.10 A diagnostic medical sonographer uses high-frequency sound waves to create images. (Courtesy Philips Medical Systems.)

certified in radiography, nuclear medicine technology (or NMTCB certified), or radiation therapy technology and meet clinical requirements. An ARRT-certified individual uses the initials *RT(CT)(ARRT)* after his or her name.

Diagnostic Medical Sonography

Diagnostic medical sonography is the visualization of structures of the body by recording the reflections of pulses of high-frequency sound *(ultrasound)* waves directed into the tissue. A person who specializes in this field is known as a *diagnostic medical sonographer* (Fig. 1.10).

Sonographers may have previous experience as radiographers, but this experience is not required. To become a sonographer, the candidate can either complete a diagnostic medical sonography program or, less commonly, be prepared on the

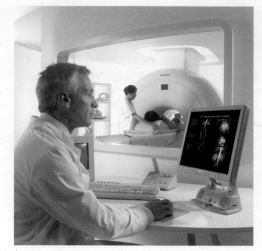

Fig. 1.11 A magnetic resonance imaging technologist uses electromagnetics, specifically radio waves and magnetism, to create diagnostic sectional images of the body. (Courtesy Philips Medical Systems.)

job. On-the-job clinical experience is typically provided only to persons who have previous experience in another health specialty, such as radiography. Individuals are eligible to take a national examination offered by the American Registry of Diagnostic Medical Sonographers (ARDMS) through a variety of pathways. A *registered diagnostic medical sonographer* uses the initials *RDMS* after his or her name. A *registered vascular technologist* uses the initials *RVT* after his or her name. A *registered diagnostic cardiac sonographer* uses the initials *RDCS* after his or her name. In addition, a *cardiovascular credentialing international organization* provides cardiac sonographers with a credential that allows them to use the initials *CCI* after their names.

In 1999 the ARRT began offering a postprimary examination in sonography. To qualify to take the examination, individuals must be ARRT certified in radiography, nuclear medicine technology (or NMTCB certified), radiation therapy, or MRI (or ARDMS certified) and meet clinical requirements. Candidates can also become eligible to take the examination by completing a formal ARRT-recognized educational program in sonography. There are approximately 165 ARRT-recognized sonography programs, primarily in the United States. Effective January 1, 2015, all candidates must have earned an academic degree to qualify for ARRT certification. An ARRT-certified individual uses the initials *RT(S)(ARRT)* after his or her name.

Magnetic Resonance Imaging

MRI uses a strong magnetic field and radio waves along with a computer to generate sectional images of patient anatomy (Fig. 1.11). Like CT, this advanced technology uses highly specialized equipment and requires specialized education. Although many MRI technologists have obtained their education through continuing education courses and on-the-job clinical experience, formal educational programs now exist with baccalaureate, associate, or certificate credentials. For the most part, MRI technologists have credentials in radiography and many are also experienced CT technologists. In 1995 the ARRT began offering a postprimary pathway for the certification examination in MRI. To qualify to take the examination, individuals must be ARRT certified in radiography, nuclear medicine technology (or NMTCB certified), radiation therapy, or sonography (or ARDMS certified) and meet clinical requirements. Candidates can also become eligible to take the primary magnetic resonance examination by completing a formal educational program in MRI approved by the ARRT. There are approximately 60 ARRT-recognized educational programs in MRI. Effective January 1, 2015, all candidates must have earned an academic degree to qualify for this certification. An ARRT-certified individual uses the initials *RT(MR)* after his or her name.

Additional Opportunities

Regardless of the area in which an individual chooses to specialize within the profession of radiologic technology, additional opportunities exist in education, management, and commercial firms.

Education. Individuals who have an interest in teaching any of the specific disciplines can find opportunities in hospitals, colleges, and universities. Careers include clinical instructor, didactic faculty member, clinical coordinator, and program director.

A *clinical instructor* teaches students primarily on a one-on-one basis in the clinical setting. A *didactic faculty member* teaches students typically through classroom lectures and laboratory activities. A *clinical coordinator* has teaching responsibilities along with administrative duties in overseeing clinical education, most often in programs using many clinical education centers. A *program director* has teaching responsibilities, as well as overall administrative responsibility for the entire educational program. Advanced coursework in education is desirable for these positions. Program directors are required to have a master's degree.

Administration. Persons who have an interest in the management of the radiology services in a given facility can specialize in a wide spectrum of supervisory and administrative positions. Many departments have supervisory positions in areas such as CT, MRI, interventional, mammography, sonography, and QM. In 1997 the ARRT began offering a postprimary examination in QM. To be eligible to take the examination, individuals must be ARRT certified in radiography, nuclear medicine technology (or NMTCB certified), or radiation therapy and meet the educational and clinical requirements. An ARRT-certified individual uses the initials *RT(QM)(ARRT)* after his or her name. The QM credential will no longer be issued after June 30, 2018. The ARRT surveyed QM practitioners, and the results indicated that in a digital imaging environment many of the previous QM tasks have now become obsolete and the exam will no longer be offered. In addition, depending on the size of the department, upper management positions are available, such as chief technologist and radiology manager or administrator. Along with experience, advanced coursework in management is desirable for these positions.

Commercial Firms. Opportunities for RTs exist in a variety of areas within commercial companies involved in the selling of x-ray equipment, image receptor systems, and related x-ray supplies. These companies need sales representatives with technical knowledge of the radiologic procedures and equipment, as well as the ability to sell. In addition, companies hire application specialists who are not directly involved in sales but who are involved with the education and training of the staff at the sites where the equipment is installed. Sales representatives and technical specialists generally have some travel requirements as part of their responsibilities.

HEALTH CARE TEAM

A wide array of specialists make up the health care team. Although not all of the various disciplines can be detailed here, some health care services that an RT encounters on a regular basis are highlighted. These services include medicine and osteopathy, nursing, and the health care careers that encompass many of the diagnostic services, therapeutic services, and health information services. Persons employed in health care find opportunities in all kinds of environments, such as hospitals, clinics, doctors' offices, long-term care facilities, schools, and industry.

Many health care workers share the titles of technologist, technician, and therapist. *Technologist* is a general term that applies to an individual skilled in a practical art. This health care provider applies knowledge to practical and theoretic problems in the field. *Technician* is a term that applies to a person who performs procedures that require attention to technical detail. Technicians work under the direction of another health care provider. The terms *technologist* and *technician* are often used interchangeably, which can create problems in disciplines in which the terms are used to denote differing levels of education. In the clinical laboratory sciences, a medical technologist (MT) has earned a 4-year degree and a medical laboratory technician (MLT) has completed a 2-year program. In general, technologists are involved in higher level problem-solving situations and have more extensive educational preparation than do technicians. Technologists and technicians work throughout all areas of health care; many provide direct patient care, whereas others serve in support roles.

Therapists specialize in carrying out treatments designed to correct or improve the function of a particular body part or system. Therapists possess varied levels of educational experiences ranging from 2-year to 4-year to graduate college degrees.

Medicine and Osteopathy

Physicians are primary care providers who promote the optimal health of their patients and who provide for patients' care during an illness. Two principal types of physicians are the medical doctor (MD) and the doctor of osteopathy (DO). MDs generally complete a baccalaureate degree program with a science major such as biology or chemistry and then complete 4 years of medical school. DOs have educations similar to those of MDs. The philosophy of osteopathic medicine differs from that of traditional medicine. In addition to

[handwritten: → lab + x-ray]

learning the important concepts of medicine, DOs are taught to do manipulations of muscles and bones as a part of the healing process. Both MDs and DOs must be state licensed to practice.

After medical school, most MDs and DOs complete additional clinical experience, known as a *residency,* in an area of specialization. Residencies are usually 3 or 4 years and may include the following branches of medicine:

- *Anesthesiology:* Study of the use of medication to cause loss of sensation during surgery
- *Cardiology:* Study of diseases of the cardiovascular system
- *Family practice:* Study of diseases in patients of all ages
- *Geriatrics:* Study of diseases of older adults
- *Gynecology:* Study of diseases of the female reproductive system
- *Internal medicine:* Study of diseases of the internal organs of the chest and abdomen
- *Neurology:* Study of diseases of the brain and nervous system
- *Obstetrics:* Study of pregnancy and childbirth
- *Oncology:* Study of the treatment of tumors
- *Orthopedics:* Study of diseases of muscles and bones
- *Pediatrics:* Study of diseases in children
- *Radiology:* Study of the use of x-rays and radioactive substances to diagnose and treat diseases
- *Surgery:* Study of the use of operative procedures to treat diseases
- *Urology:* Study of diseases of the urinary system

In addition, many physicians choose a subspecialty—for example, the primary duties of a pediatric cardiovascular surgeon include performing surgery on the heart and blood vessels of children.

Nursing

A *nurse* provides direct patient care, typically under the direction of physicians. Nurses are classified as nursing assistants, licensed practical nurses (LPNs), or registered nurses (RNs). RNs have a variety of duties, depending on their area of expertise. Nurses often choose to work exclusively in one specialty area (e.g., pediatrics, orthopedics, intensive care, the emergency department). To become an RN, the candidate must pass a state licensing examination after completion of a 2-, 3-, or 4-year program of study.

Advanced education for the nurse can lead to work as a nurse practitioner (NP), a nurse midwife, or a nurse anesthetist. An *NP* performs physical examinations, orders and interprets some tests, and, in some states, prescribes medications. A *nurse midwife* provides perinatal care and can deliver infants under the supervision of an obstetrician. A *nurse anesthetist* provides anesthesia under the supervision of an anesthesiologist.

Nursing assistants and LPNs generally work under the direction of an RN or a physician to provide basic care to patients. Nursing assistants generally have limited training, most of which is done on the job. LPNs generally complete a 1-year program and can legally administer drugs except by the intravenous route.

Diagnostic Services

Health care workers in diagnostic service areas perform tests or evaluations that aid the physician in determining the presence or absence of a disease or condition. Many health care specialists perform diagnostic procedures. For example, *cardiovascular technologists* operate equipment that records the electrical impulses of the heart, and *electroneurodiagnostic technologists* operate equipment to record the electrical impulses of the brain as a part of their responsibilities.

The clinical laboratory sciences involve a wide variety of careers in health care. An MT works in the laboratory performing tests and analyzing results. Several areas of specialization exist in the laboratory, including hematology, microbiology, clinical chemistry, immunology, and blood banking. MLTs generally work under the supervision of an MT or a physician to perform basic laboratory tests in all the various departments of the laboratory. Other laboratory personnel include the cytotechnologist, who specializes in the preparation and screening of cells, and the histologic technologist, who specializes in the preparation of tissues.

Radiology is predominantly a diagnostic service. These careers have already been detailed. Educational requirements for careers in the diagnostic services vary considerably across the disciplines, but most positions require 2 to 4 years of education beyond high school.

Therapeutic Services

Therapists provide services designed to help patients overcome some form of physical or psychological disability. Examples include *occupational therapists,* who teach useful skills to patients with physical or emotional illnesses; *physical therapists,* who help to restore muscle strength and coordination through exercise and the use of special devices such as braces or crutches; *radiation therapists,* who treat cancer patients using high-energy x-rays and gamma rays; and *respiratory therapists,* who help to treat patients with breathing difficulties. Educational requirements vary considerably across the disciplines, but most positions require 2 to 6 years of education beyond high school.

Health Information Services *[handwritten: medical records]*

Health information services involve careers that are responsible for the management of health information, such as that contained in the patient's health record. These careers do not involve direct patient contact but are essential to the efficient operation of any health care facility. For example, health information technologists are involved in the coding of patient conditions, and these codes are used to determine the amount of money a facility is reimbursed for providing care to a patient. Educational requirements for careers in health information management vary considerably across disciplines, but most positions require 2 to 4 years of education beyond high school.

Other Health Services

A vast number of other careers exist within the health care environment. Other health services include such disciplines as communication sciences, counseling, dental health, dietetics, and psychology.

SUMMARY

- *Radiation* is energy transmitted by waves through space or through a medium (matter). It is both helpful and essential for life. *Energy* is the capacity to operate or work. One form of energy is electromagnetic energy, which includes radio waves, light, and x-rays. Many forms of energy are used in medicine to help diagnose and treat patients. Some higher energy forms, such as x-rays, are capable of causing ionization. This process is capable of causing biologic damage, and caution should be exercised to prevent unnecessary exposure to ionizing radiation.

- X-rays were discovered by Wilhelm Conrad Röntgen on November 8, 1895. For his discovery, Röntgen was awarded the first Nobel Prize in physics in 1901.

- *Radiologic technology* is the technical science that deals with the use of x-rays or radioactive substances for diagnostic or therapeutic purposes in medicine. *Radiologic technologist* is a general term applied to an individual qualified to use x-rays (radiography) or radioactive substances (nuclear medicine) to produce images of the internal parts of the body for interpretation by a physician known as a *radiologist*. RTs also use x-rays or radioactive substances in the treatment of disease (radiation therapy).

- In addition to using x-rays and radioactive substances, RTs have become involved in using high-frequency sound waves (diagnostic medical sonography) and magnetic fields and radio waves (MRI) to create images of the internal anatomy of the body. Additional opportunities also exist for RTs in education, management, and commercial firms.

- The health care team comprises a wide array of specialists. RTs work as a part of the health care team and interact with many of the other health care members on a regular basis. These other members are employed in such health services as medicine and osteopathy, nursing, and the other health careers that encompass many of the diagnostic services, therapeutic services, and health information services.

- Individuals employed in health care find opportunities in all kinds of environments, such as hospitals, clinics, doctors' offices, long-term care facilities, schools, and industry.

BIBLIOGRAPHY

American Medical Association: *Health care careers directory*, ed 40, Chicago, 2012, The Association.

Carlton R, Adler AM: *Principles of radiographic imaging: an art and a science*, ed 5, Albany, NY, 2012, Delmar Cengage Learning.

Eisenberg RL: *Radiology: an illustrated history*, St. Louis, 1995, Mosby.

Gerdin JA: *Health careers today*, ed 6, St. Louis, 2016, Mosby.

Grigg ERN: *The trail of the invisible light*, Springfield, Ill, 1965, Charles C Thomas.

Gurley LT, Calloway WJ: *Introduction to radiologic technology*, ed 7, St. Louis, 2010, Mosby.

Papp J: *Quality management in the imaging sciences*, ed 5, St. Louis, 2014, Mosby.

Röntgen WC: On a new kind of rays, *Nature* 53:1369, 1896.

Simmers LM, Simmers-Narker K, Simmers-Kobelak S: *Simmers DHO: Health Science*, ed 8, Albany, NY, 2013, Delmar Cengage Learning.

2

Professional Organizations

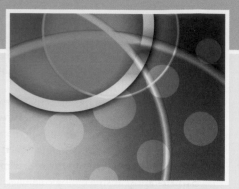

Richard R. Carlton, MS, RT(R)(CV), FAEIRS,
Arlene M. Adler, MEd, RT(R), FAEIRS

*Be active in your local, state and national organizations; never be satisfied until the highest
goal has been attained.*

Professor Ed C. Jerman
Father of Radiologic Technology, c. 1920

OBJECTIVES

On completion of this chapter, the student will be able to:
- Differentiate accreditation, certification, and representation functions of various professional organizations.
- Describe the organizations that carry out the professional aspects of a specific radiologic technology area of specialization.

- Describe the relationship of various radiologist and physicist organizations with radiologic technology.

OUTLINE

KEY TERMS

Accreditation Voluntary peer-review process through which an agency grants recognition to an institution for a program of study that meets specified criteria

Certification Voluntary process through which an agency grants recognition to an individual on demonstration, usually by <u>examination</u>, of specialized professional skills

14

Essentials and Guidelines Document specifying the minimum quality standards for the accreditation of an educational program as approved by the appropriate joint review committee sponsors

Joint Review Committee (JRC) Group of persons appointed by sponsoring organizations to oversee the accreditation process

Licensure Process by which a governmental agency (usually a state) grants permission to individuals to practice their profession

Registry List of individuals holding certification in a particular profession

Sponsoring Organization Professional organization that appoints members to a joint review committee board

Standards Document specifying the minimum requirements for accreditation of an educational program by a joint review committee

ACCREDITATION OF SCHOOLS (gold standard)

Accreditation of schools sets the conditions under which new members qualify for entry into the profession. Accredited programs have satisfactorily demonstrated compliance with educational standards developed by and for the profession. These standards are set by the organizations that sponsor the accrediting agency. Each **sponsoring organization** appoints one or more members to the board of directors known as a **Joint Review Committee (JRC).** This board is the governing body of the organization, and its members make recommendations regarding the accreditation status of schools. The sponsoring organizations of the JRCs approve a document known as either the *Essentials and Guidelines* or the *Standards,* which details the minimum requirements for how an accredited program must operate. These documents typically require a program to demonstrate its purposes, its resources, the effectiveness of its outcomes, and other elements deemed important by the sponsoring organizations.

The process of accreditation begins with an application from the program. On approval of the application, a comprehensive document known as a *self-study* must be compiled by the program according to guidelines set by the accrediting agency. On submission of this document, a team of site visitors is sent to verify the information provided in the self-study. Site visitors are volunteers from the profession who serve without pay, although the program being visited pays their expenses. The site-visiting team submits a report to the accrediting agency, and the agency staff reviews this report and presents it to the board for a vote on the recommended accreditation status. Typical accreditation award classifications include provisional, probationary, and up to 8-year status (although this may vary with the specific accreditation agency). Fees are collected for the application and the site-visit expenses, as is an annual fee from the sponsor of the program and sometimes for clinical education sites.

Accreditation is a voluntary peer-review process. Although accreditation is voluntary, few programs choose not to undergo the accreditation process. Nearly all schools value their accreditation status highly and work hard to maintain standards that meet, and often exceed, all the accreditation recommendations. A program may choose not to pursue programmatic accreditation and may rely on the accreditation awarded to a college or university under a regional institutional accrediting agency. A list of accrediting agencies, certification agencies, and professional societies is supplied in Appendix B.

Joint Review Committee on Education in Diagnostic Medical Sonography

The Joint Review Committee on Education in Diagnostic Medical Sonography (JRCDMS) was established in 1983 and is currently sponsored by the following nine organizations:

- American College of Cardiology: http://www.acc.org
- American College of Obstetricians and Gynecologists: http://www.acog.org
- American College of Radiology (ACR): http://www.acr.org
- American Institute of Ultrasound in Medicine (AIUM): http://www.aium.org
- American Society of Echocardiography (ASE): http://www.asecho.org
- American Society of Radiologic Technologists (ASRT): http://www.asrt.org
- Society of Diagnostic Medical Sonography: http://www.sdms.org
- Society for Vascular Surgery: http://www.vascularweb.org
- Society for Vascular Ultrasound: http://www.svunet.org

The JRCDMS accredits nearly 200 institutions, which may have from one to three accredited programs each. (The website address is http://www.jrcdms.org.)

Joint Review Committee on Education in Nuclear Medicine Technology

The Joint Review Committee on Education in Nuclear Medicine Technology (JRCNMT) was established in 1970 and is currently sponsored by four organizations: the ACR, the ASRT, the Society of Nuclear Medicine, and the Society of Nuclear Medicine–Technologist Section. The JRCNMT accredits approximately 100 nuclear medicine technology programs. (The website address is http://www.jrcnmt.org.)

Joint Review Committee on Education in Radiologic Technology

Radiography is considered to be the fifth oldest allied health profession because the first *Essentials* document was established in 1944, after the occupational therapy, medical technology, physical therapy, and medical records administration. Not until 1969 was the Joint Review Committee on Education in Radiologic Technology (JRCERT) established. The JRCERT board is currently nominated by the ACR, the ASRT, the Association of Educators in Imaging and Radiological Sciences, and the American Healthcare Radiology Administrators (AHRA). The JRCERT accredits more programs than any other allied health profession: approximately 700 programs in radiography, radiation therapy, medical dosimetry, and magnetic resonance imaging (MRI) programs. (The website address is http://wwwjrcert.org.)

CERTIFICATION OF INDIVIDUALS

Professional certification is a process through which an agency grants recognition to an individual on demonstration, usually by examination, of specialized professional skills. It is a voluntary process and is the responsibility of the person, not of the person's school or employer. Each certification organization sets requirements for the recognition of professionals through registration, certification, or other recognition of skills by examination. Fees are charged for these services. Especially important are the annual fees for continued recognition. Failure to pay these fees or meet other requirements, such as verification of continuing education activities, results in the removal of an individual from the registration lists of the profession. Reinstatement may involve retaking an examination or returning to school, and a special fee is often charged. In many states, loss of professional certification will include loss of the individual's state license to practice (and therefore may result in the loss of a job).

Actually, a registry is simply a list of individuals holding a particular certification. The term *registry* is commonly applied to the agency that carries out the certification function and maintains the registry list. Each registry is sponsored by appropriate professional organizations. The sponsoring organizations appoint the members of the board, and this board then determines the standards for the registry, such as eligibility requirements, examination questions, fees, and ethical standards.

Nearly all hospitals in the United States require appropriate professional certification as a condition of employment. Physicians who desire high-quality imaging also insist on appropriate professional certification for the technologists who perform radiography, ultrasonography, mammography, computed tomography (CT), MRI, and other imaging or treatment services in their offices and clinics.

Most professional societies, as well as many other professional organizations, maintain a presence on the Internet on Facebook and Twitter. Especially for students, these sites can provide valuable insight into how a professional operates on the local, state, and national stages.

AMERICAN REGISTRY OF DIAGNOSTIC MEDICAL SONOGRAPHERS

The American Registry of Diagnostic Medical Sonographers (ARDMS) offers voluntary certification through examination to eligible sonographers and vascular technologists. Since its inception in 1975, ARDMS has certified approximately 96,000 persons. ARDMS holds accreditation with the National Commission for Certifying Agencies (NCCA). ARDMS offers four credentials: registered diagnostic medical sonographer (RDMS), registered diagnostic cardiac sonographer (RDCS), registered vascular technologist (RVT), and registered physician in vascular interpretation (RPVI). Specialty areas within the RDMS

credential include abdomen, breast, neurosonology, obstetrics and gynecology, and fetal echocardiography. Specialty areas within the RDCS credential include adult, pediatric, and fetal echocardiography. Each specialty area requires two examinations, one on physics and instrumentation, and the other on the specialty procedures. (The website address is http://www.ardms.org.)

American Registry of Radiologic Technologists

The American Registry of Radiologic Technologists (ARRT) was founded in 1922 by the Radiological Society of North America (RSNA), with the support of the American Roentgen Ray Society (ARRS) and the cooperation of the Canadian Association of Radiologists and the American Society of X-Ray Technicians (now known as the ASRT). In 1936 the ARRT was incorporated, and in 1944 the ACR and the ASRT became cosponsors of the ARRT. Currently, the ASRT appoints five members to the ARRT board, and the ACR appoints four members.

The purposes of the ARRT include encouraging the study and elevating the standards of radiologic technology, examining and certifying eligible candidates, and periodically publishing a listing of registrants. This mission is accomplished through voluntary certification by examination. Once an individual has passed the appropriate examination, he or she is listed in the registry and granted the right to use an appropriate professional title. This designation is registered technologist (RT), with a specialty designation for radiographer (R), radiation therapy (T), nuclear medicine (N), cardiac interventional technology (CI), vascular interventional technology (VI), mammography (M), CT, MRI, or quality management (QM). In addition, the ARRT has added sonography (S), vascular sonography (VS), breast sonography (BS), bone densitometry (BD), and radiologist assistant (RA) examinations. For example, a registered radiographer is designated as RT(R) (ARRT). This designation is a registered trademark, and its use by non–ARRT-registered individuals is illegal.

Individuals must pay an annual fee to maintain active status with the ARRT and must adhere to the ARRT code of ethics. Members of the profession who violate the code of ethics, usually through criminal activity, may have their registration revoked. For example, former RTs who have been convicted of stealing from their employers often have their registration revoked. ARRT registrants also must certify that they have attended 24 hours of continuing education during the previous 2 years to maintain their registration status. Continuing education became mandatory for ARRT registrants in 1995.

The ARRT began offering registration in nuclear medicine technology and radiation therapy in 1962 and started postprimary examinations in 1991. Currently, the ARRT lists more than 330,000 registered technologists, many of whom have been certified in more than one professional specialty. (The website address is http://www.arrt.org.)

Medical Dosimetry Certification Board

The Medical Dosimetry Certification Board (MDCB) credentials professionals who practice medical dosimetry, one of the oncologic professions. The MDCB offers the credential Certified

Medical Dosimetrist (CMD) to those who pass their examination in medical dosimetry. (The website address is http://www.mdcb.org.)

NUCLEAR MEDICINE TECHNOLOGY CERTIFICATION BOARD

The Nuclear Medicine Technology Certification Board (NMTCB) was founded in 1977 to certify technologists in nuclear medicine and molecular imaging. Current sponsors include the Society of Nuclear Medicine, the Society of Nuclear Medicine–Technologist Section, the American Society of Clinical Pathologists, the College of Physicists, the American Society of Medical Technology, and the Association of Physicists in Medicine. The NMTCB consists of 15 persons plus an advisory council, the chair of which also sits on the board.

The purposes of the NMTCB include examining and certifying eligible candidates and periodically publishing a listing of registrants. This mission is accomplished through voluntary certification by examination. Once an individual has passed the appropriate examination, he or she becomes registered and is granted the right to use the title certified nuclear medicine technologist. The NMTCB has approximately 15,000 registrants. The NMTCB also offers three specialty examinations for nuclear medicine technologists, the nuclear cardiology (NCT), positron emission tomography (PET), and the Nuclear Medicine Advanced Associate (NMAA) examinations. (The website address is http://www.nmtcb.org.)

State Licensing Agencies

Requirements to practice the radiologic professions vary from state to state. Most, but not all, states and territories require a license, which can usually be obtained on providing proof of certification from the appropriate national certification organization (a process known as licensure). The laws in effect vary tremendously from one state to another and can vary from year to year within a state as a result of new legislation. Most radiologic and imaging sciences professionals do not experience difficulty in moving employment from one state to another because proper licensing is usually a matter of submitting the appropriate paperwork and fees. Verifying current licensing requirements is important before practicing in a new state because penalties may be assessed for practicing without a license. Many professional societies maintain current lists of contact information for all states with licensing requirements for their members. (For example, go to the ASRT website and search for "state licensing" to obtain their current list.) (See Appendix C.)

PROFESSIONAL SOCIETIES

Professional societies represent the interests of various groups to the public and to governmental bodies. The radiologic sciences have many such organizations, with new ones forming and others combining or ceasing operations from time to time. These organizations usually publish professional journals, conduct educational meetings, and represent their members to governmental bodies. They also often provide continuing education

verification, scholarships, special reports, information networking, recruitment and promotional materials, malpractice insurance, and other services for their members. Most professional societies offer significant discounts to student members and scholarships and research grants specifically designed to foster professional development of students in the professions. Some of the most important professional societies are described here.

American Association of Medical Dosimetrists

The American Association of Medical Dosimetrists (AAMD) is an international society established to promote and support the *Medical Dosimetry* profession. AAMD publishes the journal *Medical Dosimetry*, provides continuing education, and represents Medical Dosimetrists. There are currently more than 3000 members. (The website address is http://www.medicaldosimetry.org.)

American Healthcare Radiology Administrators

The AHRA was organized to promote management practice in the administration of imaging services. Membership is open to professionals engaged in the practice of radiology administration in both hospital and nonhospital settings, as well as to others in service or education who have limited management responsibilities. They have approximately 4000 members.

AHRA provides a broad range of services for its members, including the journal *Radiology Management*, a newsletter, and monographs. The association holds regular educational meetings and an annual conference. They offer the Certified Radiology Administrator (CRA) examination for radiology administrators. AHRA has strong cooperative ties with other professional associations and has spearheaded the Summit on Manpower, a consortium of radiology and health care organizations concerned with labor shortages in radiology. (The website address is http://www.ahraonline.org.) *run X-ray departments*

American Society of Echocardiography

The ASE is an organization of physicians, scientists, laboratory managers, cardiovascular sonographers, and nurses committed to excellence in cardiovascular ultrasound and its application to patient care through education, advocacy, research, innovation, and service to both members and the public. ASE was founded in 1975 and has more than 17,000 members nationally and internationally. They publish curricular and standards documents for sonographers. They publish the *Journal of the American Society of Echocardiography*. (The website address is http://www.asecho.org.)

American Society of Radiologic Technologists

The ASRT was founded in 1920. As the most prominent national professional voice for RTs, the ASRT represents individual practitioners, educators, managers and administrators, and students in radiography, radiation therapy, and nuclear medicine, as well as the many specialties within each modality. The ASRT has more than 153,000 members (nearly half of the RTs in the United States).

The goals of the ASRT are to advance the professions of radiologic technology and imaging specialties, to maintain high standards of education, to enhance the quality of patient care, and to further the welfare and socioeconomics of RTs. The ASRT publishes peer-reviewed, refereed journals (*Radiologic Technology* and *Radiation Therapist*) and produces educational curricular guides and other materials of all types. (The website address is http://www.asrt.org.)

Association of Educators in Imaging and Radiologic Sciences

The Association of Educators in Imaging and Radiologic Sciences (AEIRS) was founded in 1967. Its primary purposes are to encourage the exchange of teaching concepts, to help establish minimum standards for teaching radiologic technologies, and to advance radiologic education by encouraging educational research and technical writing by its members. AEIRS is a national association of educators. It holds meetings and publishes *Radiologic Science and Education*, *Spectrum*, and other educational data. (The website address is http://www.aeirs.org.)

Association of Vascular and Interventional Radiographers

The Association of Vascular and Interventional Radiographers (AVIR) was organized to represent radiographers and allied health care professionals specializing in cardiovascular and interventional radiology. The AVIR offers members a newsletter and regional meetings. (The website address is http://www.avir.org.)

International Society for Magnetic Resonance in Medicine–Section for Magnetic Resonance Technologists

The International Society for Magnetic Resonance in Medicine (ISMRM) was founded in 1981. Its major purpose is to further the development and application of magnetic resonance techniques in medicine and biology by promoting communications, research development applications, and the availability of information in the fields of MRI and spectroscopy. To accomplish this purpose, the ISMRM holds meetings and workshops, publishes journals and other documents, provides information and advice on aspects of public policy concerned with magnetic resonance in medicine, and otherwise performs charitable, scientific, and educational functions with respect to magnetic resonance in medicine and biology. The ISMRM's periodicals include a newsletter called *Resonance* and a journal titled *Magnetic Resonance in Medicine*. The Section for Magnetic Resonance Technologists (SMRT) publishes a newsletter and a journal, *Magnetic Resonance Imaging Technology*. (The website address is http://www.ismrm.org/smrt.)

International Society of Radiographers and Radiologic Technologists

The International Society of Radiographers and Radiologic Technologists (ISRRT) was founded in 1959 as an organization of national societies of RTs. The ISRRT is an international nongovernmental organization with official relations with the World Health Organization.

The primary objectives of the ISRRT are to facilitate communication among RTs worldwide, to advance the science

and practice of radiologic technology, and to identify and help meet the needs of radiologic technologists (RTs) in developing nations. The ISRRT holds World Congresses on a 2-year cycle. The ISRRT publishes a semiannual newsletter, proceedings of meetings, and translations of various documents of interest to the profession.

Over 70 member countries representing more than a half million radiographers belong to the ISRRT. Each member country appoints a representative to the ISRRT World Council, which serves as the governing body. The secretary-general of the organization serves as the liaison for the council, as well as the office. The ISRRT offers associate membership to individuals wishing to support the organization. (The website address is http://www.isrrt.org.)

Society of Diagnostic Medical Sonographers

The Society of Diagnostic Medical Sonographers (SDMS) is the largest professional society for sonographers, representing every specialty and level of expertise. SDMS was founded in 1970 to answer the needs of nonphysicians who were performing diagnostic sonographic procedures. Its goals are to promote, advance, and educate its members and the medical community in the science of diagnostic medical sonography and thereby contribute to the enhancement of patient care. This goal is accomplished through educational programs, scientific and professional publications, and representation and collaboration with other organizations. SDMS publishes the *Journal of Diagnostic Medical Sonography*. (The website address is http://www.sdms.org.)

Society of Nuclear Medicine–Technologist Section

The Society of Nuclear Medicine (SNM) is a multidisciplinary organization of physicians, physicists, chemists, radiopharmacists, technologists, and others interested in the diagnostic, therapeutic, and investigational use of radiopharmaceuticals. Founded in Seattle in 1954, the SNM is the largest scientific organization dedicated to nuclear medicine.

The Technologist Section of the SNM was formed in 1970 to meet the needs of the nuclear medicine technologist. It is a scientific organization formed with, but operating autonomously from, the SNM to promote the continued development and improvement of the art and science of nuclear medicine technology. Its ongoing objectives are to enhance the development of nuclear medicine technology, to stimulate continuing education activities, and to develop a forum for the exchange of ideas and information. The Technologist Section provides nuclear medicine technologists with a mechanism to deal directly with issues that concern them, such as continuing education, academic affairs, and socioeconomic issues. The organization publishes a journal called *Journal of Nuclear Medicine Technology*, or *JNMT*. (The website address is http://www.snm.org.)

Society for Vascular Ultrasound

The Society for Vascular Ultrasound (SVU) represents vascular technologists, vascular physicians, vascular laboratory managers, nurses, and other allied medical ultrasound professionals. SVU was founded in 1977 and has more than

4200 members. SVU publishes curricular and standards documents for vascular sonographers and technologists. Its journal is the *Journal for Vascular Ultrasound*. (The website address is http://www.svunet.org.)

State and Local Radiologic Technology Societies

Nearly all states and many cities and regions have local professional societies that carry out many of the functions of the larger national organizations for their states or regions. In many instances, these organizations serve as chapters or affiliates of the larger groups, although these connections may be formal or simply loose affiliations. State and local societies often make special efforts to cater to the needs of students and new members of professions with opportunities to begin a career through scholarships, student competitions, publishing, exhibits, and committee work, as well as through positions as board members.

RADIOLOGIST AND PHYSICIST ORGANIZATIONS

American Association of Physicists in Medicine

The American Association of Physicists in Medicine (AAPM) is the most prominent organization of radiation physicists, with over 8000 members. Its annual meeting is held in conjunction with the RSNA meeting each year in Chicago.

American Board of Radiology

The American Board of Radiology (ABR) was established in 1934 to conduct the certification of radiologists. The ABR has three certification divisions: radiology, diagnostic radiology, and therapeutic radiology. The basic requirement for eligibility for these examinations is a medical degree plus 4 years of residency training. A written examination must be passed before a candidate is eligible for the oral examination. The ABR also offers certification for radiologic physicists and a special competence examination in nuclear medicine.

American College of Radiology

With more than 30,000 members, the ACR is the principal organization of physicians trained in radiology and medical radiation physics in the United States. The ACR is a professional society whose primary purposes are to advance the science of radiology, improve service to the patient, study the socioeconomic aspects of the practice of radiology, and encourage continuing education for radiologists and persons practicing in allied professional fields.

American Institute of Ultrasound in Medicine

Physicians, engineers, scientists, sonographers, and other professionals involved with diagnostic medical sonography make up the AIUM. The AIUM promotes the application of ultrasound in clinical medicine, diagnostics, and research; promotes the study of its effects on tissue; recommends standards for its applications; and promotes education in the use of ultrasonics for medical purposes.

American Medical Association

The American Medical Association (AMA) was founded in Philadelphia in 1847 and is considered the largest and most active medical organization in the world. At the founding meeting, the delegates adopted the first code of medical ethics and established the first nationwide standards for preliminary medical education and the degree of Medical Doctor. More than 300,000 US physicians (approximately 70% of those practicing) belong to the AMA. The activities of the AMA include promotion and regulation of all aspects of medicine in the United States, including the allied health professions. The AMA publishes the most widely distributed medical journal in the world, the *Journal of the American Medical Association*, also known as *JAMA*, which is published weekly.

American Roentgen Ray Society

The ARRS is the oldest US radiologic society. Founded in 1900 in St. Louis, the society had approximately 7000 members by the early 1990s. Its primary objectives are educational, which are met through meetings and publication of the *American Journal of Roentgenology*.

American Society for Therapeutic Radiology and Oncology

The purpose of the American Society for Therapeutic Radiology and Oncology (ASTRO) is to extend the benefits of radiation therapy to patients with cancer or other disorders, to advance its scientific basis, and to provide for the education and professional fellowship of its members.

The society was formally incorporated in 1958 as an organization of physicians who believed that radiation, formerly used only as a diagnostic tool, had potential value as an interventional modality in the treatment of malignant disease. Today, ASTRO has more than 4000 members (including many radiation therapists) and is the leading organization for radiation oncology, biology, and physics. ASTRO publishes a newsletter and an annual membership directory. The organization also makes a major commitment to education and research through awards, fellowships, travel grants, and contributions to accredited technology programs.

International Society for Clinical Densitometry

The International Society for Clinical Densitometry (ISCD) was founded in 1993 and provides a central resource for scientific disciplines with an interest in bone mass measurement. The society has more than 4000 members and offers a technical certification examination for individuals who perform bone densitometry, as well as continuing education and accreditation for clinical sites.

Radiological Society of North America

The Western Roentgen Society was founded in Chicago in 1915 in response to a need for a national radiology organization because the ARRS had become an eastern organization. In 1920 the organization was renamed the RSNA to reflect the nature of its membership. Since 1918, RSNA has published the most influential journal in American radiology, known simply as *Radiology* and often referred to as *the gray journal* because of its traditional color, representing the shades of gray that make up the radiologic image. In 1981 a second journal, *RadioGraphics*, was added. The

helps educate

organization has more than 53,000 members from 140 countries. RSNA conducts the world's largest radiology meeting, with more than 55,000 registrants in Chicago each November. The organization also provides research grants totaling several million dollars annually to members of the professions.

Society for Imaging Informatics in Medicine

The Society for Imaging Informatics in Medicine (SIIM), formerly the Society for Computer Applications in Radiology (SCAR), was founded in 1980 to serve as a resource for imaging professionals interested in the current and future use of computers in medical imaging. The organization provides a focal point for picture archiving and communication systems (PACSs) and other radiology informatics users.

Society of Nuclear Medicine

See the discussion on the Society of Nuclear Medicine–Technologist Section.

SUMMARY

- A major part of the fabric of a profession is its organizations, especially the accrediting agencies for educational programs, the certification bodies for individuals, and the professional societies that represent the interests of the profession to the public and government.
- Radiologic technology accreditation is carried out through the various JRCs: the JRCDMS, the JRCERT, and the JRCNMT, which perform both radiography and radiation therapy accreditation.
- Individuals are certified by the various registries and by state and territorial licensing agencies. The national registries are the ARDMS, the ARRT, and the NMTCB. The ARRT offers registration in radiography, nuclear medicine, radiation therapy, cardiovascular interventional technology, mammography, CT, MRI, dosimetry, and QM.
- RTs are represented by numerous professional societies at the international, national, state, and local levels. Among the most prominent of these organizations are AHRA, ASRT, AEIRS, AVIR, ISRRT, SDMS, SMRT, and SNM–Technologist Section.
- Radiologists and physicists are also represented by numerous organizations. Among those with the strongest ties to radiologic technology are AAPM, ACR, AIUM, AMA, ARRS, ASTRO, ISCD, RSNA, SIIM, and SNM. Together, these organizations constitute the full strength of the radiologic sciences profession by their activities in accreditation, certification, and representation.

BIBLIOGRAPHY

American Medical Association: *Health care careers directory*, ed 40, Chicago, 2012, The Association, Chicago.

Eisenberg RL: *Radiology: an illustrated history*, St. Louis, 1992, Mosby.

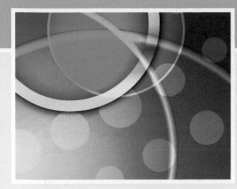

Educational Survival Skills

Arlene M. Adler, MEd, RT(R), FAEIRS,
Richard R. Carlton, MS, RT(R)(CV), FAEIRS

The real voyage of discovery consists not in seeking new landscapes but in having new eyes.

Marcel Proust

OBJECTIVES

On completion of this chapter, the student will be able to:

- Discuss the causes and symptoms of stress.
- Explain behaviors and thoughts that increase the fight-or-flight response.
- Analyze interventions that can be used to reduce or buffer stressors.
- Describe several survival techniques to reduce stress.
- Enumerate steps to manage time through organization, limit setting, and self-evaluation.
- Explain the benefit of uplifts in relation to hassles.
- Identify foods that can be eaten to supply the body nutritionally with additional vitamin C, vitamin B complex, and magnesium.
- Foster study techniques to enhance retention and to build information into complex concepts.
- List the steps for successful test taking.

OUTLINE

KEY TERMS

Buffers Activities that decrease the negative effects of stress but do not change the stressors

Fight-or-Flight Response Physiologic response resulting from anger and fear and triggered by a real or imagined threat

Hassles Unexpected negative changes or events

In-Control Language Statements that reflect an attitude of choice and evoke positive feelings

Out-of-Control Language Words or phrases that express a lack of control over a situation

Stress Demand on time, energy, and resources with an element of threat

Stressors Events, both real and imagined, that increase feelings of anxiety

Time Management Practice of self-management related to how time is used

Uplifts Planned positive activities to balance hassles

Worry Time and energy spent concerned for things over which we have little or no control

WHAT IS STRESS?

The busy world of the radiologic sciences student is filled with new ideas, concepts, demanding class and clinical schedules, and changing focus. Little thought is given to managing the stressors associated with so much change. The hope is to survive midterms and finals; to survive the changing demands of clinical instructors; and to survive work, family responsibilities, and school demands. The feeling associated with this survival effort may leave the student anxious, tired, humorless, irritable, uncreative, but on rare occasions thrilled. The path through all of these emotions provides the background for finally saying, "I'm stressed out!" The focus of this chapter is on possible interventions to manage or control stressors, including time management, study habits and test-taking strategies, and other self-care interventions.

Stress is produced by events that are perceived as demands on time, energy, or resources with the threat that not enough time, energy, or resources will be available to fulfill an obligation. Studying for an important examination is difficult when a feeling exists that not enough time is available to complete the task. The pressure is on, and the result can be overwhelming anxiety. In fact, if the threat is real enough to the individual, the heart rate increases, breathing becomes shallow and rapid, and the person may have a surge of energy that seems better handled while pacing the floor. The body is ready for a big event and does not distinguish between readiness for a 100-yard dash and readiness for a paper-and-pencil test. The chemistry of the body responds to the brain's message and prepares for physical activity. When the response of the body is to stay and continue studying, the chemicals of the body have to dissipate on their own.

Usually, we deal with more than one event at a time—home and family responsibilities, school assignments, and work activities. In combination, these events produce a compounding effect. Finally, we say, "I'm stressed out!" This declaration is the plea for help when the limits of tolerance for juggling many responsibilities have been reached.

Fight-or-Flight Response

The fight-or-flight response is the physiologic reaction to a real or imagined threat arising from emotions of both fear and anger. It is the body's way of preparing for change that is perceived as threatening. This response served our species well many years ago when our survival was threatened. It provided a way to battle the elements. The physiologic responses include the release of hormones to increase metabolism, increases in fats and sugars for energy, and increases in heart rate and respiration. Blood flows at a greater-than-normal rate to the long muscles of the extremities, and the central nervous system is stimulated. This response is the preparation for battle or escape.

An example of triggering of the fight-or-flight response is when the telephone rings at 2 AM, waking the individual from a deep sleep. All systems are *go* as soon as the ring is heard, in anticipation of bad news; the body is ready for the *battle*. The call turns out to be a wrong number. The outcome presents no emotional or physical injury, but the body has readied itself automatically for a physical response. For several minutes after such an event, a person is under the influence of the body's chemical response to the potential threat. Until the body readjusts to the nonthreatening environment, neither sleep nor relaxation will return. The same response occurs in the setting of threats such as missed deadlines, loss of self-esteem, poor test results, loss of friendship, overcommitment, and inability to set personal limits. Living in a state of constant alert over time can result in serious physical or emotional illness.

Attitudes about *self* and the role the environment plays in the ability to counter or cause a stress response are important to recognize. What is in the mind is in the body. If self-defeating, negative thoughts are predominant, then both consciously and subconsciously the body responds with an excessive release of chemicals; over time, these chemicals produce wear and tear on organs, resulting in serious illness. Positive thoughts and an optimistic viewpoint can actually decrease the potential for ill health and reduce the metabolism that chemically triggers the fight-or-flight response. Positive thoughts also serve as a self-fulfilling prophecy—attitudes that accurately predict gloom or happiness dictate whether we manage daily stressors positively or negatively.

Causes and Effects

The compounding effect of stress over several weeks to months can contribute to poor emotional and physical health. Examples include repeated colds, ulcers, muscle stiffness, elevated cholesterol, excessive sleeping, irritability, and headaches. Stress-related symptoms are often discounted and are not considered serious, but these problems are early warnings and can have both physical and emotional consequences.

Stress can be caused by such factors as a deadline; a goal of achieving all As in school; family problems, including unsupportive partners or over-demanding parents; overcommitment; poor organizational skills; health problems; a lack of self-confidence or poor self-esteem; financial problems; traffic; and car troubles. These events are stressors. What is stressful to one person may not affect someone else because of perspectives, life experiences, and personal circumstances. Stress is individual, and interventions used to reduce or buffer stress can be effective only when individually identified. What is helpful for one person may not be helpful for another. The important points are to recognize your stressors, to develop interventions, and to recognize the need for taking responsibility for yourself.

INTERVENTIONS

Change

For most people, major life events are stressful and in some cases overwhelming. Most people have observed others experiencing and coping with major changes, such as divorce, death of a family member or friend, marriage, job loss, or career change. By observing these major events, the observer makes decisions about how he or she would handle a similar situation if confronted. What has not been learned is how to handle minor changes, or hassles. In a busy life, these minor changes have great impact. Examples are an unexpected detour in the normal travel route to work or school, a last-minute change in examination time, a family argument, and car trouble. These unexpected events create great stress, and the body responds in the fight-or-flight mode. Once again, the body produces a chemical response, and these chemicals dissipate slowly through increased respiration, increased heart rate, muscle tension, and occasionally digestive upset. Response to these stressors may occur frequently enough that the body does not have enough time to get back to a homeostatic condition. In other words, the body can be constantly on alert as a result of the back-to-back changing conditions that are so much a part of a busy, responsible existence.

Minor changes can be countered by balancing unexpected change with planned positive activity. The minor changes often elicit negative responses in the form of anger, depression, poor self-concept, frustration, or defeat. Planned positive activities provide opportunities to experience joy, happiness, positive self-concept, optimism, and a sense of well-being. These activities, or uplifts, are often simple and easy to carry out. Examples include complimenting someone, watching a favorite television program, taking a walk, being efficient and organized, relaxing, having fun, hugging, and laughing.

In your chosen field of study, new concepts will be introduced, the language of the art will have to be mastered, and deadlines will need to be met both for the welfare of the patient and for the efficiency of the department. As goals are accomplished, great relief and joy are experienced, but reaching these goals without some planned positive activities will take an emotional and physical toll.

Survival Technique for Change. Plan positive activities, called *uplifts*, to balance unexpected negative change, or *hassles*.

Language

Stress tends to be contagious. When someone is in a period of great stress, such as around the time of final examinations, his or her words often clearly express the fear and frustration felt as a result of the concern that time, energy, or resources will be insufficient to get everything accomplished. The expression of this concern may alarm others, as well as augment the individual's feeling of frustration.

Many factors influence how we feel about events occurring around us every day. Internal events (fight or flight) happen even as a result of the out-of-control language we use. The use of words or phrases that express a lack of control promotes this feeling of being out of control, which is apparent in such statements as "I *have* to study for a test" and "I *never* get to do what I want to do." Statements used to express a feeling of not having any control include "I have to," "I must," "I never," "it's awful," and "it's unfair."

These examples of language express not only loss of control but also much emotion that is tied to each phrase. Saying words such as "never," "must," "have to," "awful," and "unfair" without some strong emotion associated with each is virtually impossible. Just saying each of these words awakens feelings of anger, frustration, or despair in the speaker.

If out-of-control words can evoke negative feelings, then using in-control language will produce positive feelings.

Substitute terminology that produces feelings of more control and less of a fight-or-flight response includes statements such as "I decided," "I choose," "I want to," "I like," and "I can." It is difficult to have strong negative feelings when uttering statements such as "I have decided to study this evening for my test" and "I choose to use this method to complete this procedure." Each statement reflects an attitude of choice and evokes positive feelings. These statements produce the expectation of reaching an attainable goal, as well as feelings of determination, self-control, and pleasure.

In many instances, terms that maximize stress responses are used when, in fact, personal choices have been made, but they are expressed negatively: "I have to go to class." The hope is that the unsaid portion is "I chose this field of study, and I have to go to class to reach my goal." Not only can we express such choices negatively, but also we often lose sight of the goal. The vision of whom or what we will become drives our choices; with practice, our language can reflect these decisions positively.

Survival Technique for Language. Practice language that reflects choice and expresses control over a situation. In-control language reduces the flight-or-fight response.

Worry

During high-stress times, everyone tends to be overly concerned about outcomes and to engage in a mental activity of "What will I do if ... ?" This activity is worry. "What will I do if I fail this examination?" "What if I do not complete all my clinical competencies in time?" "What if my family feels neglected?" "What if my car does not last until I graduate?" "What if I lose my job? How will I pay for tuition?" Each circumstance is a real possibility for many students, but until it is a reality, unnecessary energy is being expended through "borrowing trouble."

Worry robs energy! Less than 5% of the events about which we worry actually happen. Part of worry consists of time and energy spent being concerned about things over which we have no control. We often have little control over the mechanical functioning of our cars, especially when preventive maintenance is practiced. We worry about situations that do not involve us directly, such as a classmate passing an examination. We worry about possibilities that might be removed from our thoughts by taking some action. Taking no action is procrastination. If we could stop putting off an unpleasant or overly challenging activity because of laziness, poor management of time, or the fear of not being perfect, a significant part of worry would be eliminated. The big problem with procrastination is that a constant feeling of guilt accompanies putting off unpleasant tasks. The best news about procrastination and the worry it causes it is that we have full control over them. Do something to reduce the anxiety! Doing something wrong may be better than doing nothing at all!

Consider worry this way. Most of the things about which we worry never happen or turn out better than we thought they would. A small portion of what worries us is the result of procrastination, which can be eliminated by taking action. A minor part of worry is concern over matters that do not directly concern us and that may involve the worries that other people have.

Survival Technique for Worry. When worrying, use the following checklist to anticipate the degree of control you have over the situation:

- It probably will not happen.
- It will turn out better than expected.
- Taking action can change the outcome.
- It is not my concern.
- I have no control over the outcome.
- Am I making a mountain out of a molehill?

Managing Time

An important part of managing stress is learning to manage time. Commonly people believe that not enough time is available to accomplish all that needs to be done or all that we want to do. Because the amount of time available cannot be controlled, practicing time management becomes necessary; time management is self-management related to how time is used.

Many external interruptions are thieves of time. These interruptions include telephone calls, texts, e-mails, social networks, mistakes and incomplete information about assignments or jobs, and outside activities. These factors can be controlled by setting limits on the length of telephone calls if you choose to receive calls, limiting time spent on social media, getting a full understanding of assignments by taking a few extra minutes to clarify, and limiting outside activities temporarily.

Setting parameters on available time is also important. In many instances, too many tasks are attempted at once. This failure to set parameters regarding time happens to the student who has responsibilities that include not only school assignments, but also work, home, or family responsibilities. In addition to attempting too much at once, we may be faced with other compounding issues, including setting unrealistic deadlines, failing to say "no," procrastinating, and having a general lack of organization.

The biggest thief of time is indecision. The fear of making a mistake or of being imperfect prompts indecision. With much to be done in a limited time, loss of energy through worry and indecision is destructive and wasteful. If indecision is the product of fearing a mistake, consider thinking of a mistake as an opportunity to learn and improve on future activities and decisions.

Setting deadlines can provide opportunities to schedule time for study, make and take telephone calls, assist family members, and socialize. Scheduling activities gives some assurance of being able to meet obligations without slighting anyone. A potential problem associated with scheduling activities is that of being trapped by the schedule. Deadlines can give rise to feelings of desperation and helplessness, especially when the number of activities that can be accomplished within the allotted time frame has been overestimated—for example, allowing 3 hours in an evening to study for a test along with doing some other, minor activities, only to discover that the 3-hour time frame was not enough. The individual is then trapped into having to meet the other obligations and yet still finding time to complete the studying.

Although scheduling activities is wise, realistic time frames must be set. Unrealistic estimates of the time needed to complete a paper, study for an examination, or travel to class can give rise to feelings of panic. This panic can trigger the fight-or-flight response, which then defeats the purpose of time management. The best way to combat the result of underestimating time needed is to build in contingency plans. "If a paper takes longer to write than expected, what alternatives do I have?" "Can I take another route to school if the street repair ties up traffic?" Providing a way out reduces feelings of panic and the negative effects of the fight-or-flight response.

The best way to manage time is to practice self-management. This goal involves four steps:

1. *Know yourself.* Evaluate your personal style, and recognize the times when you are in peaks and valleys of effectiveness. Capitalize on your peak times, and plan to do the activities that are most demanding. Ask yourself if you are a morning person or a night owl. When do you think most clearly, and for how long can you concentrate on one activity? Generally, the best results come from studying for 50 to 60 minutes in one block of time, then breaking for 10 minutes. Repeating this cycle reduces fatigue and allows more productive use of time.

2. *Prioritize responsibilities.* Identify all the roles you have that involve responsibility—that is, student, employee, or housekeeper. Prioritize all these roles from highest to lowest priority. Evaluate time available after classes and after personal needs and obligations are met. Careful evaluation of activities and responsibilities should be done to determine which items can be realistically continued and which need to be delegated to someone else.

3. *Prioritize activities.* Set priorities according to goals and the length of time that will be needed to complete an activity. Setting a plan for a full week, month, or term and scheduling study, research, and social activities during these blocks of time may be helpful. By looking at a long-term plan, rushing at the last minute can be avoided, and social obligations can be met. Goals such as graduating, completing a semester, or getting a B in a course must be set so that activities will be driven by the goal.

4. *Plan for self-care.* Because we all have a need for relaxation, which includes exercise, games, rest, and socializing, this time should be anticipated and planned. For some people, planning for self-care is necessary because they learned the work-before-play ethic. Chances are that all of the work will never be done; consequently, little attention is given to social activities, leading to a negative view of life in general. For other people, the opposite may be the norm. The lack of discipline to complete work may lead to disappointing results educationally. A balance is required between work and play so that the goals can be met successfully and with enthusiasm.

Survival Technique for Managing Time. Plan your time, and set goals by the following actions:

- Knowing when you are most effective
- Prioritizing and delegating responsibility when additional resources exist
- Planning and scheduling activities as far in advance as possible to avoid last-minute rushing
- Scheduling time for relaxation and fun

BUFFERING STRESSORS

Even when all the positive steps to reduce stress are taken, stress cannot be eliminated. Because much of the stress experienced on a daily basis cannot be changed, the next best intervention is to buffer the effects of stress. Just as a mute muffles the harsh notes of a brass instrument, buffers are necessary to reduce the harmful effects of the fight-or-flight response.

Exercise

The fight-or-flight response readies the body for action. Circulation increases in the long muscles, and the heart rate and respiration rate increase to supply more oxygen to the muscles. Sugars and fats are dumped into the system to supply the needed energy for physical activity. If you are berated in front of your peers, anger, rage, fear, and indignation boil in your system and can be felt immediately. A chemical, norepinephrine, is released into the body during preparation for action. This chemical heightens the emotional response that the stress causes. If irritation by someone or something is the cause, the response is anger, which is often out of proportion to the magnitude of the event. If the person feels threatened, the result may be unreasonable fear. This response accounts for the extreme reactions often elicited in the form of irritability and loss of sense of humor when someone has been under stress for prolonged periods without proper interventions. Participation in regular aerobic activity—continuous, rhythmic activity that involves large muscles—is necessary to dissipate the undesirable chemicals in the system resulting from stress. *Aerobic* means using air to perform the activity. Examples are running, walking, biking, and other noncompetitive exercise. Because of the desire to win, exercise during a competitive event may increase tension rather than decrease it.

Exercise is not only necessary to dissipate undesirable chemicals produced by the body, but it can also be a means to prevent negative physical and emotional responses. A minimum of 30 minutes of aerobic exercise three to five times per week can have some positive health benefits. Some physical benefits are reduced risk for heart disease, decreased blood cholesterol levels, and reduced muscle tension.

Many of our efforts in society are directed at getting and keeping the competitive edge. Ego-involved activities almost never result in feelings of reduced stress. In fact, they may have the reverse effect. The noncompetitive forms of exercise are the most beneficial mentally. Exercising is done because it feels right. A sense of well-being is produced as a result of the activity. This sense of well-being after exercising is a result not only of reducing harmful chemicals produced under stress, but also of releasing *happy* chemicals in the brain that produce a sense of pleasure; the most notable of the latter chemicals are the endorphins. Endorphins released in the brain during physical activity have a relaxing effect on the body and provide a sense of well-being. This feeling contributes to what is commonly called the *runner's high*. People who exercise regularly look forward to the relaxing benefits of the aerobic activity, which usually promotes improved sleep patterns, increased energy and stress tolerance, and suppressed appetite.

If possible, find a friend to participate with you. You will give encouragement to each other. Time spent walking with a friend provides some social time as well. Sharing a mutual interest is a rewarding and satisfying experience.

Survival Technique for Buffering Stress. Exercise aerobically three to five times per week for a minimum of 30 minutes as a buffer to the chemicals produced in the body as a result of the fight-or-flight response.

Nutrition

When we are busiest, we are least able to provide good nutrition for ourselves. Stress can be buffered by eating three well-balanced meals each day. When our body undergoes the fight-or-flight response on any regular basis, levels of three nutritional substances that are important to us both physically and mentally—vitamin C, vitamin B complex, and magnesium—are greatly reduced.

Vitamin C is needed for the growth and repair of the tissues in the body and has been shown to be important in supporting the immune system. Research has shown that vitamin C has not reduced the risk for getting a common cold but it might decrease the length of the cold and/or result in milder symptoms. Frequently, when someone experiences a stressor, such as getting through final examinations, he or she may develop a cold and sore throat at that time. As vitamin C is depleted, our resistance is decreased. One way to replace the depleted vitamin C is to start a diet that includes dark-green leafy vegetables, fruits, broccoli, Brussels sprouts, potatoes, and tomatoes.

The complex of B vitamins seems to support and provide necessary energy to sustain us from day to day. When under a great deal of stress, we may oversleep or feel groggy much of the time. Lost vitamin B complex can be replaced by eating bananas, green leafy vegetables, lean meat, poultry, milk, eggs, and whole grains.

Magnesium supports the immune system. Replacement of magnesium comes from eating bananas, fish, nuts, and whole grains. A diet rich in carbohydrates (e.g., white bread) and simple sugars tends to cause sudden rises and falls in blood sugar levels. This fluctuation can cause sleepiness, sluggishness, and mental lethargy. In addition, because of the response of insulin to the introduction of sugar into the digestive tract, blood sugar levels fall sharply. This rapid decrease in blood sugar levels provides the physiologic conditions that can lead to misinterpreting information or making mountains out of molehills. Vending machine foods and fast foods are often major sources of carbohydrates and need to be avoided or at least carefully selected.

Good nutrition includes a diet that provides appropriate servings from all food groups (Fig. 3.1). The US Department of Agriculture (USDA) has updated the historical food pyramid with *MyPlate*, which emphasizes the importance of healthy food choices and being active every day. The dietary guidelines begin by emphasizing the importance of building a healthy plate consisting of five food groups: fruits, vegetables, grains, protein foods, and dairy. Recommendations include making half of your plate fruits and vegetables, switching to skim or 1% milk,

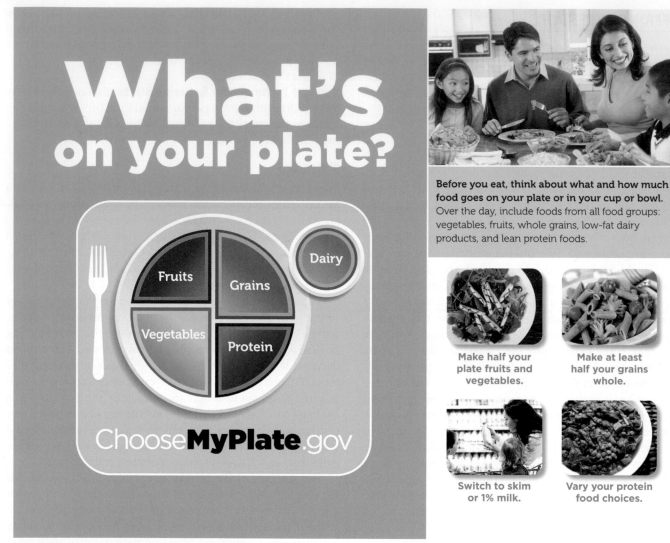

Fig. 3.1 US Department of Agriculture's MyPlate.

making at least half of your grains whole grains, and varying your protein food choices. Additionally, it is recommended that individuals choose foods and drinks with little or no added sugars, to watch for the salt in foods, and to eat fewer foods that are high in solid fats. Identifying your personal calorie limit and staying with it is important to maintain a healthy weight, as is being physically active. Maintaining a good nutritional balance will not change your stressors, but it will place you at an advantage for staying both physically and mentally healthy during stressful events. For more detailed information from the USDA, visit its website at http://www.choosemyplate.gov. This website provides a tremendous variety of resources including online tools and tips designed for college students. In addition, at https://health.gov/dietaryguidelines/2015/guidelines/, a very comprehensive set of dietary guidelines are provided which are designed to promote a healthy diet and prevent diet-related chronic diseases.

Survival Technique for Buffering Stress. Eat three nutritionally balanced meals each day to replace vitamins and minerals lost through stress.

Visualization and Meditation

Other buffers to stress include visualization and meditation. Through visualization, the individual can take a mini-vacation by mentally revisiting a pleasant experience for 10 or 15 seconds. Maybe you recall the peace of sitting on a beach and hearing the waves lap the shore. It might be the silence and coolness of getting up early and witnessing a sunrise. Maybe it is the remembrance of a campfire, including the smell of wood burning, the sound of wood snapping, the feel of the heat from the flames, and the joy of sharing the experience with friends. Each of these mental events actually provides an opportunity to escape and relax by reliving the events momentarily. It also reduces the feeling of stress and the fight-or-flight response, thus providing a brief but real opportunity to get in touch with feelings of relaxation. This activity helps buffer day-to-day stresses.

Meditation also provides a mechanism to escape stress by emptying the mind of all thoughts and focusing on only one word or one statement. In Christian meditation, it may be the process of sharing the weight of responsibility or the blessing of support through God's love and acceptance.

Vegetables	Fruits	Grains	Dairy	Protein Foods
Eat more red, orange, and dark-green veggies like tomatoes, sweet potatoes, and broccoli in main dishes. Add beans or peas to salads (kidney or chickpeas), soups (split peas or lentils), and side dishes (pinto or baked beans), or serve as a main dish. Fresh, frozen, and canned vegetables all count. Choose "reduced sodium" or "no-salt-added" canned veggies.	Use fruits as snacks, salads, and desserts. At breakfast, top your cereal with bananas or strawberries; add blueberries to pancakes. Buy fruits that are dried, frozen, and canned (in water or 100% juice), as well as fresh fruits. Select 100% fruit juice when choosing juices.	Substitute whole-grain choices for refined-grain breads, bagels, rolls, breakfast cereals, crackers, rice, and pasta. Check the ingredients list on product labels for the words "whole" or "whole grain" before the grain ingredient name. Choose products that name a whole grain first on the ingredients list.	Choose skim (fat-free) or 1% (low-fat) milk. They have the same amount of calcium and other essential nutrients as whole milk, but less fat and calories. Top fruit salads and baked potatoes with low-fat yogurt. If you are lactose intolerant, try lactose-free milk or fortified soymilk (soy beverage).	Eat a variety of foods from the protein food group each week, such as seafood, beans and peas, and nuts as well as lean meats, poultry, and eggs. Twice a week, make seafood the protein on your plate. Choose lean meats and ground beef that are at least 90% lean. Trim or drain fat from meat and remove skin from poultry to cut fat and calories.

For a 2,000-calorie daily food plan, you need the amounts below from each food group.
To find amounts personalized for you, go to ChooseMyPlate.gov.

Eat 2½ cups every day	**Eat 2 cups every day**	**Eat 6 ounces every day**	**Get 3 cups every day**	**Eat 5½ ounces every day**
What counts as a cup? 1 cup of raw or cooked vegetables or vegetable juice; 2 cups of leafy salad greens	**What counts as a cup?** 1 cup of raw or cooked fruit or 100% fruit juice; ½ cup dried fruit	**What counts as an ounce?** 1 slice of bread; ½ cup of cooked rice, cereal, or pasta; 1 ounce of ready-to-eat cereal	**What counts as a cup?** 1 cup of milk, yogurt, or fortified soymilk; 1½ ounces natural or 2 ounces processed cheese	**What counts as an ounce?** 1 ounce of lean meat, poultry, or fish; 1 egg; 1 Tbsp peanut butter; ½ ounce nuts or seeds; ¼ cup beans or peas

Cut back on sodium and empty calories from solid fats and added sugars

Look out for salt (sodium) in foods you buy. Compare sodium in foods and choose those with a lower number.

Drink water instead of sugary drinks. Eat sugary desserts less often.

Make foods that are high in solid fats—such as cakes, cookies, ice cream, pizza, cheese, sausages, and hot dogs—occasional choices, not every day foods.

Limit empty calories to less than 260 per day, based on a 2,000 calorie diet.

Be physically active your way

Pick activities you like and do each for at least 10 minutes at a time. Every bit adds up, and health benefits increase as you spend more time being active.

Children and adolescents: get 60 minutes or more a day.

Adults: get 2 hours and 30 minutes or more a week of activity that requires moderate effort, such as brisk walking.

USDA U.S. Department of Agriculture • Center for Nutrition Policy and Promotion
August 2011
CNPP-25
USDA is an equal opportunity provider and employer.

Fig. 3.1, cont'd

Other buffers to stress include progressive relaxation, deep-muscle relaxation (usually guided by audio recordings), biofeedback, and guided imagery. It is also important to rely on school and community resources, such as a campus counselor, tutors, and financial aid advisors, whenever needed.

Survival Technique for Buffering Stress. Regularly practice visualization or some form of meditation and utilize school and community resources.

STUDY SKILLS AND TEST TAKING

Study Skill Techniques

During the next few years of college and advanced-level study, you will be required to learn technical information that is tested during each term. In addition, you will have to recall pieces of learned information much later and add them to new, more advanced concepts. Because of the building of information into complex concepts, higher-level learning, not simply a brief regurgitation of facts, must take place. An excellent way to increase the effectiveness of study time is to apply the concept

BOX 3.1 Study Skill Techniques

Review the material soon after it is introduced.
Use as many senses as possible.
Plan a regular schedule of study.
Study in a group.
Attitude helps remembering!

of time management to develop good study skills. This process involves five techniques (Box 3.1):

1. *Review the material soon after it is introduced.* Most information introduced in class is forgotten within 24 hours unless steps are taken to reinforce learning it (Fig. 3.2). Students often do not begin to study for a test before the week of the test. Usually, a great deal of time has elapsed, and much of the material has been forgotten. A common theme expressed during last-minute study is, "The instructor didn't explain very well," or "The instructor never told us that!" If material is reviewed immediately or within a short time after class, the information can be reinforced and remembered longer. This practice also helps identify questionable areas in which understanding is lacking.

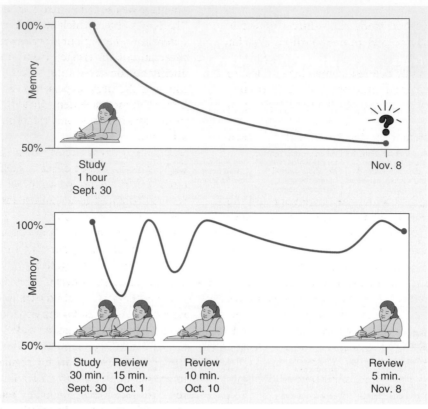

Fig. 3.2 *Top,* Massed study. *Bottom,* Spaced reviews.

2. *Use as many senses as possible.* In review of information, writing key elements or words has been shown to be beneficial. This visual stimulation through writing imprints additional and longer lasting information in the brain, which enhances recall later. Besides writing the information, recite the material aloud. Saying the words helps formulate another dimension of the concept and allows practice at saying unfamiliar terms. The combination of seeing, saying, and hearing—using several senses—has been shown to provide opportunities for increased retention of information and recall. Developing a mnemonic can also be helpful. A mnemonic is a device used as an aid for remembering. For example, to remember the heart valves, think left atrium bicuspid, right atrium tricuspid (LAB RAT).

3. *Plan a regular schedule of study.* Waiting until the last minute to study increases anxiety to a point that it actually may interfere with the ability to learn and recall information. Frustration sets in as the time ticks away. Studying or cramming for a test at the last minute may lead to confusion about details. Cramming provides only short-term recall. Plan regular review and study of all subjects from the time the material is first introduced. This action may be as simple as planning to reread notes every other day for a short time. Studies have shown that short, regular periods of study and review result in greater recall than a long period of study followed by a long period of no exposure to the information. Studying for 1 hour/week before a test with no review in between can result in a 50% loss of recall.

4. *Study in a group.* Studying in small groups of no more than five helps test your understanding of the material. The variety of perceptions offers opportunities to conceptualize the information from more than one viewpoint. If a large amount of material has to be covered, divide it among the group, each person preparing an area that may be within the individual's interest and expertise. Working in a group provides an opportunity to feel supported and encouraged, thus enhancing a personal expectation of success. The study group needs to focus on a goal with mutual agreement on the purpose of meeting and the task to be accomplished. This approach is necessary to avoid the temptation to use the time for socializing rather than studying. Once the business of study is completed, relaxing and enjoying the company of the group is important and appropriate.

5. *Attitude helps remembering.* Having a positive attitude about the reason for studying enhances your ability to learn and remember. You have set a goal for your professional future. Approach it with enthusiasm and a *can-do* attitude. Become part of the self-fulfilling prophecy that says you are in control of your successes and failures. A feeling of control, in turn, reduces the stress response and enhances your chances for a healthy period of learning.

Survival Technique for Study Skills. Plan your time and prepare by the following actions:

- Review new material soon after introduction.
- Use as many senses as possible—seeing, saying, and writing.
- Plan a regular study schedule.
- Study with a group occasionally.
- Develop a positive *can-do* attitude.

Test-Taking Tips

In addition to possessing good study skills, following a few *test-taking strategies* is also helpful. Here are some useful tips for test-taking success:

1. Take the day off from study before a comprehensive test to relax and prepare both mentally and physically. Last-minute cramming adds to anxiety and the possibility of *freezing* on the test.

2. Wear bright-colored clothes for the test. Color has great effect on moods and alertness; it also reflects feelings about the individual. Bright colors promote positive and optimistic feelings.

3. Avoid a diet full of carbohydrates the day before and the day of the test. *Carb loading* may be helpful to a runner preparing for a long-distance race but not for a person sitting and taking an examination. The carbohydrates convert to sugar, providing the runner with extra energy as he or she runs. Carbohydrates and sugars leave the nonrunner sluggish and sleepy because of the need to metabolize all the sugar without exerting much energy. A well-balanced diet that includes proteins and carbohydrates provides improved mental alertness necessary when taking a test.

4. Get a good night's sleep before the examination. Rest allows clear thinking and improved interpretation.

5. Get to the test early to allow yourself time to relax before beginning. Rushing at the last minute increases anxiety, which can decrease your mental effectiveness.

6. Scan the test, and answer all the questions you are sure you know. Do not waste time initially on questions that are problematic for you. Go back and repeat the procedure, allowing yourself a little more time to answer. Leave questions whose answers are difficult to recall until the last. This way, if it is a time-limited examination, most questions will be answered even if you are caught short of time.

7. Review your test when done, and make corrections as needed. Do not be afraid to change answers. Some recall may have occurred during the test; some questions provide a key to answers for other questions. Make certain you have answered all the questions. If you are recording answers on an answer sheet that requires blackening circles or boxes, be certain that the number of the question corresponds with the number on the answer sheet.

8. When the test is over, put it behind you. Use the results as an opportunity to enhance your knowledge in the future. Now, begin the study process all over again. Think positively!

SUMMARY

- Stress is a demand on time, energy, and resources, with some fear of not being able to meet goals or obligations. Change is a large component of stress, and managing an ever-changing environment is the way to survive. The language we use can increase or decrease feelings of control. The issues about which we worry need to be evaluated to determine whether our worries are within our control. Are these mountains created from molehills, or can the worry energy be converted into action to diminish the problem? Much of the stress experience can be altered by practicing better time management, including prioritizing by setting limits, making decisions, establishing goals, and managing self-care.

- Buffering of stress occurs when the effects of the fight-or-flight response can be offset through other activities. Most of our stressors will not go away, but we can exercise regularly, eat well-balanced meals and snacks, and use some form of meditation or visualization to reduce temporarily the physical and emotional effects of stress. These activities will not change our stressors, but they can offer an opportunity to balance some of the negative.

- For students, a great deal of stress is the result of the physical and emotional effort of preparing for classroom and clinical tests. Successful test taking depends on good time management and appropriate study skills, as well as on good nutrition and rest. Developing individualized study skills involves managing time to allow for regular review, periodic study in groups, and practicing methods to enhance learning and remembering. Letting as many senses as possible reinforce information assists in imprinting information on the brain. This approach is especially important as concepts are *built* from course to course. A systematic approach to taking the test prevents running out of time before all questions have been considered. Complete all the easiest questions first, and return to more difficult questions later. This method helps you relax and build confidence, and it helps trigger recall because questions are often interrelated.

- Most of all, maintain a positive *can-do* attitude. Attitude becomes a self-fulfilling prophecy. If you believe you can achieve your goals, you will. Associate with others who think positively. A positive attitude is contagious and needs to be fostered by you and by people around you.

BIBLIOGRAPHY

Dietary Guidelines for Americans 2015-2020: Eight Edition. Available at: https://health.gov/dietaryguidelines/2015/guidelines/ Accessed November 27, 2017.

Ellis D: *Becoming a master student*, ed 15, Stamford, Conn, 2014, Cengage Learning.

Girdano DA, Everly GS, Dusek DE: *Controlling stress and tension*, ed 9, San Francisco, 2012, Benjamin Cummings.

Haroun L: *Career development for health professionals: success in school and on the job*, ed 3, St. Louis, 2011, Saunders.

Kirtbawski PA: Test-taking skills: giving yourself an edge, *Nursing* 90(20):6, 1990.

U.S. Department of Agriculture: ChooseMyPlate.gov. Available at http://www.choosemyplate.gov/.

4

Critical-Thinking and Problem-Solving Strategies

Tracy Herrmann, PhD, RT(R), Angie Arnold, MEd, RT(R)

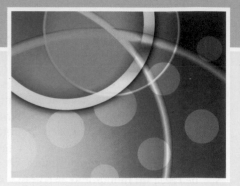

Education is not the filling of a pail, but the lighting of a fire.
William Butler Yeats

OBJECTIVES

On completion of this chapter, the student will be able to:
- Define critical thinking and problem solving.
- Discuss the importance of critical thinking and problem solving in the radiologic sciences.
- Describe the role of critical thinking in clinical, ethical, and technical decision making.
- Use the steps involved in problem solving.
- Apply teamwork and self-reflection in critical thinking and problem solving.

- Analyze and determine appropriate actions for situations that require critical thinking.
- Identify professional situations that use critical-thinking and problem-solving skills.
- Develop critical-thinking and problem-solving skills as a radiologic sciences professional.

OUTLINE

KEY TERMS

Analysis Careful examination of the components of a complex situation or problem

Case Studies Real-life patient situations that are studied and assessed for learning purposes

Critical Thinking Creative action based on professional knowledge and experience involving sound judgment applied with high ethical standards and integrity

Critique Type of evaluation that provides feedback on the quality of a work or creation in the form of an opinion or review

Evaluation Judgment or determination of the quality of a work or creation

Laboratory Experiments Exercises or activities used to reinforce cognitive concepts through the performance of planned steps, usually involving the analysis of data and answering of questions

Portfolio Collection and self-assessment of representative student work and accomplishments

Practice Standards Defining statements of the professional role and performance criteria for a practitioner

Problem Solving Answering questions in a methodic manner to resolve a challenging situation

Reflection Use of recording in a journal and personal review of current and past practices to improve future decision-making processes

Role Playing Acting out a situation in a realistic manner in the classroom or laboratory

Synthesis Combining multiple areas of knowledge to create a new work or understanding

Teamwork Collaboration with others on the health care team to provide quality patient care

WHAT ARE CRITICAL THINKING AND PROBLEM SOLVING?

In the broadest sense, critical thinking is the art of reflecting on and evaluating your thought process for the purpose of improving it. In the radiologic sciences, critical thinking is a reflective decision-making process that is necessary because every patient presents a new situation or challenge. No two procedures or treatments are the same. Each patient is an individual who must be cared for in a unique and often creative manner. A patient's individuality or pathologic condition can create a situation that requires a quick and inventive response from the radiologic sciences professional. This creative action, when performed appropriately based on professional knowledge and experience, is considered critical thinking. Critical thinking involves sound professional judgment applied with high ethical standards and integrity.

Critical thinking is required in most health care situations. An uncomfortable or difficult decision that must be made about a patient's care likely involves critical-thinking skills. Identifying inappropriate actions or situations and correcting them also involve critical thinking. Challenges with communication, modifying procedures or treatments from the normal routine with regard to patient condition, and solving equipment malfunctions or technical problems are just a few examples of situations that involve problem solving and critical thinking.

Why Learn to Think Critically and Solve Problems in the Radiologic Sciences?

Professional standards of the radiologic sciences support and define problem-solving and critical-thinking skills expected in the workplace. Credentialing agencies such as the American Registry of Radiologic Technologists (ARRT) publish codes of ethics (see Appendix D). These codes address the expected conduct of radiologic sciences professionals to perform procedures while providing the highest quality of care and to act in the best interest of the patient in an ethical manner. Professional societies such as the American Society of Radiologic Technologists (ASRT) also publish practice standards (see Appendix A) that define specific professional expectations and responsibilities. Inherent in these professional standards are the elements of appropriate decision-making skills associated with problem solving and critical thinking. Future employers will expect graduates to have developed skills in these areas.

To prepare students for the workforce, educational programs reinforce the expectations of the professional standards described previously. In addition, the programmatic and institutional accrediting agencies that guide educational institutions require the preparation of students for thinking and decision making that goes well beyond memorization. For example, the Joint Review Committee on Education in Radiologic Technology *Standards for an Accredited Program in the Radiologic Sciences* requires that radiologic sciences programs assess the problem-solving and the critical-thinking skills of their students. The goals and objectives of the student program may include elements of critical thinking, including analysis, synthesis, evaluation, and critique. Development and assessment

of these goals may be accomplished in a variety of unique ways for each accredited program. Students are likely to encounter role playing, case studies, scenarios, clinical skill assessments, laboratory experiments, complex calculations, multifaceted multiple-choice questions, team-based problems, and many additional forms of learning experiences, all designed to evaluate students' critical-thinking skills. Students may be asked to create products of learning or demonstrate learning through a portfolio, self-evaluation, or reflection through recording in a journal. Students must be open to unique learning experiences that require this higher order of thinking.

STEPS IN CRITICAL THINKING AND PROBLEM SOLVING

The key to mastering critical thinking is to extend learning beyond memorization of the concepts of the radiologic sciences profession. Students should pursue a deep long-term understanding of professional concepts and standards. Students may learn effectively by creating a scaffold of knowledge that will allow them to make additions and revisions as the students' mastery of the profession develops. Students should consider each element of their education a building block or puzzle piece that they may need to use later to solve a complex clinical problem. After all, the knowledge base of the profession will grow with or without the student. Table 4.1 lists the steps in problem solving and critical thinking and associated questions that are answered during the process.

Identify the Problem

A key element of critical thought is problem solving. The first step in problem solving is to identify the problem. This step can be challenging, given that problems are often difficult to define. An unclear problem can cause frustration and discomfort. A situation or technique may not be working for you, and, as a student, you may have difficulty determining the cause.

Investigate the Problem

The next step is to investigate by undergoing an objective examination of a problem. What do you already know about the problem? Review and examine all aspects of the problem and the factors that might influence the outcome. What are the key elements of the problem? Who or what is or may be affected by this problem? What are the implications of the problem that might result in safety risks and liability? What are the technical considerations? Will more than one solution or type of solution be needed? Identifying the elements of the problem is important so that you can proceed with finding the solution.

Formulate Viable Solutions to the Problem

Consider, develop, and formulate all possible viable solutions to a problem. Be objective and base decisions on professional knowledge, ethics, and standards. Look to these professional standards, and modify them to fit the unique situation that the problem presents. Acquire any additional information or expertise as needed. Have you experienced similar problems that can guide you to possible solutions?

TABLE 4.1	Steps in Critical Thinking and Problem Solving	
Steps in Order	**Potential Questions**
Identify the problem	• Does a problem exist? • What is the problem? • What is the cause of the problem? • Solving the problem is whose responsibility?
Investigate the problem	• What is known about the problem? • What are all of the aspects of the problem, and how will these factors influence the outcome? • What are the key elements of the problem? • Who or what is or may be affected by this problem? • What are the safety, risk, and liability implications? • What are the technical considerations? • Will more than one solution or type of solution be needed?
Formulate viable solutions to the problem	• Are your decisions regarding the problem objective and based on professional knowledge, ethics, and standards? • How will these professional standards be applied and modified to fit the unique situation presented by the problem? • What additional reliable information or expertise is needed? • Do any similar problems exist that have been successfully solved that can guide you to possible solutions? • Will a creative solution be needed for this unique problem?
Select the best solution	• Which solution will allow for the best care of the patient and is within professional ethical standards? • Does this solution correspond with the procedures and protocol for your institution? • How quickly must the solution be enacted? • How does your solution affect the patient's outcome?

Be sure to refer to your professional references or consult with an expert when necessary. Make sure your sources of information are reliable. Be creative and keep safety in mind when creating solutions.

Select the Best Solution

Finally, select and enact the best solution and action plan. Which solution will allow for the best care of the patient and is within professional ethical standards? Make sure that the chosen solution corresponds with the procedures and protocol for your institution. The most challenging problem solving and critical thinking occur when an immediate decision is required, when more than one appropriate solution to the problem exists, or when no clear viable solution exists. Be sure to follow up on the problem to see how your choices affected the outcome. Reflect on this experience for use in solving future problems.

Critical Thinking in the Classroom and Laboratory

The classroom and the laboratory provide valuable experiences that allow the student to develop critical-thinking and analysis skills that involve cognitive and psychomotor learning. *Cognitive* and *psychomotor* refer to thinking and doing, respectively. In the classroom or laboratory, students are given the freedom to develop alternative ideas, test the classics, solve new problems, and increase their understanding of old problems without endangering the health of a patient. Students can also repeatedly experiment to find the answer or examine *what if* questions without irradiating a human being. The classroom and laboratory are the best places for students to begin developing the ability to apply previous knowledge to new situations (Fig. 4.1). The classroom and laboratory also allow students to begin formulating independent judgments needed for critical thinking in the rapidly changing health care environment.

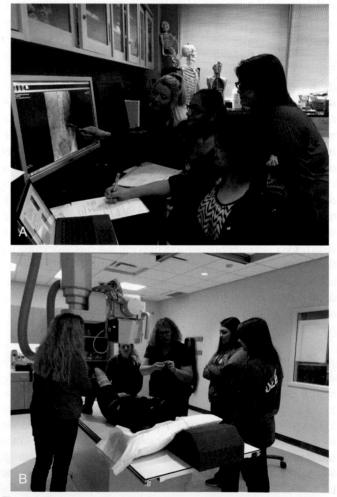

Fig. 4.1 The classroom and laboratory settings allow the students to develop critical-thinking and analysis skills such as image critique and digital imaging concepts. Students can examine *what if* questions without radiation exposure to a human being.

Development of critical-thinking skills often involves problem-based learning (solving real-life complex problems) and team-based work. Formal **teamwork** is most effective with the establishment of group rules and group roles to foster effective group processes. Peer evaluations may also be part of the process. Research that supports evidence-based practice should be integrated in the decision-making process. Evidence-based practice involves an approach in which scientific evidence and expertise are used to provide improved patient care. These activities are effective in helping students develop alternative and creative modes of inquiry.

Critical Thinking in the Clinical Setting

The clinical setting is where the student can transfer knowledge into action in a *real-world* environment. Students are exposed to unique real-life experiences that can be reinforced by the supervising radiologic sciences professional. Understanding the *why* behind a standard procedure is the key to making future decisions when a situation is not routine. Making decisions based on professional knowledge as applied to the clinical situation is important. Clinical experience provides a variety of critical-thinking situations and allows for student learning to extend well beyond *button pushing,* it permits the student to demonstrate the ability to respond when the correct decision is not clear and obvious, and it may involve recognizing when a situation is inappropriate and determining how to proceed in a professional manner.

Students who are new to the clinical setting must consider that radiologic sciences professionals use many variations of the standard procedures taught in the laboratory and classroom. Each radiologic sciences professional has developed his or her own style based on experience. These variations in practice can create a sense of frustration for the student. The student must focus on combining the best elements of each supervising radiologic sciences professional and then develop his or her own appropriate practice habits and professional style.

At the beginning phases of clinical experience, critical thinking may involve decisions made by the student regarding which role models to emulate or when to go to program officials with concerns or problems. Early critical-thinking decisions may also involve determining whether to make independent judgments or to ask for help, or it may involve deciding when making a joke is appropriate and when not to do so. With experience and education, the student will be prepared to handle critical-thinking situations that may affect the life and well-being of a patient under the student's care.

Affective Critical Thinking

Analyzing personal values and feelings and managing uncomfortable ethical situations are components of affective critical thinking. Students must value the professional knowledge that serves as the foundation for their chosen profession. Students benefit by examining the ways they learn best and then taking charge of their own education. Being a creative and active learner is important in the radiologic sciences. Students often have overwhelming feelings when they first enter the health care setting. They may observe and be involved in many situations they have not previously experienced. Feelings can be expressed through journal writing or discussions with program faculty, other students, or clinical supervisors. Students must be conscientious about maintaining patient confidentiality at all times during these types of discussions. Affective

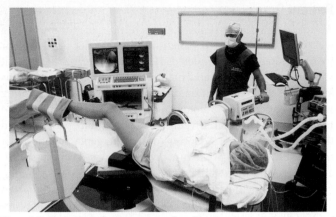

Fig. 4.2 Radiologic sciences professionals must use advanced critical-thinking skills when performing procedures and treatment such as those in the operating room.

critical-thinking skills are also important when dealing with the patient and his or her family, communicating in challenging situations, and working as part of the health care team. Students also may need to apply problem-solving and critical-thinking skills to manage their personal problems and issues to ensure that these do not affect their educational progress or, more important, patient care in the clinical setting.

CLINICAL APPLICATIONS OF CRITICAL THINKING AND PROBLEM SOLVING

Ethics

Many situations arise that require a radiologic sciences professional to make a decision based on professional ethics. These situations require the radiologic sciences professional to act appropriately regarding patient safety and radiation safety of patients and other health care personnel. At all times the radiologic sciences professional is expected to act within the guidelines of the ARRT Code of Ethics (see Appendix D). Chapter 24 provides specific examples and information about problem solving for ethical dilemmas, including potential situations that a radiologic sciences professional may face.

Technical Skills

A patient rarely arrives in the department prepared and able to cooperate as needed for a procedure or treatment. Some patients cannot stand for an upright procedure, or they cannot lie face down (prone) for an examination that requires them to be in that position. A treatment plan may need to be altered to accommodate a patient's condition or ability. In these situations, the radiologic sciences professional must evaluate and adjust the procedure or treatment according to the patient's ability and still produce the same outcome—adequate treatment or a diagnostic radiographic image. Radiologic and imaging sciences professionals may use advanced technical critical-thinking skills when performing procedures in areas such as trauma, critical care, or surgery as well as in situations where they evaluate the appropriateness of procedures and treatments (Fig. 4.2). The development of technical critical-thinking skills is an ongoing process that requires extensive knowledge of the profession. Students must learn the foundation of professional knowledge to develop future technical critical-thinking skills for use in practice.

Patient Care

A radiologic sciences professional is responsible for interacting with and caring for each patient until his or her procedure or treatment has been completed. He or she observes the patient and looks for physical and mental changes that may occur as a result of the treatment or procedure. While communicating with the patient, the radiologic sciences professional will need to consider any human diversity issues that may play a part in the care of the patient. Adapting to any emergency situation that may arise during the procedure or treatment is also necessary to ensure safe and successful completion.

The following decision-making scenarios have been created as examples of situations that call for critical thinking and problem solving. Keep in mind that these are only a few examples of situations that a radiologic sciences professional may encounter on a day-to-day basis. The first case scenario provides an example of how the steps are used.

Case 1: Human Diversity. *"Your next patient does not understand English."* You need to escort the patient from the waiting room and give her instructions for the procedure, including removing all clothing from the waist up and any metallic objects from the chest and abdomen area. You then need to take the patient into the examination room and place her in the correct position for the procedure. After completing the procedure, you need to give the patient exit information.

Identify the problem. You speak only English, and your patient does not.

Investigate the problem. What instructions will need to be given to the patient? What technical considerations must be evaluated? Does the patient speak any English? What are the cultural considerations?

Formulate possible solutions. You will need to develop a creative way to communicate your instructions to the patient. Can you identify someone else who can speak the language? Does anyone in the department speak the same language as the patient? Does the health care institution have an interpreter available? If the answer to all of these questions is "no," what do you do next?

Select and enact the best solution. In this case, no interpreter is available, and the patient understands minimal English. You will need to use a variety of methods of communication, such as demonstration and pantomime, as well as maintain your composure and patience while performing the procedure. All aspects of cultural diversity education and communication skills must be used in this instance. This type of situation occurs often; therefore keep in mind that it is just as frustrating for the patient as it is for the radiologic sciences professional.

Case 2: Patient Interaction. *"Is this elder abuse?"* As you wait for your next patient to arrive, you hear some voices in the adjacent examination room. Bob, a seasoned radiologic technologist, is speaking loudly to an older male patient. "Put your arms up! I don't have time for this! Can you hear me?! I said keep your arms up, you old fart!" he yells. Then you hear a loud thump and a groan. As you run into the room to help, you see the patient up against the wall with his head slumped to the side and Bob's hands are against the patient's chest. You notice that the patient has a

hearing aid and is in a state of fright, pain, and confusion. The patient says, "My leg gave out, why are you hurting me like this?"

Identify the problem. Was appropriate care provided? Were Bob's actions appropriate to prevent a fall? What issues are associated with Bob's communication style? Do you think Bob abused the patient because he was uncooperative?

Investigate the problem. What should you say to Bob? What questions should you ask the patient? What did you see and hear that might make a difference in your actions? What are the appropriate actions to take when a patient is falling?

Formulate possible solutions. Are you obligated to act in this situation? Can you solve the problem by yourself, or should you contact a supervisor? What possible actions on your part are appropriate?

Select and enact the best solution. What is the right thing to do when you have not witnessed the actual occurrence? Was this elder abuse that should be reported against your fellow technologist? Which solution is in the best interest of the patient?

Case 3: Patient Assessment. *"Your patient is unable to stand for x-rays."* Your patient has arrived from the emergency department for an acute abdominal series. The history provided on the requisition states that the patient is having sharp abdominal pain in his abdomen. When you ask the patient if he is able to stand for the upright abdominal radiograph, he replies, "Yes, I'll try."

Identify the problem. Should you permit the patient to stand? Could the patient's condition cause him to be weak or lightheaded if he stands? Could he have been given medication for his pain, and, if so, could it further affect his ability to stand? Even though he said that he would try to stand, should you allow him to do so?

Investigate the problem. What might happen if the patient is forced to stand? What are the ethical and legal implications if you have the patient stand when he really should not? If the patient falls, is the patient at fault for telling you he would try to stand, or are you at fault for allowing him to try?

Formulate possible solutions. Do you allow the patient to stand? What are the other alternatives to the upright abdominal radiograph? Does the alternative projection demonstrate the same anatomic structures as shown on the upright radiograph?

Select and enact the best solution. Keeping in mind that patient safety is always the first and foremost concern, if an alternative to the upright projection exists, should you use it? In the end, the decision you make must result in high-quality radiographs to aid in the patient's diagnosis but must also be in the best interest of the patient and his safety.

Case 4: Emergencies. *"Ma'am, are you feeling OK?"* Your patient is in the department receiving a scheduled radiation treatment to her skull for a pituitary tumor. Because of the nature of the treatment and the fact that the patient's head must remain perfectly still throughout the treatment, an immobilizing mask is being used. While the radiation is being administered, the immobilizing mask is placed over the patient's head and secured to the treatment table. While watching the patient on the monitor during the treatment, you notice that she appears pale and her eyes are watering. By the look on her face, you recognize that she is extremely nauseous, and her head is locked in place flat on the table within the immobilizing mask.

Identify the problem. What is your first course of action? The patient is nauseous and needs assistance quickly, but her head is clamped to the table. What medical concerns do you have at this time?

Investigate the problem. What might happen if you run immediately into the room? What will happen if the patient actually becomes ill while immobilized with her head flat on the table?

Formulate possible solutions. Do you run into the room and immediately remove the patient from the mask and assist her? Do you call for another radiation therapist or perhaps a physician to come and help you? Should anything else be done, or should anyone else be called before you assist the patient? What about the radiation treatment currently being administered? What about the treatment itself? Do you continue if her condition stabilizes?

Select and enact the best solution. Should the patient's need for immediate assistance be the first priority in this situation? Should the fact that the patient is receiving radiation treatment be considered? Should the radiation oncologist assess the patient and decide if the treatment can be continued, or should the procedure be rescheduled for another day? Do you need to contact the physician to consider whether future treatments are to be performed with some type of antinausea medication? After the decision has been made about the treatment, should the physicist be consulted to compensate for the missed dose? The immediate assessment and follow-up attention to the situation by the radiologic sciences professional are critical in situations such as this.

Case 5: Diagnosis. *"Is this an emergency?"* You are working the night shift in the emergency department, and as your images appear on the screen you notice that there is a 1-inch gap between the apex of the lung and the rib cage on the chest image for Mrs. Green. A few hours later you notice to your surprise that Mrs. Green is in the process of being discharged. You fear there has been a mistake and that the patient needs continued medical attention. The emergency department physician is busy with several other emergency patients, and the radiology resident is asleep.

Identify the problem. What is your obligation to the patient after you have completed the procedure? Should you act on the patient's behalf even though you are not responsible for the diagnosis of the patient's condition?

Investigate the problem. Should you speak to the patient or the nurse about the care the patient received? Can you look at the patient's chart, or is this a Health Insurance Portability and Accountability Act (HIPAA) violation?

Formulate possible solutions. Should you address the emergency department physician or go to another source? What questions should you ask? What is the best way to question an authority figure in this case?

Select and enact the best solution. What aspects of the ARRT code of ethics might apply to this scenario? Is there a solution that will allow you to maintain a good working relationship with the physicians while still acting in the best interest of the patient?

Case 6: Radiation Protection—Pregnancy. *"Does any chance of pregnancy exist?"* You are taking a history from a female patient who has been sent to your department for radiation treatment, and one of the first things you ask is whether she is pregnant. The patient hesitates when asked about pregnancy, then finally states, "No, there is no chance I'm pregnant—it really doesn't have anything to do with my treatment, right?"

Identify the problem. Do you take the patient at her word? Does her hesitation in answering raise a red flag? Considering what you have learned about radiation protection, is knowing whether she is pregnant really necessary?

Investigate the problem. What are the implications if you continue with treatment as scheduled and you find out later that the patient actually is pregnant? What risks would you take by administering treatment without knowing for sure? Can you be held liable for any damage caused? After all, the patient denied that she was pregnant when initially asked.

Formulate possible solutions. Do you go ahead with treatment? Do you decide not to administer treatment? Do you have any other choices?

Select and enact the best solution. Can you find any guidance in the ARRT code of ethics regarding your responsibility to the patient, specifically in the area of radiation protection? Which principle, if any, applies to this situation, and does this principle help you in enacting your final solution? Does a solution exist that will help you accomplish your goals without compromising patient safety? What solution is in the best interest of the patient?

Case 7: Radiation Protection—Supervision. *"Where did everyone go?"* You are a second-year student in a radiography program and are excited to be just a couple of weeks from graduation. One day while participating in a clinical education course at a local imaging center, word is sent to the control area that a patient has arrived for a chest x-ray examination. You tell the radiographers you will go get the patient, and they say they will meet you in the x-ray room in case you need help with the patient. Once the patient has changed into a gown and entered the x-ray room with you, she mentions she is weak and light-headed from her most recent chemotherapy treatment. You help her sit down in the chair while you go out to the control area to ask for help with the patient. When you are unable to find anyone, a secretary tells you that all the radiographers have gone to lunch because they have an early afternoon meeting.

Identify the problem. Should you go ahead and perform the examination because you have already completed many competencies and are nearing graduation? Will the patient be able to tolerate the procedure in her weakened state? If you wait for the radiographers to return, the patient will have to wait at least 45 minutes before her examination can be performed.

Investigate the problem. What might happen if you were to go ahead and perform the procedure? Are there legal and/or ethical considerations regarding performing the examination without the supervision of a radiographer? Could your decision in any way jeopardize your graduation from the program? Is the patient's weakened condition an important consideration?

Formulate possible solutions. If you perform the procedure without supervision and something happens to the patient, who is at fault? Because you are a student, are there program-specific policies that need to be considered? If the patient has to wait a long time, what do you tell her and the family members waiting for her in the lobby? Do you contact the radiographers at lunch and risk them being mad and possibly affecting your upcoming job interview for a position in the department after graduation?

Select and enact the best solution. Radiation protection rules and regulations exist regarding student supervision in the clinical setting, but you are also concerned about a sick patient waiting a long time for her radiographic examination. Students are often unfairly placed in situations such as these in the clinical setting, but your decision must follow patient safety guidelines and the program and institutional policies regarding student supervision.

Case 8: Confidentiality. *"Can you get a copy of my x-ray report?"* Your mother has been proudly telling all of your neighbors that you are currently in a radiologic technology program and are doing your clinical education at the trauma center in your town. Your next-door neighbor, whom you have known since you were a small child, tells you he had an x-ray examination performed at the trauma center over a week ago and he has not yet received a report. Because he knows you are doing your clinical education at that same hospital, he asks you to look up his report and print it for him so he can take it to his family practice physician at his follow-up appointment.

Identify the problem. Can you look up a medical report for a patient who is not under your care?

Investigate the problem. Do you have access to the reports in the computer system? What harm would it do to look up the report and print it for your kind neighbor? What ethical and/or legal implications are involved from the hospital's perspective? Are there any policies related to your radiologic technology program that must be considered? What are the implications for your family's friendship with your neighbor if you decline to get his report?

Formulate possible solutions. Do you print the report? Do you ask someone at your hospital what to do? Should you check with your program officials to see what they think? Is there some reference you have learned about in school that you could review to help you decide what to do?

Select and enact the best solution. Can you find any guidance in the ARRT code of ethics regarding patient confidentiality? Do the HIPAA policies of the institution give you guidance regarding situations such as this? In this situation is it possible for you to assist your neighbor and stay within the HIPAA guidelines of your program and the institution? Is there a different way of assisting your neighbor without printing the actual radiographic examination report?

After completing a radiologic sciences program, students will have practiced addressing scenarios such as these in the laboratory, classroom, and even clinical setting and will be prepared to handle challenging situations. Providing students with all potential challenges that may arise while working in the field of radiologic sciences is impossible for a radiologic sciences program. However, providing each student with the tools and information necessary will prepare him or her to act appropriately when faced with this type of situation.

MAINTAINING CRITICAL-THINKING SKILLS

Radiologic sciences professionals are an integral part of the health care team. Many critical-thinking skills revolve around working cooperatively and effectively with other members of the health care team. These skills may involve decisions related to working within your scope of practice and supporting other health care professionals. Students must learn to work cooperatively and "in sync" with physicians, physicists, nurses, and other allied health professionals.

The continuing professional development of radiologic sciences professionals is essential to maintaining and improving their critical-thinking skills. Keeping up with the changing technology and developments in medicine is a professional obligation for those working in the radiologic sciences. Continuing education is a key element to ensure application of up-to-date technology that allows the radiologic sciences professional to practice problem solving and critical thinking that will result in the best patient care. Continuing education can take on many forms. Additional formal education can be obtained in the college or university setting and can count toward the completion of advanced degrees. Another form of continuing education involves attending educational sessions and networking with other radiologic sciences professionals at local, state, and national conferences. Continuing education can also be acquired through directed journal readings and via online educational modules. In addition to participating in continuing education, radiologic sciences professionals must support the future of the profession by teaching and mentoring students to be competent future radiologic sciences professionals.

SUMMARY

- Radiologic sciences professionals are presented with unique and challenging ethical, technical, and patient care situations every day. Critical-thinking and problem-solving skills are essential to provide high-quality patient care, diagnosis, and treatment in these situations. The student must learn and value the basic knowledge of the profession to develop technical critical-thinking skills for use in future practice. The steps in critical thinking involve identifying and clarifying the problem, objectively examining the problem, considering and developing all possible viable solutions, and selecting and enacting the solution with the best outcome for the patient. Professional and ethical standards, such as cultural sensitivity and communication methods, must be considered when selecting the appropriate solution. The classroom and laboratory serve as a practice field for students to develop critical-thinking skills. The clinical setting allows the student to take classroom and laboratory learning into the real world. Critical-thinking and problem-solving skills may also be used to manage personal concerns and issues. Because the technology associated with the radiologic sciences is ever changing, continued professional development is an integral part of ongoing critical-thinking and problem-solving skills development.

BIBLIOGRAPHY

American Registry of Radiologic Technologists: *ARRT Standards of Ethics*, St. Paul, 2017, Minn. Available at: https://www.arrt.org/docs/default-source/Governing-Documents/code-of-ethics.pdf?sfvrsn=10.

American Society of Radiologic Technologists: *Practice standards for medical imaging and radiation therapy*, Albuquerque, 2017, NM. Available at: https://www.asrt.org/main/standards-regulations/practice-standards/practice-standards.

Boulder T, Liotta C: The integration of team-based learning in an advanced exposure course, *Radiologic Science and Education* 17:3–11, 2012.

Bugg N: Teaching critical thinking skills, *Radiol Technol* 68:433, 1997.

Cohen TF, Keith RF, Dempsey MC: Perceptions of clinical preparedness among radiography and radiation therapy baccalaureate students in JRCERT accredited programs, *Radiologic Science and Education* 22:3–13, 2017.

Davison HC, Kudlas MJ, Mannelin LR: Portfolios and critical thinking (teaching techniques), *Radiol Technol* 74:509, 2003.

Durand KS: *Critical thinking: developing skills in radiography*, Philadelphia, 1999, FA Davis.

Greathouse GF, Dowd SB: Using critical thinking to teach empathy, *Radiol Technol* 67:435, 1996.

Hamilton J, Druva R: Fostering appropriate reflective learning in an undergraduate radiography course, *Radiography* 16:339, 2010.

Jackson M, Ignatavicius DD, Case B: *Conversations in critical thinking and clinical judgment*, Pensacola, Fla, 2004, Pohl.

Kowalczyk N, Leggett T: Teaching critical-thinking skills through group-based learning, *Radiol Technol* 77:24, 2005.

Kowalczyk N, Hackworth R, Case-Smith J: Perceptions of the use of critical thinking teaching methods, *Radiol Technol* 83:226–236, 2012.

Lozano R: Needs, practices and recommendations of active learning for today's radiation therapy student, *Radiologic Science and Education* 6:17–28, 2001.

Pearce CE, Dowd SB: An exercise in critical thinking, *Radiol Technol* 67:526, 1996.

Ruggiero VR: *The art of thinking: a guide to critical and creative thought*, New York, 2004, Pearson Education.

Savin-Baden M, Major CH: *Foundations of problem-based learning*, Berkshire, UK, 2004, Society for Research into Higher Education and Open University Press.

Stadt R, Ruhland S: Critical-thinking abilities of radiologic science students, *Radiol Technol* 67:24, 1995.

Standards for an Accredited Educational Program: Joint Review Committee on Education in Radiologic Technology. Available at: http://www.jrcert.org.

Stone J: The staff therapist's role in clinical education, *Radiat Ther* 11:1, 2002.

Tanenbaum BG, Tilson ER, Cross DS, et al.: Interactive questioning: why ask why? *Radiol Technol* 68:435, 1997.

Werderman DS: An experiment in team-based learning in radiologic physics, *Radiologic Science and Education* 16:21–26, 2011.

Yates JL: Collaborative learning in radiologic science education, *Radiol Technol* 78:19–27, 2006.

PART II

Introduction to the Clinical Environment

Introduction to Clinical Education

Angie Arnold, MEd, RT(R), Tracy Herrmann, PhD, RT(R)

Tell me and I forget. Teach me and I may remember. Involve me and I learn.

Benjamin Franklin

OBJECTIVES

On completion of this chapter, the student will be able to:

- Define terms that relate to the clinical education of medical imaging radiologic science professionals.
- Explain the purpose of the clinical education in medical imaging and radiologic sciences.
- Describe the steps students may experience in the development of their clinical education skills.
- Identify the types of supervision necessary to assure safety in the clinical setting.
- Describe aspects of assessment used to measure and document student performance during clinical education.
- Explain the importance of adherence to clinical education policies regarding supervision and patient safety.
- Explain the communication strategies and steps taken by health care workers in the clinical setting to assure continuity of care and patient safety.
- Describe aspects of Team STEPPS and SBAR as they support teamwork and positive patient outcomes in the clinical setting.

OUTLINE

KEY TERMS

Affective One of the three major categories or domains of learning; includes behaviors guided by feelings and emotions that are influenced by an individual's interests, attitudes, values, and beliefs

Assist Activities in clinical that aid or support the performance of radiographic procedures and therapeutic treatments

Clinical Procedures and activities that occur in outpatient and inpatient health care settings

Clinical Coordinator Program official responsible for coordinating clinical education and evaluation of its effectiveness

Clinical Instructor Program official responsible for clinical instruction, supervision, and evaluation of students in the clinical setting

Clinical Staff Health care professionals employed in the clinical setting where students participate in clinical education and provide clinical supervision and guidance

Cognitive One of the three major categories or domains of learning; includes various levels of thought, such as knowledge, understanding, reason, and judgment

Competency Observable and documented successful achievement of performance objectives

Didactic Informational and instructional activities that may occur in formal or informal settings, typically in the classroom, laboratory, or online

Direct Supervision Oversight of clinical procedures or treatment by a qualified professional present in the exam or treatment room with the student

Indirect Supervision Oversight of clinical procedures by a qualified professional immediately available to the student

Learning Outcomes Program level measurable expectations for student learning

Objectives Topical concise descriptions of an observable behavior to be achieved by students as a result of their educational experiences within a course or educational module

Observe Activities in clinical where students watch and listen to the performance of radiographic procedures and therapeutic treatments

Program Director Program official
that provides leadership for the
program and ensures program
effectiveness

Perform Activities in clinical where
students complete radiographic

procedures and therapeutic
treatments with appropriate
supervision of a qualified
professional

Psychomotor One of the three major
categories or domains of learning;

includes behaviors involving
physical actions, neuromuscular
manipulations, and coordination

Transfer of Learning Learning in
one context and applying it to
another

CLINICAL EDUCATION

Students must participate in planned and structured learning experiences and activities in a variety of clinical settings in order to gain the procedural and therapeutic skills required to provide quality patient care. For the student to fully appreciate the health care environment, they must observe, assist with, and perform medical imaging procedures and therapeutic treatments in a real-life setting. The clinical setting allows the student to integrate the knowledge gained from didactic courses into clinical practice while caring for patients. Educational programs and health care facilities partner to provide clinical education for students.

Purpose of Clinical Education

In order to become competent health care professionals, medical imaging and radiologic science students must invest much time in the clinical setting in order to develop and refine the skills they initially learn in their didactic courses. Hospitals, clinics, specialty imaging centers, orthopedic centers, surgical centers, and cancer centers are just a few of the locations that fulfill this need. Clinical practice provides students with real-life opportunities to experience competency-based education. Competency-based clinical education is based on professional practice standards defined by professional associations and competency requirements are defined by accrediting and certifying agencies in order to support the development of quality patient care skills.

The American Society of Radiologic Technologists (ASRT) is the professional organization that provides a curriculum articulating educational guidelines to ensure that entry-level medical imaging and radiologic science professionals possess the necessary skills and knowledge for practice. The curriculum must be comprehensive and sequenced appropriately to include current information and to provide for the evaluation of student achievement. The ASRT also establishes the practice standards for medical imaging and radiologic science professions (see Appendix A). These standards define practice and establish general criteria to determine compliance with the standards. The Joint Review Committee on Education in Radiologic Technology (JRCERT) is the programmatic accrediting body that establishes supervision and safety standards for student participation in clinical education. The American Registry of Radiologic Technologists (ARRT) is the professional certifying agency that identifies the minimum educational and clinical competency requirements for certification. The ARRT standards of ethics (Appendix D) reflect the rules and standards that govern the conduct of professional technologists who hold current or former registration from the ARRT, and persons applying for

examination and certification by the ARRT. Medical imaging and radiologic science students should strive to understand, appreciate, and value these standards.

In order to master clinical skills, students must practice performing the procedures and treatments in a variety of situations, and for different patient conditions, as they continually refine their skills in order to achieve competency. As part of an educational program, students must demonstrate competency in a wide range of clinical skills, procedures, or treatments. The competencies required are specific to the medical imaging or radiologic science profession. In radiography, procedural competencies for imaging of the chest and thorax, musculoskeletal system and trauma, cranium, spine and pelvis, abdomen, fluoroscopic studies, surgical and mobile studies, and pediatrics are required. In radiation therapy, the skills required include quality control procedures, simulation procedures, dosimetry, treatment accessory devices, participatory procedures, and radiation treatment procedures. In both disciplines competence in general patient care skills, such as cardiopulmonary resuscitation, vital signs, sterile and medical aseptic technique, venipuncture, patient transfer, and care of patient medical equipment, are required. To be eligible to sit for the ARRT credentialing examination, all required clinical skills and competencies must be met and documented by program officials. A detailed list of competency requirements necessary to be eligible for the ARRT examination can be found on the ARRT website at http://www.arrt.org.

Learning Clinical Skills

Transfer of learning entails learning in one context and applying it to another. The principle of **transfer of learning** is exemplified in the clinical education component of medical imaging and radiologic sciences education, with the student recalling prior knowledge learned and using this knowledge in performing diagnostic or therapeutic procedures to develop both the skills and the confidence to work with a wide variety of patients. Thus prior learning affects the new learning within the clinical performance.

Most educational researchers agree that learning can be organized into three major categories or domains. The **cognitive** domain includes behaviors requiring various levels of thought: knowledge, understanding, reason, and judgment. The **psychomotor** domain includes behaviors involving physical actions, neuromuscular manipulations, and coordination. The **affective** domain includes behaviors guided by feelings and emotions that are influenced by an individual's interests, attitudes, values, and beliefs.

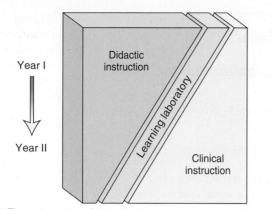

Fig. 5.1 The articulation of didactic, laboratory, and clinical instruction.

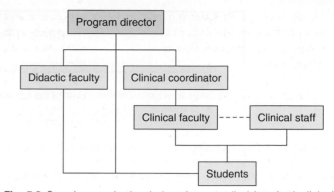

Fig. 5.2 Sample organizational chart for a medical imaging/radiologic science program.

A learning **objective** is a concise description of an observable behavior achieved by students, which is relevant to a specific topic within a course or educational module. Objectives must be measurable and achievable. They describe what behavior the student is to display, how well the student is to perform the behavior, and under what circumstances the behavior is to be achieved. Closely related to performance objectives is **competency,** the observable, successful achievement of the performance objectives. Competencies must be documented and competence must be maintained by the student. **Learning outcomes,** assessed at the program level, are measurable expectations for student learning. Learning outcomes are components of a program's assessment plan, which are used to document the effectiveness of the program.

Didactic education occurs in formal settings such as the classroom, the laboratory, and online. Didactic courses provide students with experiences designed to support conceptual learning as well as to provide an opportunity for students to gain hands-on skills in a simulated environment. A mannequin, fellow student, or another person, takes the place of the actual patient during simulations. When a fellow student or another person is involved, no radiation exposure is utilized.

In the early phases of the educational program, additional time is spent in didactic instruction. Students then progress to an increasing amount of time in the clinical setting. The laboratory setting serves as a bridge to connect classroom with clinical activities (Fig. 5.1). Within the didactic and laboratory areas, students learn the theoretic foundation of knowledge. Clinical education enables medical imaging and radiologic science students to transfer the learning from the textbooks, classroom, and laboratory environments to practical learning with real-life situations.

A large number of individuals work together to assist the student in learning clinical skills. The program officials who assist in the clinical education of the student are the program director, the clinical coordinator, the clinical instructor, and the clinical staff. Fig. 5.2 illustrates a sample organizational chart for a medical imaging/radiologic science program. The **program director** works full time in organizing, administering, and assessing the radiography program. This person is responsible for the didactic and clinical effectiveness of the program. The **clinical coordinator** works closely with the program director in ensuring program effectiveness through a regular schedule of coordination, instruction, and evaluation. The **clinical instructor** works directly with the student in the clinical setting. These program officials must possess current knowledge regarding diagnostic and therapeutic procedures, as well as competence in clinical instruction and evaluation techniques. Members of the **clinical staff** are employees of the health care institution and provide student supervision and guidance.

Clinical Progression

During the **clinical** component of the medical imaging and radiologic science program, students participate in the observation and performance of procedures and activities that occur in the clinical settings. Prior to performance of diagnostic or therapeutic procedures, students typically undergo an orientation to both the program's educational requirements and site-specific safety requirements and protocols. Prior to participation in clinical experiences, students must typically provide documentation of cardiopulmonary resuscitation certification and immunizations for communicable diseases, and may be required to undergo drug screening or a criminal background check. A sample of clinical requirements is provided as Fig. 5.3. These steps are necessary to meet the specific requirements of each clinical setting and to assure safety.

Clinical experiences include direct patient contact, which requires communication (verbal and nonverbal) and touch. Patients may be of different cultures, socioeconomic levels, age, race, ethnicity, ability, sexual orientation, etc. As such, all patients must be cared for in a unique manner. Students in the clinical setting will interact with patients that are inpatients, outpatients, emergency patients, and terminally ill patients. Students may witness birth and death and every health care experience in between, and these experiences may be heartwarming, traumatic, or saddening at times. As such, students must make every effort to take care of themselves and find ways to express concerns and feelings in a constructive way. During these times, students should consider the importance of patient confidentiality and refrain from violating Health Insurance Portability and Accountability Act (HIPAA) standards. HIPAA mandates the confidentiality of health information and establishes the requirements for the privacy, security, and transmission of health information. Details regarding HIPAA are provided in Chapter 25 (Health Information Management).

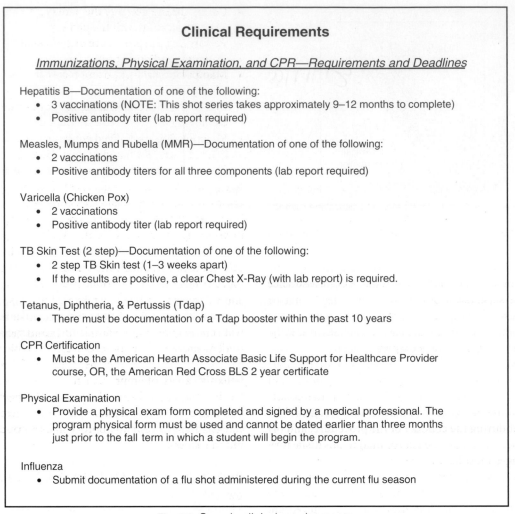

Clinical Requirements

Immunizations, Physical Examination, and CPR—Requirements and Deadlines

Hepatitis B—Documentation of one of the following:
- 3 vaccinations (NOTE: This shot series takes approximately 9–12 months to complete)
- Positive antibody titer (lab report required)

Measles, Mumps and Rubella (MMR)—Documentation of one of the following:
- 2 vaccinations
- Positive antibody titers for all three components (lab report required)

Varicella (Chicken Pox)
- 2 vaccinations
- Positive antibody titer (lab report required)

TB Skin Test (2 step)—Documentation of one of the following:
- 2 step TB Skin test (1–3 weeks apart)
- If the results are positive, a clear Chest X-Ray (with lab report) is required.

Tetanus, Diphtheria, & Pertussis (Tdap)
- There must be documentation of a Tdap booster within the past 10 years

CPR Certification
- Must be the American Hearth Associate Basic Life Support for Healthcare Provider course, OR, the American Red Cross BLS 2 year certificate

Physical Examination
- Provide a physical exam form completed and signed by a medical professional. The program physical form must be used and cannot be dated earlier than three months just prior to the fall term in which a student will begin the program.

Influenza
- Submit documentation of a flu shot administered during the current flu season

Fig. 5.3 Sample clinical requirements.

The initial stage of clinical education involves extensive observation. This tapers off as the new student gains confidence and can effectively integrate the appropriate cognitive, psychomotor, and affective behaviors. Throughout the length of the program, clinical situations will arise that are new to the student. After gaining knowledge of the various procedures in a didactic setting, and practicing the performance of the procedures in the laboratory setting, the student is ready to watch and give critical attention to all that is occurring in the clinical setting, noting the role of the various participating health professionals. As medical imaging and radiologic science professionals perform various diagnostic and therapeutic procedures, they serve as role models for the new student. The inquisitive student makes mental notes of how the procedure or treatment is being performed and begins to emulate the actions seen.

When the student feels confident, he or she can then proceed to assistance, the next phase of clinical education. In this phase, the student begins aiding and supporting the medical imaging and radiologic science professional in the performance of diagnostic and therapeutic procedures. The student is now gaining hands-on experience—literally placing a hand on the patient to assist the patient as they move to the table or helping them to assume a specific position for the diagnostic or therapeutic procedure. Students should take the initiative to participate in many aspects of the diagnostic or therapeutic procedure in order to develop their skills. Students should take an increasingly more active part in the procedure or treatment as they gain confidence. Questions and discussion about the procedure should not be conducted in the presence of the patient to maintain a comfortable patient environment.

After assisting the medical imaging or radiologic science professional with various aspects of the diagnostic or therapeutic procedure, the student develops confidence and proceeds to the performance of the entire procedure or treatment independently and with appropriate supervision from the medical imaging or radiologic science professional. During the performance of the procedure or treatment, the student should accurately demonstrate all necessary tasks at the required skill level based on his or her experience.

Clinical Supervision

In order to assure the safety of patients, students, staff, and the general public present in the health care environment, students should be supervised at all times while in the clinical setting. Medical imaging and radiologic science programs accredited by the JRCERT are

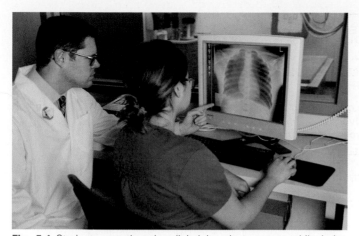

Fig. 5.4 Student operating the digital imaging system while being directly supervised.

required to abide by accreditation standards that require assurance of the appropriate supervision of students. For example, until a radiography student achieves and documents competency in any given procedure, all clinical procedures are carried out under the direct supervision of a qualified radiographer.

The parameters of direct supervision require that the qualified radiographer (1) review the request for examination in relation to the student's achievement, (2) evaluate the condition of the patient in relation to the student's knowledge, (3) be physically present during the conduct of the procedure, and (4) review and approve the procedure and/or image. Unsatisfactory radiographic images must be directly supervised by a qualified radiographer, regardless of the student's level of competency. Radiation therapy students must be directly supervised in the performance of treatments for the duration of the program. Fig. 5.4 shows the student operating the digital imaging system while being directly supervised.

The parameters of indirect supervision require that the qualified radiographer reviews, evaluates, and approves the procedure as for direct supervision, and is immediately available to assist students regardless of the level of student achievement. "Immediately available" is interpreted as the physical presence of a qualified radiographer adjacent to the room or the location where a radiographic procedure is being performed. This availability applies to all areas where ionizing radiation equipment is used for medical imaging procedures, including mobile and operating room procedures. Indirect supervision is not permitted for radiation therapy students. *not directly w/ you, but within shouting distance*

CLINICAL ASSESSMENT

Clinical performance is assessed in each clinical course (Fig. 5.5). Assessment of students' knowledge or comprehension of clinical education involves the ability to apply, analyze, synthesize, create, and evaluate. Numerous cognitive, psychomotor, and affective behaviors are involved in performing a diagnostic or therapeutic procedure, including the following:

- Assessing the request
- Preparing the room for performance of the procedure or treatment

- Caring for the needs of the patient
- Communicating with the patient
- Performing the procedure or treatment
- Providing radiation protection
- Manipulating the exposure factors or settings for the treatment plan
- Evaluating the radiographic image or ensuring the appropriate treatment
- Manipulating specialized equipment
- Appropriately discharging the patient

These behaviors are assessed through the use of direct, objective observation and are documented via rating scales, checklists, critical incident forms, and anecdotal notes. Affective behaviors involving attitudes and values are also among those considered in assessing the progress of the student's clinical development. Evaluators may also assess the student's ability to (1) communicate effectively with staff and patients, (2) perceive patient needs, (3) display maturity and confidence, and (4) follow through with clinical responsibilities in a reliable and conscientious manner.

In the assessment of their clinical performance, the student will routinely receive feedback and constructive criticism. This feedback will include descriptive information of how student clinical performance has been successful and will identify potential areas of improvement. Students should utilize this feedback from professionals to maintain their competent skills and refine those that need improvement. Accepting and using constructive criticism to improve skills is critical to clinical education success.

CLINICAL POLICIES AND DISCIPLINARY PROCEDURES

In order to assure quality care and safety, all parties involved in clinical education must understand and abide by policies established by both the program and the clinical site. Program faculty members develop timely policies, procedures, rules, regulations, and guidelines that are applicable to clinical education. A clinical education handbook or guide is vital in providing consistent written information for all parties. The resultant benefit is improved integration of the didactic, clinical, and affective aspects of the radiography curriculum. Student failure to follow policies may result in disciplinary action that ranges from oral or written warnings to program suspension or dismissal.

Medical imaging and radiologic science clinical policies typically involve radiation safety and pregnancy (see Chapter 9), attendance requirements, professional appearance and behavior, drug and alcohol, infection control (see Chapter 17), nondiscrimination, social media, HIPAA/patient confidentiality (see Chapter 25), supervision, immunizations, and electronic devices. Students must be knowledgeable of their program and clinical site policies in order to practice competently and successfully in the clinical setting. For example, medical imaging and radiologic science students must become knowledgeable about HIPAA and follow confidentiality mandates. Confidentiality of patient information is an ethical standard that must be maintained by the student during the course of their education. The failure of students to abide by HIPAA mandates may result in disciplinary

Student Clinical Evaluation Form

Name: _____   Date:_____

Rotation/Area: _____   Term:_____

Clinical Performance Standards *(Defines the clinical performance, standard activities of the student in the care of the patient and delivery of procedures, which includes patient assessment and management with the procedural analysis, performance and evaluation)*

	Acceptable	Needs Improvement	Unacceptable	Not Observed
1. Demonstrates humanist approach to the patient (concern for patient)				
2. Is responsible and prompt towards duties in assigned area.				
3. Shows enthusiasm with regard to educational opportunities				
4. Appears to be self-confident				
5. Is able to recall pertinent details with regard to assigned area and performance				

Quality Performance Standards *(Defines activities of the student in the technical areas of performance including equipment. Material assessment, safety standards, and total quality management)*

1. Accuracy of work				
2. Consistent quality of work				
3. Application of knowledge				
4. Shows appropriate level of efficiency				
5. Organization of work				

Professional Performance Standards *(Defines activities of the student in areas of education, interpersonal relationships, personal and professional behaviors and ethical behavior)*

1. Speaks respectfully to team members (i.e., Dr.'s, Technologist, RN, Transport)				
2. Shows appropriate level of versatility (adjusts to change)				
3. Works in synchronous manner as a team member				
4. Ability to follow directions				
5. Accepts instructional criticism				

Comments:

Clinical Instructor Signature: _____

Fig. 5.5 Sample clinical evaluation.

procedures, such as reprimand, probation, or program dismissal, depending on the severity of the situation. In addition, program policy regarding professional appearance will outline the acceptable uniform for the student. Identifying name badges, patches, and radiation-monitoring devices are also a part of the professional uniform. Because students can only learn hands-on skills when they are present in the clinical setting, attendance policies may be emphasized in clinical policies and in grading of clinical education. The program provides clinical schedules that indicate the actual dates and times for all clinical experiences. Absenteeism and tardiness are often documented and may result in disciplinary procedures.

Students in medical imaging and radiologic science programs are required to abide by the policies and procedures of the sponsoring institution, the program, and the clinical education centers. Students are also expected to abide by the standards of ethics of the ARRT. Failure to adhere to these requirements may result in disciplinary procedures or academic sanctions. The specific steps in the disciplinary procedure are detailed in the student clinical education handbook and may include oral and written warnings. A repetition of infractions may result in suspension or dismissal from the program. Serious infractions, including, but not limited to, a threat to patient safety, gross insubordination, disclosure of confidential information, falsification of records, cheating, theft, willful damage of property, and substance abuse, may result in immediate dismissal from the program. In all cases, students have the right of due process as defined by the sponsoring institution and the program policies.

TEAMWORK AND COMMUNICATION

In the clinical setting, patient safety is of the utmost importance. Health care institutions use different approaches to assure patient safety. One such approach is Team Strategies and Tools to Enhance Performance and Patient Safety (TeamSTEPPS). TeamSTEPPS is an evidence-based teamwork system used in many health care institutions to improve the quality, safety, and efficiency of health care. The purpose of utilizing the TeamSTEPPS approach is to create highly effective teams necessary to assure the best patient outcomes. The five key principles to TeamSTEPPS include team structure coupled with skills in communication, leadership, situation monitoring, and mutual support. Team structure must be established to assure that team members work effectively together to ensure patient safety. Communication amongst team members must be structured to assure clarity and accuracy. Leadership ensures that teams are knowledgeable of changes and have the resources they need to best care for the patient. Situation monitoring is a process of being attentive to the functions of the team and the surrounding circumstances to assure team effectiveness. Mutual support is the ability of teams to understand their responsibilities and the responsibilities of others, and to provide the necessary support to others.

A key element to teamwork in the clinical setting is communication. Health care workers must communicate effectively with each other in order to assure quality patient care and safety. One example of a communication method used to assure an effective handoff of patients from one health care worker to the other is SBAR (situation, background, assessment, and recommendation). Patient handoff occurs when a patient is transferred from one health care worker to another for different types of care, procedures, or treatments. SBAR is a structured communication process that provides for accurate sharing of patient information between health care workers when patient handoff occurs. Since medical imaging and radiologic science professionals frequently participate in patient handoffs, SBAR is an important skill for them to hold as it supports the communication of vital information that may save a patient's life. The steps in SBAR include describing the situation and the clinical background, assessing the situation, and making recommendations. Table 5.1 shows the questions that would be asked when considering SBAR in a clinical situation.

TABLE 5.1 Steps in SBAR

Situation	What is the situation?
Background	What is the clinical background?
Assessment	What is the problem?
Recommendation	What do I recommend/request be done?

The following example illustrates one way a radiographer might experience SBAR when communicating with a nurse as a patient is transferred from the emergency department for an x-ray.

S: A chest x-ray has been ordered for Bertha Smith.

B: Bertha Smith is a 56-year-old with congestive heart failure and multiple ED (emergency department) visits. She looks pale and diaphoretic. Her BP (blood pressure) is 90/65 verified with a manual cuff. Her pulse is 110. We've got her on O2 (oxygen).

A: I think she may be having an MI (myocardial infarction, heart attack).

R: Bertha needs a chest x-ray STAT (immediately). Is a mobile x-ray in order due to the severity of her condition?

Interprofessional education (IPE) is one approach to teaching students and health care workers how to interact and work with each other in the clinical setting. IPE allows for health care and social care workers or students, from two or more professions, to engage in learning with, from, and about each other. This interprofessional learning environment cultivates professional collaborative practice to support patient-centered health care. Students in medical imaging and radiologic science programs may participate in IPE activities to support the development of clinical skills that translate to professional practice after graduation (Fig. 5.6A–C).

SUMMARY

- Clinical education is a necessary component of the medical imaging and radiologic science curriculum. It provides a structured and ordered mechanism for the student to develop and refine the important skills needed in a variety of one-on-one, direct interactions with the patient. A correlation and transfer from the didactic and clinical portions of the curriculum must occur for clinical education to be successful. This correlation includes a successful weaving and integration of cognitive, psychomotor, and affective behaviors during the observation, assistance, and performance of actual radiographic procedures.

- Students progress in their clinical skills by first observing, then assisting, and finally performing diagnostic or therapeutic procedures. Appropriate supervision during performance is necessary to assure safety. Students are assessed via competency evaluations for specific procedures or treatments. Clinical learning experiences must be objectively and promptly assessed with improvements made as a result of constructive feedback.

- In an effort to ensure a complete and accurate understanding of the clinical education process, a large number of clinical education policies and procedures are developed and implemented by program officials. These policies and procedures

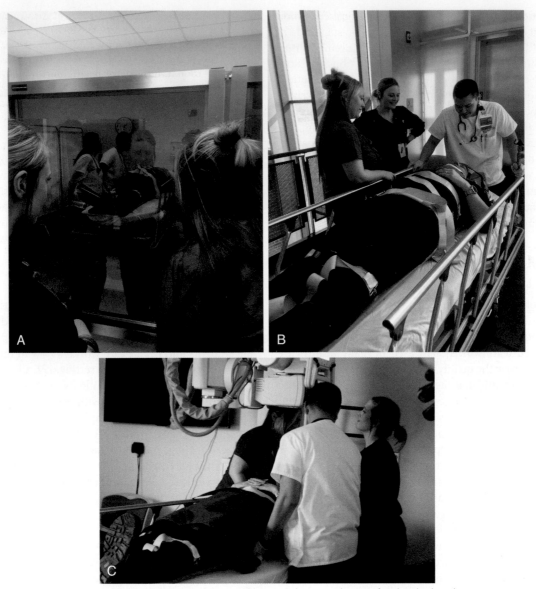

Fig. 5.6 Health care profession students working together at an interprofessional education event.

typically involve appropriate supervision, procedure performance, assessments, radiation protection practices, professional ethics, HIPAA, attendance, and pregnancy. If policies and procedures are not followed then disciplinary action may be taken.

- Teamwork and communication are important aspects of collaboration in providing quality patient care. TeamSTEPPS, SBAR, and IPE are approaches that focus on standardization and safe practice in providing quality patient care.

BIBLIOGRAPHY

Agency for Healthcare Research and Quality: TeamSTEPPS 2.0. https://www.ahrq.gov/teamstepps/instructor/index.html.

American Registry of Radiologic Technologists: ARRT standards of ethics. Published 2017. https://www.arrt.org/docs/default-source/Governing-Documents/arrt-standards-of-ethics.pdf?sfvrsn=12.

American Registry of Radiologic Technologists: Didactic and clinical competency requirements. https://www.arrt.org/arrt-reference-documents/by-document-type/didactic-and-clinical-competency-requirements.

American Society of Radiologic Technologists: Practice standards. Published 2017. https://www.asrt.org/main/standards-regulations/practice-standards/practice-standards.

American Society of Radiologic Technologists: ASRT curricula. Published 2017. https://www.asrt.org/educators/asrt-curricula.

Dawson EM: A qualitative study of minority radiologic science students' clinical experiences, *Radiol Technol* 89(6):666–674, 2017.

Eberhardt S: Improve handoff communication with SBAR, *Nursing* 44:17–20, 2014.

Giordano S: Improving clinical instruction: comparison of literature, *Radiol Technol* 79(4):290–296, 2008.

Hawking N: Teaching and the profession: effective communication affects student achievement and retention, *Radiol Technol* 76(3):234–236, 2005.

Holmström A, Ahonen S: Radiography students' learning: a literature review, *Radiol Technol* 87(4):371–379, 2016.

Joint Review Committee on Education in Radiologic Technology: Accreditation standards. Published 2018. https://www.jrcert.org/programs-faculty/jrcert-standards/.

Jones TL: Creating an effective student learning environment in the imaging sciences: a theoretical perspective, *Rad Science Ed* 20(1):21–29, 2015.

Lee SY, Dong L, Lim YH, Poh CL, Lim WS: SBAR: Towards a common interprofessional team-based communication tool, *Med Educ Online* 50(11):1167–1168, 2016.

Macaulay C, Cree V: Transfer of learning: concept and process, *Soc Work Educ* 18(2):183–194, 1999.

Mann KV: Thinking about learning: implications for principle-based professional education, *J Contin Educ Health Prof* 22(2):70–76, 2002.

Roberts GH, Carson J: The roles instructors play in clinical education, *Radiol Technol* 63(1):28–31, 1991.

U.S. Department of Defense. *Health.mil. Situation, Background, Assessment, Recommendation (SBAR) toolkit.* Access-Cost-Quality-and-Safety/Quality-And-Safety-of-Healthcare/Patient-Safety/Patient-Safety-Products-And-Services/Toolkits/SBAR-Toolkit>http://www.health.mil/Military-Health-Topics/ Access-Cost-Quality-and-Safety/Quality-And-Safety-of-Healthcare/Patient-Safety/Patient-Safety-Products-And-Services/Toolkits/SBAR-Toolkit. Accessed January 12, 2018.

Wentworth L, Diggins J, Bartel D, Johnson M, Hale J, Gaines K: SBAR: Electronic handoff tool for noncomplicated procedural patients, *J Nurs Care Qual* 27:125–131, 2012.

Vilvens H, Henderson C, Maloney B, Roman T, Trotta D: Improving health care collaboration and communication: integration of inter-professional education opportunities for undergraduate students, *J Res Pract Coll Teach* 1:1–8, 2016.

Yates JL: Collaborative learning in radiologic science education, *Radiol Technol* 78:19–27, 2006.

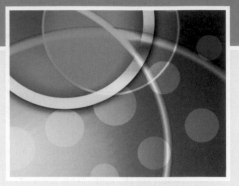

6

Radiology Administration

Rebecca Lamberth, MJ, MS, RT(R)(MR), CRA, FAHRA

*Digital imaging has untied our hands with regard to technical limitations.
We no longer have to be arbiters of technology; we get to participate in the interpretation of
technology into creative content.*

John Dykstra, Scientist

OBJECTIVES

On completion of this chapter, the student will be able to:

- Provide an overview of the administration of a hospital radiology department and the structure of hospital organization.
- Describe how the radiology department fits into and complements the hospital environment.
- Understand the role of the radiology administrator.
- Describe the functions of management, including planning, organizing and facilitating, staffing, directing, controlling, coordinating, and project management.
- Discuss the transition from traditional functions of management to the requirements of managing radiology in the current health care environment.
- Describe regulating agencies that affect radiology.
- Discuss the characteristics of desirable applicants for employment in radiology.

OUTLINE

KEY TERMS

Adverse Drug Events (ADEs) Injuries, large or small, caused by the use (including nonuse) of a drug; can be as harmless as a drug rash or as serious as death from an overdose; the two types of ADEs are those caused by errors and those that occur despite proper use

Board of Directors or Governing Board Group of people authorized by law to conduct, maintain, and operate a hospital for the benefit of the public and whose legal and moral responsibility for policies and operations of the hospital are

not for personal benefit of the members

Centers for Medicare & Medicaid Services (CMS) Federal agency that administers the Medicare program and partners with states to administer Medicaid

Certificate of Need (CON) Certificate approved by a local (state) review board permitting hospitals to construct new or additional facilities, open new services, or make large purchases—a condition required for reimbursement by Medicare

Certified Radiology Administrator (CRA) Professional who has demonstrated skill and knowledge in asset management, financial management, operations management, human resource management, and communication and information management in radiology

Chief Executive Officer (CEO) Person appointed by the board of directors who has full accountability for the entire hospital or health care organization

Clinical Support Services Services providing the components of patient care that collectively support the physician's plan for diagnoses and treatments

Continuous Quality Improvement (CQI) System of development in the workplace for daily improving performance at every level in every operational process by focusing on meeting or exceeding customer expectations

Department Unit of the hospital with specific functions or specialized skills such as housekeeping, surgery, radiology, or accounting

Department Chair Physician who represents a department or service and sits as a formal member of the executive medical staff committee; responsible for all of the medical operations of a hospital department and may also oversee a residency training program

Human Resources Department Ancillary department of the hospital responsible for recruiting, selecting, supporting, and compensating employees; developing and maintaining skills, quality, and motivation; collective bargaining; and occupational health and safety

The Joint Commission (TJC) Independent not-for-profit organization that evaluates and accredits more than 17,000 health care organizations and programs in the United States and is the nation's primary standard-setting and accrediting body in health care; TJC standards focus on improving the quality and safety of patient care provided by health care organizations

Medical Director Physician responsible for the medical operation and quality of a hospital department or service; also responsible for providing input regarding policies and procedures and day-to-day operations of the department

Medical Error Failure to complete a planned action as intended or the use of a wrong plan to achieve an aim; can be related to an incorrect diagnosis, equipment failure, infection, or a misinterpretation of an order

Medical Staff Formal organization of physicians authorized to admit and attend to patients within a hospital; have authorized privileges, bylaws, elected officers, and various committees and activities (see Medical Director, Department Chair, and Service Chief)

Mission Statement Statement of an organization that summarizes its intent to provide service in terms of the services it offers, the intended recipients of services, and a description of the level of cost

Occupational Safety and Health Administration(OSHA) Federal agency that enforces standards for safety in the workplace, conducts inspections, and directs determination of fines for noncompliance with policies and regulations

Performance Improvement (PI) Process of identifying and analyzing important organizational and individual performance gaps, planning for future performance improvement, designing and developing cost-effective and ethically justifiable interventions to close performance gaps, implementing the interventions, and evaluating the financial and nonfinancial results

Radiology (Medical Imaging) Department Organization of a hospital or medical clinic that provides diagnostic imaging through medical technologies such as x-ray examination, fluoroscopy, computed tomography, interventional radiography, magnetic resonance imaging, mammography, nuclear medicine, and ultrasonography

Service Chief Physician responsible for overseeing a component or subdepartment of a hospital service— for example, a radiologist who is chief of the nuclear medicine service

Third-Party Payers Insurance companies, Medicare, Medicaid, and other commercial companies that are the payers of inpatient and outpatient medical expenses for the patient

Total Quality Management (TQM) Management of quality in the workplace from a perspective of total involvement of every employee, with a strong focus on process measurement and control

THE HOSPITAL ENVIRONMENT

Hospital Organization

Hospitals are a central part of one of the nation's largest industries, the health care industry, and offer a broad range of services provided by highly educated and trained personnel, using highly sophisticated equipment and technology. The complexity of a hospital can be compared with that of a town or city in which people work together in mutually supportive functions—for example, the building, or plan, of a hospital provides space, electricity, plumbing, and roadways that require upkeep and maintenance. A hospital employs people in 20 or more different professions and an equal number of trades; these people require physical supports such as food service and payroll services. Supplies are needed, which are purchased from vendors or suppliers outside the hospital or produced from within the organization. Similar to a city, a hospital requires policies, procedures, administrative staff, rules, regulations, and plans.

The hospital-city analogy can be carried further to compare the governance and organization of a hospital with that of a city. Citizens are central to a city, and patients are central to a hospital. To ensure that its citizens are protected and to provide services necessary to living and conducting business, a city is organized through its governmental body. In a similar fashion, the hospital is organized through a board of directors and administrative staff to carry out the hospital's mission.

Hospitals have a direct relationship with the community in which they are located, comparable to the relationship a city has with the county or state where it is located. This relationship should be mutually supportive and beneficial. Single hospitals have merged into multihospital groups, or systems, similar to the way nearby cities merge activities first and later combine governance.

The medical staff and employees of a hospital show a parallel with the city's skilled and trained persons who provide services to other citizens. Volunteers in both scenarios enable many tasks to be performed at a reasonable cost to the central customers. In the hospital setting, volunteers and the auxiliary service organizations provide many hours of service, compassion, and assistance in an embodiment of the spirit of cooperation central to the best in human living.

If the citizens of a city can be compared with a hospital's patients, the city's elected officials, magistrates, and other civil servants might be compared with the various hospital employees who provide services. However, this is where the comparison between a hospital and a city stops. Not every citizen of a city is charged with carrying out the city's mission or fully understands its meaning. An organization's **mission statement** is the defining and guiding force that outlines the reason for existence. "The mission statement summarizes the hospital's intent to provide service in terms of the intended recipients of service, the type of care or services, and the level of quality and cost expected. Because every function of a hospital should be focused on what the organization wants to accomplish, all of its members should be familiar with the mission."

The organizational chart of a hospital demonstrates how managers and employees carry out the functions within the institution in an organized and logical manner. In its basic definition, it demonstrates who reports to whom in the organization. Governance of a hospital begins with the **board of directors** or **governing board**, which is authorized by law to operate a hospital. The board employs a **chief executive officer (CEO)** or president, and defines how the operation of the hospital is maintained and conducted. The primary restriction imposed on individual board members is that their governance may not afford them personal benefit. The CEO or president then sets in place a formal reporting structure for the organization and interacts with the medical staff to ensure coordination and quality of patient care and services.

In the organizational chart in Fig. 6.1, the line of communication between the medical staff and CEO is a dashed line, indicating direct communication but not directly controlled. The **medical staff** is the formal organized structure of physicians

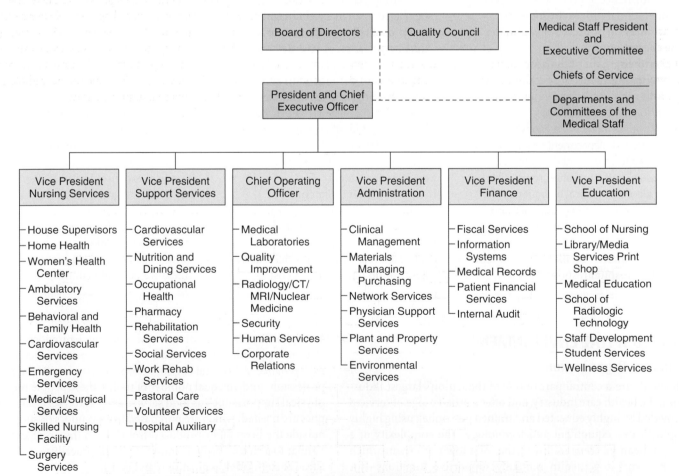

Fig. 6.1 Organizational chart. *CT,* Computed tomography, *MRI,* magnetic resonance imaging.

within a hospital with authorized privileges, bylaws, elected officers, committees, and organized activities. Radiologists fit into the formal structure of the medical staff; they either perform on a contractual basis to provide and supervise specific services or serve as paid employees of the health care organization.

A hospital is made up of many departments and services organized to provide care and clinical support services to its patients and clients. Most of a hospital's departments are interrelated, and some of these departments and services are directly dependent on each other. For example, all patient care services depend on the admissions department for information regarding the patients being served. Nursing areas, ancillary clinical departments, the medical staff, billing offices, and other departments rely on the health information management (HIM) department for maintaining and retaining the patient's medical record. The human resources department is responsible for the recruitment, retention, benefits, and compensation of all employees who work in the hospital. Business offices handle the financial functions of the hospital, including billing patients and insurance companies, paying for equipment and supplies, and maintaining strict accounting practices.

The radiology or medical imaging department plays an important role in the care of the patient. The quality of care provided to the patient by radiology (or any department) is directly related to the quality of the coordination and cooperation that exists between the department and all the other departments and services that make up the health care organization.

Organizational Transition in the 1990s and 2000s

Social and economic conditions of the late 1980s and early 1990s caused vast changes in health care organizations, forcing them to alter their organizational structures. The development of new technologies, changes in reimbursement, and a greater focus on utilization review processes contributed to a decline in inpatients during the 1980s. In the 1990s, managed care growth played a significant role in further decreasing inpatient utilization. Economic hardships and total quality management both have been influential in eliminating middle and lower management positions in many hospitals and radiology departments. These changes have continued throughout the 1990s and 2000s, and into the 2010s as changes in reimbursement and the introduction of the *Patient Protection and Affordable Care Act* escalated further cost reductions and subsequent downsizing. Figs. 6.2 and 6.3 demonstrate the vertical and horizontal organizational structures that represent changes occurring in health care, as well as other industries, in the last 20 years. The vertical structure depicted in Fig. 6.2 demonstrates a top-heavy organization, with additional layers of senior administration staff. After reorganization, many hospital organizations resemble the flat horizontal structure in the example in Fig. 6.3. An example of continued downsizing can be seen as positions in Fig. 6.1 are altered to eliminate positions such as the chief operating officer, vice president of support services, and vice president of administration. In Fig. 6.3, radiology administrators are becoming responsible for departments outside imaging, such as the laboratory or cardiopulmonary services. Similarly, it is no longer uncommon for a business manager, laboratory manager, or other administrator to inherit responsibility for a radiology department.

The matrix structure pictured in Fig. 6.4 has been useful in some hospitals, as well as other industries attempting to strategically manage the products and services that cross departmental boundaries. For example, the women's services manager would likely consult with the radiology manager about gynecologic and obstetric ultrasonography and mammography. The outpatient services manager would consult with the radiology manager on patient wait time and the flow of patients from one department to the next (e.g., emergency department, electrocardiography, laboratory, radiology); other managers would consult in a similar manner.

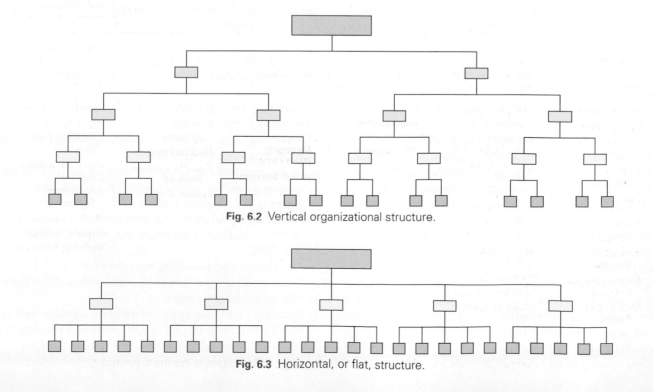

Fig. 6.2 Vertical organizational structure.

Fig. 6.3 Horizontal, or flat, structure.

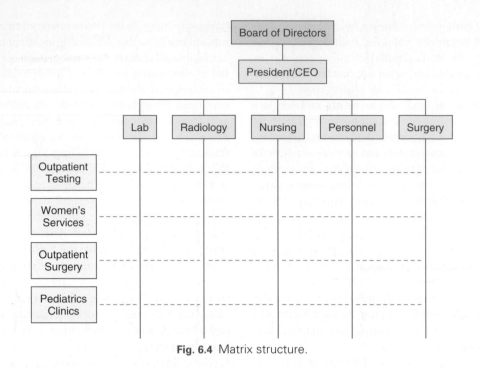

Fig. 6.4 Matrix structure.

Radiology Organization

Similar to the organization of a hospital, the formal structure of a **radiology (medical imaging) department** is a subset of the larger organization. The radiology department has the same focus on the hospital mission to serve patients and has needs similar to those of the larger organization—personnel, information, supplies, equipment, space, electricity, plumbing, and maintenance.

Subdepartments of Radiology. Larger radiology departments are often divided into subdepartments, modalities, or sections such as diagnostic radiography, ultrasound (US), nuclear medicine (NM), positron emission tomography (PET), computed tomography (CT), magnetic resonance imaging (MRI), mammography, and interventional radiology (IR), which is sometimes referred to as special procedures. In some health systems, radiation therapy and oncology is also a subsection of radiology (Fig. 6.5). Depending on the size of the facility, each of the subdepartments may be organized as a department within itself, with separate budgeting, reporting structure, and staffing. Examples of this could include nuclear medicine and ultrasonography departments or emergency radiologic services that may be independent of the main radiology department. Both centralized and decentralized radiology services have advantages and disadvantages. Each facility develops its reporting structure to best meet the apparent needs of the patients and physicians while attempting to maximize the potential of its managers and technologist staff.

Another important subsection to any department's operations is support services. Examples of these areas are registration, scheduling, informatics, and patient transportation services. To operate any imaging department properly, these subsections must also be carefully managed and focused on providing optimal patient care.

Administrative Director of Radiology. Organization of the radiology department begins with an administrative director, who reports to senior hospital administration and has direct responsibility and authority for operation and organization of the department. Key traditional responsibilities include staffing, planning, educating, supervising, organizing, coordinating, communicating, maintaining safety, and minimizing hazards in the workplace.

The many changes facing the health care industry in the 21st century have brought to all administrators, and specifically those in radiology, new challenges that require new skills and responsibilities, including the following:

- Managing limited resources
- Leading
- Coaching and staff development
- Managing cultural diversity and a multigenerational workforce
- Managing and facilitating change
- Analyzing opportunities
- Analyzing market needs and developing market strategies
- Analyzing administrative data
- Negotiating and managing contracts for purchase of equipment and supplies and for maintaining equipment
- Creating and justifying budgets
- Managing capital assets and contracts
- Planning facilities to maximize use of space, efficiency, and technology
- Recognizing and managing legal risks
- Understanding regulatory compliance with multiple agencies
- Managing customer relations
- Specifying and managing information systems and computed tomography (CT), magnetic resonance imaging (MRI) picture archive and communication systems (PACSs)
- Understanding organizational politics

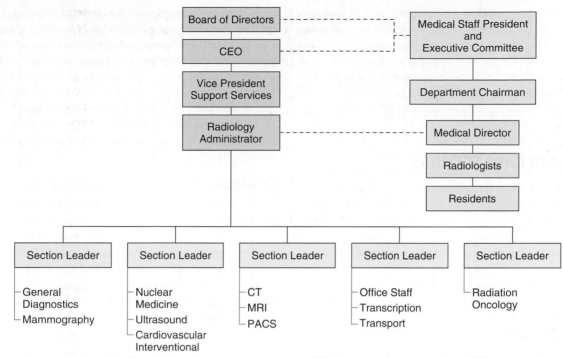

Fig. 6.5 Example of radiology department structure. *CT*, Computed tomography, *MRI*, magnetic resonance imaging; *PACS*, picture archive and communication systems.

- Recruiting, retaining, and developing qualified employees in the face of shortages of radiology professionals
- Delegating responsibilities effectively
- Networking with other departments and professional organizations
- Maintaining technical proficiency
- Strategic planning, including technology assessment
- Managing and improving patient and staff safety
- Effective project management skills

In 2002 the Radiology Administration Certification Commission established the **Certified Radiology Administrator (CRA)** designation in order to elevate the professionalism of radiology administrators. The CRA credential identifies those who have proven skills and knowledge in medical imaging management, specifically focusing on human resource management, asset resources, fiscal management, operations, and communication.

Medical Director. The radiology administrator has a responsibility to communicate with the medical director, department chairman, and/or service chief to ensure the coordination of medical staff activities with the activities and policies and procedures of the medical imaging department. Considerable variation occurs from one hospital to another in the relationship between the administrative director and the medical director of radiology. In some institutions the administrator reports directly to the medical director; in others the medical director has little responsibility for day-to-day operations, staffing, and organization. In most cases, the **medical director** has responsibility for overseeing the quality of patient care, approving clinical protocols, reviewing policies and procedures, and recommending improvements to quality and safety of care, equipment purchases, and technology acquisition. According to **The Joint Commission (TJC)**, the medical director is responsible for

all quality-improvement activities, although he or she may delegate responsibilities to the administrative director.

Department Chair. The medical director of radiology may also serve as department chair. The **department chair** of radiology is the department's link to the formal organization of the medical staff. He or she serves on the executive committee and other standing and ad hoc committees. Whereas a medical director has responsibility for a department or subdepartment, in some facilities the chair has responsibility for the full range of services and is directly responsible for participation in the medical staff organization. Considerable variation occurs from institution to institution in the title and responsibilities of the medical head of radiology services and its subdepartments. Whether the title is medical director, chair, or **service chief,** the primary responsibility is high-quality patient care and clinical oversight.

Radiologists. Radiologists may practice alone as individual physicians or in groups. Within groups, the larger the number of radiologists, the more formal the group's own organizational structure will be and the more specialized the services they can provide. Partnerships may or may not include all of the radiologists working together by agreement. When radiologists first become part of a practicing group, they may work as employees or junior partners before becoming full partners. The function of the group's organization is to run the business of the group, which includes billing patients for professional services such as radiology examination results, managing and paying their group employees, managing group investments and benefits plans, and serving as a mechanism for decision making. Improving the quality and safety of patient care may also be a function of the group's management processes.

Radiation Safety Office. The radiation safety officer (RSO) is the person delegated within an organization that is responsible for the safe operation and use of radiation and radioactive materials, as well as implementing the radiation protection program. An organization is required to designate an RSO in writing if licensed for the use of radioactive materials and the individual must meet specific requirements by either the Nuclear Regulatory Committee (NRC) or the Agreement State. Typically organizations employ a physicist or have a radiologist fulfill the role of the RSO.

OTHER HEALTH CARE SETTINGS

In recent decades, radiology services have transitioned from being primarily hospital based to other health care settings. Among these settings are clinics, physicians' offices, freestanding imaging centers, manufacturing plants, research centers, outpatient surgical centers, mobile imaging centers, veterinary medicine settings, and teleradiology services.

Clinics

Imaging services in the health clinic setting may include a range of modalities, from radiography for orthopedic services to all modalities for larger outpatient health care settings. Technologists may perform a variety of procedures and other functions, or may specialize in specific procedures. Clinics may be owned or operated by physicians or by university medical centers, hospitals, health systems, or private and for-profit organizations.

Physician Offices

Physician offices may be similar to clinics, but they are organized as the primary base of a single physician or a group of physicians. Radiologic services may vary from basic x-ray procedures to a full range of services, including ultrasonography, CT, nuclear medicine, MRI, mammography, bone densitometry, and vascular or interventional procedures.

Imaging Centers

Imaging centers may be owned by hospitals, medical centers, radiologists, other physicians, or nonmedical investors or corporations. They may be freestanding or associated with a clinic, physicians' office, or other medical center. It is also possible for an imaging center to be a joint venture between a health care facility and a physician group, in which both parties have a vested interest. The difference between a clinic and an imaging center is primarily that a clinic provides patient care by nonradiologist physicians as its primary function. The imaging center's primary function is diagnostic imaging; however, some imaging centers provide basic laboratory tests, electrocardiographic examinations, and other diagnostic testing, in addition to imaging procedures.

Mobile Imaging

The 1980s saw the development of a large array of mobile imaging modalities. Mobile services provide increased access to care in remote areas and, in the case of high-priced technologies such as MRI and PET, allow facilities to share the expense of providing access. Although the same basic skills are required of technologists and sonographers in these settings, new challenges are presented in the constant travel and interaction with medical facilities with diverse expectations and personalities. In addition, because of the remote nature of their services, patient care staff members are required to provide high levels of independent judgment. Mobile services are also used to support sites or regions until volume can be established to justify fixed site replacement services. Mobile mammography units offer an added convenience of providing screening services in other locations such as health clinics, corporations, and department stores.

Emergency or Urgent Care Centers

In the 1980s a variety of freestanding emergency and urgent care centers sprang up in the United States to provide quick access in non–life-threatening emergent situations. Shopping centers were among the many locations in which these centers were developed. Although many did not survive, some centers remain and meet important health care needs in their locations. Most of these centers provide basic general diagnostic radiographic procedures.

Outpatient Surgical Centers

During the 1990s, managed care and other forces influencing reduced costs in health care stimulated movement toward reduced inpatient hospital care and increased outpatient services. Many surgical procedures are now performed outside the traditional hospital setting, usually in stand-alone surgery centers. Radiology services performed in surgery centers may provide additional opportunity for technologists who are interested in surgical radiography.

Industry and Research

Lesser-known settings providing radiology services are those in industry and research. In recent years, health care services, including radiography, entered industry to protect the health of workers and lower the cost of health care. Some workplaces have their own clinics to monitor and safeguard the health of the workers. Employers are also seeking to reduce the cost of their employees' health care by negotiating lower costs with preferred hospitals, clinics, and physicians. Other industrial settings include the use of CT, x-ray, or ultrasound to examine the interiors of manufactured or used parts such as munitions or aircraft parts. Museums and archeologic facilities also use imaging to examine historical artifacts such as mummies removed from grave sites.

MANAGEMENT FUNCTIONS

The primary functions of management include *planning, organizing and facilitating, staffing, directing, controlling,* and *coordinating.* In the course of performing these functions, the radiology administrator communicates with a wide range of clients, customers, employees, service providers, manufacturers, other departments, senior administrators, and medical staff, as well as the community at large. As organizational transitions occur, the skills of communication take on a far greater significance. In the past, an administrator of any department or service could operate independently while focusing primarily on his or her own department. In the 2000s, new skills of communication were required to improve quality, enhance coordination, and lower the costs of doing business. Similarly, the functions of management are evolving from the traditional roles of directing and controlling employees to leading, coaching, and supporting employees. The influence for this change comes from the movement toward **continuous quality improvement (CQI)**, **total quality management (TQM)**, or **performance improvement (PI)**.

The concept of quality improvement moved from industry to health care in the 1980s. The impetus was derived from both the need to reduce the costs of providing health care and the rising expectations of patients, physicians, and **third-party payers**. When an institution focuses on quality or safety process improvement, it undergoes a cultural transformation, evolving over several years into a customer-focused organization. Employees are organized into multidisciplinary work teams and trained to evaluate their work processes to reduce errors or adverse medical events and simplify the work. *Doing the right things right the first time* and *meeting and exceeding the customer's expectations* become facility-wide objectives under the quality or patient safety mission. The cost savings resulting from CQI are discovered through in-depth analysis of work processes and elimination of redundant, unnecessary, and outdated work details. Improvements in productivity and efficiency have proved to reduce the costs of doing business and encourage employee ownership in the workplace.

Radiology departments involved in TJC patient safety goals or process improvement study the work functions within the department, such as patient wait time, report turnaround time, or methods for preventing medication errors. Perhaps even more significant to the overall success of the hospital are the interdisciplinary CQI or patient safety process improvement activities conducted among multiple departments. An example of this concept would be the review of emergency services to reduce the length of stay in the emergency department. Laboratory, radiology, admissions, and nursing services all have an impact on the time required to diagnose and treat a patient in the emergency department. As these departments begin to look at one another as internal customers, they begin the cultural change of a quality and patient safety focus.

Planning

A primary management function is the process of deciding in advance what is to be accomplished. *Planning* charts a course of action for the future that enables coordinated and consistent fulfillment of goals and objectives. Planning focuses attention on objectives and emphasizes efficiency and consistency. It also offsets uncertainty and change through thinking about the future and creating contingencies for what can be imagined or foreseen, as well as promoting economical operation and minimizing costs. Without planning, activities occur at random. With planning, activities are assigned to specific employees with the skills and knowledge to achieve results.

Planning is also critical in maintaining a sufficient number of properly qualified technologists to accomplish a variety of procedures in many different subspecialties. Starting new services,

efficiently managing growing or changing procedure volumes, and managing work during leaves of absence (e.g., maternity leaves, vacations) involve considerable planning skills, which vary directly with the size of the facility.

Additional examples in which planning is critical include developing and educating radiology employees; orienting new employees; replacing expensive radiology equipment; ongoing construction and renovation projects; and developing policies, procedures, guidelines, and methods for carrying out goals and objectives of the hospital and department.

Organizing and Facilitating

Once objectives, policies, procedures, and methods are defined through planning, administrators must implement ways of carrying out those objectives. *Organizing* is the development of a structure or framework that identifies how people do their work. The division of work is essential to efficiency because it defines responsibility and authority. Through the organizing function, the administrator communicates what activities are to be performed, how they are grouped together, who has the responsibility, and who has the authority for carrying out the work. The framework created by the organizing function can be demonstrated through organizational charts such as those in Figs. 6.2 to 6.5 for a hospital and a radiology department. *Facilitating* describes what management does in the way of helping, assisting, and expediting processes. The manager can help expedite the carrying out of the objectives and can remove obstacles that might get in the way of implementation of improvement processes.

Staffing

Work cannot be accomplished without people, and because the quality of work is directly related to the quality of skills of the people involved, staffing is viewed as a critical function. *Staffing* involves getting the right people with the right skills to do the work and developing their abilities so they can do the work better. Staffing functions include recruiting and retaining qualified employees, orienting and developing competent employees, identifying short-term and long-term labor needs, and developing specifications for job qualifications. The tools that administrators use to carry out their staffing functions are job descriptions and qualifications, structured interviews, defined competencies, performance appraisals, the budget, wage or salary scales, orientation programs, and support from the human resources department.

Directing

The transition in management previously described also affects the function of directing. Under the old concept of directing, some administrators or supervisors *barked* orders or issued directives. Under the new concepts of management, administrators and supervisors employ the tactics of influencing, guiding, persuading, and coaching employees. *Directing* involves the stimulation of effort needed to perform the required work. An administrator or supervisor uses communication skills to clarify and ensure understanding of the work to be accomplished, as well as the rationale of why and how it should be accomplished.

An example of how supervisors direct through good communication is in discussing policies and procedures. When employees understand the rationale for policies, they are more likely to enforce and support them. In addition, it is important for leaders to supervise activities by training, developing, and guiding employees. Through the function of leading, an administrator or supervisor inspires or influences employees to contribute toward the accomplishment of goals and objectives. Motivating encourages independent participation.

While directing, an administrator or supervisor often encounters the need to delegate work to others. The ability to delegate well is a learned skill that includes informing, guiding, educating, reviewing, evaluating, and giving feedback. Student radiologic technologists learn their clinical skills through a form of delegation. Work performed by others is assigned to them, and they are entrusted with technical accuracy, patient safety, and a measure of efficiency necessary to complete radiologic procedures. The clinical instructor or registered technologist in charge of the student must understand the educational development and proficiency of the student being assigned to complete a procedure. The supervisor of a delegated task must achieve a balance that permits independence of student action to maximize the learning experience while maintaining the quality and safety of the procedure for the patient.

For students being delegated work in patient care settings, the issue of responsibility versus authority is often perplexing. Unless it is well defined for students in the clinical setting, the fact that a certain measure of authority is also delegated with the responsibility of caring for patients may be unclear. Examples of situations in which this concept is important include the student's authority to direct patients to follow instructions for activities such as procedure preparation, movement through the department, and radiation safety. Students also should be instructed in their authority to solve problems, to report potential errors, and to adhere to ethical standards.

Controlling

Just as students need instructors to observe, test, measure, and guide their educational progress, the hospital needs administrators to review daily, weekly, monthly, and annually the activities and resources used to provide care to patients. *Controlling* defines performance standards or guidelines used to measure progress toward the goals of the organization. Once the plans and goals of the hospital are formed, measures must be developed to determine whether each department or section is achieving success toward these goals. Key performance indicators (KPI) allow the administrator the ability to create a formal process of feedback and flow of information to the department and organization. The information from the KPIs can then be used to make adjustments if needed to keep operations or expenses moving in the right direction. In a typical radiology department, key performance indicators may include monitors such as monthly expense and revenue reports, weekly reports of employee performance, employee turnover rate, inventory of supplies, radiation safety, and quality of equipment operation.

The controlling process can be described in four steps: (1) establishing methods of achieving planned goals and objectives, (2) defining standards and measures to give feedback on progress, (3) measuring and reporting progress, and (4) taking action to correct variations from the expected standards. An example of controlling for radiologic technology students is the use of testing in the educational program:

1. One of the goals is the successful completion of the registry examination.
2. Defining standards is the development of curriculum, and measures are the tests used to check student progress in learning.
3. Test taking and reporting define student progress.
4. Taking action to correct deficiencies in learning helps the student move toward the successful registry examination.

Standards of controlling are often discussed as either managerial or technical. The standards used to control managerial functions include policies and procedures, rules, and other reports of operations or *people functions.* Standards for hiring personnel with specific job skills and credentials fall into this category. *Technical standards* refer more to safety and equipment operation; technical standards would include standards that govern the more technical functions such as equipment operation (quality control), radiation control, and specific routines for radiographic positioning and exposure.

Coordinating

Coordinating is a process by which the manager achieves orderly group activities and unity of effort by workers who are fully aware of a common purpose (the organization's mission). In carrying out coordinating activities, an administrator communicates with other areas to facilitate work information and flow. Representing the department and being a spokesperson for the department are critical administrative functions requiring political sensitivity to the needs of both the department and the hospital.

Optimal coordination requires superior skills in the critical areas of presentation, debate, analysis, and articulation. For example, the coordination required to bring a new service such as mobile imaging (e.g., MRI, PET) to a community hospital includes at least the following departments or individuals:

- Financial management department for assistance or approval of the proposed financial plan for the project
- Hospital executive administration for project approval
- Board of directors for project approval
- Physicians for referring cases to the new service
- Marketing or public relations staff, who must be kept informed of the arrival of the new service
- Human resources department if new employees are needed or if changes in job descriptions, competencies, or salaries are involved
- Supervisors to inform and train employees for the new service requirements
- Plant services to plan for the location and docking of the mobile imaging truck on the hospital campus and provision of electrical, water, network, and telephone connections
- Service providers to coordinate the schedules of arrival and departure for the purpose of scheduling patients
- Surgical services if anesthesia is to be provided and monitoring equipment is required

- Nursing services for required assistance with patient care
- Postanesthesia recovery services to care for patients after treatment
- Materials management services to ensure availability of new supplies

Project Management

Project management involves organizing and managing resources for a project to be carried out within a specified period with defined costs and expected outcomes. The success and speed with which a new service is developed are directly related to the project management skills of the administrator and team members. Coordinating the project and instilling a cooperative spirit with the interacting departments require a special set of skills. Good project management methodology defines outcomes, builds a plan, manages the risks of the plan, and communicates progress and results according to a schedule developed by a consensus of the group.

REGULATING AGENCIES AND COMMITTEES

The operation of a radiology department is regulated by external agencies, as well as by the governing body of the hospital. External regulating agencies include both voluntary and required regulation. Whereas government agencies usually impose required regulations on health care institutions, other regulating groups such as TJC are voluntary, paid regulators that apply guidelines to measure quality and safety. An example of an involuntary regulating activity tied to reimbursement is accreditation of mammography services for payment by Medicare and other insurance providers. Although participation in some external regulating agencies is voluntary, reimbursement is becoming increasingly dependent on satisfactory compliance with their guidelines and individual state guidelines.

External Agencies

External regulators and agencies that affect radiology operations today include the entities described in the following sections.

The Joint Commission. TJC regulates the quality and safety of care provided to patients and the way a health care organization is supervised and operated. TJC guidelines include the assignment of responsibilities within the hospital, the development of policies and procedures for national patient safety goals, and the management of continuously improving quality. Hospitals voluntarily participate in TJC accreditation, and the organization conducts onsite visits to check hospital compliance with established guidelines and national safety goals. Although voluntary, several other regulatory agencies and payers require the health facility be TJC accredited for reimbursement of services.

There are several standards outlined by TJC, specifically related to safe operations in radiology departments. Although TJC provides updated or revised elements annually, many of the standards outline practices for measuring and monitoring radiation dose, maintaining safety in and around MRI units, inspection and testing requirements to ensure safe equipment operations, requirements for facility physicist services, and defining training and continuous education for technologists.

Previously (JCAHO) if they pass - get gold standard

State Health Departments. State regulatory agencies such as state boards of health define rules to protect the health and safety of the patients or clients of a health care facility or provider. Although states vary considerably, most health departments provide oversight into licensing requirements and regulations related to radiation programs. In addition, 36 US states currently maintain a **certificate of need (CON)** program. The CON is a certificate of authority or permission granted by a state review board allowing a hospital or other health care entity to construct new facilities, develop new services, or purchase expensive equipment or technologies (e.g., MRI, PET). The rules for cash expenditures, which vary from state to state, were developed in an attempt to control the rising costs of health care through control of duplication of services.

→ IDPH - Iowa Department of Public Health

Nuclear Regulatory Commission. Radiation-regulating agencies include the Nuclear Regulatory Commission(NRC) and state licensing agencies for control of equipment and technologists. A state board of health may require licensure of radiologic technologists or may leave the regulation of users of ionizing radiation to the voluntary jurisdiction of the individual health care facility. These regulating groups conduct inspections and levy fines for noncompliance with regulations, which vary from state to state. In most states (referred to as Agreement States), NRC duties have been phased into state agencies such as the department of health or department of radiation safety. Noncompliance with these regulations also could force a health care facility to shut down any operations that involve ionizing radiation.

controls radiation

Occupational Safety and Health Administration. The **Occupational Safety and Health Administration (OSHA)** is the federal agency that establishes standards for safety in the workplace. Some of the critical concerns of OSHA in radiology include handling and disposal of hazardous materials, standard precautions for protection of employees from infectious diseases, and eye protection from processing or disinfecting chemicals.

outside agency

Accreditation Organizations and the *Mammography Quality Standards Act*. The American College of Radiology (ACR) and the Intersocietal Accreditation Commission (IAC) are professional organizations that offer accreditation in modalities such as CT, MRI, ultrasound, and nuclear medicine. The ACR and IAC award accreditation to departments and facilities that demonstrate a high standard of practice through peer-reviewed submission of data from that modality. Although equipment accreditation has traditionally been voluntary, the **Centers for Medicare & Medicaid Services (CMS)** now requires suppliers of the technical component of advanced diagnostic imaging services (CT, MRI, and NM) to be accredited in order to receive Medicare reimbursement. Currently this requirement does not apply to hospitals or critical access hospitals.

The ACR is also the accrediting body for mammography services. All facilities providing mammography must be ACR accredited to be certified by the U.S. Food and Drug Administration (FDA). The *Mammography Quality Standards Act* (MQSA) was developed in 1992 to ensure that all women have access to high-quality mammography services. The FDA and various state health department programs are the regulatory arm of this act, and MQSA certification is required for reimbursement by Medicare. Many states have the authority to inspect on behalf of the FDA.

Health Insurance Portability and Accountability Act

The *Health Insurance Portability and Accountability Act* of 1996 (HIPAA) established a set of national standards for the protection of certain personal health information. The Privacy Rule within the guidelines addresses the use and disclosure of a person's health information by organizations subject to this rule. These standards of HIPAA were developed to increase public trust in the protection of health care information, hold providers and payers accountable, facilitate the adoption of secure electronic management of medical data, and increase data integrity and availability. Many health care organizations have appointed a privacy officer to develop HIPAA policies and procedures, and ensure compliance with them throughout the health care system. Health care information cannot be obtained or shared without the express permission of the individual or designee. An example of this would be if a technologist or student accessed the health information of a friend to read the report or look at the images. This is considered a breach of confidentiality, and the student could be subject to disciplinary actions, including termination of employment or expulsion from a radiography program. All external persons or entities that use or disclose personal health information but are not employees of the provider must sign a business associate agreement that further protects confidentiality of the patient.

Internal Agencies

In addition to external agencies, internal committees also regulate operations in a hospital or health care facility.

Safety Committee. Hospitals are required by TJC to establish a safety committee that directs education of employees on safety policies and procedures, and ensures safe operation of the facility for patients and employees. Safety committees regulate such activities as storage and removal of hazardous or contaminated materials; physical control of chemical, radiation, and biologic hazards; special cleaning and emergency procedures; inspection of facilities to identify hazards; and correction of hazardous conditions. In the early 2000s, hospitals began to broaden the scope of the safety committee to include monitoring clinical patient safety issues such as **adverse drug events (ADEs)** and **medical errors**. Examples of monitoring and reducing medical errors include reduction of medication administration errors, adverse drug events, and patient falls.

Infection Control Committee. The infection control committee regulates infection control policies and procedures, and conducts epidemiologic studies for patient and employee protection.

Radiation Safety Committee. The radiation safety committee(RSC), required by the NRC or state radiation governing body and TJC, regulates hospital activities for radiation safety and nuclear medicine activities. Radiation safety committees define safe handling of radioactive materials and policies for patients and staff exposed to radiation. Policies and procedures used in the case of radiation accidents are also within the responsibilities of the RSC. The RSC has responsibility for all areas in an organization that utilize ionizing radiation equipment or radioactive materials in or outside of the radiology department, such as operating rooms, cardiac catheterization laboratories, endoscopy suites, and hospital outpatient centers.

Pharmacy and Therapeutics Committee. The pharmacy and therapeutics (P&T) committee is a required committee of hospital medical staff responsible for reviewing drugs and their use in the hospital. In most hospitals the P&T committee also reviews drugs used in imaging and their protocols for use, such as iodinated contrast media. The direct control of medication contraindications and safety in a radiology department is typically the responsibility of the radiology management team, who writes policies and procedures, keeps records, and arranges for training in appropriate drug administration for all appropriate employees in the department. Many hospitals now have contrast agents managed directly through the pharmacy department who share these responsibilities for safe medication administration.

Risk Management and Corporate Compliance. Risk management was developed to manage and control the amount of legal and financial risk to the organization and ensure that a hospital continues to remain in good standing with its reputation in the community. Its goal is to keep the organization, employees, and patients free from any risks that may hinder quality of care and to minimize safety concerns for all customers.

Corporate compliance was developed to prevent an organization from committing health care fraud. Most health care organizations work hard to be compliant with federal, state, and insurance regulations. Having a formal compliance program fosters a culture of responsibility and demonstrates that the health system is committed to doing the right thing in all situations and interactions.

Picture Archive and Communications Systems. PACSs became widely accepted as a digital alternative to film-screen imaging devices in the late 1990s. PACS is defined as a system for acquiring, archiving, interpreting, and distributing digital images throughout a health system enterprise. The most noted benefit of PACS is that it allows a health care provider to access digital imaging information anytime and anywhere care is being provided. The clinical benefits of PACSs are the availability of digital images where care is provided, faster turnaround of imaging diagnosis, simultaneous consultation ability with the radiologist, and the ability to always retrieve an examination file without fear of it being lost or misplaced. Financial benefits are the elimination of film, storage, processor, processor maintenance, and paper supply costs. The implementation of PACSs and other digital technology, such as voice recognition dictation systems, has dramatically changed the delivery of imaging services in all health care settings.

CHARACTERISTICS OF GOOD EMPLOYEES

When radiology administrators and supervisors prepare to hire new employees, two specific criteria stand out for administrators. First, the prospective radiology employee should be knowledgeable and possess the necessary technical skills to perform the required job duties. Second, they should have superior skills in interactive relationships. Many administrators believe they can assist the new employee who has a solid knowledge base to grow and acquire an increased range of technical skills, but people skills depend on long-term training, instincts, and personality development. An employee with strong interpersonal skills cooperatively enhances patient care and workflow, thereby increasing his or her value to the workplace.

One of the most important concepts that employees in any organization or business should understand is that the customer is the reason that they are employed. Even in large health care organizations, the hospital, clinic, or office cannot survive or succeed without a steady supply of customers who use the services provided and pay for these services. This includes both patients and the referring physician. In past decades, health care facilities relied on physicians to refer patients to them. In recent years, however, patients have begun to exert influence about where they will obtain their health care services, even to the point of changing physicians when they are dissatisfied. The health care consumer of today is more educated, well versed, and informed on their choices, especially with access to options based on Internet research

Payers are also evaluating satisfaction of their health plan members and holding the facility accountable through contractual arrangements. In the 1990s, health care providers began to recognize insurance companies and other third-party payers as customers looking to contract with health care providers for the best-quality, lowest-cost service. In the early 2000s, some third-party payers began paying reimbursement bonuses to facilities that demonstrated evidence of improved patient safety. In 2010, the incentive for hospitals to improve patient experience was further strengthened by the Patient Protection and Affordable Care Act by including data from patient experience surveys in the calculation for Medicare payments to hospitals. The Hospital Consumer Assessment of Healthcare Providers and Systems (HCAHPS) is a 32-item survey instrument used to measure the patient's perspective on their hospital experience and allows for comparisons between hospitals nationally.

Now that payers such as Medicare link patient experience to reimbursement, it is more important than ever to hire the right people for the organization. Finding the right candidate to work in the radiology department is a process typically facilitated by the human resources department. The initial interview may be with a recruiter who can do the screening of applicants for minimum job requirements. The next phase is generally with the hiring manager in the department of interest. The interview session may include a series of structured questions to determine the applicant's ability to perform the job duties. It may also include time to perform a series of tasks, such as having a technologist perform an exam or other relevant tasks

specific to the position for which they have applied. The management interview session may also be an opportunity for the applicant to describe situations or projects in previous positions, detailing their role and how they responded. Checking references and other background information is part of the application process that must be completed before a job offer can be made.

In the 21st century, high-quality service and communication skills are as important as technical skills in the preparation of students for future employment. High-quality service can be defined as doing things right the first time and meeting or exceeding the customer's expectations. Radiology administrators expect employees (including students as prospective employees) to take personal responsibility for their own motivation to seek out personal development in basic communication skills. Radiologic technologists and students should seek to achieve the following:

- Ability to see their work from the patient's or the physician's point of view
- Skills in handling customer concerns
- Ability to practice service with a smile
- Ability to respond as if the customer is always right
- Meet or exceed the expectations of all patients and physicians
- Critical thinking skills
- Be a team player and understand the value of a team

One opportunity for the student radiologic technologist to work on developing desirable people skills is through routine clinical practice. Although technical skills can be readily learned and proficiency can be measured, the interaction with each patient offers a new opportunity for problem solving. Each difficult patient improves the student's ability to meet or exceed the next patient's expectations. If student technologists become discouraged when performing routine chest radiographs, they should consider that the skills in interpersonal relationships are built patient by patient, and that each patient interaction offers an opportunity to do it better than before.

Another area of opportunity for developing people skills is through interaction with employees in departments outside radiology. The student technologist has the opportunity to be an ambassador of the department of radiology, a representative of the department administrator or even the hospital CEO. When an investment is made by an employee or student technologist in mutual cooperation and support, the dividends are paid back in many forms. When patients observe cooperative interactions between employees, their perception of the quality of the facility and the value they receive in the service provided is enhanced. Perhaps the most obvious payback to the technologist is in the satisfaction realized working in a supportive and cooperative environment. Every encounter or interaction between two employees is an investment—either enhancing or destroying the satisfactory environment. Each employee can make a difference.

Within the radiology department, students should be offered additional opportunities to learn the details of operations through involvement in all departmental functions. Transporting patients, performing image management, processing requisitions, assisting radiologists, and assisting technologists are all important activities that develop well-rounded perspectives of the importance of all radiology employees. Students are well advised to take advantage of every opportunity to become knowledgeable, empowered employees serving and solving problems for every customer, because it will be the hallmark of successful institutions and the sought-after employees of the future.

SUMMARY

- With an understanding of how an imaging department functions within the framework of a hospital organization, the student radiologic technologist can better relate to the cooperation and interaction required to deliver high-quality safe care to patients.

- The field of radiology has broadened in recent decades to include other health care settings such as clinics, imaging centers, and mobile imaging. Although the knowledge requirements for technologists continue to include solid technical skills, a higher demand is placed on superior interpersonal and patient care skills.

- The basic functions of management apply to all hospitals, departments, subdepartments, and work units. Each entity is required to plan, organize, and facilitate work; enlist qualified employees; direct the work to be done; control the quality and outcome; and coordinate activities of staff within the unit, as well as with others outside the work unit. The organization of workers within a health care facility, such as a hospital, is developed to provide service to its primary customers: the physicians and their patients.

- Health care facilities, providers of diagnostic services, and users of ionizing radiation and other medical devices are regulated by mandatory and state agencies, plus voluntary agencies, to ensure the safety of patients, employees, and others in the workplace. In addition to complying with external agencies, radiology departments must comply with internal committees and maintain policies and procedures for patient and employee safety.

- Because radiology departments provide a unique service in diagnosis and treatment, they are usually organized within the facility under a departmental structure in which the student radiologic technologist is expected to learn and become proficient in radiologic procedures, communication, and patient care. Each activity of the student in radiology, whether directly related to developing technical skills or indirectly related to developing interpersonal skills, is an important activity that will prepare the student for future success in his or her chosen profession.

BIBLIOGRAPHY

Arenson RL, Garzio C: *A practical guide to leadership and management in academic radiology*, Springfield, Ill, 2012. Charles C. Thomas.

Certified Radiology Administrator: *CRA Program.* Available at: https://www.ahra.org/CRA. Accessed October 19, 2017.

Deming WE: *Out of crisis*, Boston, 1986, Massachusetts Institute of Technology, Center for Advanced Engineering Study.

Foreman MS, Hubbard L, Marquez LO: *Operations management in radiology*, Sudbury, Mass, 2010, Association for Medical Imaging Management.

HCAHPS: *Fact Sheet.* 2015. Available at: http://www.hcahpsonline.org/Files/HCAHPS_Fact_Sheet_June_2015.pdf

Headrick LA: *Learning to improve complex systems of care: collaborative education to ensure patient safety*, Washington, DC, 2000, U.S. Department of Health and Human Services, Health Resources and Services Administration, Bureau of Health Professions, Division of Medicine and Dentistry.

Institute of Medicine: *Committee on Quality: To err is human: building a safer health system*, Washington, DC, 1999, National Academies Press.

Institute of Medicine: *Committee on Quality: Crossing the quality chasm: a new health system for the 21st century*, Washington, DC, 2001, National Academies Press.

Karami M, Fatehi M, Torabi M, et al.: Enhance hospital performance from intellectual capital to business intelligence, *Radiol Manage* 35:30, 2013.

Leebov W: *Effective complaint handling in health care*, Chicago, 1990, American Hospital.

Leebov W: *The quality quest: a briefing for health care professionals*, Chicago, 1991, American Hospital.

Leebov W, Vergare M, Scott G: *Patient satisfaction: a guide to practice enhancement*, Oradell, NJ, 1990, Medical Economics Books.

McLaughlin DB, Olson JR: *Healthcare Operations Management*, ed 3, Arlington, Va, 2012, Health Administration Press.

Merlino DA, Gaines SR, Gerber SW: *Asset Management in Radiology*, Sudbury, Mass, 2009, Association for Medical Imaging Management.

National Conference of State Legislatures: *Certificate of Need: state health laws and programs.* Available at: http://www.ncsl.org/research/health/con-certificate-of-need-state-laws.aspx. Accessed November 13, 2017.

Rakich JS, Longest BB, O'Donovan TR: *Managing health services organizations*, Baltimore, 1992, Health Professions Press.

Rushford M, Weinreich L: *Human resource management in radiology*, ed 2, Sudbury, Mass, 2016, The Association for Medical Imaging Management.

Shearer DA: Management styles and motivation, *Radiol Manage* 34:47–52, 2012.

The Joint Commission: *Diagnostic Imaging Requirements.* 2015. Available at: http://www.jointcommission.org/assets/1/18/AHC_DiagImagingRpt_MK_20150806.pdf.

The Joint Commission: *National patient safety goals.* 2016. Available at: http://www.jointcommission.org.

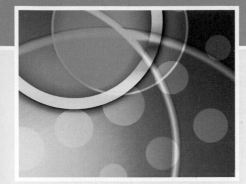

Radiographic Imaging

Vesna Balac, MS, RT(R)(MR)

Four factors … contribute to the quality of the … radiograph: First, distortion; second, detail; third, contrast; fourth, density.

Professor Ed C. Jerman, Father of Radiologic Technology
An analysis of the end-result: the radiograph. Radiology. 1926 6:59.

OBJECTIVES

On completion of this chapter, the student will be able to:

- Discuss primary, scatter, and remnant radiation.
- Describe the fundamentals of image production.
- Describe the three major categories of image receptor systems used today in radiography.
- Compare and contrast the latent image formation process for film-screen radiography, photostimulable phosphor systems, and indirect and direct capture digital radiography.
- Discuss image quality in terms of image receptor exposure, contrast, spatial resolution and distortion.
- Describe fluoroscopic imaging.

OUTLINE

KEY TERMS

Attenuation Process by which a beam of radiation is reduced in energy when passing through tissue or other materials

Automatic Rescaling Process by which images are produced with uniform brightness and contrast, regardless of the amount of exposure

Brightness Function of a display monitor; changes image lightness/darkness

Computed Radiography (CR) Cassette-based digital radiography; the digital acquisition modality that uses storage phosphor plates to produce images

Contrast Difference between adjacent image receptor (IR) exposures on a radiographic image

Data Drop Condition due to extreme overexposure, which causes digital detector elements to become overwhelmed with photon energy and leads to drop of data during image reconstruction

Density Degree of darkening or blackness of exposed and processed photographic or radiographic film

Detector Saturation Data drop that involves areas or regions of the digital detector

Digital Radiography (DR) Cassette-less image receptor systems that convert x-ray energy into a digital electronic signal for manipulation and display

Direct Capture DR Devices that convert incident x-ray energy directly into an electrical signal, typically using a photoconductor as the x-ray absorber and a thin-film transistor as the signal collection area, which then sends the electrical signal to the computer for processing and viewing

Distortion Misrepresentation of the true size or shape of an object

Exposure Indicator (EI) Numeric representation of the quantity of exposure received by a digital image receptor

Exposure Latitude Range of exposures that can be used and still result in the capture of a diagnostic-quality image

Fog Undesirable exposure to the image receptor

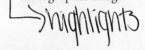

Radiation can't come through (handwritten)

Grid Device consisting of thin lead strips designed to permit primary radiation to pass while reducing scatter radiation by absorption

Half-Value Layer Amount of filtration necessary to reduce the intensity of the radiation beam to one half its original value

Image Receptor (IR) Medium used to capture the image for recording, such as x-ray film or a digital imaging plate

Indirect Capture DR Devices that absorb x-rays and convert them into light; the light is then detected by an area-charge-coupled device or thin-film transistor array in concert with photodiodes, and then converted into an electrical signal that is sent to the computer for processing and viewing

Intensifying Screen Layer of luminescent crystals placed inside a cassette to expose x-ray film efficiently and thereby significantly reduce patient dose

Inverse Square Law Mathematic formula that describes the relationship between radiation intensity and distance from the source of the radiation

→ Penetration (handwritten)

Kilovolt Peak (kVp) Measure of the potential difference, which controls the quality and affects the quantity of x-ray photons produced in the x-ray tube

Latent Image Invisible image created after exposure but before processing

Milliampere-Seconds (mAs) Measurement of milliamperage multiplied by the exposure time in seconds, which controls the total quantity of x-ray photons produced in the x-ray tube

Penetrating Ability Ability of an x-ray beam to pass through an object; controlled by the kilovolt peak of the beam

Penumbra Fuzzy edge of an object as imaged radiographically; also known as image unsharpness

Photon Quantum or particle of radiant energy *– comes out of x-ray tube* (handwritten)

Primary Radiation X-ray beam after it leaves the x-ray tube and before it reaches the object

Radiolucent Permitting the passage of x-rays or other forms of radiant energy with little attenuation

└ radiation can come through (handwritten)

Radiopaque Not easily penetrable by x-rays or other forms of radiant energy

Remnant Radiation Radiation resulting after the x-ray beam exits the object

Scatter Radiation Radiation produced from x-ray photon interactions with matter in such a way that the resulting photons have continued in a different direction

Source-to-Image Distance (SID) Distance between the source of the x-rays (usually the focal spot of the x-ray tube) and the image receptor

Spatial Resolution Degree of accuracy of the structural lines actually recorded in the image

Umbra True edge of an object as imaged radiographically

Window Level Image manipulation parameter that changes image brightness on the display monitor, usually through the use of a mouse

Window Width Image manipulation parameter that changes image contrast on the display monitor, usually through the use of a mouse

---

Radiographic imaging is an essential but complicated subject. There are many concepts that one must not only understand but also apply in the clinical environment. This chapter is intended to give an overview of the most common image receptor systems used in radiography, the image formation process, and the image quality factors essential to producing a diagnostic radiographic image. It will present many basic concepts that will be expanded in other courses. It is important to grasp the basic definitions and concepts before moving on to the more involved topics.

IMAGE PRODUCTION

When x-rays were discovered in 1895, the medical community almost immediately realized the value of this discovery. Seeing inside of the human body became possible. In the following years, capturing the image produced by x-rays in a format allowing for storage and repeated viewing had become the task of the radiologic technologist. Despite the almost daily advances within the field of radiology, the basic mechanism of x-ray production has not changed a great deal. A beam of x-rays, mechanically produced by passing high voltage through a cathode ray tube, traverses a patient and is partially absorbed in the process. A device called an **image receptor (IR)** intercepts the x-ray **photons** that are able to exit the patient. Multiple different IR systems are used in radiography, including film-screen systems, **computed radiography (CR)** cassette-based systems, **digital radiography (DR)** cassette-less systems, and fluoroscopic imaging systems.

Basically, the following four requirements exist for the production of x-rays:

1. Vacuum (tube housing)
2. Source of electrons (filament) *or Cathode* (handwritten)
3. Method to accelerate the electrons (voltage) rapidly
4. Method to stop the electrons (target) *or anode* (handwritten)

The vacuum removes all of the air, so gas molecules will not interfere with the production of x-rays. When the electrons strike the target, x-ray photons are produced; however, less than 1% of this production is actually x-rays; the remaining 99% or more is heat.

The beam of x-ray photons is generated by the careful selection of technical exposure factors by the radiographer. These photons then exit the x-ray tube during the exposure. This beam of photons, before it interacts with the patient's body, is called **primary radiation**. When the primary beam passes through a patient, the individual x-ray photons interact with the various materials that make up the human body. Depending on the characteristics of these materials, the quantities of the photons are lessened by differing degrees as they pass through matter. The resulting beam that is able to exit from the patient is called exit or **remnant radiation**. This remnant radiation produces an image in the IR.

Along the way, an x-ray photon may interact with the body's matter in such a way that the resulting photon continues its travel in a different direction. This type of radiation may or may not be able to reach the IR, but it does not carry any useful information. **Scatter radiation** is the term generally used

KVP
Penetration
Toe 50
Ankle 60
Knee 70
Hip 80

MAs
Photons
Finger - 2
hand - 4
elbow - 6
shoulder - 8

2, 4, 6, 8,
who do we
appreciate?

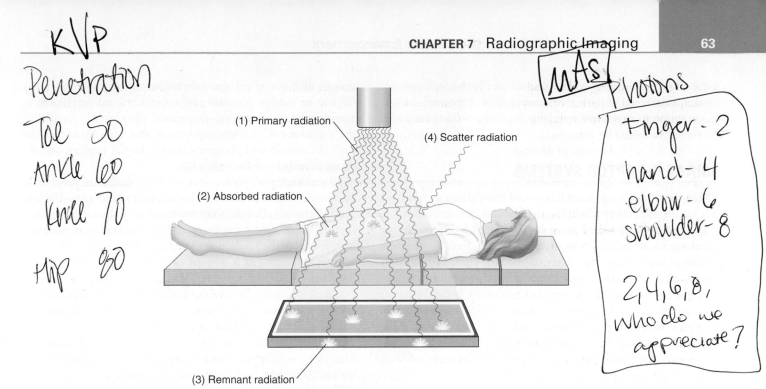

Fig. 7.1 The Path and Attenuation of a Beam of X-radiation. (1) The primary beam exits the x-ray tube. (2) The beam enters the patient, where the individual x-ray photons' energies are altered (attenuated) by their passage through body tissues of varying characteristics. (3) The attenuated, or remnant, beam exits the patient, carrying with it an energy representation of the body tissues traversed and strike the image receptor. (4) Some x-ray photons interact with matter and continue in a different direction, producing scatter radiation, which is nondiagnostic.

Penetration

to describe this type of nondiagnostic radiation. **Attenuation** is the process by which the nature of the primary radiation is changed (partially absorbed or scattered) as it travels through the patient. The x-ray beam is attenuated differently, depending on the type of body tissue irradiated. For example, bone tissue, being more densely packed and made of harder material, attenuates the beam to a greater degree than soft tissue of the same thickness. This difference in attenuation allows for the formation of radiographic images. The entire path of a beam of x-radiation is shown in Fig. 7.1.

In describing the relative ease with which x-ray photons may pass through matter of different types, two terms are commonly used. **Radiolucent** materials allow x-ray photons to pass through comparatively easily; translucent panes of glass allow the passage of light. **Radiopaque** materials are not easily traversed by x-ray photons, just as panes of tinted glass do not allow the full amount of light to pass through. Thus bone is described as a relatively radiopaque tissue, whereas air is described as relatively radiolucent.

loose - can get through it easy

lead lined walls, lead aprons

The radiographer directly controls image quality. Selection of the proper exposure factors for each individual examination is necessary to produce a high-quality diagnostic radiograph. The exposure factors under the control of the radiographer, often referred to as *technique* or *prime factors*, include the following:

1. **Milliampere-seconds (mAs)** is the parameter that controls the amount of x-radiation produced by the x-ray tube; it is the product of milliamperage (mA) multiplied by seconds. It directly controls the quantity of x-ray photons produced. mA is a measure of the electrical current passing through the x-ray tube. Time (in seconds) is a measure of the duration of the exposure and may be expressed in decimals, fractions, or millisecond values.

# of photons we need over a given time

2. **Kilovolt peak (kVp)** is a measure of the electrical pressure (potential difference) forcing the current through the tube. It controls the penetrating ability of the beam and primarily affects the quality but also the quantity of the x-ray photons produced.

3. **Source-to-image distance (SID)** is the distance between the point of x-ray emission in the x-ray tube (the focal spot) and the IR. It affects the relative intensity of the radiation that reaches the IR and affects the geometric properties of the image. This measurement has also been known as *focal-film distance* or *target-to-film distance*.

Other factors that can be controlled by the radiographer include focal spot size, primary beam configuration, quantity and quality of scatter, and speed of the IR.

central ray

Diagnostic radiography makes use of the differential attenuation of a beam of x-rays by various types of body tissue. In this way, information can be gained about the anatomy, physiology, and pathology of many of the body's organ systems. The degree to which the x-rays are attenuated depends on patient thickness and tissue characteristics, such as cell composition, relative atomic number, thickness, and cell density. In addition, pathologic conditions can change the way in which the radiation is attenuated. A thick, dense tissue with a relatively high atomic number, such as bone, attenuates the beam to a greater degree than does a thin, less dense tissue with a low atomic number, such as fat. Bone prevents the easy passage of the x-ray photons, resulting in less IR exposure; therefore, bone is represented as a lighter shade of gray (almost white in some instances), and it can be described as an area of decreased IR exposure (in CR and DR) or radiographic **density** (in film-based systems), on the image.

Because radiography is actually the investigation of tissue characteristics, attempting to standardize all other factors

degree of blackening

affecting image quality so that the subject is the only variable makes sense. Technique charts, automatic exposure control, accurate positioning, and standard imaging protocols are useful in this regard.

IMAGE RECEPTOR SYSTEMS

Once the attenuated beam has exited the patient as remnant radiation, the information it carries about the types of tissue the beam has traversed must be translated from an energy message to a visual image that can be viewed and stored. X-ray photons have the ability to produce changes in photographic film, photostimulable phosphors, and photoconductor materials, such as amorphous selenium (a-Se). Various IR systems exist, including film-screen systems, digital cassette-based systems, and digital cassette-less systems. Historically, film was the primary recording medium; however, almost all film-based systems have now been replaced with CR and DR systems.

Film-Screen Systems

Special film, manufactured to be particularly sensitive to x-radiation and certain colors of light radiation, is used to capture the energy message carried by the remnant beam and to convert it into an image. After the energy strikes it, the film must be processed before an image can be seen. A useful analogy is that of regular photographic film, in which the camera is loaded with the film, which then receives the light reflecting off the subject. When the roll of film is finished, it is rewound into a light-tight canister, developed, and printed. The printed image can then be viewed and stored. The image is not visible before processing because it is stored in a form that is not visible.

Radiographic film is similar. The remnant x-ray photons carry an energy representation of the object of interest that strikes the film emulsion, causing a transfer of energy. This image is stored in the emulsion until it is processed. This invisible image is called the **latent image**. Once the film has been processed, a visual image appears. The correct term to describe an image produced by x-ray photons on a piece of film is a *radiograph.*

Intensifying screens are thin layers of polyester plastic coated with layers of luminescent (light-emitting) phosphor crystals. The screens are mounted in a cassette, and the film is placed inside. Typically, radiographic film has an emulsion coating on both sides and is known as duplitized or double-emulsion film. Duplitized film is designed to be used with two intensifying screens for the most efficient performance. Estimates indicate that more than 99% of the photographic effect on a film-screen radiograph is from screen light, with the remaining effect caused by the direct action of x-ray photons.

Digital Cassette Systems

Photostimulable Phosphor Systems. Also known as CR or cassette-based DR, photostimulable phosphor systems make use of the digital acquisition modality in which photostimulable storage phosphor (PSP) plates are used to produce radiographic images. PSP plates are also referred to as *imaging plates* (IPs). CR can be used in standard radiographic rooms just like film-screen systems; therefore, no special changes are needed to the x-ray rooms. The new equipment that is required includes the CR cassettes and phosphor plates, the CR readers, and the image-display workstations.

The storage phosphor plates are very similar in makeup to intensifying screens used in film-screen radiography. The biggest difference is that the storage phosphor plate can store a portion of the incident x-ray energy it traps within the material for later readout. The reader releases the stored energy in the form of light and converts it into an electrical signal, which is then digitized.

The CR cassette looks like the film-screen cassette. It consists of a durable, lightweight plastic material. The cassette is backed by a thin sheet of aluminum that absorbs x-rays. Instead of intensifying screens inside, there is antistatic material (usually felt) that protects against static electricity buildup, dust collection, and mechanical damage to the plate.

In CR, the radiographic image is recorded on a thin sheet of plastic known as the *imaging plate.* The IP consists of several layers, including the protective layer, phosphor layer, conductive layer, light-shield layer, support layer, and backing layer. The cassette also contains a barcode label or barcode sticker on the cassette or on the IP (viewed through a window in the cassette), which allows the technologist to match the image information with the patient-identifying barcode on the examination request.

With CR systems, no chemical processor or darkroom is necessary. Instead, after exposure, the cassette is fed into a reader (Fig. 7.2) that removes the IP and scans it with a laser to release the stored electrons.

There is no change in how the patient is x-rayed compared with film-screen radiography. The patient is positioned using appropriate positioning techniques, and the cassette is placed either on the tabletop or within the table or upright Bucky. Proper kVp, mAs, and distance must still be employed to produce a high-quality image. The biggest difference lies in how the exposure is recorded. In CR, the remnant beam interacts with electrons in the barium fluorohalide crystals contained within the IP. This interaction stimulates, or gives energy to, electrons in the crystals, allowing them to enter the conductive layer, where they are trapped in an area of the crystal known as the *phosphor center.* This trapped signal will remain for hours, even days, although deterioration begins almost immediately. In fact, the trapped signal is never completely lost. However, the residual trapped electrons are so few that they do not interfere with subsequent exposures.

kVp, mAs, and distance are selected for reasons similar to those for conventional film-screen radiography; kVp must be chosen for penetration and somewhat for the type and amount of **contrast** desired. Early on, manufacturers stated that the minimum kVp should be no less than 70. This is no longer true. The kVp values now range from approximately 45 to 120. It is not recommended that kVp values less than 45 or greater than 120 be used, because those values may be inconsistent and produce

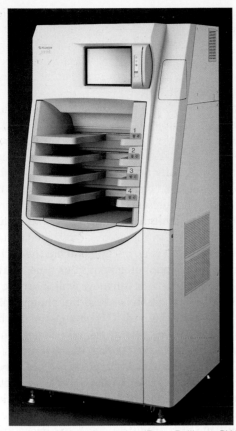

Fig. 7.2 Computed radiography reader. (From Ballinger PW, Frank ED. *Merrill's Atlas of Radiographic Positions and Radiologic Procedures.* 10th ed. St. Louis: Mosby; 2003.)

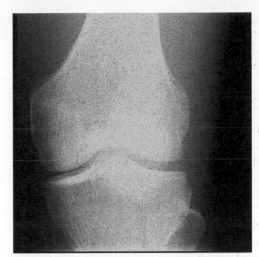

Fig. 7.3 Image with quantum mottle.

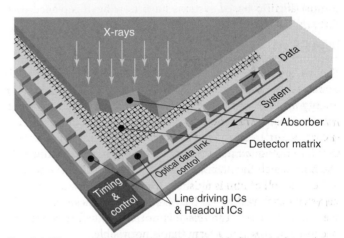

Fig. 7.4 Direct capture digital radiography thin-film transistor detector. (From Carter C, Veale B. *Digital Radiography and PACS.* St. Louis: Mosby; 2010.)

too little or too much excitation of the phosphors. Remember, the process of attenuation of the x-ray beam is exactly the same as in film-screen radiography. It takes the same kVp to penetrate the abdomen with CR systems as it did with film-screen systems.

The mAs is selected according to the number of photons needed for a particular part. If there are too few photons, regardless of the kVp chosen, the result will be a lack of IR exposure to create sufficient phosphor stimulation. When insufficient light is emitted from the phosphors, it produces an image that is grainy, a condition known as *quantum mottle* or *quantum noise* (Fig. 7.3).

Digital Cassette-less Systems

Digital cassette-less systems use various materials for detecting the x-ray signal. The detectors are permanently enclosed in a rigid protective housing. Both **direct capture DR** and **indirect capture DR** detectors are used with these systems.

Direct Capture. In direct capture, x-ray photons are absorbed by the coating material and immediately converted into an electrical signal. The DR detector has a radiation-conversion material or scintillator, typically made of amorphous selenium (a-Se). This material absorbs x-rays and converts them to

electrons, which are stored in the thin-film transistor (TFT) detectors (Fig. 7.4). The TFT is an array of small (approximately 100 to 200 μm) pixels. A pixel is a single picture element, and a matrix is a rectangular series of pixels. The degree of accuracy of the structural lines recorded, known as **spatial resolution** is determined by the individual size of each pixel in a digital image. Each pixel contains a photodiode that absorbs the electrons and generates electrical charges. More than 1 million pixels can be read and converted to a composite digital image in less than 1 second.

Indirect Capture. Indirect capture detectors are similar to direct detectors in that they may use TFT technology. Unlike direct capture, indirect capture is a two-step process: x-rays photons are first converted to light using a scintillator, and that light is then converted to an electric signal.

The scintillation layer in the IP is excited by x-ray photons, and the scintillator reacts by producing visible light. This visible light then strikes the amorphous silicon, which conducts electrons down into the detector directly below the area where

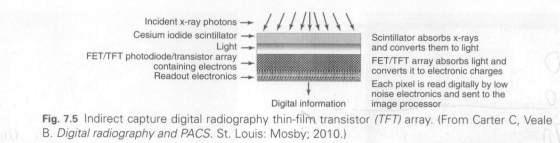

Fig. 7.5 Indirect capture digital radiography thin-film transistor *(TFT)* array. (From Carter C, Veale B. *Digital radiography and PACS*. St. Louis: Mosby; 2010.)

the light struck. There are two types of indirect conversion devices: the charge-coupled device (CCD) and the TFT array. The CCD uses a chip to convert light photons to electrical charge. The TFT array isolates each pixel element and reacts like a switch to send the electrical charges to the image processor. As with direct capture, more than 1 million pixels can be read and converted to a composite digital image in less than 1 second (Fig. 7.5).

IMAGE QUALITY FACTORS

The acceptance characteristics of a diagnostic-quality image, termed *image quality factors*, fall into two main categories: (1) photographic qualities affecting the visibility of the image and (2) geometric qualities affecting the sharpness and accuracy of the image. There are four primary image quality factors. Two of these are photographic in nature: IR exposure and contrast. As an image quality factor, *density* was the term that was used to reflect the impact of IR exposure to the radiographic film. Radiographic density is defined as the overall blackening of film emulsion in response to this exposure. With digital systems, this important image quality factor has not changed but can be expressed simply as IR exposure, because film is no longer the receptor of the image. In the digital environment, **brightness** is a monitor control function that can change the lightness and darkness of the image, but it is not related to IR exposure. Contrast is the visible difference between adjacent IR exposures, or the ratio of black to white. The two geometric quality factors are spatial resolution (also known as *sharpness* or *recorded detail*), the distinct representation of an object's true borders or edges, and **distortion**, the misrepresentation of the true size or shape of an object.

A proper balance between the photographic and geometric properties of an image results in good image quality. The geometric properties allow the size, shape, and edges of the object of interest to be accurately represented, whereas the photographic properties allow these carefully reproduced characteristics to be seen.

By way of illustration, imagine that you are trying to take a snapshot of an ornately carved stone. You want every detail to be captured, so you take extra trouble to focus carefully. To make certain of success, you make three exposures, each at a different setting. When the photograph has been processed, you examine your three photos. One photo is perfectly exposed, and you are able to see every important detail in the carving. The second is too dark, and any detail is hard to distinguish. The third is too light, and again, the details of the carving are impossible to see.

Consider the two poorly exposed photographs. Just because a photograph is too dark or too light, does that mean that good detail sharpness is not present? These problems of overexposure and underexposure affect the visibility but not the sharpness of the detail.

You return to the carving, intending to use the proper exposure setting to get more photographs. This time, you forget to focus the camera properly, or you move while pressing the shutter. The resultant photograph has beautiful photographic properties, but is fuzzy and blurred. This photograph can be said to possess good visibility but poor sharpness of detail. The desired image should have good levels of both characteristics (Fig. 7.6).

When images are evaluated, sharpness and visibility of detail must be examined to assess overall quality. The photographic factors that control visibility of detail are considered first.

Photographic Qualities

Image Receptor Exposure. In film-screen radiography, density has always been the result of IR exposure to the radiographic film. When film is replaced by a digital radiography system, IR exposure becomes the critical factor affecting image quality, and the radiographer must closely monitor the IR exposure values to ensure a good image. Radiographic density can be described technically as a comparison of the light incident on the film to the light transmitted through the film. If a digital image is printed to hard-copy film, the traditional term *density* can still be used.

When a hard copy radiograph is viewed on a viewbox, the incident light is transmitted more easily through the light gray areas than through the darker areas. The darker areas that block the transmission of light are said to have *greater radiographic density*. Although it can be easily measured scientifically with a densitometer, density is often a subjective measurement, judged by the human eye. A radiograph must possess the proper IR exposure to present adequate visibility of detail to the viewer in the same way that a photograph should not be overexposed or underexposed to do justice to its subject. In many instances, a radiologist's use of the term *density* refers to anatomic density and not to radiographic density. A report noting an increased density in the right lung field should be interpreted to mean that the lung tissue is denser than other tissues. The IR exposure, or radiographic density on a film, in such an area would therefore be decreased because the denser tissue would absorb more of the x-ray beam than the tissue that is less dense. Many variables can affect IR exposure, including mAs, patient factors, kVp, distance, beam modification, **grids**, and IRs (Table 7.1).

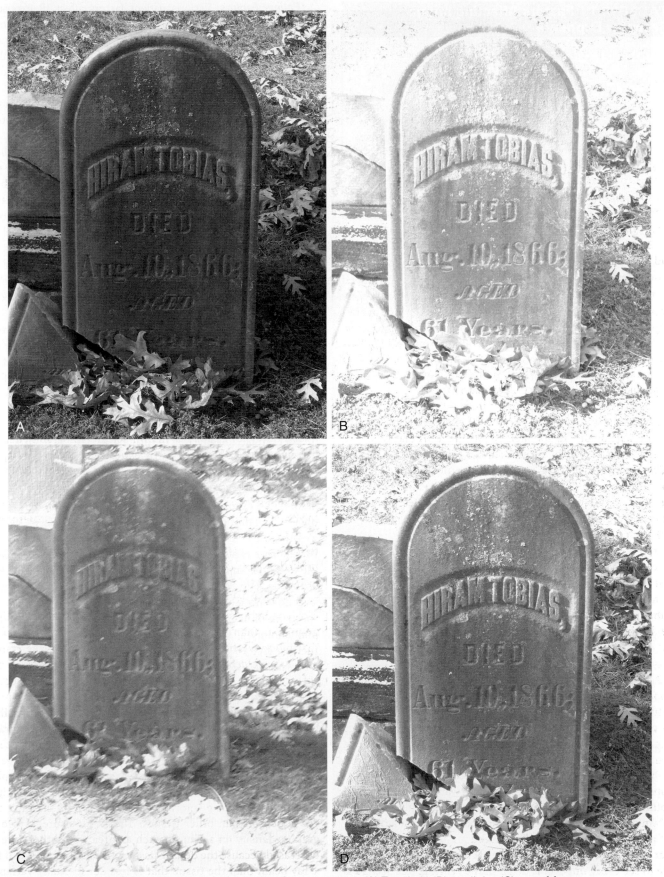

Fig. 7.6 Different-quality photographs of a gravestone. (A) Too dark, (B) too light, (C) out of focus, and (D) perfect.

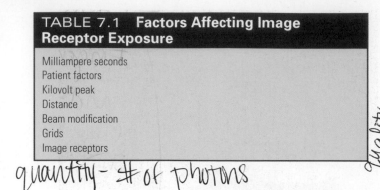

TABLE 7.1 Factors Affecting Image Receptor Exposure

Milliampere seconds
Patient factors
Kilovolt peak
Distance
Beam modification
Grids
Image receptors

[handwritten annotations: quantity - # of photons; quality; range 25-600]

Milliampere-Seconds. The number of electrons that flow from cathode to anode in the x-ray tube is controlled by mAs. This process in turn controls the number of x-ray photons produced. The greater the number of x-ray photons generated, the greater will be the resultant IR exposure. Increasing the number of x-ray photons produced increases the exposure (in milliroentgens [mR]) in a directly proportional relationship, and this results in an overall increase in IR exposure. mAs is the product of mA and time. Any combination of mA and time producing equivalent mAs values should produce equivalent IR exposures. This process is known as *mAs reciprocity.*

$$mA \times time = mAs$$

Examples

$$100 \, mA \times \frac{1}{10}s = 10 \, mAs$$

$$200 \, mA \times \frac{1}{20}s = 10 \, mAs$$

$$300 \, mA \times \frac{1}{30}s = 10 \, mAs$$

The mAs, mA, and time factors are all directly related to image receptor exposure, as well as patient exposure. These effects can also be stated as follows:

- Increasing mAs increases IR exposure and patient exposure.
- Decreasing mAs decreases IR exposure and patient exposure.

The radiographs in Fig. 7.7 illustrate these effects.

Example

$$100 \, mA \times \frac{1}{10}s = 10 \, mAs = \text{original exposure or film density A}$$

$$200 \, mA \times \frac{1}{20}s = 10 \, mAs = \text{maintains exposure or film density B}$$

$$100 \, mA \times \frac{1}{5} \, s = 20 \, mAs = \text{increases exposure or film density C}$$

Patient Factors. Various patient factors affect IR exposure. Patient size and thickness, the predominant atomic numbers of the materials (which may include contrast media intentionally introduced into the body), pathologic conditions, anomalies, temporarily compressed tissues, and a number of other techniques all change the subject density of the object being examined. As subject density increases, IR exposure decreases, and vice versa.

Kilovolt Peak. In addition to the number of x-ray photons produced, the relative strength of the photons must be considered. An x-ray photon of very low energy would have difficulty passing through dense body tissue. Conversely, this same low-energy photon would pass easily through less dense tissue. This characteristic is referred to as the **penetrating ability** of an x-ray beam. Each average body part can be shown to best advantage by using an optimal kVp setting as a guideline.

The kVp setting determines the highest energy level, or the peak, possible for the photons within that beam. Most of the photons are, in fact, below the peak kilovoltage, covering a range from zero to peak value. The x-ray beam is described as *polyenergetic* or *heterogeneous* for this reason.

The relationship between kVp and exposure is not as simple as that of mAs. As kVp increases, IR exposure increases but not in direct proportion. The general rule of thumb to account for the change in IR exposure relative to change in kVp is called the *15% rule.* Increasing kVp 15% will approximately double IR exposure. Decreasing kVp 15% will approximately halve IR exposure.

For example, imagine that the original kVp is 75. Of the original kVp (75), 15% equals 11.25 or approximately 11. If we want to double the IR exposure using the kVp, 11 kVp should be added to the original selection (75), which would result in 86 kVp. If we want to halve the IR exposure using the kVp, then 11 kVp should be subtracted from the original (75), which would then equal 64 kVp.

Using this rule to change kVp while maintaining the same IR exposure is also possible. This process is done by changing the mAs to compensate for the exposure change caused by the change in kVp. When this adjustment is made, the change in kVp does not change the quantity of the exposure—only the spectrum or energy of the photons. kVp can be changed while maintaining the same IR exposure as follows:

Increase kVp 15% and halve mAs.
Decrease kVp 15% and double mAs.

Example

To maintain the original image receptor exposure, what new value of mAs is necessary when changing from 75 kVp and 50 mAs to 86 kVp?

$$75 \times 0.15 \, (15\%) = 11.25 \, (\sim 11)$$

$$75 + 11 = 86$$

Because the kVp increased 15%, the mAs must be halved to maintain the original image receptor exposure:

$$\text{Original mAs} = \frac{50}{2} = 25 \, mAs$$

The radiographs in Fig. 7.8 illustrate these effects.

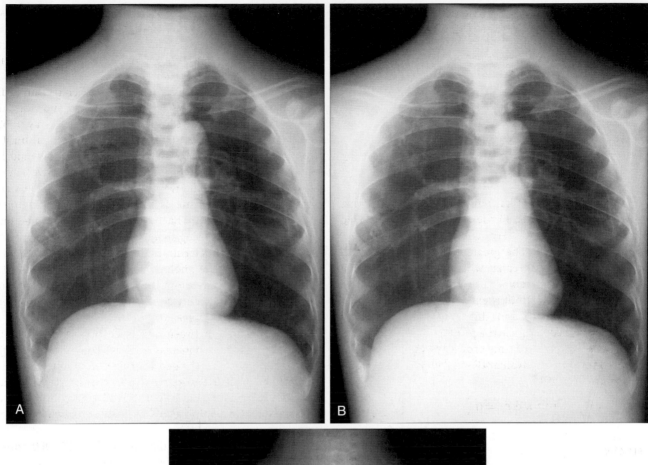

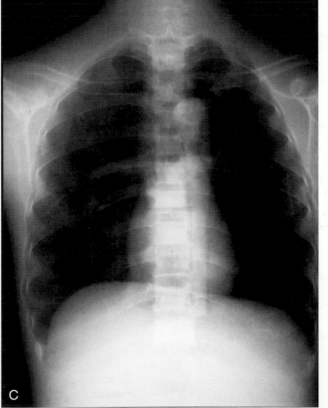

Fig. 7.7 Radiographs show the influence of milliamperage and time on image receptor exposure using film/screen imaging. (A and B) Same milliampere-seconds with different milliamperage and time settings. (C) Double the milliampere-seconds. With digital image receptors, exposure indicator values must be assessed to determine under- or over-exposure.

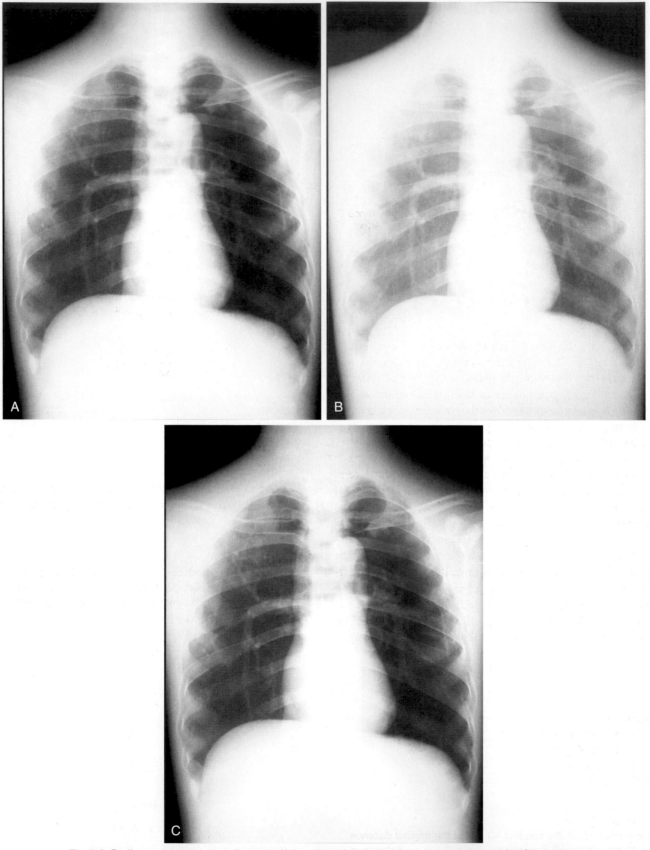

Fig. 7.8 Radiographs show the influence of kilovolt peak on image receptor exposure using film/screen imaging. (A) Acceptable radiograph. (B) Fifteen percent decrease in kilovolt peak with no change in milliampere-seconds. (C) Fifteen percent decrease in kilovolt peak with double the milliampere-seconds to maintain the same image receptor exposure as in A. With digital image receptors, exposure indicator values must be assessed to determine under- or overexposure.

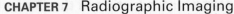

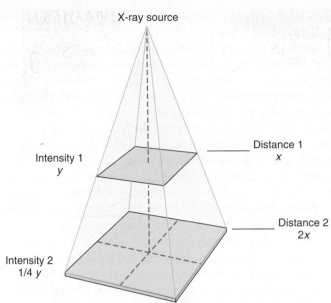

Fig. 7.9 Inverse square law.

Distance. A beam of radiation obeys many of the same laws that light does. If a flashlight beam is projected onto a wall, the relative intensity of the light increases as it is moved closer to the wall. The intensity increases as the distance decreases. As the flashlight is moved farther from the wall, the intensity of the light decreases as the distance increases. This characteristic is described as an *inverse relationship.*

The same relation holds true for an x-ray beam. If all other factors are equal, the greater the distance the photons have to travel, the less chance they have of reaching the IR because of the divergence of the beam (Fig. 7.9). This relationship means that the same exposure factors used at a greater distance would result in reduced IR exposure. The relationship between distance and exposure is described by the **inverse square law**: the intensity of radiation (as measured in mR) is inversely proportional to the square of the distance from the source. In other words, as an example, if the distance is doubled, the intensity decreases to one-fourth of the original. The mathematic expression of the inverse square law is as follows:

$$\frac{I_1}{I_2} = \frac{D_2^2}{D_1^2},$$

where
I_1 = Original intensity (mR)
I_2 = New intensity (mR)
D_1 = Original distance
D_2 = New distance

Example
If the intensity of the beam is 40 mR at the original distance of 40 cm, what will the intensity be if the new distance is 20 cm?

$$\frac{I_1}{I_2} = \frac{D_2^2}{D_1^2}$$

$$\frac{40}{x} = \frac{20^2}{40^2}$$

$$\frac{40}{x} = \frac{1^2}{2^2}$$

$$\frac{40}{x} = \frac{1}{4}$$

$$x = 160 \ mR$$

Note that decreasing the distance by half causes the intensity to increase by a factor of 4.

The inverse square law describes the effect of a change in distance on beam intensity, but the radiographer would frequently like to be able to compensate for a necessary change in distance. This compensation may be accomplished by using a conversion of the inverse square law known as the *exposure maintenance formula.* This formula is actually a direct square law. The mathematic expression of the exposure maintenance formula is as follows:

$$\frac{mAs_1}{mAs_2} = \frac{D_1^2}{D_2^2},$$

where
mAs_1 = Original mAs value
mAs_2 = New mAs value
D_1 = Original distance
D_2 = New distance
Because mAs, mA, and time are all directly proportional to beam intensity, this formula may be used to derive any of these three factors.

Example
If a radiograph produced at 72 inches SID using 20 mAs must be repeated at 36 inches SID, what new mAs setting is necessary to maintain the same image receptor exposure?

$$\frac{mAs_1}{mAs_2} = \frac{D_1^2}{D_2^2}$$

$$\frac{20}{x} = \frac{72^2}{36^2}$$

$$\frac{20}{x} = \frac{2^2}{1^2}$$

$$\frac{20}{x} = \frac{4}{1}$$

$$4x = 20$$

$$x = 5 \ mAs$$

Beam Modification. Anything that changes the nature of the radiation beam, apart from the factors already discussed, is referred to as *beam modification.* The beam may be modified before it enters the patient, in which case it is called *primary beam modification*, or after it exits the patient, in which case it is generally known as *scatter control.*

The primary beam can be adjusted by changing filtration and beam limitation. Filtration is the use of attenuating material, usually aluminum, between the x-ray tube and the patient. This substance mainly removes very-low-energy nondiagnostic x-ray photons in the primary beam to decrease patient exposure. As more material is placed in the path of the beam, the resultant intensity decreases. For example, a bare light bulb glows with a specific intensity. Placing a paper shade over the bulb filters out some of the light, thereby reducing its intensity. With all other factors equal, the same exposure factors used with 4 mm of filtration would produce less IR exposure than if used with only 2 mm of filtration.

The amount of attenuating material required to reduce the intensity of a beam to half the original value is referred to as the half-value layer. Because aluminum is the most common material used for filtration in diagnostic radiography, half-value layer is usually expressed in terms of millimeters of aluminum equivalency (mm Al/Eq).

Beam limitation is the use of devices, such as a collimator, to confine the x-ray beam to the area of interest, thereby reducing exposure to body parts other than those under examination. In addition to patient protection, beam limitation dramatically affects radiographic quality. During the transit of an x-ray photon through matter, the probability that the photon will collide with an atom is high. This collision may result in a change in direction, as well as a decrease in the energy of the photon. This scattered photon is virtually useless from a diagnostic standpoint and contributes only to patient dose. This type of photon is usually described as *scatter radiation.* If scatter radiation reaches the IR, it is not carrying useful information. Scattered photons that strike the IR degrade the quality of the image by contributing unwanted exposure known as fog.

By limiting the size and shape of the primary beam to the area of interest, we are decreasing the probability of the production of scatter radiation. Scatter can never be eliminated, but its effect can be lessened. In fact, scatter accounts for a large percentage of the IR exposure of the image. By restricting the primary beam and decreasing scatter, we are, in effect, subtracting photons from the remnant beam. Therefore a decrease in scatter causes a decrease in IR exposure.

Grids. Despite the careful use of primary beam modification, once the beam enters the patient, scatter radiation is produced. As stated previously, the more scatter that reaches the IR as fog, the poorer the appreciation of the details. A grid is a device that is designed to remove as many scattered photons exiting the patient as possible before they reach the IR. A grid consists of thin radiopaque lead strips interspersed with radiolucent spacing material. The grid is placed between the patient and the IR to intercept scattered photons, which, by definition, have been diverted from their original paths. Increasing the lead in a grid increases its ability to remove scatter from the remnant beam. Decreasing the amount of scatter enhances the radiographic contrast. However, the additional lead in the grid also requires

increased exposure factor settings, which increases the radiation dose to the patient.

Grids are generally described according to grid ratio, the ratio of the height of the lead strips to the distance between them, and grid frequency, the number of grid lines per inch or centimeter. Grid ratios commonly range from 5:1 to 16:1, with the higher ratio grid able to prevent more scattered photons from reaching the IR. Grid frequencies are generally 85 to 200 lines per inch. Because the grid reduces the number of photons reaching the IR, it also causes a decrease in IR exposure. All other factors being equal, if the same exposure factors are used with a 5:1 grid and a 10:1 grid, the 10:1 grid produces an image with less IR exposure.

Image Receptors. With digital IRs, there are several key factors that must be considered when evaluating proper IR exposure. These include exposure latitude, the exposure indicator (EI), automatic rescaling, and window leveling.

Exposure latitude refers to the range of exposures that can be used and still result in the capture of a diagnostic-quality image. The exposure latitude is greater for digital imaging receptors than for film-screen exposures. The greater exposure latitude is a result of the higher dynamic range of the receptors. *Dynamic range* refers to the IR's ability to respond to the exposure. With film-screen systems, overexposure and underexposure are quite evident and are reflected in an image on a film that is too light or too dark. In digital radiography systems, this difference, which is easy to see on film, is not evident on the display monitor. In CR and DR, if the exposure is more than 50% below the ideal exposure, quantum mottle results. The biggest difference between digital and film-screen radiography lies in the ability to manipulate the digitized pixel values, which allows for greater exposure latitude.

EI is a numeric representation of the quantity of exposure received by a digital IR. The total signal is not a measure of the dose to the patient, but rather indicates how much radiation was absorbed by the IR, which gives only an idea of what the patient received. The base EI number for all systems designates the middle of the detector operating range.

For the Fuji (Tokyo, Japan), Philips (Eindhoven, the Netherlands), and Konica Minolta (Tokyo, Japan) systems, the EI is known as the *S* or *sensitivity number.* It is the amount of luminescence emitted at 1 mR at 80 kVp and has a value of 200. The higher the S number with these systems, the lower the exposure. For example, an S number of 400 is half the exposure of an S number of 200, and an S number of 100 is twice the exposure of an S number of 200. The numbers have an inverse relationship to the amount of IR exposure.

Carestream (Rochester, New York) uses the term *exposure index.* A 1-mR exposure at 80 kVp combined with aluminum or copper filtration yields an EI number of 2000. An EI number plus 300 (EI + 300) is equal to a doubling of exposure, and an EI number minus 300 (EI − 300) is equal to halving the exposure. The numbers for the Carestream system have a direct relationship to the amount of exposure so that each change of 300 results in change in exposure by a factor of 2. This is based on logarithms, but instead of using 0.3 (as is used in conventional radiographic characteristic curves) as a change by a factor of 2, the larger number 300 is used. This is also a direct relationship—the higher the EI, the higher the IR exposure.

TABLE 7.2 Recommended Exposure Indicators

Manufacturer	Overexposure	Underexposure	Adult: Nongrid and Grid	Distal Extremities Nongrid
Carestream	>2500	<1600 tabletop <1800 Bucky	1800–2100	2200–2400
Agfa	>2.9	<2.1	2.1–2.3	2.4–2.6
Fuji/Philips/Konica Minolta	<100	>250 tabletop >400 Bucky	200–300	75–125

From Carter C, Veale B. *Digital Radiography and PACS.* St. Louis: Mosby; 2010.

TABLE 7.3 Exposure Indicator Deviation Index Control Limits for Clinical Images

DI	Range Action
Greater than +3	Excessive radiation exposure: Repeat only if relevant anatomy is clipped or "burned out" Require immediate management follow-up
+1 to +3.0	Overexposure: Repeat only if relevant anatomy is clipped or "burned out"
–0.5 to +0.5	Target range
Less than –1.0	Underexposure: Consult radiologist for repeat
Less than –3.0	Repeat

DI, Deviation index. From American Association of Physicists in Medicine. An exposure indicator for digital radiography: Report of AAPM task group 116, 2009.

TABLE 7.4 Factors Affecting Contrast

Kilovolt peak
Patient factors
Contrast media
Milliampere-seconds
Beam modification
Image receptor
Grids

The term for EI for an Agfa (Mortsel, Belgium) system is the *logarithm of the median exposure* (lgM). An exposure of 1 mR at 75 kVp with copper filtration yields an lgM number of 2.6. Each step of 0.3 above or below 2.6 equals an exposure factor of 2. For example, an lgM of 2.9 equals twice the exposure of 2.6 lgM, and an lgM of 2.3 equals an exposure half that of 2.6 lgM. The relationship between exposure and lgM is direct.

Digital imaging system manufacturers use different methods to numerically represent exposure values (Table 7.2). This lack of a universal system has been a source of confusion for technologists, and consequently there has been a need to standardize EIs. The American Association of Physicists in Medicine is actively working on solving this issue, and their intent is to establish a standard scale that would be accepted by all manufacturers. Once this scale is accepted, the users would establish a target value for each examination, based on their system. The deviation index (DI) would be used in conjunction to determine if the appropriate radiographic technique factors were used during an examination. The DI can be defined as a comparison of the target value with the actual exposure recorded by the IR (Table 7.3).

Automatic rescaling is used when exposure is greater or less than what is needed to produce a diagnostic image. Automatic rescaling means that images are displayed with uniform brightness and contrast, regardless of the amount of exposure to the IR. Problems occur with automatic rescaling when too little or too much exposure is used. Quantum mottle or noise is often seen when not enough exposure is used for a particular anatomic body part. Too much exposure can detract from image quality and lead to **data drop**. Data drop

is a condition that causes digital detector elements to become overwhelmed with photon energy, which leads to drop of data during image reconstruction. Data drop can occur over an entire area of the detector, leading to **detector saturation**. Therefore, detector saturation can be described as data drop that involves areas or regions of the detector. Data drop and detector saturation can present serious clinical issues for the interpreting physician. Therefore, rescaling is no substitute for appropriate technical factors. One should not rely on the system to scale the image into an appropriate brightness and contrast through rescaling when higher-than-recommended mAs values are used for a particular body part, to avoid repeats.

Windowing is a processing operation that controls brightness and contrast on the monitor. **Window level** controls image brightness, and **window width** controls contrast (the ratio of black to white). The user can quickly manipulate both by using a mouse. Care should be taken, because this may be a permanent change depending on the vendor, and could have a negative impact on the stored image in the picture archiving and communication system.

Contrast. The second photographic image quality factor is contrast. Contrast is the visible difference between adjacent IR exposures. An object may be accurately represented on an image, but if it cannot be distinguished from the objects surrounding it, then the eye will not adequately appreciate the object. Proper contrast enhances the visibility of detail. Contrast can be understood by recalling the story of the little boy who was asked to draw a picture in art class. After laboring for some time, he presented a sheet of completely white paper to the teacher. The puzzled teacher asked what the picture was supposed to represent, to which the little boy replied, "It's a white horse eating marshmallows in a snowstorm." Of course, because no contrast existed between the different densities, the teacher failed to see the image the child described.

Many factors affect contrast, including kVp, patient factors, contrast media, mAs, beam modification, IRs, and grids (Table 7.4).

Fig. 7.10 Radiographic contrast is demonstrated with radiographs of step wedges at various kilovolt peak settings to show variations in the number of shades of gray, also known as the *scale of contrast*.

factor of contrast- the Computer software manipulates the contrast

quality

Kilovolt Peak. The chief controlling factor of contrast had historically been kVp. Adjusting the kVp controls the penetrating ability of the x-ray beam. Higher kVp is required to penetrate bony tissue than soft tissue. It is important to understand that the relationship between the kVp and contrast has changed with the use of CR and DR technologies, and the old rules no longer apply. This is due to computer software's ability to manipulate the image by altering the amount of contrast demonstrated. Therefore, kVp does not have the impact on the final image contrast as it did with film-screen. However, it is important to note that kVp still controls the signal differences in the digital detector and should be selected for the desired level of subject contrast. Unlike image contrast, subject contrast cannot be manipulated with post-processing because it is directly influenced by the attenuation properties of the tissues.

Contrast is the difference between the range of adjacent IR exposures represented on an image. These IR exposures fall into a range from darkest to lightest gray. This range of gray tones is known as the *scale of contrast*. The fewer the gray tones present, the greater the difference between individual IR exposures. Consider the difference between maximum and minimum IR exposures. In Fig. 7.10, if the 60-kVp strip goes from dark to light in five steps, whereas the 120-kVp strip goes from dark to light in more steps, the difference between the individual IR exposure steps in the 120-kVp strip will be less than that in the 60-kVp strip.

Images with relatively few gray tones are said to possess *high contrast*, *short-scale contrast*, and *narrow latitude*. Images with greater numbers of gray tones are said to possess *low contrast*, *long-scale contrast*, and *wide latitude*. Remember that contrast is

TABLE 7.5 Terms Used to Describe Contrast Relationships

Few Gray Tones	Many Gray Tones
Minimum to maximum relatively quickly	Minimum to maximum slowly
High contrast	Low contrast
Short-scale contrast	Long-scale contrast
Narrow latitude	Wide latitude
Lower kilovolt peak value	Higher kilovolt peak value

a relative measure. No absolute standards of high or low contrast exist; only comparisons between images can be made.

A higher energy beam tends to penetrate objects in its path more easily and thus produces a wider range of gray tones. Table 7.5 outlines these relationships.

Patient Factors. As described in the section on IR exposure, the tissues that make up the human body attenuate the beam of radiation to differing degrees. This differential attenuation is the basis for image contrast. If two objects represented on an image have similar tissue densities, they produce similar IR exposures. This is often the case in radiography of the abdominal organs. Distinguishing details within these similar tissue densities would be difficult. This is an example of a body part with low subject contrast. Other body parts possess high subject contrast. In radiography of the chest, the bony tissue of the ribs has much greater tissue density than the surrounding air-filled lung tissue. The resulting IR exposures are therefore different and easily distinguishable.

Contrast Media. Enhancing the inherent contrast is sometimes possible through the use of contrast media. Contrast media are substances that attenuate the beam to a different degree than the surrounding tissue. Examples of contrast media used in radiography include barium and iodine compounds, and air. Filling the stomach and intestine with barium compound allows these structures to be visualized and examined radiographically. The kidneys filter an intravenous injection of iodine compound, allowing examination of the urinary tract as the compound is excreted. Because the contrast medium introduces an additional subject density to the body, technical factors, particularly kVp, must be adjusted for adequate penetration.

Milliampere-Seconds. mAs alters IR exposure, and therefore, influences contrast. If an image is grossly overexposed or underexposed, then contrast is affected. If exposure is maintained, then mAs will have no effect on the contrast of the image. With film, under- or over-exposure was clearly evident in the resultant image. For digital systems, the exposure indicator should be in the acceptable range to assure that the detector received the correct exposure. No increase in mAs can compensate for inadequate penetration.

Beam Modification. One of the primary purposes of beam modification is scatter control. Scattered radiation allowed to reach the IR produces nondiagnostic exposures referred to as *fog*. Removal of fog results in the loss of some specific gray tones. Decreasing the number of gray tones, by definition, causes a move toward higher contrast. Anything that decreases scatter increases contrast.

Image Receptors. With digital image detector systems, the traditional relationship between contrast and exposure variables does not exist. With digital systems, contrast is determined

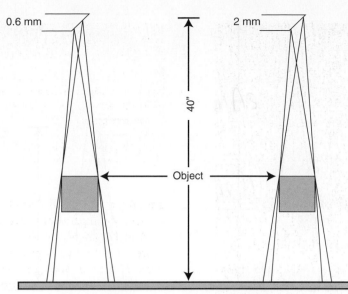

Fig. 7.11 Effect of focal spot size on sharpness.

through digital processing, which sets the range of information that will be supplied to the monitor. The information is displayed in a range of brightness, which can then be adjusted through the manipulation of the window width. Even though digital processing controls image contrast, sufficient differences in exposure to the receptor are necessary. Therefore, the radiographer still must set proper exposure factors to create an acceptable image quality with minimum exposure of the patient.

Grids. Because grids absorb scatter radiation, they function to improve contrast. Grids are available in a diverse range of ratios and frequencies. These choices allow the radiographer to select how much scatter radiation is to be eliminated, and thereby control the visible level of contrast on the image. Because of the high sensitivity of digital detectors to scatter radiation, the use of a grid is much more critical than in film-screen radiography. When possible, the highest grid frequency available should be used with digital imaging to avoid certain grid errors.

increases detail

Geometric Qualities

Spatial Resolution. The sharpness with which an object's structural edges are represented on an image is referred to as *spatial resolution.* It is also described as *sharpness of detail, definition,* and *recorded detail.* Sharpness of detail is complemented by visibility of detail. Good image quality requires a proper balance of the two.

The chief factors affecting spatial resolution include motion, object unsharpness, focal spot size, SID, object-to-image distance (OID), and digital detector characteristics.

Motion. The most common cause of image unsharpness is motion. Patient motion may be voluntary or involuntary. Voluntary motion can be controlled by the use of careful instructions to the patient, suspension of patient respiration during exposure, short exposure times, and judicious use of appropriate immobilization devices. Involuntary motion, such as that caused by the heartbeat and the peristaltic movements of the intestines, is best controlled by the shortest exposure time possible. Equipment motion, such as the vibration of the

tabletop during a table grid exposure, also can be decreased by the use of short exposure times.

Object Unsharpness. The fundamental problem in radiography, as in photography, is attempting to represent a three-dimensional object on a two-dimensional image. Objects that undergo radiography do not consist of straight edges and sharp angles. A basic unsharpness exists to the image of a three-dimensional object that cannot be eliminated. Lessening the effect of this inherent loss of detail is possible by adjusting the factors over which the technologist has control: focal spot size, SID, and OID.

Focal Spot Size. Imagine the beam from a small flashlight. The light beam is relatively narrow and causes a sharp, well-defined shadow of an object placed in its path. Compare this shadow with that of the same object produced by a floodlight. If all the distances are the same, the image produced by the smaller source will be sharper than that produced by the larger source. In the x-ray tube, the width of the beam is controlled by the selection of the small or large focal spot. In general, the small focal spot is used when fine detail is required, as in the radiography of small bones. The large focal spot is used for most general radiographic examinations. Fig. 7.11 illustrates how the focal spot size affects the sharpness of the structural edges of an object.

Source-to-Image Distance. In addition to its effect on the intensity of a beam of radiation, the distance from the focal spot to the IR is also a major influence on the size and spatial resolution of the image. Because a beam of radiation diverges from the source in the same fashion as light, the flashlight may again be used to illustrate the point. If an object is positioned close to a blank wall (the IR) and the flashlight is held at a distance from the object so that a shadow is visible, then a fuzzy unsharp edge around the true shadow becomes obvious. The fuzzy edge is called **penumbra** or image unsharpness, and it obscures the true edge, or **umbra.** If the flashlight is positioned closer to the object, then as distance decreases, the penumbra around the true shadow increases. If the flashlight is positioned farther from the object, then the penumbra decreases, causing the image to appear sharper (Fig. 7.12).

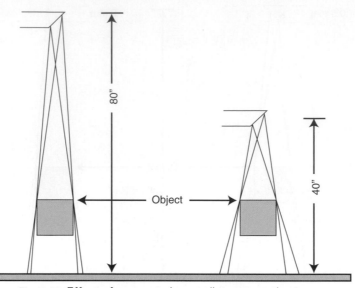

Fig. 7.12 Effect of source-to-image distance on sharpness.

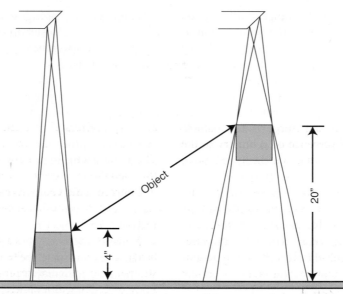

Fig. 7.13 Effect of object-to-image distance on sharpness.

In radiography, the greater the SID, the better the spatial resolution will be. Because radiographic rooms and equipment are not currently built to accommodate extremely long distances, SIDs are standardized so that the degree of penumbra is at least a known factor. The most common SID is 40 inches, but some procedures such as chest radiography use a 72-inch SID. Exceptions to these standards exist, but the SID of an examination should always be indicated to allow for the calculation of image unsharpness.

Object-to-Image Distance. The flashlight experiment is used to observe what happens to penumbra when the OID is varied. When the object is moved closer to the IR, penumbra decreases and image sharpness increases (Fig. 7.13). As the object is moved farther from the receptor, penumbra increases and sharpness decreases. Thus the smaller the OID is, the better

the spatial resolution will be. Many of the objects that must be radiographed are structures located deep within the body. Getting them close to the IR is often impossible. Thus control over OID often depends on the radiographer's knowledge of anatomy and positioning.

Digital Detector Characteristics. Digital imaging systems have characteristics inherent in their physical makeup, as well as the pixel and matrix sizes incorporated into them, that allow improvements in spatial resolution. The smaller the pixel size, the better will be the image resolution.

Distortion. Distortion is the misrepresentation of the true size or shape of an object. Size distortion is commonly known as *magnification*, and shape distortion is sometimes referred to as *true distortion*.

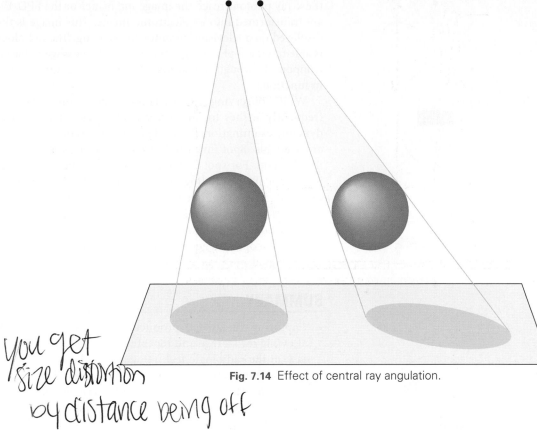

you get size distortion by distance being off

Fig. 7.14 Effect of central ray angulation.

Size Distortion. Magnification of the image is unavoidable because it is influenced by the divergence or geometry of the beam, but it may be controlled to a certain extent by the use of proper SID and OID.

The size of the recorded image varies with the SID, because the size of the light field covered by a flashlight varies with the distance from the source. If the SID decreases, magnification of the image increases. Magnification decreases as SID increases (see Fig. 7.12). The use of standardized SIDs allows the radiologist to assume that a specific magnification factor is present on all images. For this reason, noting any deviation from the standard SID is extremely important.

Varying the OID also influences the magnification of the resultant image. If a flashlight is kept at a standard distance and the object is moved closer to the receptor, the magnification of the image decreases. If the object is then moved farther from the receptor, magnification increases. Magnification decreases as OID decreases. In terms of spatial resolution and magnification, the best image is produced with a small OID and a large SID (see Fig. 7.13).

Shape Distortion. The misrepresentation of the shape of an object on an image is called *shape distortion* or *true distortion*. It is controlled by the alignment of the beam, part, and IR. Influencing factors include central ray angulation and body part rotation.

The beam of radiation diverges from the source in an approximately pyramidal shape (see Fig. 7.9). This divergence means that the photons in the center of the beam are traveling along the straightest pathway and those at the beam's periphery are traveling at a greater angle. The straight, central portion of the beam is referred to as the *central ray*. The most accurate representation of an object results from the passage of photons in a straight line through the area of interest. This characteristic is the reason for the emphasis on central ray entrance and exit points in positioning instructions.

When the central ray is angled, the relationships among the beam, part, and IR are altered. A sphere that is imaged by a straight perpendicular beam is represented as a circular image. An image of the same sphere, when imaged by an angled beam, appears as an oval. Objects may appear to be elongated or foreshortened (Fig. 7.14).

Because the structures of the body do not lie in exact 90-degree perpendicular relationships to one another, central ray angulation is used in many radiographic examinations to help demonstrate specific anatomic details.

Changing the orientation of the body part undergoing radiography also affects the relationship of the beam, object, and IR. If the object of interest is superimposed on another object, the resulting image is difficult to evaluate. By rotating or obliquing the body, the object of interest can be projected free from the interference of the overlying object. Frequently, a combination of part rotation and central ray angulation is used to best demonstrate the anatomic details free from superimposition by overlying structures (Fig. 7.15). Ideally, the goal of a radiologic technologist is to place the anatomic part parallel to the IR and have the central ray aligned perpendicular to the IR.

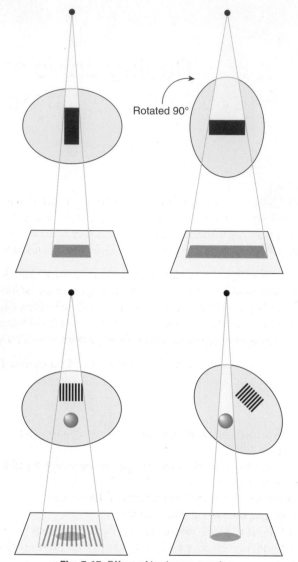

Rotated 90°

Fig. 7.15 Effect of body part rotation.

FLUOROSCOPIC IMAGING

Fluoroscopic examinations often involve a combination of imaging processes. The fluoroscopic image itself is a dynamic, or moving, image rather than a static radiographic image. An analogy is that of a movie compared with a snapshot.

The fluoroscopic examination is usually divided into two portions: (1) viewing a physiologic event in real time (as it occurs) and (2) archiving images for later review. Modern fluoroscopic units are constructed so that the x-ray tube may be located either over or under the x-ray table. Opposite the tube is the image intensifier unit or the flat-panel detector (FPD), a device that intercepts the attenuated beam as it exits the patient. The image intensifier or an FPD is the actual IR in this case, rather than the IRs previously described. When

the x-ray photons reach the image intensifier or the FPD, they are transformed into an electronic image. This image is then displayed on a television monitor for viewing. The radiologist is able to view a physiologic event (e.g., the passage of barium compound through the stomach) and observe abnormalities in function.

While observing the dynamic image, the radiologist frequently wishes to preserve an image as a record of the dynamic examination. A variety of image-archiving methods are available. Spot imaging is a common method of achieving this end. For spot images, the fluoroscopic unit changes instantaneously to radiographic mode for the duration of the exposure. These spot images are then processed, viewed, and stored, as with any other image. Digital fluoroscopy is replacing traditional filming and allowing for easy manipulation of the fluoroscopic images after they have been converted to a digital signal.

SUMMARY

- Capturing the image produced by x-rays in a format allowing for storage and repeated viewing has become the task of the radiologic technologist. The basic mechanism of x-ray production has not changed a great deal. A beam of x-rays, mechanically produced by passing high voltage through a cathode ray tube, traverses a patient and is partially absorbed in the process. A device called an IR intercepts the x-ray photons that are able to exit the patient. Various different IR systems are used in radiography, including film-screen systems, CR and DR systems (cassette-based and cassette-less), and fluoroscopic imaging systems.
- An image of good quality must possess a proper balance of photographic properties (IR exposure and contrast) and geometric properties (spatial resolution and distortion). Of the many factors contributing to image quality, the radiographer must be able to manipulate technical factors such as mAs, kVp, and SID; choose and operate appropriate imaging equipment and accessories; and use proper positioning and patient care skills to obtain high-quality diagnostic images.

BIBLIOGRAPHY

American Association of Physicists in Medicine: *An exposure indicator for digital radiography: report of AAPM task group 116*, College Park, 2009, The Association.

Bushong S: *Radiologic science for technologists*, ed 11, St. Louis, 2017, Mosby.

Carlton R, Adler A: *Principles of radiographic imaging: an art and a science*, ed 6, Clifton Park, NY, 2019, Cengage Publishing.

Carroll Q: *Radiography in the digital age: physics, exposure, radiation biology*, Springfield, 2011, Charles C. Thomas.

Carter C, Veale B: *Digital radiography and PACS*, ed 2, St. Louis, 2013, Mosby.

live x-ray
tube is under the table

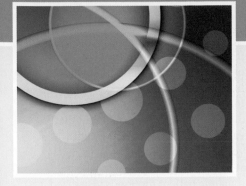

Radiographic and Fluoroscopic Equipment

Randy Griswold, MPA, RT(R)

To test further the ability of lead to stop the rays, he selected a small lead piece, and in bringing it into position observed to his amazement not only that the round shadow of the disc appeared on the screen, but that he suddenly could distinguish the outline of his thumb and finger, within which appeared darker shadows—the bones of his hand....

Correlating these observations with the shadow picture of the bones of his hand upon the fluorescent screen, he conceived another experiment for which one evening he persuaded Mrs. Roengten to be the subject.... When he showed the picture to her, she could hardly believe that this bony hand was her own and she shuddered at the thought she was seeing her skeleton. To Mrs. Roengten as to many others later, this experience gave a vague premonition of death.

Dr. W.C. Roengten by Otto Glasser 1945

OBJECTIVES

On completion of this chapter, the student will be able to:

- Discuss the role of the radiographer in maximizing diagnostic yield
- Identify the typical features of a radiographic/fluoroscopic system
- Explain the manipulation of radiographic equipment
- Explain the purpose of the collimation assembly and its importance in radiation protection
- Distinguish among the various types of radiographic tables and their functionality
- Explain the major controls on the radiographic system control console
- Differentiate between the types of x-ray tube support systems
- Explain the purpose of the upright image receptor and its functionality
- Discuss the concept of alignment of the various radiographic system components
- Briefly discuss the two classes of digital imaging detectors and future technologies resulting from digital detectors
- Distinguish between the two general classes of fluoroscopic system designs
- Discuss mobile radiographic systems and their applications

OUTLINE

KEY TERMS

Autotracking A feature of modern x-ray systems that enables simultaneous vertical movement of an upright image receptor and overhead x-ray tube.

Anode Positive electrode of the x-ray tube.

Bucky Mechanism Grid that is an integral part of the x-ray table, located below the tabletop and above a cassette receptor tray. It decreases the amount of scatter radiation reaching the image receptor, which improves image quality increases contrast. It also moves during exposure so that no grid lines appear on the image.

KEY TERMS—cont'd

Cassette Lightproof holder for the image receptor. In computed radiography, the cassette holds the reusable photostimulable phosphor imaging plate; in conventional film-screen radiography, the cassette contains intensifying screens and a sheet of film.

Cathode Negative electrode of the x-ray tube.

Collimator Diaphragm or system of diaphragms made of an absorbing material; designed to define the dimensions and direction of a beam of radiation. This device consists of four rectilinear radiopaque blades that are adjustable to control the x-ray's field size and shape.

Digital Imaging Acquisition of static images in an electronic fashion; conversion of images to a digital format for image manipulation, enhancement, storage, and networking.

Diode Electrical component that possesses polarity with a negative and positive terminal.

DR Panel Common term for a flat-panel digital image receptor using either indirect or direct digital capture technology.

Flat-Panel Detector Type of digital detector employing amorphous silicon or selenium material bonded with thin-film transistor technology for digital image creation and amplification.

Fluoroscope Device used for dynamic radiographic examinations; usually consists of an x-ray tube situated underneath the x-ray table and an electronic image detector situated over the x-ray table.

Fluoroscopy Examination by means of the fluoroscope, employing image intensification.

Goniometer Angulation scale incorporated into the x-ray tube-head assembly to indicate the degree of x-ray tube angle relative to the image receptor.

Hard Copy Radiographic image created on a polyester film medium.

Latent Image Invisible image created after x-ray exposure and before image processing.

Longitudinal Lengthwise, or along the long axis.

Orthogonal A perpendicular relationship between the x-ray beam central ray (CR) and image receptor.

Overhead Tube Crane Mechanical support for suspending the x-ray tube and collimator assembly from the ceiling of the radiography room.

Picture Archival and Communication System (PACS) Computer network for the transmission, viewing, and archival storage of medical images; often integrated into a larger hospital information system (HIS) and radiology information system (RIS).

Positive Beam Limitation (PBL) Form of x-ray beam collimation of field size ensuring that the x-ray exposure field is no larger than the receptor size.

Postprocessing Manipulation of medical images after they have been acquired through x-ray exposure in order to improve image quality and diagnostic yield.

Pyrex Glass Special type of glass that can withstand very high temperatures from the x-ray tube anode.

Primary Barrier A receptor of x-radiation that intercepts the primary beam and prevents exposure if not interlocked with the central ray of the x-ray beam. In fluoroscopy, the fluoroscopic digital panel or image intensifier tube are primary barriers.

Radiolucent Describes a material that easily transmits x-ray energy with very little absorption.

Real-Time Images Images in which dynamic patient motion is visualized instantly as fluoroscopic imaging is occurring.

Remnant Radiation All radiation exiting the patient during exposure and ultimately striking the receptor.

Soft Copy Visualization of x-ray images using a video monitor for display and interpretation.

Spot Film Equipment that permits the acquisition of static images during a dynamic fluoroscopic examination; images are recorded using film or are acquired digitally and stored electronically.

Tether Electrical wire connection between a digital detector and the x-ray generator and computer.

Transverse Placed crosswise; situated at right angles to the long axis of a part.

Trendelenburg Tilt Table tilt angle in which the patient's head and thorax are lower than his or her legs.

Tube Angulation Pivoting the tube at the point where it is attached to its support.

Vertical Perpendicular to the plane of the horizon.

X-Ray Tube Device that produces x-rays.

X-Ray Tube Head Equipment consisting of the x-ray tube, collimator, and operator controls; permits manipulation of the x-ray tube in many directions for proper positioning.

DIAGNOSTIC YIELD AND EFFICACY

The purpose of any medical imaging procedure is to provide accurate information about the patient's medical condition or disease. When a physician orders a diagnostic study, he or she has an array of procedures to choose from to help determine what is wrong with the patient. These studies may range from simple x-ray studies to medical sonograms or complex computed tomography (CT) or magnetic resonance imaging (MRI) examinations. All diagnostic procedures have an expected yield of medical information regarding the patient's condition. When physicians choose one procedure over another, many factors are considered in making the selection. These may include radiation dose, risk to the patient, the patient's medical condition and tolerance of the procedure, costs and insurance coverage, and timeliness. As an exercise, ask a physician to share the many factors he or she considers in ordering a diagnostic study. The list may be surprising and will help you to understand why physicians expect radiographers to maximize the diagnostic yield of clinical information from images taken of their patients.

The accuracy with which a diagnostic study reveals a patient's medical condition is its diagnostic efficacy. Image artifacts such as jewelry, clothing, tubes, lines, and so on do not truly represent the patient's medical condition and lower diagnostic efficacy. The amount of clinically useful medical information about the patient is the procedure's diagnostic yield. When one factors in the reasons for ordering a medical study, it is expected that the diagnostic yield of information will clearly outweigh the input considerations for doing the study. A competent imaging professional seeks to produce the highest image quality and diagnostic efficacy using only the necessary input factors to maximize the diagnostic yield. When this is done consistently, employers, physicians, nurses, and colleagues will develop respect for the technologist's value as a health team member.

MANIPULATION OF RADIOGRAPHIC EQUIPMENT

A primary role of a radiographer is the manipulation of expensive, high-technology x-ray equipment. The new student must learn to master the mechanical aspects of a radiographic examination early. Becoming as comfortable as possible with maneuvering the x-ray equipment is important. Once this task has been accomplished, the beginning radiographer can concentrate on learning to master other important skills, such as patient care, positioning, technique selection, and image quality. Generally speaking, the earlier a student masters the essential skills of equipment manipulation, the more success he or she will have in the other professional aspects of radiography. On the other hand, a student who does not learn to handle the x-ray equipment early will have trouble moving on to advanced skills. To the employer, the equipment used is an investment in patient care, costing many thousands of dollars, and it is important that radiographers not lose respect for these investments in medical practice.

Regardless of the manufacturer, all x-ray systems have the same basic design features. These components include an x-ray tube and support system, collimator assembly, x-ray table, x-ray generator, control console, and upright image receptor holding devices. All components combine to form an x-ray imaging system. Newer technologies have allowed the images to be recorded digitally and manipulated to optimize appearance and quality. Traditionally our profession has been a film-based (analogue) medium, but with the advent of high-speed computers and software, images are now recorded using digital detectors. Over the last 20 years or so, the greatest technologic innovations have occurred primarily with digital detector technology. The basic components of the x-ray system, however, have remained essentially unchanged.

The first step in mastering equipment manipulation is being able to identify the generic components of a radiographic system. A beginning radiographer who has visited a radiology department can be overwhelmed by the many different radiographic room designs. The design of radiographic equipment allows the radiographer to position the x-ray tube and collimator assembly

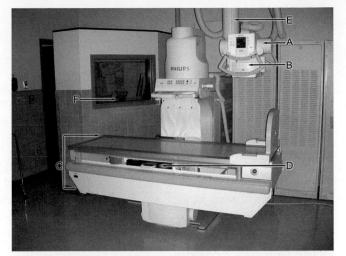

Fig. 8.1 The generic components of diagnostic radiographic equipment include the x-ray tube (A), collimator (B), radiographic table (C), and receptor tray (D). The overhead tube crane support (E) is suspended from ceiling-mounted rails, and the generator control console is behind a leaded control booth (F).

around the patient in any number of orientations. Patients are typically recumbent on a radiographic table or upright in front of an image receptor. The image receptor may be a computed radiography (CR) cassette or digital flat-panel detector. The radiographer directs the x-ray tube and collimator toward the patient at prescribed distances and angulations according to established departmental procedures.

The new student should be able to identify the generic components of a radiographic system: x-ray tube, collimator assembly, radiographic table, control console, and x-ray tube support (Fig. 8.1).

X-Ray Tube

The **x-ray tube** is the component of the radiographic system that produces the x-rays. It is made of **Pyrex glass** and encased in a sturdy, lead-lined metal housing with large high-voltage electrical cables attached at each end. The x-ray tube's primary components are the **anode** and **cathode** (see Fig. 9.1). A tube stand or **overhead tube crane (OTC)** suspension supports the x-ray tube and allows the radiographer to position it as needed over and around the patient.

Electrical energy is supplied to the x-ray tube through two large electrical cables. By design, x-ray tubes possess electrical polarity in that one side of the tube is positive (anode) and the other negative (cathode). This **diode** polarity is critical to its operation as a large electrical potential is created between its poles during exposure. The potential difference, expressed as kilovoltage peak (kVp), causes the rapidly accelerating electrons to pass through the tube from cathode to anode, creating x-radiation. The tube converts this electrical energy into x-rays and heat in a manner similar to energy conversion in a light bulb.

The cathode filament is typically a tightly wound tungsten wire helix, similar to the filament in an incandescent light bulb. As electrical current passes through the filament wire, its temperature increases to the point of "boiling off" electrons through a process known as *thermionic emission*. At the precise

tube stand - supports the tube

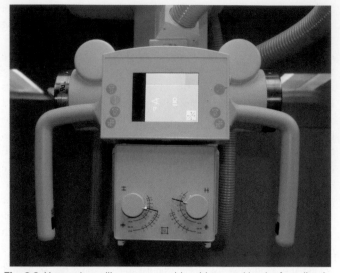

Fig. 8.2 X-ray tube collimator assembly with control knobs for adjusting the dimensions of the x-ray field.

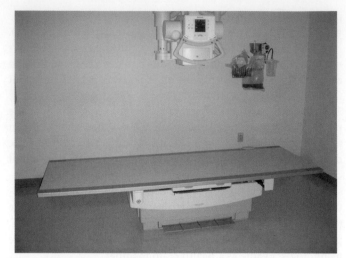

Fig. 8.3 Radiographic system with variable-height radiographic table. The table is in a lowered position.

moment of exposure, a large electrical potential is applied across the dipoles of the x-ray tube, causing the liberated electrons to accelerate at tremendous speed from cathode to anode. As the electrons collide with the positively charged anode, the kinetic energy of the electron stream is converted into heat and x-radiation. In most modern-day x-ray tubes used for medical diagnosis, the anode assembly is a rotating disc of tungsten. Rotating anode tubes, as they are typically called, can withstand huge anode heat buildup and permit high milliamperage exposures with extremely short exposure times that minimize patient motion.

With an x-ray tube, the radiographer controls the number and energy of the x-rays produced by adjusting the amount of electrical energy going into the tube. This adjustment is made at the radiographic system's control console.

Collimator Assembly and Positive Beam Limitation. Attached directly below the x-ray tube is an x-ray beam–limiting device called a collimator (Fig. 8.2). The collimator controls the size and shape of the x-ray field coming out of the x-ray tube. The radiographer determines the size of the rectangular x-ray field by adjusting two controls on the front or sides of the collimator, one for length and one for width.

Manipulation of the collimator blades is inherent in every radiographic procedure and becomes second nature. The process of "coning down," as it is commonly called, implies increased collimation and a smaller x-ray field size. In addition, a retractable tape measure for measuring the source-image distance (SID) is conveniently built into the collimator cover, as is a tube-head angulation scale (goniometer).

Engineered into the collimator assembly is a high-intensity light bulb with a mirror. Turning the light field on involves a simple push of a button, which projects a light field onto the patient, and this illuminated area is representative of the x-ray field's exposure area. Keep in mind that this is a high-intensity bulb that can become very hot to the touch. Manufacturers have protected such bulbs in heat shrouds, and the light turns off after a preset time

interval. Newer collimator designs are now using light-emitting diodes (LEDs) instead, which last much longer and do not get hot. Equipment designers have placed a Plexiglas "shadow shield" on the underside of the collimator to project a shadow of crosshairs marking the beam's central point. In some cases additional shadow lines that indicate the position of exposure detectors, known as *automatic exposure controls* (AECs), will also have been added.

Most x-ray machines are equipped with an automatic collimation system that performs positive beam limitation (PBL). This feature allows the x-ray unit to detect the size of the image receptor the radiographer is using and automatically collimates to a size not larger than the image receptor. Federal law no longer requires a PBL system, but permitting the x-ray beam to expose patient tissue larger than the image receptor is poor professional practice and a violation of ethical practice standards. In systems with flat-panel digital radiography (DR) detectors, often the collimation assembly is manually controlled without a PBL. A good radiographer is diligent in the use of proper collimation and is respected by colleagues.

Newer collimation designs are using a sensing mechanism to ensure a proper perpendicular relationship between the x-ray beam's central ray (CR) and the radiographic grid; this is particularly challenging with the use of portable radiography. To avoid undesirable grid cutoff in these situations, it is important that the x-ray beam and grid be in the correct orientation. This new technology has integrated sensors on a grid encasement that encloses the receptor; when the CR and grid are orthogonal to each other, indicators ensuring correct alignment are displayed.

Radiographic Table. The radiographic/x-ray table is the most obvious and recognizable component of the radiographic system. The size, shape, and location of the table controls vary among manufacturers. X-ray tables are classified as tilting or nontilting, having a free-floating or stationary tabletop, and having adjustable or nonadjustable height. Adjustable-height tables permit lowering of the tabletop to a comfortable and safe height, enabling patients to get on and off the table more easily (Fig. 8.3). To permit an x-ray exposure, typically the table must be raised to a working height. Care must be taken in lowering a

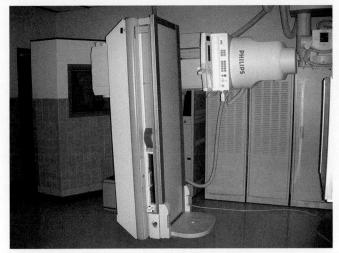

Fig. 8.4 Tilting tabletop in the upright (vertical) position. Note the attached footboard.

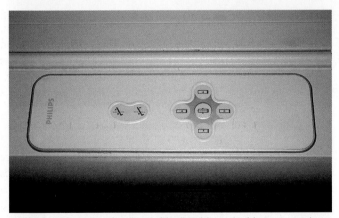

Fig. 8.5 Closeup of radiographic tilt table and tabletop controls.

table to make sure that nothing is under the top as it descends. Many a technologist has caused tabletop damage through inattentiveness, costing the employer thousands of dollars in repairs. In addition, care must be taken in cleaning tabletops, and only approved nonabrasive cleansers should be used.

Tilting tables are available in basically two types. A 90-90 table can tilt from the horizontal position to a complete vertical position in either direction. A 90-45 table can tilt to a complete vertical position in one direction and to a 45-degree tilt in the other direction. A footboard for patient safety is usually attached to a tilting tabletop. A tabletop in the upright position with a footboard attached is shown in Fig. 8.4. Table tilt is controlled by a switch located at table or floor level on the long side of the table. Depressing the switch tilts the table to a desired degree. Both tilting and nontilting tables may have additional features, including a moving tabletop, a receptor or cassette tray (often called a *Bucky tray*), and controls for tabletop movement and tilt (Fig. 8.5).

X-ray tabletops are **radiolucent** and movable in any combination of two directions. These movable tabletops may be motorized or free-floating and permit the radiographer to move the tabletop rather than the patient. Floating tabletops have a switch that controls an electrical locking mechanism. If the

locking mechanism is deactivated, the radiographer can move the top manually in any combination of motions including diagonal or circular ones. Motorized tops have switches that drive the tabletop in the direction desired. The controls for the tabletop or table tilt are usually located at the end or center of the working side of the x-ray table. The **Bucky mechanism** is located directly beneath the tabletop and is designed to hold the image receptor stationary during the x-ray exposure and to keep it centered to the x-ray beam's central ray. It also serves as the holder for the radiographic grid, which moves back and forth during an exposure and is positioned underneath the tabletop, creating a top to the Bucky tray when it is pushed completely into the table (Fig. 8.6). The tray is pulled out from the table, and the cassette is placed in the tray and locked into place. The Bucky mechanism can be manually moved the entire length of the table and then locked into place. Newer digital detector systems have replaced the cassette tray, and some designs even permit cross-table lateral imaging by swinging the detector up into a vertical position, adjacent to the lateral edge of the table (Fig. 8.7). A beginning radiographer should take time to practice operating the various x-ray tables and Bucky trays before attempting to position patients.

Control Console. The x-ray generator is the workhorse of the total system. It consists of two main components: an electronics cabinet and operator console. The power of an x-ray system is rated in kilowatts and expressed numerically, typically ranging from 30 to 100 kW. To the radiographer, the console is the electrical interface between the operator and the equipment. Generator console designs vary but all have some key features (Fig. 8.8). All systems will allow the radiographer to turn the system on and off, select the x-ray exposure factors, initiate and terminate the exposure, and provide an audible and visual indication of x-ray exposure.

The console has five generic controls that the new student must learn: the main power, kilovolt peak (kVp), milliamperage (mA), timer, and x-ray tube rotor-exposure switch. The selection of kVp, mA, and time is collectively referred to as *technique selection*. On many units, mA and time are combined into a factor known as *milliampere-seconds* (mAs), which is simply mA multiplied by time in seconds (s). Additional controls typically include selections for anatomic body parts, AEC, receptor exposure, and x-ray tube focal spot size.

Power. The main power switch supplies power to the radiographic system. Turning the power on does not activate x-ray production. The power device should be clearly marked on the control console and is usually either a switch or a pushbutton device. Some x-ray units require power to be activated both at the control console and at a main power box equipped with a high-voltage circuit breaker.

Kilovoltage Peak. The penetration power of an x-ray beam is determined by its voltage and is expressed as kVp. As kVp increases, so does penetration; 1000 volts (V) of electrical power equal 1 kV, and the kilovoltages in radiography can range from 30 to 150 kVp. The kVp is user selectable and digitally displayed

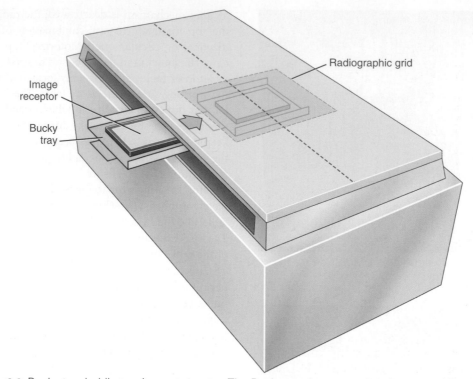

Fig. 8.6 Bucky tray holding an image receptor. The Bucky tray is centered to the x-ray table underneath a radiographic grid.

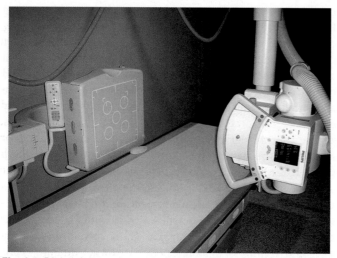

Fig. 8.7 Digital detector in cross-table lateral position centered to x-ray tube.

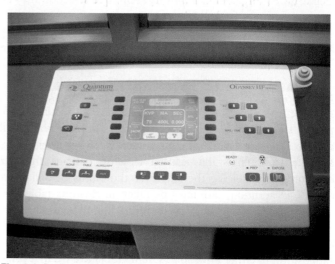

Fig. 8.8 Radiographic generator operator's control. Exposure controls are convenient pushbuttons with visual display of selected exposure factors. In this version, exposures may be made using prep and expose buttons or a two-position switch firmly attached to the control (*upper right corner*).

on the control console (Fig. 8.9). The correct kVp can vary based on patient thickness, body part, and examination type, and increasing or decreasing the kVp can be as simple as holding the kVp selection up or down or entering a numeric value on a keypad. The correct combination of mAs and kVp ensures the lowest patient dose and highest image quality, particularly with digital image detectors.

Milliampere-Seconds. One milliampere is equal to one thousandth of an ampere (A). The milliamperage indicates the amount of current supplied to the x-ray tube. With most pieces of radiographic equipment, the radiographer can select the mA

setting and the exposure time separately or can select the total mAs. On control consoles the mA setting generally ranges from 50 to 1000 mA and is selectable in increments of 100 (i.e., 200, 300, 400 mA) up to the maximum value. Most routine diagnostic radiography is done at 50 to 400 mA.

Just as with a digital camera, picture quality is determined by the amount of time during which the camera allows light into the detector. This is often controlled electronically, and the user gives it no thought when taking photographs. Similarly, radiography requires an x-ray exposure time that will be automatically

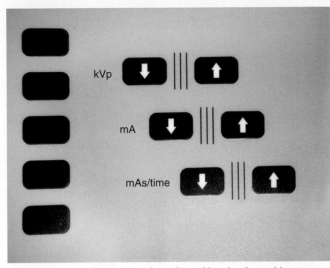

Fig. 8.9 Exposure factors may be selected by simple pushbutton operation. This control permits independent control of milliamperage (mA), kilovolt peak (kVp), exposure time, and exposure milliampere-seconds (mAs).

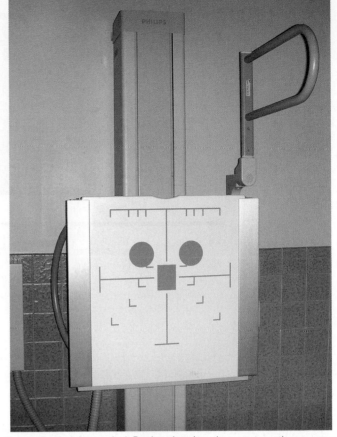

Fig. 8.10 Upright vertical Bucky showing three automatic exposure control (AEC) detector chamber positions. Detectors may be selected separately, in tandem, or as a triad.

terminated. Time is expressed in seconds and commonly in fractions of seconds or milliseconds (the latter is 1/1000 second). The timing of an exposure is initiated by the operator, and the duration of the exposure is controlled by a sophisticated electronic timing circuit. Exposure technique selection may be done in the mAs mode or time mode. When the mAs mode is selected, the generator is programmed to use the highest allowable milliamperage to achieve the shortest exposure time. In select cases the time mode is used for breathing studies.

When the mA is multiplied by the total exposure time(s), the total quantity of x-ray exposure or mAs is the result. This mAs value directly affects the amount of x-ray exposure of the patient and ultimately the image receptor. Most generators will calculate mAs and display it. *The radiographer still must understand the mAs calculation and what it means in terms of patient exposure and image quality.*

Example
300 mA × 0.020 s = 6 mAs

Exposure. After the x-ray exposure factors have been selected and the patient, x-ray tube, and other equipment for the examination have been properly prepared, an exposure can be made. The device that begins the exposure is called the *rotor-exposure switch*. It may be a pushbutton or trigger-type switch that is part of the control console. The rotor-exposure switch actually contains two different switches that are mechanically interlocked so that one must be activated before the other. The first switch that is activated is the rotor, or *prep*, switch. The rotor switch causes the anode to rotate and prepares the x-ray tube for the selected exposure factors. The preparation process usually takes 1 to 2 seconds. After the tube has been properly prepared, the second switch is activated to begin the exposure. A sophisticated electronic timer automatically ends the exposure. According to federal regulations, termination of the exposure must be indicated both audibly and visually.

The duration of an x-ray exposure may be established manually or automatically. Manual exposures are typically used with *tabletop* procedures such as extremity examinations, cross-table radiography, examination of patients on carts or in wheelchairs, and examinations of small infants. The length of the exposure is a function of the total mAs chosen and the amount selected. Generally the shortest exposure time possible is used to minimize motion on images. For many procedures, exposures are terminated using AEC circuitry. The technology of AEC has simplified exposure technique selection and improves the consistency of image quality. Using AEC requires that the selected anatomy be correctly positioned over the AEC detectors to achieve optimum image quality at the lowest patient dose. Most AEC systems use three solid-state detectors, with each detector activated separately or in any combination (Fig. 8.10). The radiographer will position patients properly using AEC technology and select the correct combination of detectors for a given examination. As more generators are integrated with DR technology, exposure technique selection is now done by way of a computer interface through the DR software. The basic principles of technique calculation and selection still apply, however. mAs controls total x-ray beam quantity, and kVp controls x-ray beam quality.

It is important to understand what is occurring when the x-ray tube is "prepped." The anode begins to spin at a high rate,

center anatomy of interest to photocell

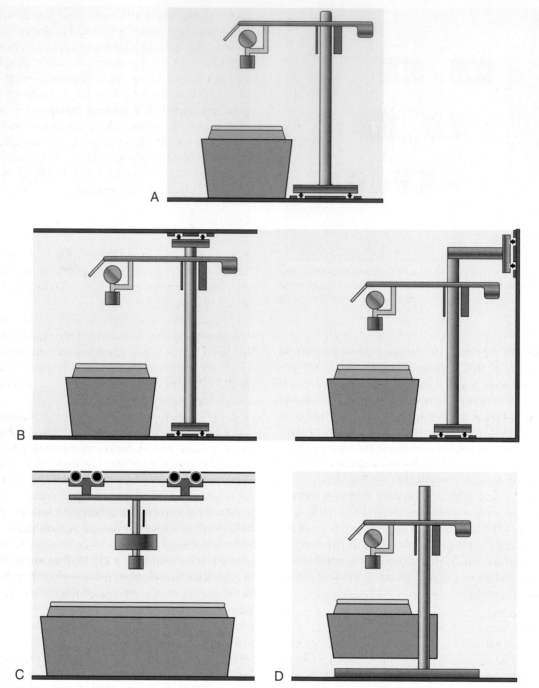

Fig. 8.11 X-ray tube support systems come in two basic designs: floor-mounted tube stands (A, B, and D) and ceiling-suspended tube crane systems (C).

and the cathode filament heats up to its selected mA. During the second step of the exposure sequence, a large potential difference (kVp) is applied across both electrical poles of the x-ray tube, causing electrons to travel from the cathode to the anode at high speed, producing x-radiation. Repeatedly prepping the tube unnecessarily can damage the x-ray tube and shorten its useful life. The radiographer clearly needs to understand proper exposure control operations and use extended "anode prep" times *only* when clinically appropriate. Much like a car has its own normal sounds of operation, x-ray units do also, and it is important to pay attention to unusual sounds and report them to appropriate personnel.

X-Ray Tube Support Designs

X-ray tube support systems come in two distinct designs: floor-mounted tube stands (Fig. 8.11A, B, and D) and ceiling-suspended OTCs (see Fig. 8.11C). Both designs are intended to permit easy, flexible positioning of the x-ray tube toward the patient. Tube-stand systems are typically found in clinic settings and consist of a vertical column that runs along a longitudinal rail mounted to the floor. The length of longitudinal travel is determined by the rail length. In addition, these systems permit some limited transverse travel across the patient, vertical travel, and x-ray **tube angulation**. Some designs allow for tube-stand rotation around a vertical axis, permitting cross-table exposures

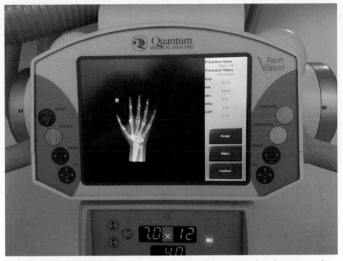

Fig. 8.12 Overhead tube crane controls demonstrating image review for assessment. Exposure conditions can also be set from the tube crane controls on a different display. (Courtesy of Shimadzu Europa.)

and extended x-ray tube vertical travel to about 10 to 12 inches above the floor. With proper applications training, these systems afford nearly complete x-ray tube positioning, similar to an overhead suspension system at considerably less cost. Their key limitation involves the radiography of patients on carts.

OTC systems are the most sophisticated type and the standard of care in hospitals and large clinics. As one might expect, they are more costly to purchase and install, as the x-ray room must have a rigid rail system in the ceiling to attach the overhead x-ray tube suspension. The versatility of x-ray tube positioning is unmatched in an OTC system and permits all radiographic projections of even the most complex angulations on patients who are recumbent, on a cart, in a wheelchair, or standing. Manufacturers have gone to considerable lengths to make these systems lightweight and aesthetically pleasing, ergonomically friendly, and solid in design and functionality. The newer OTC designs now include the capability to set exposure factors at the tube head as well as to review the completed digital images (Fig. 8.12). This is particularly valuable in trauma cases, where time and efficiency are critical. Performing the radiographic exposure must still be done behind the control booth, however. A competent radiographer will quickly become familiar with OTC features and movements, much like getting to know the inside of a favorite automobile. Deliberate, efficient movement of the x-ray tube-head assembly is the mark of a good radiographer and does not go unnoticed by coworkers.

Controls for Tube Movement

Most x-ray tube heads have a set of handles located between the x-ray tube and the collimator. The radiographer grips these handles and releases the appropriate locks to move the x-ray tube in the direction desired. For the longitudinal, transverse, vertical, and tube angulation movements, a corresponding switch is located between or on the handlebars; each switch locks or unlocks the corresponding movement. For example, if the radiographic system is energized and all the tube movement switches are in the locked position, the tube cannot be moved. If the vertical switch is moved to the unlocked position, the tube

can be moved toward the ceiling or the floor. Locks for each of the tube movements are controlled independently, allowing the operator to make adjustments in one plane at a time. Some units also have a single switch that takes all the locks off. It is extremely important not to force the movement of the tube with the locks on. If the tube does not move easily, the proper lock must be released. A beginning radiographer should get a feel for x-ray tube movement by practicing moving, aligning, and locking the tube before attempting any radiographic procedure. Patients may quickly lose confidence in a student's abilities if they observe that he or she has difficulty in handling a simple task such as moving the x-ray tube.

Wall-Mounted Bucky Systems and Cassette Holders

Many radiographic rooms have an upright holder that allows the technologist to obtain radiographs of standing patients. The two primary devices are a simple wall-mounted cassette holder and a wall-mounted Bucky system.

A simple wall-mounted cassette holder is a mechanical device that allows the radiographer to place a cassette in an adjustable holder. The cassette holder mechanism is attached to a two-rail system that permits the cassette to move up and down. A locking mechanism controlled by a knob secures the cassette at the appropriate height.

A wall-mounted Bucky unit is commonly found in hospitals and clinics and is supported by a vertical column attached to the floor and wall. It has a surface similar to a tabletop with the Bucky tray mechanism just under the surface. The tray is manually pulled out, and the receptor is placed in the tray and locked into place. The entire Bucky mechanism can be manually moved after release of a locking mechanism that permits the radiographer to move it along a vertical plane. A control knob or lever operates an electrical locking mechanism that permits vertical movement (Fig. 8.13). Wall-mounted Bucky units typically permit only vertical movement, although some units can be tilted into a horizontal position for radiography of the head and extremities.

Alignment Concepts

The major responsibility of the radiographer is proper manipulation of the various components of the radiographic system to provide a high-quality image or radiograph of the anatomic area of interest. This task is accomplished by proper alignment of the various components of the radiographic system to the anatomic area of interest. Equipment manufacturers have gone to great lengths to make their products intuitive and user-friendly. Controls and features have been strategically positioned to eliminate ergonomic injuries and enable fast and efficient operation. Newer systems now offer an autotracking feature that synchronizes the upright Bucky and vertical movement of the overhead x-ray tube. It is the radiographer's responsibility to become proficient with equipment features. Among these challenges is the efficient alignment of the patient's anatomy to the x-ray tube and image receptor. All designs provide predetermined locking positions (détentes) for the x-ray tube, table, and upright wall holder. These détentes are unique to each room layout and are set up by the service engineers during room installation.

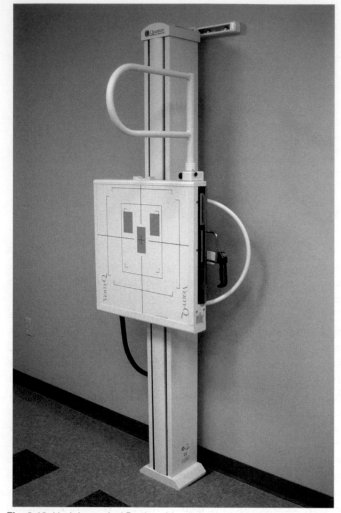

Fig. 8.13 Upright vertical Bucky with a "pistol-grip" locking mechanism.

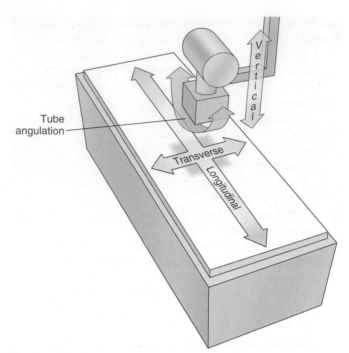

Fig. 8.14 The basic movements of a typical diagnostic radiographic tube: longitudinal, transverse, vertical, rotational, and tube angulation.

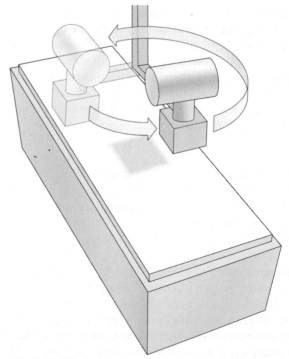

Fig. 8.15 Tube rotation around the vertical tube column.

An effective method for proper alignment is to bring the x-ray tube into the locked position with the longitudinal and transverse axis of the receptor (Fig. 8.14). The x-ray tube and receptor are now aligned and centered to each other. The patient can now be positioned properly in the center of the x-ray field using a four-way floating tabletop. This minimizes patient movement and shifting and provides for a quicker, safer examination. It is important to set up the room equipment before escorting the patient into the room. Fine-tuning of the equipment is done with the patient in the final position before exposure. An additional set of tube movements provides rotation around the vertical axis, permitting convenient cross-table lateral imaging (Fig. 8.15). Please remember that this equipment can be very intimidating to patients, particularly children. Minimizing equipment motion in front of the patient eases patient apprehensions and makes the procedure move more quickly, presenting a more professional image.

IMAGE RECEPTOR SYSTEMS

An x-ray beam comprises a countless variety of electromagnetic energies. The photons or *quanta* that make up the beam have both electrical and magnetic properties but no mass or charge. The purpose of an image receptor is to absorb the energies of the x-ray beam and convert this energy into a form that can be stored, processed, and ultimately viewed by someone for medical interpretation. Historically, the medium of choice for recording this x-ray energy was a polyester film sandwiched between two intensifying screens in a light-tight cassette. This screen-film (analogue) combination was the gold standard for medical imaging for over 60 years. With the advent of microprocessor technology and computers, analogue imaging has been replaced by **digital imaging** technologies. Regardless of the receptor technology, the basic principles of radiation exposure still apply, and professional radiographers are obligated to practice the ALARA principle—*as low as reasonably achievable.* Overexposure that is 100% above the optimal exposure should be considered an ALARA violation. Underexposed images will result in *noisy* or grainy images, and overexposure will produce images with low contrast.

Image receptors are classified as either cassette-less or cassette-based. Cassette-less systems are true digital receptors their technology for converting the energy of the x-ray beam to a digital computer signal is either direct or indirect. Cassette-based systems employ a photostimulable storage phosphor (PSP) screen in a light-tight cassette. Referred to as *CR,* the technology of PSP plates affords an economical transition toward digital imaging technology.

All radiation detected by the receptor is referred to as **remnant radiation** and consists of primary beam radiation, scatter, and secondary radiation. It is important to remember that *the only radiation that is of clinical value to us in medicine is radiation that is absorbed by the detector material.* With CR and DR technologies, the energy of the beam is captured by a detector material, converted to electrons as an analog signal, which is the **latent image,** and then changed into a digital signal through computer software and an analog-to-digital (A/D) converter. Computers handle only digital signals and therefore require this A/D conversion. The data set is now applied to any number of computer programs (algorithms), and for analysis the resultant image is displayed on a viewing monitor (**soft copy**) and/or printed to laser film (**hard copy**). Present-day systems use very little laser film for printing, because most digital images are sent by way of a computer network to be archived in a sophisticated **picture archival communication system (PACS)** or copied to a digital video disk (DVD) or compact disk (CD) for storage and transport.

Photostimulable Phosphor Technology PSP

Commonly referred to as *CR,* PSP imaging uses a reusable imaging plate that is flexible and coated with an alkali-earth halide material. The imaging plate is enclosed in a light-tight cassette. PSP detectors capture the energy of the remnant beam and store it for a period in electron traps. These electron traps represent the latent image. The cassette with plate is then inserted into a sophisticated reader device, which opens the cassette, removes the PSP plate, and scans the plate with a precise low-energy laser beam. The laser light energy stimulates the stored energy in the PSP material, typically a barium fluorohalide, and forces the fluorescent emission of light energy from these atomic stored energy electron traps. This stimulated, fluorescent light makes up the signal from the PSP plate. Signal strength is directly proportional to the x-ray energy that created it and represents radiation exposure to the plate. The light is gathered up by a light guide assembly and directed into a photomultiplier tube device for signal amplification. This stronger electrical signal runs through an A/D conversion and is sent to a computer for analysis and image processing.

After the plate has been scanned by the laser beam, remaining electron traps must be atomically cleared by passing in front of an intense white light source, a process known as *conditioning.* The erased PSP plate is then reinserted into a cassette for reuse. CR plates and PSP technology offer an economical transition to digital

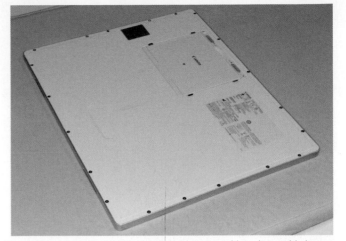

Fig. 8.16 A wireless digital radiography detector with rechargeable battery.

imaging but are becoming less attractive owing to changing medical insurance reimbursements for this type of medical imaging.

CR plates have some interesting characteristics, of which the radiographer who uses them routinely must be aware. After exposure to radiation, the plate is very sensitive to additional exposure, particularly low-energy x-rays. In addition, the plate will begin to lose its stored energy after exposure and should be placed in the reader in a timely fashion. Image fading can occur as fast as 10 minutes after exposure. Within 8 hours of exposure, the plate may lose as much as 25% of its original signal, resulting in suboptimal image quality. If a plate has not been processed within 24 hours of exposure, it should not be considered suitable for clinical use and should be erased. Proper placement of the anatomy on the receptor and symmetric beam collimation are critical to creating a good image. Finally, the best spatial resolution with CR receptors is achieved with smaller receptors. The difference in resolution can be as much as two line pairs per millimeter (lp/mm) between cassette sizes.

Digital Radiography Technology

True DR receptors fall into one of two categories: direct or indirect. Often called **flat-panel detectors,** both use thin-film transistor (TFT) technology for electronic readout of the signal created from x-ray exposure. Unlike CR technology, no reader is required and conditioning of the receptor is unnecessary. The greatest advantages of DR technology are its lower dose, quicker image presentation, and better spatial resolution. DR receptors are typically more expensive by comparison and sensitive to mechanical abuse such as dropping the DR cassette or fluids getting into the DR circuitry. Special care must be taken by the radiographer to ensure that DR plates are protected from abuse and inattentive handling, including fluids. Many departments routinely wrap DR panels in plastic bags to prevent fluid invasion and for improved patient hygiene.

DR detectors require the application of electricity in preparation for an x-ray exposure. To achieve this, manufacturers have designed DR panels that are electrically connected to a power source through a flexible cable (**tether**) or rechargeable battery pack (Fig. 8.16). Often, battery-powered panels are provided with extra batteries in a charging station, sometime referred to as a "toaster" (Fig. 8.17). In using these panels, it is critical that

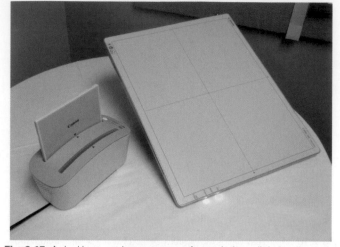

Fig. 8.17 A dual battery charger system for a wireless digital radiography detector.

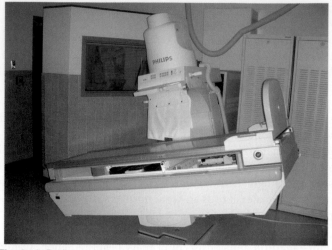

Fig. 8.18 Radiographic and fluoroscopic unit in Trendelenburg tilt position. Note the fluoroscopic tower with large field-of-view image intensifier, permitting larger fluoroscopic coverage.

the battery strength be checked regularly and before each use. Naturally if it is low, a replacement battery should be inserted.

Additionally, DR detectors require a connection between the panel and a computer for image reconstruction and processing. This is achieved either through the tether or in a newer system, whereby a wireless radiofrequency (RF) transmitter connects to the computer using RF technology. This technology is increasingly popular with technologists for its convenience and positioning flexibility. As your radiography career grows, these DR detectors will be increasingly likely to be wireless, lighter in weight, and more durable.

Direct DR detectors use the semiconductor material amorphous selenium (a-Se) as the detector material. The energy of the x-ray beam is captured by this material and is *directly converted* into an electronic digital signal to be used by the computer. A-Se offers excellent x-ray photon capture efficiency and outstanding spatial resolution.

Indirect DR detectors work a bit differently and use the semiconductor amorphous silicon (a-Si) as the material of choice. a-Si cannot convert the direct action of the x-ray beam and relies on a scintillator such as cesium iodide or gadolinium to capture the energy of the x-ray beam. The scintillator material emits light on x-ray stimulation, and this light is then captured by the a-Si to convert to electrons and then to a digital signal. The fact that an intermediate step is used for this type of x-ray energy conversion makes the process that of an indirect digital detector, and thus its classification. Indirect DR is more popular in the marketplace for various reasons, such as cost, stability, and manufacturing consistency; it is the technology of choice for flat-panel fluoroscopy, which has replaced the traditional image intensifier tube.

MANIPULATION OF FLUOROSCOPIC EQUIPMENT

The largest number of images one creates as a radiographer most likely will be static images of patients. Remember, each of these images reflects the patient's anatomy at that moment in time and, when interpreted in a timely fashion, should accurately portray

the patient's condition. For study of the dynamic action of the human body, **real-time images** are created, showing internal activities and processes. Known as **fluoroscopy,** this method is used to create images that are continuous and demonstrate vital processes such as gastrointestinal (GI) movement and structure, blood vessels, genitourinary functionality, and joint mobility, among others. As the technology of interventional medicine progresses, fluoroscopy is increasingly being used for the placement of tubes, catheters, and vascular lines. Traditional fluoroscopic studies such as stomach (upper GI) and colon (lower GI) examinations are decreasing, being replaced by CT and MRI studies, whereas interventional fluoroscopic studies are on the increase. There is no reason to expect this trend to change; as a result, the role of the fluoroscopic technologist continues to evolve. The basic design of fluoroscopic equipment, however, has not changed significantly. This equipment consists of a fluoroscopic image receptor (image intensifier or flat-panel fluoroscopic detector) and separate fluoroscopic x-ray tube.

Commonly referred to as *R/F systems,* fluoroscopic equipment is available in two different designs: the fluoroscopic x-ray tube above the patient or below the patient. With the fluoro tube below the patient, the detector is orthogonally fixed above the patient (Figs. 8.18 and 8.19) This design has been popular for many years and looks very similar to radiographic units, with the addition of a **fluoroscope** in a tower on the back of the table (see Fig. 8.18). The tower consists of a sophisticated image intensifier tube or digital detector (see Fig. 8.19) attached to a carriage platform. During fluoroscopy the fluoroscopic tower is locked into position with the fluoroscopic x-ray tube so that both are centered to each other. The image receptor is considered a **primary barrier** to the x-ray beam, and fluoroscopic exposures are allowed only when the fluoroscopic x-ray tube and image receptor are locked in place and centered. Generally the fluoroscopic tower and tube are positioned over the patient in a vertical orientation and the patient is rotated within this vertical image plane. At the conclusion of fluoroscopy, the image receptor assembly is pushed toward the back of the table and locked into the park position.

radiation comes up from tube (under table) to intensifier

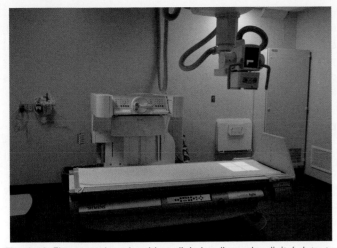

Fig. 8.19 Fluoroscopic unit with a digital radiography digital detector used for fluoroscopy. Note the replacement of an image intensifier with a large-area digital fluoroscopic flat-panel detector.

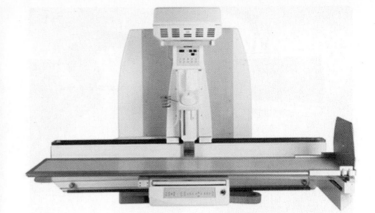

Fig. 8.21 A single-panel digital radiographic/fluoroscopic system design with the x-ray tube above the patient for fluoroscopy. Many of these designs now offer a height-adjustable table for patient convenience (http://www3.gehealthcare.co.uk/en-gb/products/categories/radiography_and_fluoroscopy/connexity#.)

R/F = Radiographic/Fluro

An alternative R/F system design positions the x-ray tube above the patient and fluoroscopic detector below (Fig. 8.21). A principal advantage to this approach is that a single detector can perform both fluoroscopic and static imaging. These systems provide a variable SID from 40 to 72 in and many of the fluoroscopic and radiographic controls can be operated remotely, behind a control booth or using a mobile pedestal control in the exam room (see Fig. 8.21). The expandable SID permits improved image resolution and a lower patient skin dose during fluoroscopy. An important consideration, however, is that with this design, the scatter radiation coming from the patient during fluoroscopy is more intense at the waist level and above. Because of this, persons standing next to the patient during fluoroscopy should be aware of exposure to their necks and eyes particularly and use appropriate lead protection.

R/F tables are capable of various degrees of tilt ranging from 90 degrees vertical to 15 to 90 degrees of **Trendelenburg tilt**. Most have at least a 90/15 tilt range, with controls located tableside or with a floor switch. Tilting is motor driven and activated only while the control is pushed. Often, tilt tables come with an attachable foot board and in some cases shoulder restraints for extreme Trendelenburg tilt angles. Additionally, newer systems offer an adjustable, variable-height table to accommodate patients who have difficulty stepping up. Easing patient anxieties during height adjustment and table-tilt movements is the mark of a good radiographer and is best accomplished by *simple communication with the patient.*

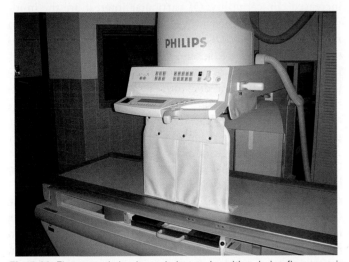

Fig. 8.20 Fluoroscopic lead curtain in usual position during fluoroscopic study.

The development of digital detector technology has replaced the conventional image intensifier tube for fluoroscopic imaging. Image intensifiers have historically been known for image quality drawbacks, such as blooming, peripheral fall-off, and higher dose in the magnification modes of operation. Flat-panel fluoroscopic detectors do not have these weaknesses, and newer systems now place a sophisticated digital a-Si flat-panel detector in a fluoroscopic carriage above the patient, replacing the conventional "tower" design (see Fig. 8.19). These new detectors have outstanding image quality characteristics that make them clinically very desirable by radiologists and interventionalists. Hanging from the front of the fluoroscopic carriage is a removable lead apron or *fluoroscopic drape* (Fig. 8.20). This is an extremely effective barrier for reducing radiation exposure to the radiologist and technologist during procedures and *should remain in position during fluoroscopy* unless the clinician requests its removal to improve the success of the examination. It is good practice to reattach the fluoroscopic drape after the procedure in preparation for the next examination.

Some designs have attached the image receptor and fluoroscopic tube on a C-arm support, permitting angulation around the patient instead of moving the patient (Fig. 8.22). This is particularly useful for sophisticated interventional procedures. Regardless of the design, the principles of fluoroscopy remain the same. The patient is positioned between a fluoroscopic x-ray tube and image receptor, and live, dynamic images are viewed and recorded to assess the patient's function and structure. The competent imaging professional will thoroughly understand the unique features of an R/F system design, particularly with regard to clinical use and radiation exposure to staff.

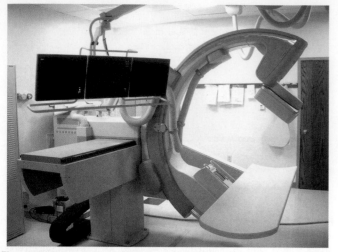

Fig. 8.22 Interventional fluoroscopic system illustrating the C-arm design with flat-panel digital detector technology.

During fluoroscopy, images are viewed in the examination room on a flat-screen television monitor that is hanging from the ceiling or on a mobile floor stand. All R/F systems provide a last image hold (LIH) function, which *freezes* the last video image on the monitor for detailed study by the viewer. Please note that this is a stored image and not a live image, and therefore no additional dose is administered to the patient. At the conclusion of the examination, all stored images should be erased from the viewing monitor to protect patient privacy and comply with Health Insurance Portability and Accountability Act (HIPAA) regulations.

Recording images during fluoroscopy is done electronically though digital recorders, and no cassettes are required. Current digital technology enables the operator to record fluoroscopic images, as well as the images taken during the **spot image** mode. Fluoroscopic images are recorded at a much lower patient dose than with spot images. The compromise with dose reduction is always image quality, and fluoroscopic images are typically more grainy or *noisy* than digital spot images. Manufacturers have added features such as LIH, dose modulation, spatial frequency processing, pulsed fluoroscopy, and electronic shuttering in an effort to reduce patient dose. However, the choice between fluoroscopic and spot imaging is made by the clinician based on diagnostic yield and dose.

Digital spot images are taken at a higher dose, yielding better image quality. Image acquisition can involve single on-demand images as well as series images at rates of 1 to 15 frames per second (fps). Images are stored and may be manipulated in a computer system, allowing the operator to enhance their appearance and clinical value. Radiographers need to become proficient in these **postprocessing** functions, which can include operations such as image reversal, image annotation, spatial filtering (edge enhancement), magnification, and windowing of brightness and contrast (level and width), among others.

Images taken during fluoroscopic procedures are enhanced by the radiographer for optimum clinical value and electronically sent to a PACS for long-term storage and physician viewing. The PACS is a complex computer network that is typically part of a larger hospital information system (HIS). Hospitals are now filmless, and all images are recorded electronically by digital imaging technology. Images are acquired, enhanced, stored, and viewed by way of this PACS network and communicated worldwide, if necessary, for consultations and completeness of patient care. Becoming proficient with PACS technology is important to the radiographer's success.

FUTURE DIGITAL TECHNOLOGIES

As digital receptors improve, we can expect improved spatial resolution and reduced patient doses. In addition, vendor software developments will enhance system functionality and ease of use with intuitive user interfaces, miniaturizing of components, and higher throughput. Occurring simultaneously will be the inherent increase of computer network transmission speeds and computer capacity. This technologic trend has been in place for over 20 years and will continue.

The development of DR detectors has opened the door for increased clinical utility. Of particular interest are the innovations of digital tomosynthesis and dual-energy subtraction radiography. Because DR detectors can acquire an x-ray exposure and convert it to digital data so quickly, it now becomes possible to perform rapid exposures back to back in just a matter of milliseconds. *The diagnostic yield of these two advancements will no doubt have a profound impact on the practice of radiography.*

Tomosynthesis

One of the greatest challenges for a radiologist is to visualize human anatomy in a three-dimensional fashion with a two-dimensional radiograph. This two-dimensional image naturally creates superimposition of anatomic structures. Along with this is the simple fact that a radiograph is a single view of the patient. Many procedures require at least two perpendicular views of patient anatomy to give the viewer a depth perspective. CT scanners acquire hundreds of views of patient anatomy as they rotate around the patient during a CT acquisition. Each of these views is sent to a computer for analysis, and challenges of superimposition of anatomy are no longer an issue. Tomosynthesis is a radiographic procedure that acquires as many as 60 low-dose projection images during a single x-ray tube–detector sweep of the patient and with a single breath-hold. These 60 images are then sent to a computer workstation for analysis. To the radiologist, the multiple views of the patient's anatomy are much like those of CT scan, with a significantly lower dose and cost, and small pathologic findings can become more visible. This technology holds tremendous potential for chest lesions and breast disease. Without DR detector technology, tomosynthesis would not be possible (Fig. 8.23).

Dual-Energy Subtraction Radiography

DR detectors working with high-frequency x-ray generators permit rapid switching of kVp values in only a few milliseconds. This feature permits two exposures to be taken of a patient's anatomy, one at a very low kVp and the other at a higher kVp. The degree of differential absorption is markedly different between the two exposures. The lower kVp exposure

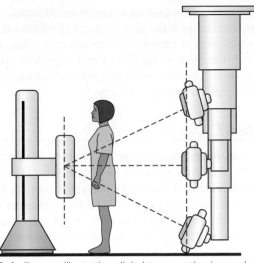

Fig. 8.23 A diagram illustrating digital tomosynthesis employing digital detector technology to achieve multiple views of patient anatomy during image acquisition.

will allow better visualization of calcifications. The higher kVp exposure penetrates dense patient anatomy more uniformly and demonstrates soft tissue structures. When the two different data sets are compared through computer analysis, the two images are subtracted and the net result is the visualization of calcified anatomy, particularly pulmonary nodules. The presence of calcium deposits in pathologic processes aids greatly in the characterization of the pathology. DR detectors that can acquire two images quickly, in a matter of a few milliseconds, have also enabled this exciting new technology.

MANIPULATION OF MOBILE EQUIPMENT

Performing mobile radiography is commonplace in radiology departments. Not all patients can travel to the radiology department, and in many cases radiography is required in locations such as the emergency department, surgery suite, or intensive care unit. Numerous types of mobile units are available in both radiographic and fluoroscopic modes (Fig. 8.24). The systems are similar to fixed units in the department except for the feature of mobility and the fact that in mobile radiographic units the exposure control is at the end of a coiled wire so as to maximize distance from the patient during exposure. Mobile units may be motor-driven for travel convenience, but the other equipment motions are manual.

As use of interventional radiologic procedures increases, an increasing number of fluoroscopic procedures are being performed in the surgical suite. Portable fluoroscopy is accomplished through the use of a mobile C-arm design (see Fig. 8.24B) and consists of a fluoroscopic x-ray tube and image receptor assembly centered to each other. Most designs now use a flat-panel digital fluoroscopic detector, which has reduced the weight and size of the C-arm designs. The inherent strengths of flat-panel fluoroscopy, as previously discussed, make portable C-arms popular for interventional procedures such as pain management, orthopedic surgeries, vascular line placements, and so on (Fig. 8.25).

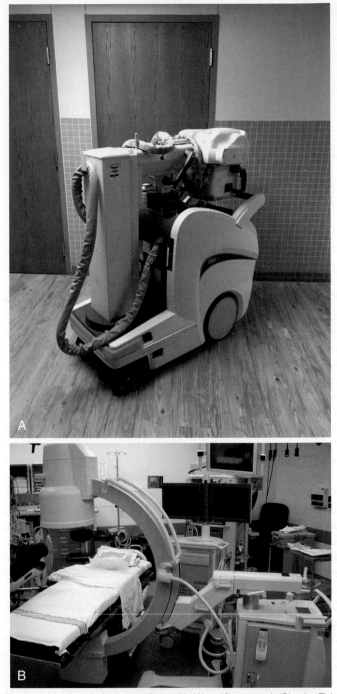

Fig. 8.24 Mobile units include radiographic (A) and fluoroscopic (B) units. This radiographic unit has a collapsible vertical column for safer operator mobility. (Source:http://medicaldealer.com/carestream-drx-revolution-portable-x-ray.)

Modern mobile C-arm systems consist of the C-arm assembly and a video monitor cart for image display. The monitor cart also contains a sophisticated computer for image processing and enhancement. Mobile C-arm units offer features such as pulsed fluoroscopy, LIH, and high-level fluoroscopy to enhance their value in difficult surgical cases. The radiographer must become comfortable with the system's many features to perform successfully in the stressful environment of surgery.

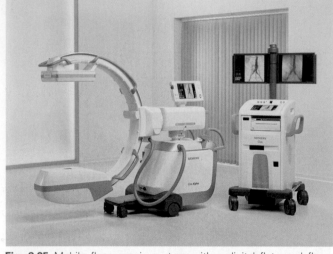

Fig. 8.25 Mobile fluoroscopic system with a digital flat-panel fluoroscopic detector. (Source: Siemens Healthcare https://static.healthcare. siemens.com/siemens_hwem-hwem_ssxa_websites-context-root/ wcm/idc/groups/public/@global/@imaging/@c-arms/documents/image/ mda1/ndk3/~edisp/mobile_c_arm_cios_alpha_1-02444086/~renditions/ mobile_c_arm_cios_alpha_1-02444086~10.jpg)

In addition, the technology of portable DR detectors has evolved to permit DR portable radiography. These detectors are very expensive and fragile and should be handled with great care. Manufacturers have gone to considerable lengths to make these detectors light in weight, durable, and fluid-resistant but no vendor has yet developed the "perfect" DR detector panel. Wireless DR panel systems have gained considerable popularity and use an on-board battery or capacitor to provide a small "trickle charge" to the TFT layer of these panels. The charge is placed on the TFT layer just prior to and during the x-ray exposure; therefore an electronic communication between the panel and generator is required. Following exposure, the radiographic image is quickly available for review and acceptance. It is important to remember that with wireless detectors, the charge level of the battery should be inspected before setting out to perform the mobile study. These detectors provide excellent image quality and a quicker, more convenient process for obtaining high-quality images and sending them to a PACS system.

SUMMARY

A beginning radiographer can be overwhelmed initially by the complexity of radiographic and fluoroscopic equipment. New students must master the components of the radiographic system and how they operate to achieve the highest diagnostic yield. Familiarity with the x-ray tube, collimator, x-ray table, control console, and x-ray tube support is important. An understanding of the mechanical aspects of collimation, control console operation, and manipulation of the Bucky mechanism as well as the tube support, table, and image receptor systems is essential; it is among the skills that must be mastered early by a beginning radiographer. As the medical imaging profession continues to evolve into a digital environment, the complexity and cost of imaging equipment will continue to increase. This necessarily requires the radiographer to become competent with computers, various image detector technologies, exposure dose indicators, and image processing features. Without a doubt the importance of imaging will be paramount in more interventional procedures, and the demands of fluoroscopy and digital radiography will be greater than ever. The student must become as comfortable as possible with the technologic aspects of the x-ray examination process. Students who do well in the clinical aspects of radiography are those who master the mechanics of equipment manipulation early and learn to respect the level of technology used in delivering medical images, thus enhancing the standard of care in medicine.

BIBLIOGRAPHY

American Association of Physicists in Medicine: *Acceptance testing and quality control of photostimulable storage phosphor imaging systems: report of AAPM Task Group 10*, AAPM rep no. 93. College Park, Md, October 2006, The Association. 2006.

Bushong SC: *Radiologic science for technologists*, ed 10, St. Louis, 2012, Mosby.

Carlton R, Adler AM: *Principles of radiographic imaging: an art and a science*, ed 5, Albany, NY, 2012, Thomson Delmar Learning.

Carroll Quin B, Bowman Dennis: *Adaptive Radiography with Trauma, Image Critique and Critical Thinking, Delmar Cengage Learning Pub.*, 2Albany, 2014, NY.

Carroll Q: *Radiography in the digital age: Physics, Exposure, Radiation Biology*, Springfield, Ill, 2011, Charles C. Thomas.

Carter C, Veale B: *Digital radiography and PACS*, ed 2, St. Louis, 2013, Mosby.

Curry TS, Dowdey JE, Murry RC: *Christensen's introduction to the physics of diagnostic radiology*, ed 4, Philadelphia, 1990, Lippincott Williams & Wilkins.

Drafke Michael, Nakayama Harry: *Trauma and mobile radiography*, ed 2, Philadelphia, 2001, F.A. Davis Co. Pub.

Fauber TL: *Radiographic imaging and exposure*, ed 3, St. Louis, 2008, Mosby.

Glasser, Otto, Dr. W.C. Roengten, 1945 Charles C. Thomas Publisher, Springfield, IL

Selman J: *The fundamentals of imaging physics and radiobiology*, ed 9, Springfield, Ill, 2000, Charles C Thomas.

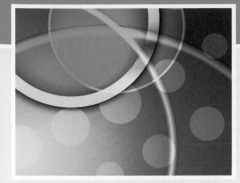

Basic Radiation Protection and Radiobiology

Kelli Welch Haynes, EdD, RT(R)

> *Today I was reading about Marie Curie*
> *she must have known she suffered from radiation sickness*
> *She died a famous woman denying her wounds*
> *denying her wounds that came from the*
> *same source as her power*
>
> *Adrienne Rich*
>
> *"Power," The Dream of a Common Language: Poems 1974–77*

OBJECTIVES

On completion of this chapter, the student will be able to:

- Identify the sources of ionizing radiation.
- List the units used to measure radiation exposure and their correct use.
- Describe the sources of radiation exposure.
- Explain the ways in which ionizing radiation interacts with matter.
- List the permissible limits of exposure for occupational exposure and the general public.
- Explain the reason for the varying sensitivity of human cells to ionizing radiation.
- Describe the ways in which the entire body responds to varying amounts of radiation.
- Discuss the various practices used to protect the patient from excessive radiation.
- Discuss the various approaches used to protect an occupational worker from excess radiation.
- Describe several devices used to detect and measure exposure to ionizing radiation.

OUTLINE

KEY TERMS

Air Kerma SI quantity used to measure energy transferred from radiation to matter, which may be at the surface of a patient's or radiographer's body

ALARA Mnemonic meaning to keep all radiation exposure as low as reasonably achievable

Becquerel (Bq) Unit of radioactivity in the International System of Units, equal to one disintegration per second

Classic Coherent Scattering Interaction with matter in which a low-energy photon (below 10 kiloelectron volts) is absorbed and released with its same energy, frequency, and wavelength but with a change of direction

Compton Scattering Interaction with matter in which a higher energy photon strikes a loosely bound outer electron, removing it from its shell, and the remaining energy is released as a scattered photon

Curie (Ci) Unit of radioactivity defined as the quantity of any radioactive nuclide in which the number of disintegrations per second is 3.7 × 10^{10}

Germ Cells Cells of an organism whose function is to reproduce the organism (e.g., ovum, spermatozoa)

Gray (Gy) Unit in the International System used to measure the amount of energy absorbed in any medium; 1 Gy = 100 radiation absorbed doses

International System (SI) of Units System of units based on metric measurement developed in 1948 and having units used to measure radiation

Kiloelectron Volts (keV) Units of energy equal to 1000 electron volts

Pair Production Interaction between matter and a photon possessing a minimum of 1.02 million electron volts of energy producing two oppositely charged particles, a positron and a negatron

Photodisintegration Direct interaction with the nucleus of the atom, causing a state of excitement within the nucleus, followed by the emission of a nuclear fragment

Photoelectric Interaction Interaction with matter in which a photon strikes an inner shell electron, causing its ejection from orbit with the complete absorption of the photon's energy

Radiation Forms of energy emitted and transferred through matter

Radiation Absorbed Dose (rad) Unit used to measure the amount of energy absorbed in any medium; equal to 100 ergs of energy absorbed in 1 g of material

Radiation Equivalent Man (rem) Unit of dose equivalence; equal to the product of absorbed dose in rad and a quality factor

Roentgen (R) Unit of exposure in air; that quantity of x-radiation or gamma radiation that produces the quantity 2.08 × 109 ion pairs per cubic centimeter of air

Sievert (Sv) Unit in the International System used to measure the dose equivalence, or biologic effectiveness, of differing radiations; 1 Sv = 100 rem

Somatic Cells All of the body's cells except germ cells

X-rays Form of electromagnetic radiation traveling at the speed of light, possessing the ability to penetrate matter

IONIZING RADIATION

Whenever a radiographer is applying ionizing radiation to produce a diagnostic image for the radiologist, he or she should remember the great responsibility this entails. Ionizing radiation is energy capable of penetrating matter and possesses sufficient energy to eject orbital electrons along its path, thus ionizing atoms. Exposure to radiation always involves a risk for biologic changes that cannot be ignored. The benefits of improved diagnosis of disease outweigh the risk, however, as long as the radiographer is using sound judgment and always works to minimize the quantity of radiation the patient receives. The radiographer must act to protect all persons from unnecessary radiation exposure, including himself or herself, the patient, and others within the clinical environment.

Sources of Ionizing Radiation

Although humans are exposed to radiation in everyday living, it is rarely given much thought. The two basic sources of ionizing radiation exposure are natural (or background) radiation and human-made (artificial) radiation sources. Background sources occur spontaneously in nature and are not affected by human activity. These forms include cosmic radiation from the sun and other planetary bodies and naturally occurring radioactive substances present on earth (such as uranium and radium), which can be inhaled or ingested through food, water, or air (radon). Sources of human-made radiation include the nuclear industry, radionuclides, medical and dental exposures, and some consumer products. The nuclear industry has contributed fallout from aboveground weapons testing, from accidents in nuclear power stations, and from the disposal of by-products from these plants. Exposure to radionuclides results from products containing radioactive elements, such as smoke detectors, and radiopharmaceuticals used in the diagnosis and treatment of disease. Medical and dental exposures constitute the greatest source of human-made radiation. In addition, certain consumer products such as video monitors, suntan beds, and microwave ovens contribute slightly to the annual US exposure. Because the radiographer is primarily responsible for the application of medical ionizing radiation to patients, understanding the process by which x-rays interact with matter is important.

Human-Made Radiation

Human-made ionizing radiation, or x-rays as they are more commonly called, is a form of electromagnetic radiation that travels at the speed of light. Unlike particulate radiation, which

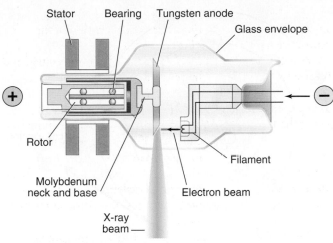

Fig. 9.1 Rotating anode tube.

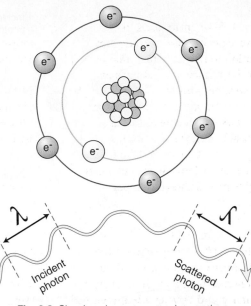

Fig. 9.2 Classic coherent scatter interaction.

is a liberated portion of a radioactive atom capable of traveling for short distances and reacting with matter, x-rays are bundles of energy moving as waves in space, depositing their energy randomly. For x-rays to be produced, three things must be present: (1) a source of electrons, (2) a means to rapidly accelerate the electrons, and (3) something to rapidly stop this movement. These conditions are all met by the x-ray tube and its electrical supply (Fig. 9.1). The tube itself is composed of a *cathode*, or negative terminal, and an *anode*, or positive terminal, enclosed in a special heat-resistant glass envelope to maintain the vacuum necessary for optimal x-ray production. The filament in the cathode assembly is composed of thoriated tungsten, which provides the source of electrons. When milliamperage *(electric current)* is applied to the filament, it responds by boiling off electrons through a process known as *thermionic emission.* Once kilovoltage (high voltage) is applied to the tube terminals, the electrons resulting from thermionic emission instantaneously accelerate toward the anode end of the tube. X-rays are produced when the electrons strike the anode, undergoing an energy conversion that produces both x-rays and heat. The resultant x-ray beam is heterogeneous—that is, it has many energies, measured in **kiloelectron volts (keV)**. These x-rays, also known as the *primary or useful beam,* are directed toward the patient through a window in the tube. Once the x-rays strike matter, three possibilities exist: (1) they can be absorbed, (2) they can transfer some energy and then scatter, or (3) they can pass through unaffected.

Interactions of X-Rays With Matter

X-rays interact with matter in five ways: (1) **classic coherent scattering**, (2) **photoelectric interaction**, (3) **Compton scattering**, (4) **pair production**, and (5) **photodisintegration**. Classic coherent scattering, photoelectric interaction, and Compton scattering occur within the diagnostic range of x-ray energies, whereas pair production and photodisintegration occur in the therapeutic range of energies. Both Compton scattering and photoelectric interaction directly influence patient and occupational worker exposure. They are the way in which x-rays transfer their energy to living tissue. They constitute the basis for all patient exposure and the reason behind the need for protective measures.

Classic Coherent Scattering. X-rays that possess energy levels below 10 keV can interact with matter through classic coherent scattering (Fig. 9.2). Also known as *coherent, Thomson,* or *unmodified scattering,* classic coherent scattering occurs when an incoming x-ray photon strikes an atom and is absorbed, causing the atom to become excited. The atom then releases the excess energy in the form of another x-ray photon possessing the same energy as the original photon, but proceeding in a different direction. This change in direction is known as *scattering.* Most of these scattered photons travel in a forward direction, stopping when they strike anything in their path. More importantly, classic coherent scattering results in no energy transfer to the patient.

Photoelectric Interaction. The second common interaction of x-rays with matter in the diagnostic range is the photoelectric effect (Fig. 9.3). The photoelectric effect occurs when an incoming x-ray photon strikes an inner shell electron and ejects it from its orbit around the nucleus of the atom, creating an ion pair. The atom, having lost an electron, is positively charged, and the released electron, referred to as the *photoelectron,* continues to travel until it combines with other matter. All the energy from the photon is completely consumed in this interaction; it is said that the energy is absorbed by the atom. As outer shell electrons transition to fill vacancies in inner shells, they release excess energy in the form of x-rays. X-rays originating within the body as a result of the photoelectric effect are collectively known as characteristic radiation and are the source of secondary radiation. Because complete energy absorption takes place in photoelectric interactions, this constitutes the greatest hazard to patients in diagnostic radiography.

Compton Scattering. The last interaction common to the diagnostic x-ray range is the Compton effect (Fig. 9.4). The Compton effect, also known as *modified* or *Compton scattering,* occurs when an incoming x-ray photon strikes a target atom

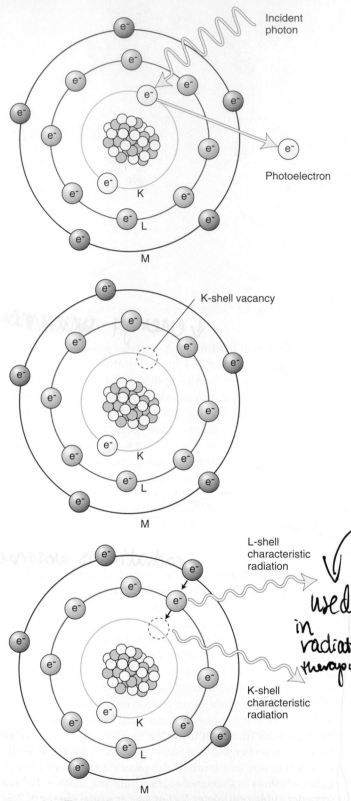

Incident photon

Photoelectron

K

L

M

K-shell vacancy

K

L

M

L-shell characteristic radiation

used in radiation therapy

K-shell characteristic radiation

K

L

M

Fig. 9.3 Photoelectric absorption interaction.

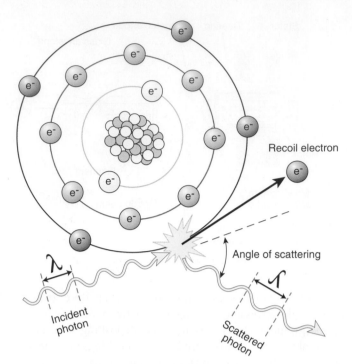

Recoil electron

Angle of scattering

λ

Incident photon

Scattered photon

Fig. 9.4 Compton scatter interaction.

energy that can react with the patient through further Compton or photoelectric interactions, or that can exit the patient and reach imaging equipment or the occupational worker. This interaction is also referred to as modified scattering, because the original photon possesses less energy after the interaction. The Compton effect is extremely important because it is responsible for a majority of occupational worker exposure to radiation.

Pair Production. The last two interactions that occur between ionizing radiation and matter require high-energy photons above 1 million electron volts (MeV). They are less relevant to diagnostic radiography, because the equipment used in the production of x-rays cannot produce photons that possess this energy, but they are of particular importance in radiation therapy.

For pair production to occur, an incoming x-ray photon must possess a minimum of 1.02 MeV of energy (Fig. 9.5). This photon does not interact with the surrounding electron orbits; instead, it approaches the nucleus of the atom and interacts with its force field. The photon disappears, and two particles emerge to replace it: a *positron* and a *negatron*. A positron is a positively charged particle, and a negatron is negatively charged. Each particle possesses half the energy (minimum, 0.51 MeV) of the original x-ray photon. The particles continue to travel, causing ionization, until the positron interacts with another electron, annihilates it, and produces two photons moving in opposite directions. Because the energy level necessary for pair production is at least 1.02 MeV, it does not occur in the diagnostic x-ray range.

Photodisintegration. X-ray photons possessing a minimum of 10 MeV of energy can interact directly with the nucleus of the atom, causing a state of excitement within the nucleus, followed

used in atomic bombs

and uses a portion of its energy to eject an outer shell electron. The remainder of the photon's energy proceeds in a direction different from that of the incoming photon. This process results in a Compton or recoil electron ejected from the outer shell, which travels until it combines with matter, and a photon of less

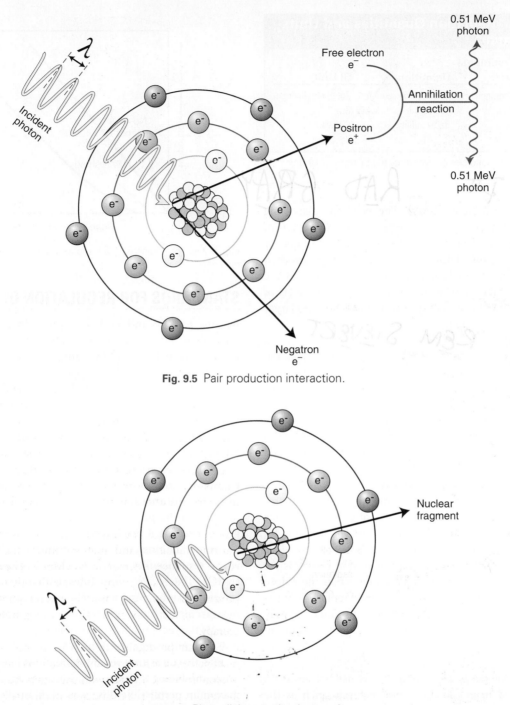

Fig. 9.5 Pair production interaction.

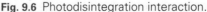

Fig. 9.6 Photodisintegration interaction.

by the emission of a nuclear fragment (Fig. 9.6). This process is referred to as *photodisintegration*. It does not occur in diagnostic radiography, but does occur in the nuclear industry.

Units of Measure

To quantify the amount of radiation a patient or occupational worker receives, a system of units has been developed. The units most commonly used since the 1920s are listed in Table 9.1. In 1948 the International Committee for Weights and Measures developed a system of units based on metric measurement. The SI units system (Système International d'Unitès, or **International System [SI] of Units**) was officially adopted in 1985.

Roentgen (Coulombs per Kilogram). The **roentgen (R)** is the measure of ionization in air as a result of exposure to x-rays or gamma rays. It is defined as the quantity of x-radiation or gamma radiation that produces the quantity 2.08×10^9 ion pairs per cubic centimeter (cc) of air, for a total charge of 2.58×10^{-4} coulombs per kilogram (C/kg; coulomb is a quantity of electric charge). The roentgen is restricted to measuring photons with energy below 3 MeV and only exposure in air. It does not indicate actual exposure to individuals when absorbed. The roentgen has no equivalent in the SI units because exposure may be expressed directly as coulombs per kilogram, so the roentgen is being phased out as a unit of measure.

TABLE 9.1 Radiation Quantities and Units of Measurement

Quantity	Traditional Unit	Definition	SI Unit
Exposure in air	Roentgen	2.08×10^9 ion pairs/cc	Coulomb/kilogram
Absorbed dose	Rad	100 ergs/g	Gray
Dose equivalent	Rem	Rad × quality factor	Sievert
Activity	Curie	3.7×10^{10} dps	Becquerel

SI, Système International d'Unités (International System of Units).

Radiation Absorbed Dose (Gray). The need for discussing absorbed dose resulted in the development of the **radiation absorbed dose (rad)**. The rad measures the amount of energy absorbed in any medium, defined as 100 ergs of energy absorbed in 1 g of absorbing material. The rad has been replaced by the **gray (Gy)** in the SI system, which is defined as 1 joule (J) of energy absorbed in 1 kg of material. The Gy is 100 times larger than the rad; 1 Gy = 100 rad.

Radiation Equivalent Man (Sievert). Not all types of radiation produce the same response in living tissue. Alpha particles, neutrons, and beta particles may produce a different degree of biologic damage than x-rays and gamma rays. To express accurately the biologic response of exposed individuals to the same quantity of differing radiations, the rem was developed. The **radiation equivalent man (rem)** is the unit of dose equivalence, expressed as the product of the absorbed dose in rad and a quality factor.

The quality factor varies, depending on the type of radiation being used. For example, the quality factor for x-rays is 1; therefore 1 rad of x-ray exposure equals 1 rem of dose equivalence (1 rad × 1 = 1 rem). The quality factor for fast neutrons is 10; thus 1 rad of fast neutron exposure equals 10 rem of dose equivalence (1 rad × 10 = 10 rem), meaning that neutrons are 10 times as biologically damaging as x-rays when their dose equivalents are compared. The rem has been replaced by the **sievert (Sv)** in SI units, which is defined as the product of the Gy and the quality factor. The sievert is 100 times larger than the rem; 1 Sv = 100 rem.

Air Kerma. **Air kerma** is an SI unit that is used to measure energy transferred from radiation to a material, such as the patient's body. Air kerma is replacing the traditional quantity exposure to express radiation exposure. Kerma is an acronym for "kinetic energy released in matter." Air kerma is the total kinetic energy released in a unit mass (kilogram) of air and is measured in joules per kilogram (J/kg).

Curie (Becquerel). The measure of the rate at which a radionuclide decays is referred to as *activity*. The **curie (Ci)** is the unit of activity, equal to 3.7×10^{10} disintegrations per second (dps). The SI unit of activity is the **Becquerel (Bq)**, defined as 1 disintegration per second (dps). Therefore 1 Ci = 3.7×10^{10} Bq. These units are commonly employed in nuclear medicine and radiotherapy.

The traditional and SI units are compared in Table 9.1.

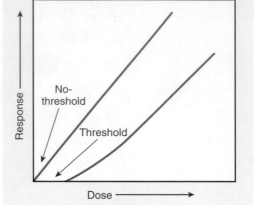

Fig. 9.7 Graph indicates no-threshold versus threshold response to radiation.

STANDARDS FOR REGULATION OF EXPOSURE

Because patients and workers exposed to radiation are at risk for biologic effects, limits must be set to ensure safe practice for both the patient and the radiation worker. Guidelines and standards set by regulatory agencies must be followed. The Center for Devices and Radiological Health (CDRH), under the direction of the US Food and Drug Administration, sets and regulates the standards for radiation-producing equipment; it also continues to research possible ways of minimizing exposure to ionizing radiation. The National Council on Radiation Protection and Measurements (NCRP) is a not-for-profit organization formed by Congress in 1964 to collect and distribute information regarding radiation awareness and safe practice to the public. The NCRP is considered an advisory group, because it does not have the authority to enforce the recommendations contained within its reports. Enforcement is the responsibility of the Nuclear Regulatory Commission (NRC). The NCRP cooperates with other organizations to review, on an ongoing basis, the latest data on radiation units, measurements, and protection. The following information reflects the recommendations made by the NCRP, in cooperation with other organizations.

Effective dose limit recommendations have been set to minimize the biologic risk to exposed persons. The concept of a maximum permissible dose was traditionally used to describe the maximum dose of ionizing radiation that, if received by an individual, would carry a negligible risk for significant bodily or genetic damage. Currently the term *effective dose limits* is used, which takes into account various types of radiation exposure and tissue sensitivities. Dose limits were established for both the occupational worker and the general population. These recommendations follow two theories: nonthreshold and risk versus benefit (Fig. 9.7).

Nonthreshold indicates that no dose exists below which the risk of damage does not exist. *Risk versus benefit* governs the exposure of individuals when physicians ordered radiographic procedures. The benefit to the patient from performing those procedures must outweigh the risk of possible biologic damage. Because current studies indicate that an individual's dose should

TABLE 9.2 Effective Dose Limit Recommendations

Population and Area of Body Irradiated	DOSE LIMITS	
	SI Unit	Traditional Unit
Occupational Exposures		
Effective Dose Limits		
Annual	50 mSv	5 rem
Cumulative	10 mSv × age	1 rem × age
Equivalent Dose Annual Limits for Tissues and Organs		
Lens of eyes	150 mSv	15 rem
Skin, hands, and feet	500 mSv	50 rem
Public Exposures (Annual)		
Effective Dose Limit		
Continuous or frequent exposure	1 mSv	0.1 rem
Infrequent exposure	5 mSv	0.5 rem
Equivalent Dose Limits for Tissues and Organs		
Lens of eye	15 mSv	1.5 rem
Skin, hands, and feet	50 mSv	5 rem
Embryo-Fetal Exposures (Monthly)		
Equivalent dose limit	0.5 mSv	0.05 rem
Education and Training Exposures (Annual)		
Effective dose limit	1 mSv	0.1 rem
Equivalent Dose Limit for Tissues and Organs		
Lens of eye	15 mSv	1.5 rem
Skin, hands, and feet	50 mSv	5 rem

SI, Système International d'Unités (International System of Units). National Council on Radiation Protection and Measurements (NCRP). *Limitation of Exposure to Ionizing Radiation.* NCRP Report No. 116. Bethesda, MD: The Council; 1993.

be kept *as low as reasonably achievable* (ALARA), and that no dose is considered permissible, the term *maximum permissible dose* is no longer acceptable. Instead, NCRP has recommended certain *effective dose* limits, summarized in Table 9.2.

The annual whole-body effective dose limit for the occupational worker is 50 mSv (5 rem). Currently the recommended maximum accumulated whole-body effective dose limit is 10 mSv × age in years (or 1 rem × age in years). With this formula, a 40-year-old radiation worker may accumulate 1 rem × 40, or 40 rem (400 mSv) in his or her lifetime.

Anyone exposed to ionizing radiation not as a radiation worker is considered a member of the general population for radiation protection purposes. The whole-body dose-equivalent limit for the general population is one-tenth the occupational worker's annual limit, or 5 mSv (0.5 rem).

BIOLOGIC RESPONSE TO IONIZING RADIATION

Ionizing radiation, absorbed by matter, undergoes energy conversions that result in changes in atomic structure. These changes, when considered in light of living tissue, can have major consequences on the life of any organism. To understand

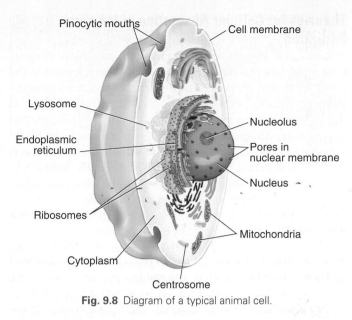

Fig. 9.8 Diagram of a typical animal cell.

the necessity of protecting oneself and the patient from exposure to radiation, a basic review of cellular biology and how radiation interacts with cells is important.

Basic Cell Structure

The cell is the simplest unit of organic protoplasm capable of independent existence. Simple organisms are composed of one or two cells; complex organisms are *multicellular*—that is, made of many cells. Although cells may differ from one another depending on their primary function, their structures are similar. Most cells are divided into two parts: (1) the nucleus and (2) the cytoplasm (Fig. 9.8). The nucleus is separated from the rest of the cell by a double-walled membrane called the *nuclear envelope.* This membrane has openings, or *pores,* that permit other molecules to pass back and forth between the nucleus and the cytoplasm. Most important, the nucleus contains the *chromosomes,* which are made up of genes. *Genes* are the units of hereditary information, composed of DNA, which is a double-stranded structure coiled around itself as a spiral staircase. It is one of the molecules at risk when a cell is exposed to ionizing radiation.

The cytoplasm of the cell is separated from its environment by the cell membrane. It contains several organelles responsible for the metabolic function of the cell. The cytoplasm itself is primarily water, which can undergo changes when struck by ionizing radiation.

Cell Types

Cells are of two types: (1) somatic cells and (2) germ cells. **Somatic cells** perform all the body's functions. They possess two of every gene on two different chromosomes. Their chromosomes are paired, but each pair is different. Somatic cells possess a total of 46 chromosomes, or 23 pairs. They divide through the process of mitosis. **Germ cells** are the reproductive cells of an organism; they possess half the number of chromosomes as the somatic cells, for a total of 23. Germ cells reproduce through the process of meiosis.

Theories for Cellular Absorption of Ionizing Radiation

When a cell absorbs ionizing radiation, two basic theories exist to explain this interaction. The first theory, known as the *direct hit theory*, proposes that any type of radiation transfers its energy directly to the key molecule it has struck, resulting in the formation of ion pairs or elevation to an increased, excited energy state. Although any important structure can be hit by radiation, serious consequences arise when radiation interacts with DNA. Breaks in the bases or phosphate bonds can result in rearrangement or loss of genetic information, which can injure or kill the cell as it continues through its life cycle.

The other interaction with ionizing radiation is by indirect hit. Key molecules are affected by radiation depositing its energy elsewhere in the cell. Because cells are approximately 80% water, indirect action occurs when water molecules are ionized. This action produces chemical changes within the cell that alter the internal environment, injuring the cell, which can result in eventual cell death. With x-radiation and gamma radiation, the vast majority of cellular damage is the result of indirect hits.

Target Theory of Absorption of Ionizing Radiation

Both direct and indirect interactions with ionizing radiation apply to the target theory of absorption of ionizing radiation. Simply stated, certain molecules existing within a cell are key to the continued viability or life of that cell. Some of these molecules exist in great number; others in limited supply. If damage occurs to a molecule in abundant supply, the effect on the cell may not be as detrimental because others exist to maintain the function of the cell. Injury to a molecule in limited supply, however, can be life threatening, because no immediate replacement is available. The term *target* is used to describe any critical molecule, in this case the nucleus of a cell, that has undergone some interaction with ionizing radiation, either directly or indirectly. The target whose damage has serious consequences to the life of the cell is DNA.

Radiosensitivity of Cells

To study the cell's response to radiation, a method of classification according to sensitivity was developed by Bergonie and Tribondeau in 1906. These researchers determined that mitotic activity and specific characteristics of each cell affected how the cell exhibited radiation damage. Cells are most sensitive to radiation during active division, when they are primitive in structure and function. Examples of radiosensitive cells include the basal cells of the skin, crypt cells of the small intestine, and germ cells. Cells resistant to radiation, being more specialized in structure and function, do not undergo repeated mitosis. These cells include nerve, muscle, and brain cells.

Ancel and Vitemberger, who modified this theory, stated that all cells possess the same sensitivity to radiation; the time of expression of injury is the factor that differs. This factor depends on mitosis and the external conditions in which the cell is placed. Therefore rapidly dividing cells demonstrate the injury sooner and only appear as though they are more sensitive to radiation than those whose mitotic rate is slower. Organs composed of parenchymal cells that rapidly divide, such as skin or the small intestine, exhibit injury sooner than the esophagus or muscle, whose cells divide more slowly.

Response of Cells to Radiation

Cells respond to radiation in many ways. They die before beginning mitosis, delay entering mitosis, or fail to divide at their normal rate. Fortunately, cells also try to repair the damage sustained through absorption of ionizing radiation. This possibility depends on how sensitive the cell is to radiation, the type of damage sustained, the kind of radiation (particulate or electromagnetic), the exposure rate, and the total dose given. Incomplete repair can result in adverse biologic effects occurring after time has elapsed.

Total Body Response to Irradiation

The total body response of any organism to radiation depends on the effect on all the systems of the body. Because every system is different in its sensitivity or resistance, the total body response at a particular dose is defined by the system most affected. This response, known as *acute radiation syndrome*, occurs only when the organism is exposed fully (total body) to an external source of radiation given in a few minutes. Only then does the organism develop the full set of signs and symptoms that define each syndrome, which depends on the dose received.

Early Effects of Radiation Exposure. Three general stages of response exist for each acute radiation syndrome. The first is the *prodromal stage*, commonly referred to as the *nausea, vomiting, and diarrhea* stage. The second stage is the *latent period*, in which the organism feels well; however, during this time, the body is undergoing biologic changes that will lead to the final period, the *manifest stage*. Now the organism feels the full effects of the exposure, leading to either recovery or death (Table 9.3).

TABLE 9.3 **Biologic Response to Ionizing Radiation: Total Body Response to Irradiation Acute Radiation Syndrome**			
	Bone Marrow (Hematopoietic) Syndrome	**Gastrointestinal Syndrome**	**Central Nervous System Syndrome**
Dose required	2–10 Gy (200–1000 rad)	10–50 Gy (1000–5000 rad)	50+ Gy (5000+ rad)
Manifest symptoms	Infection, hemorrhage, anemia	Massive diarrhea, nausea, vomiting, fever	Seizures, coma, eventual death
Cause of symptoms	Inability to produce blood cells in bone marrow	Damage to epithelial lining of the GI system	Brain edema, intracranial pressure, CNS failure
Mean survival*	6–8 weeks (or recovery in 6 months)	3–10 days	Few hours to 2–3 days

*Varies with actual dose received.

Three radiation syndromes are (1) bone marrow syndrome, (2) gastrointestinal (GI) syndrome, and (3) central nervous system (CNS) syndrome. Bone marrow syndrome, or *hematopoietic syndrome*, occurs at doses of 2 to 10 Gy (200 to 1000 rad). Total body exposure results in infection, hemorrhage, and anemia. GI syndrome results from doses of 10 to 50 Gy (1000 to 5000 rad). Individuals experience massive diarrhea, nausea, vomiting, and fever when subjected to these doses. CNS syndrome occurs at doses above 50 Gy (5000 rad), with the individual experiencing seizures, coma, and eventual death from increased intracranial pressure. Although these syndromes indicate serious, even lethal, consequences from exposure to radiation, an important point to remember is that these doses are far greater than those received by the occupational worker or patient.

Late Effects of Radiation Exposure. Other effects of radiation exposure termed the *late effects* are equally important; these can develop over a long period after exposure. These effects result not only from high doses of radiation, but also from low doses administered over a longer time. Late effects are divided into two groups: (1) *somatic effects*, which develop in the individual exposed, and (2) *genetic effects*, which occur in future generations as a result of damage to the germ cells.

The two most frequently induced somatic effects are cataract formation and carcinogenesis. The lens of the eye is extremely sensitive to radiation, and studies have demonstrated the high incidence of cataract formation in laboratory animals exposed to radiation. In addition, survivors of the explosion of the atom bomb developed cataracts.

The most important late somatic effect is cancer development. The first documented case was the hand of a radiographer in 1902. Early radiologists, technologists, and researchers developed skin cancer and leukemia from prolonged exposure to ionizing radiation. Watch-dial painters developed osteosarcoma from ingesting radium when they put their paintbrushes in their mouths to draw the tip to a point. Miners who inhaled radioactive dust while digging for uranium developed lung cancer. All of these cases led to today's strict limitations on radiation exposure.

Long-term genetic effects result from germ cells whose DNA has been altered by radiation exposure, meaning the effects are not seen in the exposed individual; instead, if an affected cell is fertilized and develops, the effects show up in future generations. These mutations—alterations in the DNA coding of the chromosome—are recessive. They appear only if the mutated cell is fertilized by another reproductive cell carrying the same mutation. This fact of genetics acts to minimize the appearance of possible radiation-induced changes.

PROTECTING THE PATIENT

Although the patient must be exposed to ionizing radiation for a diagnostic image to be produced, care must be exercised to minimize the quantity of radiation exposure. The radiographer has the responsibility of maximizing the quality of the radiograph while minimizing the risk to the patient. Consequently, the concept of ALARA—as low as reasonably achievable—is used to guide technical factor selection when performing examinations of the patient. In particular, the cardinal principles of protection—time, distance, and shielding—are used to minimize patient exposure.

Time   *Short time*

When the radiographer minimizes the length of time a patient remains in the path of the x-ray beam, he or she is applying one of the primary rules of protection. This goal is accomplished when the radiographer accurately applies the rules of radiographic technique to produce diagnostic images and uses technique charts to help determine the correct amount of radiation to direct toward the patient. The chances of repeated exposures are minimized, reducing the patient's time in the path of the x-ray beam.

Distance   *Maximum distance*

Another way to lessen patient dose is to maximize the distance between the radiation source and the patient. This increased distance lessens the entrance or skin dose to the patient. This action is not the most reasonable method to minimize patient dose, because the patient must be in the path of the ionizing beam for an image to be created. In addition, increasing distance requires an increase in technical factors to create an acceptable image.

Shielding

The last rule of protection is to shield by placing some material over the reproductive organs (gonads) of the patient whenever they are within 4 to 5 cm of the primary beam. Gonadal shielding is used only when it will not interfere with the anatomy of interest. This precaution is particularly important when performing radiography on children and adults of reproductive age. Shields are made of lead, which has an atomic number of 82. Lead absorbs x-rays through the process of photoelectric effect, thereby minimizing patient exposure. The three basic types of shields are (1) flat contact shields, (2) shaped contact shields, and (3) shadow shields.

Flat contact shields are made of a combination of vinyl and lead, and are placed directly over the gonads of the patient (Fig. 9.9). They are made in various sizes to accommodate the age of the patient. *Shaped contact shields* are cup-shaped and designed

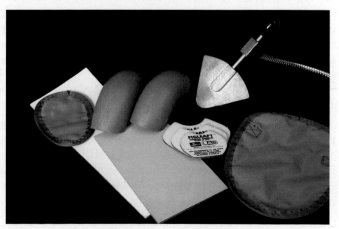

Fig. 9.9 Gonadal shields.

specifically to protect the gonads of male patients. Because of their shape, they can remain in place securely, even when the patient must turn to accommodate the examination. *Shadow shields* are mounted to the side of the collimator of the x-ray tube on a flexible extension arm. They can be manipulated to extend into the path of the beam and cast a shadow on the patient, indicating the area being protected. *Lead rubber blockers* also are used in some situations. *Lead aprons* should be used for additional patient shielding whenever the apron will not interfere with the anatomy of interest. It is highly recommended that patients be provided with a lead apron whenever feasible.

Additional Methods of Protection

Other factors specific to the production of x-rays can be manipulated with the purpose of minimizing patient exposure. These factors include beam restriction, image receptor speed, technical factor selection, and filtration. The radiographer always must restrict the primary beam to the anatomic area of interest, never exceeding the size of the image receptor used to capture the information. This restriction limits the exposure to the area undergoing radiography and does not increase the overall patient dose. Through the use of high-speed image receptors, a diagnostic image can be produced with reduced radiation, which minimizes patient exposure. In addition, selecting technical factors that use high kilovoltages increases the probability that Compton interactions will occur. This method results in a reduction of the energy being directly absorbed by the patient, creating a decrease in patient exposure. When reduced kilovoltage techniques are selected, an increased quantity of the radiation is completely absorbed within the patient, adding to the dose. Finally, filtration material in the path of the x-ray beam absorbs the low-energy x-rays that only add to the patient's entrance dose. Eliminating their presence in the primary beam does not affect the finished image, because most do not exit the patient to reach the image receptor. Aluminum is the most common material used in filtration. Its atomic number and K-shell binding energies encourage photoelectric absorption of the low-energy x-rays.

PROTECTING THE RADIOGRAPHER

The same principles of time, distance, and shielding are used to reduce the occupational worker's exposure to radiation. This reduction is accomplished by minimizing the time spent in the room when ionizing radiation is being produced, using the greatest possible distance from the source of exposure and placing a shield between the worker and the radiation source.

Time

The radiographer should always spend the least amount of time possible in a room when a source of radiation is active. This risk exists only when exposures are being made; once the exposure is terminated, no radiation remains within the room or the contents of the room. The amount of dose received is directly related to the length of time spent with the source. During fluoroscopy, in which radiation is used for imaging dynamic structures, x-rays are emitted for longer periods. Therefore most

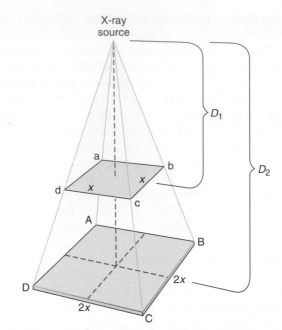

Fig. 9.10 The Inverse Square Law. The intensity of radiation at a given distance from a point source is inversely proportional to the square of the distance.

units are equipped with 5-minute timers to alert the operator when the time has elapsed.

Distance

Distance is the best measure of protection for an occupational worker. The principle of the inverse square law states that the intensity of radiation varies inversely with the square of the distance. Simply stated, increasing the distance from the source of the x-ray beam greatly reduces the quantity of radiation that reaches the radiographer (Fig. 9.10). This reduction occurs because the x-rays leaving the tube spread out *(diverge)* and cover a much larger area, which in turn lessens their intensity. The following formula can be used to determine the exact exposure reaching the worker:

$$\frac{\text{New intensity}}{\text{old intensity}} = \frac{\text{Old distance}^2}{\text{New distance}^2}$$

For example, if the intensity of radiation received by the radiographer were 20 mR at a distance of 1 m from the tube, what then would the intensity be at a distance of 2 m from the tube, all other factors remaining the same? Solving for the new intensity, we get:

$$\frac{\text{Newintensity}}{20 \text{ C/kg}} = \frac{1^2}{2^2}$$

$$\text{Newintensity} = 1 \times \frac{20 \text{ C/kg}}{4} = 5 \text{ C/kg}$$

Doubling the distance between the radiographer and the source of radiation reduces the exposure by a factor of 4 (now ¼ the dose at the original distance). Conversely, if the distance

(handwritten margin note) good. communication telling them good manners

TABLE 9.4   Radiation Protection Measures for Patients and Technologists

Cardinal Principle	Patient	Technologist
Time	Minimize the length of time they are in the primary beam.	During fluoroscopy, spend the least amount of time in the room that is practical.
	Consult technique charts and use shorter exposure times to avoid repeat exposures.	
	During fluoroscopy, less beam "on" time.	
Distance	Maximize distance between the patient and the source of radiation.	Increase the distance from the source of scatter (the patient) during fluoroscopic and mobile studies.
	SID should be at least 40 inches (100 cm).	
Shielding	Collimate the beam to the area of interest only.	Wear lead aprons and thyroid shields during fluoroscopic and mobile studies.
	Use gonadal shielding whenever possible.*	
	Provide a lead apron to the patient when extremities are radiographed.*	Stand behind fixed or mobile barriers.

*If the shield will not interfere with visualizing the anatomy of interest.
SID, Source-to-image receptor distance.

from the source of radiation is reduced by ½, the exposure will increase to 4 times the original. Therefore distance is an extremely important factor in radiation protection.

A radiographer should not make a practice of holding a patient who cannot cooperate during a radiographic procedure. This circumstance places the radiographer closer to the beam and to the patient, who is a source of scatter radiation from Compton interaction, and increases the time a radiographer is near the source of radiation. Whenever possible, immobilization devices such as sandbags or restraint bands should be used. If these devices are ineffective or unavailable, assistance should be obtained from a nonoccupational worker such as a nurse, physician, or relative of the patient. The person who assists the patient must wear shielding devices to minimize his or her exposure.

Shielding

The radiographer must use shielding whenever time and distance alone cannot satisfactorily protect the worker. Lead is the material used in both fixed protective barriers and accessory devices such as aprons and gloves. Lead aprons and gloves should be worn when taking advantage of fixed barriers is impossible. They are constructed of lead-impregnated vinyl, with a content of 0.25 to 1.0 mm of lead equivalency. However, it is recommended that aprons worn by personnel during fluoroscopic procedures be 0.5 mm of lead equivalency. The greater the amount of lead used, the better the protection offered to the worker. The greatest drawback to increased lead content is the increase in weight. The minimum permissible amount of lead equivalency for aprons used when the peak kilovoltage is 100 is 0.25 mm. Gloves usually possess the same minimum amount.

The shielding garments must be in good condition; cracked aprons and gloves do not successfully attenuate radiation. Protective apparel must be stored properly on specially designed racks so that cracks do not develop. To determine whether aprons or gloves adequately protect the wearer, they should undergo fluoroscopy at least once per year to check for damage.

Fixed protective barriers are part of the radiographic room construction and can be divided into primary and secondary barriers. *Primary barriers* are those that can be struck by the primary beam exiting the x-ray tube. *Secondary barriers* are those that can be struck only by secondary, scatter, or leakage radiation. A diagnostic radiologic physicist who considers the design and use of the room determines the exact quantity of lead or the equivalent thickness of concrete (Table 9.4).

Pregnant Student

Student pregnancy is covered under NRC regulations regarding the declared pregnant worker. Radiologic science programs accredited by the Joint Review Committee on Education in Radiologic Technology (JRCERT) must publish and make these regulations known to accepted and enrolled female students. Although guidelines for the exposure of pregnant women have been in place for many years, in 1994 the NRC in the United States became the first regulatory agency to limit the absorbed radiation dose to the unborn child. The dose limit is 0.5 rem (5 mSv) for the declared pregnant woman for the duration of her pregnancy. In addition, the NCRP recommends that once pregnancy is known, a limit of 0.05 rem (0.5 mSv) per month should apply. Should a pregnant student voluntarily disclose her pregnancy in writing to her program officials, a second monitor (fetal dosimetry badge) is issued and worn during energized laboratory sessions and clinical assignments.

Studies of average exposures of radiologic technologists indicate it is unlikely that the exposure of a pregnant student would exceed these limits. Consequently, little reason exists for the pregnant student to decide not to declare her pregnancy or to substantially alter her clinical assignments. Deciding what the risk to her fetus may be and taking precautions to avoid excessive radiation exposure are the responsibilities of the pregnant woman. Careful attention to the ALARA concepts of time, distance, and shielding are an important part of this decision.

As a result of US Supreme Court litigation designed to end sex discrimination against pregnant women in the workplace, American employers may not bar women of childbearing age from jobs because of potential risk to their fetuses. Essentially the ruling upholds the Title VII *Civil Rights Act of 1964* as forbidding sex-specific fetal-protection policies. Consequently, the NRC requires that all persons frequenting any portion of a restricted radiation area be instructed

most common

in the risks of radiation exposure to the embryo and fetus. (Restricted areas include diagnostic radiologic rooms, nuclear medicine laboratories, and any other area where ionizing radiation is applied to humans.) These instructions must include the right to declare or not declare pregnancy status. A declared pregnant woman is one who has voluntarily elected to declare her pregnancy. She is not under any regulatory or licensing obligation to do so. If a declaration is made, it must be in writing, be dated, and include the estimated month of conception. Acknowledgment of a pregnancy verbally or by visual observation does not meet the requirements of these regulations. Furthermore, the woman has the right to revoke her declaration of pregnancy. Until the proper declaration has been made, the total exposure dose limit is 5 rem (50 mSv).

Current recommendations in the literature discourage moving a newly declared pregnant woman to an area of lower radiation exposure, because reassignments have the potential to increase the exposure of others who are not yet aware they are pregnant. ALARA radiation protection philosophy supports a schedule that evenly distributes exposure risk to all students at a relatively uniform monthly exposure rate to avoid substantial variations among individuals.

The NRC regulations require that a personnel monitor be used if the declared pregnant student could potentially receive 10% of the embryo or fetal dose limit. This amount would be 0.05 rem (0.5 mSv) for the entire pregnancy, or 0.005 rem (0.05 mSv) per month. In addition to the collar monitor, a second dosimeter (fetal badge) must be worn at waist level. During fluoroscopic procedures when a lead apron is worn, the fetal badge is worn at waist level under the lead apron.

RADIATION MONITORING

Any occupational worker who is regularly exposed to ionizing radiation, who may potentially be exposed to 10% or more of the effective dose limits, must be monitored to determine estimated exposure. Monitors (dosimeters) measure the quantity of radiation received based on conditions in which the radiographer was placed. The most common personnel-monitoring devices are the optically stimulated luminescence (OSL) dosimeter, film badge, thermoluminescent dosimeter (TLD), and pocket dosimeter.

Students entering clinical rotations or an energized laboratory will also be issued a dosimeter. This device should always be worn at collar level, outside of leaded apparel, facing forward. Each month, an exposure report will be received by the educational program, indicating the amount of exposure for the monitoring period. This report is maintained on file as part of the student's permanent record. Programs accredited by the JRCERT are required to inform students of their radiation exposures in a timely manner.

Optically Stimulated Luminescence Dosimeters

The Luxel OSL dosimeter (Landauer) is the most common method used to monitor personnel exposure (Fig. 9.11). This

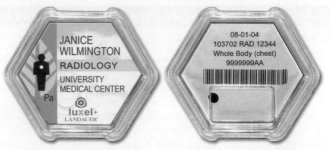

Fig. 9.11 Luxel OSL dosimeter. (Courtesy Landauer, Inc.)

type of dosimeter consists of a strip of aluminum oxide, a copper filter, an open window, a tin filter, and an imaging filter. The device is heat-sealed within a laminated, light-tight paper wrapper. The entire package is then sealed in a tamper-proof plastic blister pack. The front of the dosimeter provides information identifying the person wearing it, the name of the department, and a badge placement icon. To determine the individual's exposure, the aluminum oxide is exposed to a laser light, which stimulates the aluminum oxide after use, causing it to become luminescent in proportion to the amount of radiation exposure, which determines the occupational worker's exposure.

The OSL dosimeter can detect x-rays and gamma radiation in the range of 5 keV to in excess of 40 MeV. The dose measurement range is from 1 mrem to 1000 rem. Doses less than 1 mrem are not detectable and reported as *M*, or minimal. Typically the OSL dosimeter is worn for 2 months, but may be exchanged on a monthly basis. The holder should be worn between the collar and waist, on the front of the occupational worker. An advantage of this personal radiation monitoring device is that, because of the blister packaging, it is unaffected by heat, moisture, and pressure. The main disadvantage of this device is the inability to get an immediate reading of the worker's exposure; the dose can be determined only when the aluminum oxide is analyzed by the dosimetry company.

Thermoluminescent Dosimeters

A third device used to monitor personnel exposure is the TLD. It consists of a plastic holder containing crystals that absorb a portion of the energy they receive from a radiation exposure. When the device is exposed, the absorbed energy causes the outer valence electrons to be trapped in the forbidden zone, the region immediately past their resting orbit. The number of electrons elevated to this state depends directly on the amount of radiation received. When the time comes to determine the dose, these crystals are heated so that the trapped electrons return to their original resting state. This process results in a release of the extra energy in the form of a light photon. The light is collected and analyzed to determine the quantity of the dose received by the TLD.

The crystal most commonly used in TLDs is lithium fluoride. Once the lithium fluoride crystals have been heated (*annealed*), they can then be reused—a feature that is not possible with

TABLE 9.5	Commonly Used Dosimeters in Diagnostic Radiography	
	Optically Stimulated Luminescence Dosimeters	**Thermoluminescent Dosimeters**
Construction	Plastic holder containing sensing material, tin and copper filters, and an open window	Plastic holder containing crystals of sensing material
Sensing material	Strip of aluminum oxide crystals	Lithium fluoride crystals
Processing	Crystals are heated; light emitted is proportional to the dose received	Crystals are heated; light emitted is proportional to the dose received
Maximum wear time	Up to 2 months	Up to 3 months
Sensitivity	1 mrem (0.01 mSv)	5 mrem (0.05 mSv)

a film badge. The TLD provides readings as low as 5 mrem (0.05 mSv; Table 9.5).

Pocket Dosimeters

The last dosimetry device is the pocket dosimeter, which appears similar to a pen flashlight and is constructed of a central metal electrode surrounded by air and enclosed in a metal holder. The electrode is positively charged; as the dosimeter is exposed to ionizing radiation, the air in the dosimeter is ionized. Negative ions moving toward the electrode combine with some of the positive charges, neutralizing the electrode. This loss in charge is proportional to the amount of radiation, and a pointer on a scale moves upward relative to the loss in charge. The pocket dosimeter is used when an immediate reading of occupational dose is desired; however, it is subject to false readings and does not provide a permanent record. Pocket dosimeters are not commonly used to monitor the exposure of medical imaging personnel.

Field Survey Instruments

Other types of instruments are used to detect the presence of radiation and give the user an indication of the intensity of the source. These devices are known as *field survey instruments*. A common instrument used to detect x-radiation, gamma radiation, and beta radiation is the Geiger-Müller counter, which is an ionization chamber constructed of an electrode housed within a chamber. The walls of the chamber are negatively charged, and the electrode is positive. When x-rays pass through the chamber and interact with the air, ionization occurs. Free electrons are attracted to the positively charged electrode, where they can be measured. The number of free electrons is directly proportional to the radiation exposure and can be displayed on a special meter that interprets this information and determines the exposure in roentgens or coulombs per kilogram.

SUMMARY

- Medical ionizing radiation is a form of electromagnetic radiation capable of penetrating matter and depositing energy as it travels. Although ionizing radiation can interact with matter in five ways, of particular importance to imaging are the photo-electric interaction and Compton effect. Both of these interactions contribute to

the creation of the diagnostic radiograph, and both contribute to the radiation exposure of the patient and the radiographer.
- The quantities of radiation important in radiography are exposure, absorbed dose, and dose equivalence. The traditional units used to measure these quantities were the roentgen, rad, and rem, and the corresponding SI units are coulombs per kilogram, gray, and sievert.
- Biologic changes that occur as a result of exposure to radiation begin at the cellular level. The effects depend on what type of cell was struck, how the energy was transferred, the type of radiation, and the sensitivity of the cell. The immediate response of the cell is to repair itself. However, when this self-repair is not possible, other changes begin to take place. These changes have an impact not only on the cells struck but also on all the systems that are composed of the cells. The effects resulting from exposure are either *somatic*, affecting the individual exposed, or *genetic*, affecting future generations through changes in germ cells. To minimize these changes, appropriate protective measures must be used.
- To minimize patient exposure, the radiographer must keep in mind all of the principles of image production that play a role in patient exposure. Examples of these factors are kilovoltage, image receptor speed, collimation, filtration, and repeated exposures. Whenever possible, shields must also be applied to protect the reproductive organs of the patient, provided the examination is not compromised. The radiographer must also protect himself or herself from unnecessary radiation through the use of the cardinal rules of protection—time, distance, and shielding. Finally, a record of the amount of radiation the occupational worker receives or to which he or she is exposed can be obtained by using monitoring devices such as OSL dosimeters, film badges, TLDs, and pocket dosimeters.

BIBLIOGRAPHY

Bushong C: *Radiologic science for technologists: physics, biology, and protection*, ed 11, St. Louis, 2017, Elsevier.

Carlton RC, Adler AM: *Principles of radiographic imaging: an art and a science*, ed 6, Albany, NY, 2019, Cengage.

Dorland's Illustrated Medical Dictionary, ed 31, Philadelphia, 2007, Saunders.

Hall EJ, Giaccia AJ: *Radiobiology for the radiologist*, ed 7, Philadelphia, 2012, Lippincott Williams & Wilkins.

National Council on Radiation Protection and Measurements: *SI units in radiation protection and measurements, NCRP Rep no. 82*, Bethesda, 1985, The Council.

National Council on Radiation Protection and Measurements: *Recommendations on limits for exposure to ionizing radiation, NCRP Rep no. 91, 1987*, Bethesda, Md, 1987, The Council.

National Council on Radiation Protection and Measurements: *Limitation of exposure to ionizing radiation, NCRP Rep no. 116*, Bethesda, Md, 1993, The Council.

Statkiewicz-Sherer MA, Visconti PJ, Ritenour ER, Haynes KW: *Radiation protection in medical radiography*, ed 8, St. Louis, 2017, Elsevier.

U.S. Food and Drug Administration: *Radiation emitting products*, Washington, DC, n.d., The Administration.

U.S. Nuclear Regulatory Commission: *Instruction concerning prenatal radiation exposure, Regulatory guide 8.13, rev 2*, Washington, 1987, The Commission.

U.S. Nuclear Regulatory Commission: *Standards for protection against radiation, 10 CFR Part 20*, Washington, DC, 1994, The Commission.

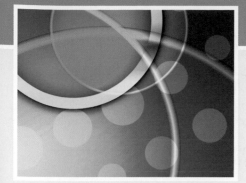

Human Diversity

Bettye G. Wilson, MAEd, RT(R)(CT), ARRT, RDMS, FASRT

Give me your tired, your poor,

Your huddled masses yearning to breathe free,

The wretched refuse of your teeming shore.

Send these, the homeless, tempest-tost to me,

I lift my lamp beside the golden door.

**Excerpted from the base of Statue of Liberty inscription,
"The New Colossus," a poem written by Emma Lazarus**

OBJECTIVES

On completion of this chapter, the student will be able to:
- Define human diversity.
- List some of the human diversity characteristics.
- Describe the human diversity traits of age, ethnicity or national origin, race, gender or sexual orientation, and mental and physical ability.
- Name the values that are prescribed to US mainstream culture.
- List the elements associated with cultural competency.

- Discuss valuing diversity.
- Know the empathetic practices that help foster cultural insight and produce improved outcomes.
- Describe the six areas of human diversity that health care providers need to understand to provide high-quality and effective care.
- Discuss ways in which professional medical imaging organizations have expressed valuing human diversity.

OUTLINE

KEY TERMS

Assimilation Process by which people of diverse backgrounds slowly give up their original cultural language and identity and melt into another, usually larger, group

Bias Prejudice; thinking negatively of others without any or significant justification; generally a combination of stereotyped beliefs and negative attitudes

Biculturalism Being able to negotiate two or more different cultures competently, individual and mainstream

Cultural Of or relating to culture

Cultures All of the socially transmitted behavior patterns, arts, beliefs, institutions, and all other products of human work and thoughts by particular classes, communities, or populations

Discrimination Actions involved in the unequal or prejudicial treatment of people because they belong to a certain category, group, or race. May also include disability, ethnicity, and sexual orientation.

Diverse Differing from one another; made up of distinct characteristics, qualities, or elements

Diversity Fact or quality of being diverse, different (all of the ways in which human beings are both similar and different)

Ethnic Designating any of the basic groups or divisions of humankind or of a heterogeneous population, as distinguished by customs, characteristics, language, and common history; national origin

Ethnicity Ethnic affiliation or classification

Ethnocentrism Tendency toward viewing the norms and values of the individual's own culture as absolute and using them as a standard against which all other cultures are measured

Gender Chromosomal designation of female or male being

Homophobia Irrational fear of and hostility toward homosexuality

Mental and Physical Abilities Capacity to perform cognitive and psychomotor tasks

Race Population that differs from others in the relative frequency of some gene or genes; any of the different varieties of humankind, distinguished by type of hair, color of eyes and skin, stature, bodily proportions, or other characteristics

Racism Belief in racial superiority, leading to discrimination and prejudice toward races considered inferior

Religion Belief in a divine or superhuman power or powers, to be obeyed and worshipped as the creator(s) and ruler(s) of the universe

HUMAN DIVERSITY

At the beginning of the 21st century the issue of human **diversity** was enjoying widespread importance throughout the United States and globally. The new millennium was perhaps the impetus for social change and acceptance, and understanding human diversity is at the heart of this issue. Human diversity, also called **cultural** diversity, addresses the variety of human societies and cultures and examines their similarities and differences. Taken literally, *human diversity* simply means the differences inherent among people. Studies indicate that these differences are what make each person unique and valuable in his or her own right. Humans are divided into different **cultures.** Cultures develop behaviors, norms, and values that are suited to a specific environment and over time take on the strength of tradition. Even when conditions or environments change, cultures often do not. Lifelong habits are, in fact, a form of conditioning that is difficult to overcome.

Throughout history the world has been composed of different nations and thus people of different cultures. Because of this composition, surprisingly, human diversity has only recently become an issue of utmost importance. Theories suggest that human diversity is more important today than ever before because of increased globalization. *Globalization* simply means that people now cross borders into other countries to work, go to school, receive medical care, visit, and live. This increase in globalization means that nations, societies, and businesses have become increasingly cross-cultural or multicultural.

Evidence of multiculturalism is everywhere—in cities, businesses, communities, educational institutions, and health care systems. With the influx of differing cultures, the need exists to understand, at least broadly, human diversity and to develop strategies to negotiate and mediate conflict caused by cultural differences. Colleges, universities, and businesses, as well as health care providers, institutions, and organizations, have taken the lead in fostering cultural diversity dialogue, education, understanding, and conflict resolution. Indeed, many educational institutions and businesses have developed positions and offices that deal only with diversity issues. Vice presidents for equity and diversity, offices of equity and diversity, diversity programs for employees, and other initiatives can be found that are meant solely to foster a positive **diverse** environment. Professional health care providers, including physicians, nurses, and technologists, have addressed human diversity issues through their professional organizations. The American Society of Radiologic Technologists (ASRT), the American Society of Diagnostic Medical Sonographers, and the Society of Nuclear Medicine–Technologist Section have all made positive steps in addressing diversity issues within their disciplines by establishing minority scholarships, mentoring programs, and other initiatives. In fact, these organizations, through their ethical codes and standards, prohibit discrimination by those practicing under their domains. Most of these initiatives begin with trying to get people to understand themselves and their own cultural biases first and then to understand, accept, and value the contributions of persons from other cultures. Health care institutions and organizations are also doing the same. In these institutions and organizations, the realization exists that patients and workers alike are becoming increasingly diverse, and the key to providing high-quality patient care to a diverse population, by a diverse health care work force, is through organized cultural diversity initiatives. A concerted push toward cultural competency can be found throughout the United States.

Cultural competency is defined as possessing a set of attitudes, behaviors, and policies that come together in a system, or among individuals, to enable effective interactions in a cross-cultural framework. Understanding and accepting the types of diversity are core to this process.

UNDERSTANDING HUMAN DIVERSITY

Characteristics

People have many differences, making them diverse as a whole. It has been said that no two people are exactly alike and that this uniqueness is what makes us individuals. Although the differences are intrinsic, extrinsic differences exist that further mark our diverse natures. Diversity includes many human characteristics that affect our perceptions of ourselves and others, individual values, opportunities, and acceptance. Some of the most prevalent characteristics are age, disability, economic status, education, **ethnicity,** family status, first language, gender, geographic location, lifestyle, organizational level, physical characteristics, political affiliation, religious preference, sexual orientation, work style or ethic, and many others.

Everyone has at least one personal **bias.** These biases, whether based on reason or simply perceptions of human characteristics, are real. Personal biases, even without conscious thought, play a major role in how individuals perceive others. Seemingly, the impact of some biases can be lessened through knowledge. The more that is known about a subject, the better the understanding of the subject will be. Examining all of the diverse human characteristics is not in the purview of this book or this chapter. Although there are many others, the following diversity topics will be addressed because of their designation as the common and significant human diversity traits within a society:

- Age
- Ethnicity and national origin
- Race
- Gender and sexual orientation
- Mental and physical ability
- Religion

Age. Some cultures and individuals assign different values based on age. For example, some Asian cultures specifically have an attitude of deference toward older adults. These cultures note that the advances in their society occurred because of the contributions made by their elderly citizens. European and Western cultures generally do not regard older adults in this manner. In fact, older adults are sometimes regarded as burdens on society. An upsurge in the reporting of cases of elder abuse may be considered a sign of a disregard of senior citizens.

Consider the latest (2010) US Census data:

- There has been an increase in individuals over the age of 60 years since 2000.
- There are 57,085,908 people over the age of 60 (18.5%), with 40,267,984 (13.0%) of those being over 65 years of age.
- In addition, 27,832,721 (9.0%) of the population is over the age of 70.
- There are 5,493,433 (1.8%) people 85 years of age or older.

Combined, these groups make up more than 40% of the total population, rivaling the population 18 to 44 years of age. As this so-called baby boomer generation ages, persons considered to be seniors will by most accounts overtake the current majority population. Therefore age biases must be corrected, and older individuals must be regarded for the value of the experiences and knowledge they have and continue to contribute to mainstream American business, cultural, economic, and social settings.

Americans have given names to subsets of the population. The term *baby boomer,* the most discussed subset because of sheer numbers, is applied to individuals born from 1946 to 1964. *Generation X* includes persons born from 1965 to 1980, and the *Generation Y* designation is applied to those born from 1981 to 1999. The term *Generation Z* (New Silent Generation) refers to those born from 2000 to the present.

The most significant subset, because of the impact they will have on the population, is the baby boomer group. Seventy-five million babies were born from 1946 to 1964. In the year 2006 the first of these individuals turned 60 years of age. This fact gives notice that in the coming decades a significant increase in the number of senior citizens and their proportion will occur in the total US population. In fact, projections are that the older adult population will increase substantially over the next three decades, with persons 85 years of age or older being the fastest growing segment of the population. Recent research suggests that this may not be true, since baby boomers are dying at a faster rate than projected and immigration of those in that generation has not kept pace. Some say that *Generation Y,* also termed *the Millennial Generation,* will soon, if not already, overtake the baby boomers as America's largest generation.

What must not be forgotten is that the baby boomer generation is considered to be generally healthy and well educated. These individuals are expected to stay in the workforce longer because they are expected to live longer than previous generations. In general, the graying of America is expected to transform many areas, including banking, health care, labor, politics, retirement systems, social services, and the stock market. This expectation forces an overview and overhaul of social mores and prejudices regarding older adults in the job market through their end-of-life care.

Time is not on the side of American society to address these issues. In 2000, Americans over the age of 85 outnumbered those at the beginning of the previous century by 26 times. At the beginning of 2010, more than 53,000 Americans were over the age of 100. Projections suggest that more than 1 million baby boomers will also live to see that age.

National policies geared toward baby boomer research and development have encountered heavy opposition because of many societal biases. Some of these biases include the following:

- Valuing youth over age
- Viewing of aging as something undesirable or bad
- Placing little value on the contributions of senior citizens
- Favoring reactive instead of proactive approaches to policy development and implementation
- Considering all senior citizens to be mentally inferior

Continued age bias exists within the United States, especially in the realm of employment. The *Age Discrimination in Employment Act,* 29 USC §§621-634, was passed with the intent of preventing employers from exhibiting **discrimination** based solely on age in hiring, promotion, job assignment, compensation, and termination. US society, and the institutions contained within, must work to eliminate biases associated with age. This goal must be an essential element of any cultural diversity initiatives. People of all ages make positive contributions to society.

Ethnicity, National Origin, and Race. Ethnicity relates to a person's distinctive racial, national, religious, linguistic, or cultural heritage. The term *race* also may be used to denote ethnicity. In the United States, the term *race* is most often used to distinguish between African Americans and Caucasians. The United States has long considered itself a melting pot of people with diverse **ethnic** heritages. Indeed, the Statue of Liberty beckons all people to our shores, although governmental practices during the last few years have restricted our acceptance of all people. Many people throughout the world still consider America the land of freedom and opportunity. Some of those who now call America home came to pursue the promised opportunities, others came to escape persecution and oppression, and still others were brought to this country under servitude. Whatever the reason that individuals come to and remain in America, all are considered Americans. A special debt of gratitude is owed to the Native Americans who inhabited this land before its existence was *discovered.* Native Americans played an instrumental role in the successful colonization of this great nation through their assistance and friendship. The settlers and the natives were the first diverse ethnic groups in the United States. From that point on, numerous other ethnic

TABLE 10.1   2010 US Census Data Report on the Ethnic and Racial Makeup of the Population (1000)

US Population (1000)	2005	2007	2008	2009
Caucasian alone	237,251	240,947	242,685	244,298
African American/black alone	37,813	38,742	39,205	39,641
Native America/Alaska Native alone	2,924	3,038	3,095	3,151
Asian alone	12,571	13,307	13,655	14,014
Native Hawaiian/other Pacific Islander alone	527	553	566	578
Combination (≥2)	4,666	4,993	5,159	5,324
Hispanic or Latino origin (may be of any race)	42,552	45,508	46,979	47,655

groups have joined the ranks of American culture, although many were not born in this country. The 2010 US Census data provide interesting statistics on the ethnic and racial makeup of the population. Table 10.1 contains growth trends among the groups for 2005 through 2009.

The census also addresses trends in growth, projecting that the US Hispanic population will grow at a faster rate than all other minority groups. Further projections include data suggesting that the current majority ethnic group will lose that designation within the current century because of the combined growth among the now minority groups and immigrants. This projection means that the US population will become increasingly diverse, and the need to understand and accept human diversity as a fact of life is more important than ever. To understand and accept human diversity and to create and maintain a society that is mutually inclusive, ethnocentrism and racism must be eliminated. **Ethnocentrism** is regarded as the tendency of some individuals to view norms and values of their own culture as the only acceptable ones and to use them as the standard by which all other cultures are measured. **Racism** is the belief that one race or culture is superior to others and the use of this belief to discriminate against races that the believer considers to be inferior. When ethnocentrism and racism are allowed to exist within a society, discrimination, prejudice, and oppression are often also evident and expressed. For individuals to live and work together for the mutual good of everyone, people must learn to value the contributions of all individuals, respect all cultures, and live together as one race: human.

In the past, the interaction of culturally different individuals with mainstream (majority) culture has been that of either assimilation or biculturalism. **Assimilation** is described as the process by which persons of a diverse (different) culture, over time, give up their original cultural language and identify with, and try to merge into, another culture (usually the majority). **Biculturalism** is the ability of individuals to be able to competently negotiate two or more cultures: the mainstream culture and the individual's own culture.

Assimilation, by definition, promotes a loss of the contributions and customs of a minority culture as individuals try to become accepted by the majority or mainstream culture. Members of the US mainstream culture are said to value and identify with the following:

- Activity and hard work
- Personal achievement and success
- Individualism
- Efficiency and practicality

TABLE 10.2   Some Core Values Exhibited by the More Prevalent Ethnic Cultures Within the US Population

Ethnic Group	Core Values
African American	Extended family
	Cooperation
	Spirituality
	Interdependence
Latino	Extended family
	Father as patriarch
	Respect
	Hierarchical relationships
Mexican American	Extended family (close-knit)
	Curanderism (Mexican folk healing)
	Frequent contact with native country (Mexico)
	Respect
Native American	Extended family
	Spiritualism
	Collectivism
	Unified whole universe
US mainstream	Individualism
	Affluence (material comfort, consumerism)
	Competition
	Personal achievement and success

- Affluence, consumerism, and material comfort
- Competition
- Openness, directness, and being well informed

Assimilation diminishes the accomplishments, contributions, and values of one culture in favor of those of the mainstream. People of different ethnicities may have different core values, although people who reside in the United States also generally prescribe to core values of the mainstream. This tendency means that most US residents are bicultural. Some of the core values of individuals within the prevalent ethnic groups within the United States are listed in Table 10.2.

As may be learned from the information in Table 10.2, many differences exist among cultural values. Cultural values are simply socially shared ideas about what is good, moral, and right and what is bad, immoral, and wrong. What must be understood so that generalizations and stereotyping about an ethnic group are not fostered is that not all members of a specific cultural group share the values of the group as a whole and not all members show absolute compliance with their defining culture.

Ethnic and racial cultural differences are often accompanied by linguistic differences. This difference has become evident as the US population grows increasingly diverse. Linguistic differences cause problems with communication. Speaking to and understanding people whose language is not the same as the majority of individuals in the mainstream culture of a society are difficult. In the United States, linguistic differences have provided fodder for controversy. Several groups in this country, which are quite vocal, have taken the position that, because the United States is an English-speaking country, policies should be adopted that require English to be spoken by every resident. What these groups may have failed to realize is that the United States has never adopted an official language. What these groups are essentially seeking is assimilation, which generally does not come easily. Many people believe that *when in Rome, one should do as the Romans do,* meaning if you are in the United States, you should speak English. The answer to the linguistic cultural barrier may not be known for some time. What is known is that to communicate with people from diverse cultures, a common method of communication must be developed. This concept is particularly important in the delivery of services, especially education and health care.

The quality of health care delivery depends to a great extent on communication between providers and consumers. Individuals who are limited in English proficiency pose a real challenge to the delivery of high-quality health care. This cultural barrier subrogates patient rights and responsibilities, as well as the rights of providers. If a patient does not or cannot understand his or her health care providers, and vice versa, essential information cannot be communicated. Simple commands or questions can be difficult for a provider to convey. Table 10.3 contains some common commands and questions used in medical imaging in English with translation into Spanish, French, German, Italian, and Japanese. Although the content in this table is as accurate as the sources from which it was retrieved, there are words and phrases in other languages that vary in their meaning and intent.

One of the major concerns of linguistic differences is informed consent. A patient cannot be truly informed if he or she does not understand what is attempted to be communicated to them. This failure places health care providers at great liability and serves as a barrier to medical treatment decisions. To provide improved medical care to individuals without or with limited English proficiency, many health care institutions are striving to overcome linguistic barriers to high-quality health care by doing the following:

- Hiring additional bilingual and bicultural staff
- Providing medical interpreters
- Providing translators
- Encouraging employees to become bilingual or multilingual
- Providing medical documents (e.g., consent forms) in different languages

These measures are a good start in significantly improving the quality of health care for people who do not speak or understand English, the majority language of the US culture; however, more measures will probably need to be undertaken as additional linguistic barriers to health care are encountered. Believing that every health care provider will be able to competently communicate with every person who does not speak English is unreasonable. Complete linguistic competency may be an elusive goal but is one toward which increasing progress must be

TABLE 10.3	Common Commands and Questions Used in Medical Imaging
English	Hello, what is your name?
Spanish	¿Hola, cuál es su nombre?
French	Bonjour, quel est votre nom?
German	Hallo, was ist ihr name?
Italian	Ciao, che cosa é il vostro nome?
Japanese	こんにちは、お名前は何ですか。
English	Take a deep breath.
Spanish	Tomar una respiración profunda.
French	Prenez un soufflé profound.
German	Nehmen Sie einen tiefen Atem.
Italian	Prenda un alito profondo.
Japanese	深呼吸してください。
English	Hold your breath.
Spanish	Contenga La respiracion.
French	Tenee votre soufflé.
German	Halten Sie ihren Atem.
Italian	Tenga il rostro alito.
Japanese	呼吸を止めて。
English	Breathe.
Spanish	Respirar.
French	Respirez.
German	Atmen Sie.
Italian	Respiri.
Japanese	呼吸してください。
English	Show me where you hurt.
Spanish	Muestrame donde daeles
French	Montres moi oûvous blessez.
German	Zeigen Sie mir Sie verletzen.
Italian	Mostrimi dove danneggiate.
Japanese	痛いところはどこですか。
English	Radiology
Spanish	Radiologia
French	Radiologie
German	Radiologie
Italian	Radiologia
Japanese	放射線学
English	x-ray
Spanish	Radiografia or rayos X
French	Rayon-x
German	Röntgenstrahle
Italian	Raggi X
Japanese	x線

made. Discrimination is often fostered in part by the inability to understand people who do not look, act, or speak the same as most of the members of the majority culture.

In the book *What Language Does Your Patient Hurt In? A Practical Guide to Culturally Competent Patient Care* the authors attempt to provide information that health care professionals may use when interacting with patients from different cultures. Although not all cultures are addressed, African American, American Indian, Asian, Hispanic, Middle Eastern, and former Soviet Bloc cultures are.

To lessen the impact of discrimination based on ethnicity and race, the 19th-century Civil Rights Acts, amended in 1993, ensures that all persons have equal rights under law. In addition, it provides an outline of the damages available to people receiving actions under the *Civil Rights Act* of 1964, Title VII, the *Americans with Disabilities Act* of 1990, and the *Rehabilitation Act* of

1973. Although government statutes exist to protect individuals based on ethnicity and race, such laws may not be necessary if people understand that individuals from all ethnicities and races have contributed positively to the growth and development of humankind and continue to do so. Understanding this concept is a giant step toward respecting and valuing human diversity.

Sometimes I feel discriminated against, but it does not make me angry. It merely astonishes me. How can anyone deny themselves the pleasure of my company? It's beyond me.

Zora Neale Hurston

Gender and Sexual Orientation. Human beings are genetically divided into two groups according to sex: female or male. **Gender** describes the biologic or chromosomal sexual identity of an individual. Gender identity can be described as an inner sense of maleness or femaleness that may be influenced by several factors, including culture. US mainstream culture has progressively come to realize and include contributions made by females outside of the home and in child rearing. In the early 1900s, traditional female roles outside of the home were in the areas of teaching, clerical work, and nursing. By the end of that century, women had permeated and became accepted as executive officers of corporations, physicians, lawyers, politicians, and other professionals. However, women within these fields still often face what is known as a *glass ceiling,* in which they are precluded from being promoted to high-level positions because of their gender. Just as discrimination based on age and ethnicity still exists, discrimination based on gender also exists. This tendency exists in spite of the fact that women are as capable and as educated as many men.

Historically, women have often been called *the weaker sex,* and some people have even considered women incapable of performing certain tasks at all, or at least not as well as men. Even some research studies reported in the news media have erroneously suggested that women also do not have the intellectual capacity to solve complex analytic problems and are therefore not suited for some professions such as engineering and research. Regardless of data to the contrary, these misconceptions still persist into the 21st century.

Although the genetic makeup of men and women differs, both are equally capable. From birth, boys and girls are often treated differently. Many adults are predisposed in their thinking as to what boys should do and what girls should do. Even the types and colors of clothes worn by an infant indicate whether the child is a boy or a girl (i.e., pink for girls, blue for boys). Little girls play with dolls and have tea parties; little boys are steered toward playing with cars, trucks, footballs, and basketballs. This steering is called *gender role stereotyping.* Gender role stereotyping is the expectation of how people should behave based solely on whether they are male or female beings. These stereotypes have nothing to do with the individual's capabilities, but they limit his or her alternatives. Only by recognizing, promoting, and valuing the capabilities and contributions of individuals, male or female, can society embrace gender diversity as one of the essential elements for embracing human diversity.

Sexual orientation is another area of diversity often found under the topic of gender. This topic includes heterosexuality,

homosexuality, and bisexuality. Heterosexual individuals are persons who are mentally, physically, and sexually attracted to individuals of the opposite gender. Homosexual, lesbian, or gay individuals are persons who are mentally, physically, and sexually attracted to persons of their same gender. Bisexual people are persons who are mentally, physically, and sexually attracted to members of both genders. These three groups have coexisted in society throughout history, but heterosexuality is generally the most accepted practice. However, in the latter part of the last century, homosexual and bisexual individuals sought acceptance and recognition. They also sought to end discrimination based on sexual orientation and to seek equal treatment for themselves and their partners. This effort has been met with some societal resistance, but some successes have been reported in the area of gay rights. As of the writing of the last edition of this text, 17 states and the District of Columbia had legalized same-sex marriages, either by court decision, by state legislatures, or by popular vote.

In June of 2015, the Supreme Court of the United States reached a landmark decision regarding this issue. The Court decided that same-sex couples have the constitutional right to marry. This 103-page ruling made same-sex marriages legal in all states. Citing the Fourteenth Amendment's Due Process Clause, the justices reminded us that the clause as a part of the Amendment provides protection of fundamental liberties. These liberties extend into certain personal choices, such as intimate choices that define an individual's personal identity and belief. These liberties are at the core of a person's dignity and autonomy.

Although the legalization of same-sex marriages represents a huge step in acceptance of these unions, individuals leading *alternative lifestyles*—including those described as homosexual, lesbian, gay, or bisexual—live, work, and make positive contributions to society and deserve equality. What is problematic is that numerous individuals do not like these members of society and are in fact considered homophobic.

Homophobia is the irrational fear of homosexuality, accompanied by hostility toward individuals who are or are perceived to be homosexual, gay, lesbian, or bisexual. Although homophobia remains, the impetus for change in the way individuals in society think about homosexual and bisexual individuals began early in the 1900s.

The history of homosexuality reveals that these individuals have had a long struggle in their quest for acceptance. They have experienced and continue to experience isolation, alienation from loved ones and compatriots, ridicule, and abuse. Not until the 1930s did research on homosexuality begin to be conducted in earnest and on a large scale. In 1938, Dr. Alfred Kinsey initiated what would become an unsurpassed analysis of human sexuality. Dr. Kinsey's research lasted for 20 years, with the release of his first findings occurring at midpoint in 1948. Dr. Kinsey's work is credited with providing statistical documentation and validation of homosexuality within the populace. Dr. Kinsey developed a scale that included six parameters of sexual tendencies within the population. The publication of the *Kinsey Scale,* or *KSix,* is considered a landmark in the study of homosexuality, providing the beginning of a reversal of negative connotations associated with homosexuality. Box 10.1 describes the Kinsey rating scale of sexual orientation.

BOX 10.1 Kinsey Scale of Heterosexuality and Homosexuality (KSix)

- **0:** Exclusively heterosexual experience(s)
- **1:** Predominantly heterosexual experience(s), only incidentally homosexual
- **2:** Predominantly heterosexual experience(s), but more than incidentally homosexual
- **3:** Equally heterosexual and homosexual experience(s)
- **4:** Predominantly homosexual experience(s), but more than incidentally heterosexual
- **5:** Predominantly homosexual experience(s), but only incidentally heterosexual
- **6:** Exclusively homosexual experience(s)

NOTE: Kinsey used this scale in the original report of his findings on heterosexual and homosexual behavior within the population. Kinsey found that American male individuals fell in the category of 1 to 2 but that the majority fell within 1 to 5, and at least appeared to be somewhat bisexual. He also reported that 10% of American males were exclusively homosexual.

As may be noted in Box 10.1, KSix provides data on the prevalence of individuals with homosexual and bisexual tendencies compared with those having strictly heterosexual tendencies. For the first time, research suggested that homosexuality and bisexuality were not as rare as many people thought. People began to realize that they were working and interacting with homosexual and bisexual individuals and that these individuals were making positive contributions to society. This type of forward thinking has led to an increasingly accepting climate for persons leading alternative lifestyles within society and fosters a better understanding of human diversity, although hate crimes against these individuals continue to occur.

Mental and Physical Ability. Mental and physical abilities vary across the spectrum of the population as a whole. The intelligence quotient is used to determine if individuals have normal, superior, or inferior intellectual capability. Physical and mental parameters are used to judge whether individuals are able to perform tasks that are considered essential to everyday life at the level of persons who are considered normal. Certainly, people do not have the same mental and physical abilities. However, the majority of people can just as certainly make some positive contribution to society in some form.

Throughout history, people with what are considered as less-than-normal physical or mental capacity and those having certain medical diseases have often been shunned by society. In some instances these individuals were kept away from mainstream society for fear that they would be ridiculed, shunned, or worse. They were also seen as objects requiring assistance, protection, and treatment, rather than subjects of human rights. This thinking often led to these individuals being denied the equal access to the basic freedoms and rights that most people take for granted (e.g., education, employment, health care, participation in cultural and social activities).

More than 600 million individuals, accounting for approximately 10% of the world's population, have some type of disability. Some of these individuals have severe disabilities; others have moderate or mild disabilities. Some enjoy favorable living

TABLE 10.4 Four Core Values of Human Rights Law and How Each Relates to Individuals With a Disability

Value	Relationship to Disabled
Autonomy	Provides respect for the right of persons with a disability to have self-directed actions and behaviors and requires that the individual be the ultimate consideration and at the center of all decisions that affect her or him
Dignity	Provides mechanisms that recognize and support the inestimable value of, because of her or his inherent self-worth, every individual, regardless of ability
Equality	Relates to the fair and equal treatment of everyone, regardless of perceived differences, including a disability
Solidarity	Requires society to support and maintain the freedoms of individuals with application of the appropriate social mechanisms

conditions, whereas others do not. Many are well taken care of, and others are not. Regardless of their level of disability, living condition, or level of care, these individuals often share a common bond—discrimination and social exclusion.

During the last three decades, a shift in perspective has taken place regarding people with disabilities. Disabled individuals have been accorded the same rights as those without disabilities. Many nations have addressed this issue, including the United States. This profound shift in the way disabled people are treated has also been endorsed by the United Nations.

The *Americans with Disabilities Act* of 1990 was a profound and necessary step in preventing discrimination against persons with disabilities. It provides protection, under the law, for people with mental or physical disabilities. It also directs institutions, especially those receiving federal funds, to make *reasonable accommodations* for persons with disabilities. Facilities are required to be accessible to all individuals.

In addition to efforts in the United States, the United Nations and other conventions have addressed the issues of persons with disabilities and have kept these issues at center stage since the UN General Assembly proclaimed 1981 as the International Year of the Disabled. In 1993 the UN General Assembly adopted a resolution: Standard Rules on the Equalization of Opportunities for People with Disabilities. The aim of the Standard Rules is to ensure that people with disabilities, as members of their societies, be allowed to exercise the same rights and obligations as all others; it also requires states to remove obstacles to equal participation.

Also in 1993 the Vienna Declaration for Human Rights reaffirmed the commitment of the world to eradicate discrimination based on disability. The declaration states that *all human rights and fundamental freedoms are universal and thus unreservedly include persons with disabilities.* This declaration placed the treatment of persons with disabilities in a human rights context.

All of these efforts are directed at enhancing, promoting, and protecting the human rights of persons with disabilities. Four essential core values of human rights law are particularly important when thinking about people with disabilities: (1) autonomy, (2) dignity, (3) equality, and (4) solidarity. Table 10.4 lists additional information on these core values.

Worldwide, many nations, including the United States, are committed to promoting equality and full participation in society for persons with disabilities. Although the process may seem slow, reform in the way individuals with disabilities are viewed is underway. Nondiscrimination, equal access, and the equally effective enjoyment of all human rights by people with disabilities are long overdue. Disabilities are just one of the many diverse areas among human beings. Discrimination, inequality, and injustice applied to persons with disabilities deprive society of their active participation, as well as significant contributions. Avoiding the term *disabled,* which tends to provoke a negative mindset because of the prefix *dis* (meaning "to deprive of"), and instead thinking of these individuals as being differently *abled,* might promote a different mindset and alter society's perception. These differences are the core element of human diversity.

Religion. Religion is a very important part of culture. Its existence must not be ignored in the quest to provide equal and quality health care services to a diverse group of consumers. Hundreds of different religions exist, and just as many differing beliefs even within the same religion. This realization has led to some medical schools offering courses on medicine and spirituality. Health care providers, like their patients, have their own religious or spiritual beliefs, and sometimes these beliefs differ totally. Some people believe that their beliefs are the only ones that are correct and try to persuade others to change theirs. It must be remembered that to embrace cultural diversity, we must embrace cultural differences in religious beliefs and practice. The study of world religions will help in understanding differing beliefs, practices, and taboos.

Not all individuals have religious beliefs; some are atheists and some are agnostics. Still others consider themselves to be spiritual without subscribing to a specific religion. When dealing with any of these individuals, the radiologic technologist or radiation therapist must be careful not to offend the patient by ignoring or insulting their beliefs or lack thereof. In the preface to the book *World Religions for Healthcare Professionals,* the editors make the statement, "Regardless of the context from which you offer healthcare, providers must also be purposeful in this day and age to attend to matters of religion. The religious diversity that healthcare providers face in the lives of their patients is unprecedented in world history. North America is the most religiously diverse culture to ever appear and our healthcare providers must deal with this fact routinely." Health care providers would be wise to heed their advice.

EMBRACING DIVERSITY

As mentioned in each of the preceding sections, individuals from all different cultures have contributed positively to society. A realization that everyone should learn to live and work with people who may be culturally different should also exist. In addition, goods and services are consumed and provided by people from different cultures. By recognizing, accepting, and learning about cultures that may be different from their own, people can learn ways of avoiding conflict among cultures and enjoy a more inclusive, representative, nondiscriminatory society. Only then can human diversity be fully embraced and valued.

Living and working in a diverse society is challenging. Civility and respect for others, in both areas, is expected. This respect comes from individuals and begins with first learning about other cultures. Many misconceptions exist about other groups of individuals. These misconceptions may have been developed and fostered by the beliefs and experiences of others and not as a result of personal contact. By learning ways to accommodate diversity, people can become increasingly adept at dealing with others.

A good example of the application of respect is the #MeToo movement that began in late 2017 to empower women through empathy, especially the experiences of young and vulnerable brown or black women. The phrase was designed to help reveal the extent of problems with sexual harassment and assault by showing how many people have experienced these events themselves. After millions of people started using the phrase, and it spread to dozens of other languages, the purpose changed and expanded, as a result there is also a focus on determining the best ways to hold perpetrators responsible and break the cycle. It has been estimated by the World Health Organization that sexual harassment affects a third of all women worldwide. A 2017 poll found that 54% of American women report receiving "unwanted and inappropriate" sexual advances with 95% saying that such behavior usually goes unpunished. In addition, #MeToo underscores the need for men to intervene in situations when they see demeaning behavior. The #MeToo movement is helping society understand the magnitude of the problem. It requires men to take a stand against behavior that objectifies women. This means changes in laws and building a culture that respects women's right to object and be taken seriously.

> *Diversity transcends race and gender, affirmative action, and equal employment opportunity. It must encompass a fundamental appreciation of one another and a respect for both our similarities and our differences. It must include a heartfelt respect in attitude and in behavior toward those of different race, gender, age, sexual orientation, and those with disabilities. All the facets that make each individual the unique and precious resource that each of us is.*
>
> **Ronald Brown, Former Secretary of Commerce**

Learning is the essential element of knowledge. Understanding and accepting cannot take place if a refusal to learn exists. Interacting with different cultures personally, socially, and on a business level assists in the learning process. Knowledge itself does not automatically transcend into better outcomes; other steps also need to be taken. Policies and practices must also be put in place to allow forward thinking, acceptance, and inclusion of differing cultures. Knowledge about individuals and groups of people should be integrated and transformed into standards, policies, practices, and attitudes that are used in the appropriate cultural settings so as to increase the quality of services. A better quality of care occurs when an atmosphere is provided in which everyone acquires knowledge and skills that can be shared by all.

DEVELOPING CULTURAL COMPETENCY

Cultural competency is defined as possessing a set of attitudes, congruent behaviors, and policies that come together in an agency, in a system, or among professionals that enable effective interactions in a cross-cultural or multicultural environment. Many elements may contribute to the ability of an agency or institution to become culturally competent. Five of these elements are the following:

1. Valuing diversity
2. Possessing the capacity for cultural self-assessment
3. Having a consciousness of the dynamics of cross-cultural interaction
4. Institutionalizing cultural knowledge
5. Developing adaptations of service delivery that reflect an understanding of a multicultural environment

These five elements will not work in isolation within an agency or organization. They must be demonstrated at every level within the institution, including administration, policy making, and services. Becoming culturally competent does not happen overnight; it is an ongoing process that requires reevaluation of the ways things are done within an agency or organization and how those things influence the environment and the services rendered.

For total cultural competency to be achieved, consideration must be given to all of the areas of human diversity, including language. Linguistic competency means providing readily available, culturally appropriate oral and written language services to individuals with limited English proficiency. This goal may be accomplished through the use of bicultural and bilingual individuals or interpreters.

In health care, including medical imaging and radiation therapy, human diversity has always been evident. To provide health care consumers (patients) with high-quality patient care, diagnosis, and treatment, clear and unimpeded communication must occur. Health care providers must not demonstrate bias toward any patient for any reason; rather, they must strive to understand and accept the cultural differences of patients because of their age, ethnicity, physical and mental abilities, gender and sexual orientation, and illness or disease.

Certified and registered medical imaging technologists and radiation therapists are governed by professional codes and standards that preclude discriminatory practices and provide for delivery of high-quality patient care with disregard for cultural differences. The standards of ethics and the incorporated code of ethics of the American Registry of Radiologic Technologists (ARRT) (see Appendix D) specifically address non-discriminatory professional practice by persons holding ARRT credentials. The ASRT has also developed initiatives to increase cultural diversity among members of the profession. One of the more notable initiatives is the establishment of the Royce Osborne Minority Student Scholarship. The scholarship fund, endowed by the ARRT, provides scholarships to minority imaging and therapy students in educational programs throughout the country. The ASRT has also issued several position statements in support of cultural competency and has incorporated ethical and professional attributes into documents governing those practicing in medical imaging and radiation therapy. The ARRT and ASRT, as well as many other professional imaging organizations, have tried to make it clear that they value human diversity and the contributions made to the profession by the diverse population of administrators, clinicians, educators, and managers alike.

Medical professionals are embracing diversity and striving toward cultural competency, but they face unique challenges. Although they have become increasingly knowledgeable about issues of diversity in health care, medical professionals have not necessarily become effective. They know that patients, whatever their cultural background, require dignity and respect and need to feel seen and heard as individuals. Knowledge of different cultures and empathy toward all patients are two ways that providers can become culturally competent in providing care. Empathy may be the core skill needed in health care intervention. Three critical empathetic practices help bridge cultural insight and produce better outcomes:

- Making quick, powerful connections with patient (communication)
- Gathering culturally relevant information (assessment and communication)
- Working with patients to form strategies that meet their individual needs, the needs of the provider, and the needs of the medical facility or practice (negotiating)
- The application of empathy skills accomplishes the following:
- Promotes better health care outcomes overall
- Increases patient satisfaction
- Decreases health care costs
- Decreases provider liability

Health care providers need information, and one of the best ways of obtaining culturally relevant information is by emphasizing empathy through intense listening and curiosity. The core of empathetic communication is accurately understanding patient feelings and communicating this understanding back to them effectively. Empathy is therapeutic in that it provides the patient with a feeling of being understood by the health care provider, makes the patient feel less isolated by illness or disease, and gives the patient a sense of individuality.

To provide high-quality and effective care for all patients, health care providers need to understand the following six areas of human cultural diversity and how these areas influence the delivery of care:

1. Communication
2. Space
3. Time
4. Environmental control
5. Biologic variations
6. Social organizations

Table 10.5 provides a definition for each of these areas.

Becoming culturally competent is no easy task, but it is an essential one. Society is becoming more diverse on a daily basis. We can no longer ignore the impact of our multicultural society. Members of society must learn to value human diversity and become culturally competent. This knowledge can only enrich society as a whole.

TABLE 10.5 Six Areas of Human Cultural Diversity Related to Health Care and Their Impact on Care Delivery

Area	Definition and Impact on Health Care
Communication	The ability to convey and receive information. Knowing the norm within a culture will facilitate understanding and lessen miscommunication. Miscommunication is a frequent problem among different cultures.
Space	Distance extending in all directions. Proximity to personal boundaries and comfort level—eye contact, distance, and touch practices—vary among cultures. Failure to understand and respect different cultural practices, including space, may cause miscommunication and lessen regard for health care providers.
Time	Period of duration; indefinite, unlimited duration in which things are considered as happening (e.g., past, present, future). Cultures have different time orientations—for example, England and China seem to be oriented in the past, valuing tradition and doing things as they have always been done; people from these countries may be hesitant to try new medical procedures or treatments. Present-oriented cultures (e.g., Latin American, Native American, Middle Eastern) may neglect preventive care measures because they focus on the here and now. Health care providers must work with these cultures in an attempt to get these individuals to understand that medicine is focused on both prevention and treatment and that everyone can live a healthy and long life.
Environmental control	Ability of people to control nature. Differences in health practices and definitions of health and illness are evident in the different cultures. These variations need to be understood so that the appropriate actions can be undertaken to preserve the health of individuals and provide adequate treatment while preserving cultural concepts.
Biologic variations	Ethnical or racially related differences in body structure, skin color, hair texture, and other physical characteristics; the term also addresses genetic variations, susceptibility to certain diseases, nutritional preferences and differences, and psychological characteristics, among others. Health care providers must understand how these biologic variations affect the health of individuals within the different ethnic cultures, and they must secure diagnosis and provide treatment based on some of these variations.
Social organizations	Patterns of behaviors related to cultures learned through the process of enculturation. Health care providers must recognize these differences and accept them. Providers need to know that in some cultures great value is placed on the decisions made by the elders. In others, the expectations and roles of children are strictly defined.

SUMMARY

- Human diversity is a topic of global importance. The people of the world have noticed that their societies are becoming increasingly diverse. Individuals need to learn to accept multiculturalism so that all people can believe that they are an integral part of the society in which they live. For acceptance of human diversity to develop, the concept of human diversity itself must first be understood. Inherent biases may hinder this understanding, but knowledge about the various cultures may help erase some of these biases. In addition, learning about the laws and statutes that help protect some cultures from discrimination is helpful as individuals in a society learn to embrace and value human diversity. That these laws and statutes were developed as a direct result of past discrimination and inequality also must be remembered. Many countries throughout the world, including in the United States, are seeking ways to teach their citizens to be accepting of multiculturalism. Corporations, industry, education, and health care institutions are in the midst of a cultural diversity awareness and competency movement. Health care institutions, organizations, and professionals are taking a strong lead in recognizing that patients, as well as workers, are culturally diverse. Patient care hinges on understanding, communication, and empathy, and health care is fostering the development of these skills in every practitioner, because doing so will directly benefit society (US culture) as a whole. Human diversity has positively influenced society, and the recognition of this influence through cultural competency can only have greater positive impacts on society.

Always remember that you are unique, just like everybody else.
Anonymous

BIBLIOGRAPHY

29, USC §§621-634: Age Discrimination Employment Act.
42, USC Chapter 21: Civil Rights Act of 1964.
42, USC §§1981, 1981a, 1983, 1988: Nineteenth Century Civil Rights Acts.
42, USC §§102: Americans with Disabilities Act of 1990.
American Registry of Radiologic Technologists: Ethics Division: Standards of Ethics. Available at: http://www.arrt.org. Accessed November 1, 2015.
American Society of Radiologic Technologists: Scholarships. Available at: www.asrt.org. Accessed January 10, 2017.
Bonder B, Martin L, Miracle A: Achieving cultural competence: the challenge for clients and healthcare workers in a multicultural society, *Generations* 25:35, 2001.
Culturaldiversity.org: *Transcultural nursing: basic concepts and case studies: assessment measures.* Available at: http://www.culturediversity.org/assesmnt.htm. Accessed February 19, 2014.
Dictionary.com translator. Available at: http://dictionary.reference.com/translate/text.html. Accessed November 2, 2009.
Fourteenth Amendment – Legal dictionary: Available at: https://legal-dictionaty.the free dictionary.om/FourteenthAmendment. Assessed October 21, 2017.
Freeman Institute: *Diversity: the value of mutual respect.* Available at: www.freemaninstitute.com/diversity.htm. Accessed January 2, 2014.
Gilanti GA: *Caring for patients from different cultures.* Philadelphia, 2008, University of Pennsylvania Press.
Radu, S. "How #MeToo has awoken women around the world," 2017, US News. Archived from the original on January 6, 2018. Retrieved January 6, 2018.
Salimbebe S, Eason C, Burch P, et al.: *What language does your patient hurt in? A practical guide to culturally competent patient care,* ed 2, St. Paul, Minn, 2006, ECM/Paradigm Publishing.
Scotus Gay Marriage Decision: Available at: https://govtsearches.com/Scotus Rulings. Assessed Oct 2, 2017.

Shams-Avari P: Linguistic and cultural competency, *Radiol Technol* 76:437, 2005.

Sorajjkool S, Carr MF, Nam JJ, editors: *World religions for healthcare professionals*, New York, 2010, Routledge.

Spanish translation of English Medical terms: Available at: https://translate.google.com. Assessed October 1, 2017.

Townsley-Cook D, Young T: *Ethical and legal issues for medical imaging professionals*, St. Louis, 2007, Mosby.

University of Alabama at Birmingham, Office of the Vice President for Equity and Diversity: Diversity. Available at: http://www.uab.edu/equityanddiversity. Accessed December 10, 2013.

U.S. Department of Commerce: *U.S. Census Bureau: Statistical abstract of the United States*, Washington, DC, 2011, U.S. Government Printing Office.

Wilson BG: *Ethics and basic law for medical imaging professionals*, Philadelphia, 1997, FA Davis.

Zillman, C: *A new poll on sexual harassment suggests why 'Me Too' went so insanely viral*, 2017, Fortune. Archived from the original on January 13, 2018. Retrieved January 13, 2018.

PART III

Patient Care

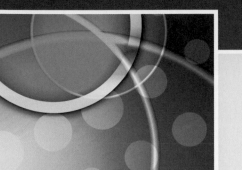

Patient Interactions

Bettye G. Wilson, MAEd, RT(R)(CT), ARRT, RDMS, FASRT

Once one learns to cut himself off from his feeling, it is sometimes frightening to realize how difficult it seems to get back in touch with them. This cannot always be done at 5:00 pm on schedule, and the student soon learns, like Dr. Jekyll, that the potion doesn't always wear off when it's time to go home.

David Reiser and Andrea Schroder
Patient Interviewing: The Human Dimension

OBJECTIVES

On completion of this chapter, the student will be able to:

- Identify qualities needed to be a caring radiologic technologist.
- Specify needs that cause people to enter radiologic technology as a profession.
- Discuss general needs that patients may have according to Maslow's hierarchy of needs.
- Relate differences between the needs of inpatients and those of outpatients.
- Explain why patient interaction is important to patients, as well as their family and friends.

- Analyze effective methods of communicating with patients of various ages.
- Explain appropriate interaction techniques for various types of patients.
- Discuss considerations of the physical changes of aging with regard to radiologic procedures.
- Discuss appropriate methods of responding to terminally ill patients.

OUTLINE

KEY TERMS

Advance Directive Legal document prepared by a living, competent adult to provide guidance to the health care team if the individual should become unable to make decisions regarding his or her medical care; may also be called a living will or durable power of attorney for health care

Communication Exchange of information, thoughts, or messages; includes interpersonal rapport; also includes the accurate conveyance of information, clear self-expression, and transmission of information and ideas to others. Medical charting and documentation is a form of communication between health care professionals.

Emotional Intelligence (EI) Ability to evaluate, perceive, and control emotions

Gerontology Pertaining to the study of older adults

Inpatient Someone who has been admitted to the hospital for diagnostic studies or treatment

Maslow's Hierarchy of Needs Model of human needs developed by Abraham Maslow, original hierarchy identifies two types of needs: deficiency and growth needs were further divided into seven levels, four at the deficiency needs level (physiologic, safety, belongingness and love, and esteem) and three in the upper growth needs

level (need to know and understand, aesthetic, and self-actualization)

Nonverbal Communication Exchange of information, thoughts, or messages using methods other than the actual words of speech—for example, tone of voice, speed of speech, facial expressions, and position of the speaker's extremities and torso (body language)

Outpatient Patient who comes to a health care facility for diagnosis or treatment but does not usually occupy a bed overnight

Palpation Application of light pressure with the fingers

Paralanguage Music of language; cadence and rhythm of speech

Patient Assessment Objective evaluation and determination of the status of a patient

Patient Autonomy Ability and right of patients to make independent decisions regarding their medical care

Verbal Communication Messages sent using spoken words; the exchange of information or thoughts; can be dramatically shaped by vocabulary, clarity, tone, pitch of voice, and even the organization of sentences

PERSONAL UNDERSTANDING

Radiologic technology is a people-oriented, hands-on profession that requires proficiency in a wide variety of communication techniques. Educational programs in the radiologic sciences should strive to assist students in developing effective methods of patient contact early. This approach will assist them in achieving a successful and enjoyable career. One of the best ways to learn to communicate effectively with others is to first learn to understand emotions. Emotions are a part of everyone's personality—it is a personality trait. Patients exhibit a wide range of emotions, and the way technologists handle those emotions relies on how well they understand not only the emotions exhibited by their patients but also how well they understand their own. That understanding is one of the concepts involved in emotional intelligence (EI).

Although numerous definitions of EI exist, broadly defined, it simply means the ability to look at yourself and at others in an effort to recognize and understand emotions, and to use that recognition and understanding to manage those emotions in both arenas. Patients come to be imaged in various states of emotion. Some are depressed, some are in pain, some are angry, and some are genuinely hostile. It is very important that radiologic technologists recognize the exhibited emotions, and communicate with patients in a way that is appropriate for their emotional state. However, before communicating with the patient, the technologist must examine his or her own emotional state. For example, a patient presents crying because she has been given bad news concerning her health status. Before meeting the patient, the technologist was quite happy, having just had his yearly evaluation and been given a hefty 10% raise. As the technologist in this situation, when you meet the patient, you immediately recognize her state of emotion and then reflect on your own. How do you communicate with this patient? Should you continue your jovial state, begin to cry as well, or recognize that you must communicate in a way that is empathetic to the patient and effective in calming her present state of emotion? Of course, the answer is to communicate using care and empathy. Empathy is a valuable part of EI and an essential value in a health care professional. EI has

only been studied in depth during the last three decades. People have differing levels of EI, but these levels can be increased. There are numerous sources and tools for evaluating and increasing EI. Individuals with high EI are said to be more successful on and off the job. In health care, this translates into more effective communication and patient care.

The importance of interacting effectively with diverse patients is critical to the radiologic technologist, as well as to the patient. These techniques greatly improve the quality of medical images, as well as patient care. Obtaining the patient's cooperation is one of the most challenging parts of a radiologic technologist's role. The most seasoned radiologic technologist will sometimes have to repeat images if the patient does not understand the procedure or does not cooperate because of poor communication.

The communication skills of the radiologic technologist often determine the patient's overall opinion of the medical imaging department. Because hospitals and clinics depend heavily on reimbursement for patient services, the use of effective interactive skills can make the patient's visit pleasant and meaningful, and it might encourage his or her return for additional medical care.

Words of Comfort, skillfully administered, are the oldest therapy known to man.

Louis Nizer

Students and technologists alike also have needs to satisfy their career ambitions, which often include the following:

- Helping others
- Working with people
- Making a difference
- Thinking critically
- Demonstrating creativity
- Achieving results

A career in radiologic technology is capable of fulfilling all of these needs and many more. When personal needs are met, experiencing increased confidence in technical abilities as well is not unusual. The patient often perceives this confidence as competence because the external appearance is that of a self-assured individual capable of professionally and effortlessly carrying out procedures.

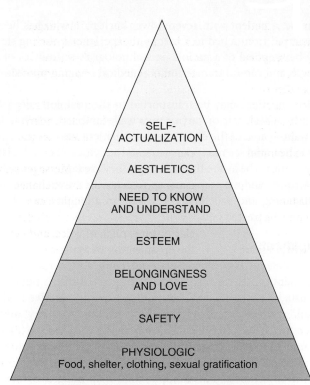

Fig. 11.1 Maslow's hierarchy of needs.

The pyramid, from bottom to top, reads:

PHYSIOLOGIC
Food, shelter, clothing, sexual gratification

SAFETY

BELONGINGNESS AND LOVE

ESTEEM

NEED TO KNOW AND UNDERSTAND

AESTHETICS

SELF-ACTUALIZATION

Maslow's hierarchy of needs provides insight into this type of behavior for all persons, professionals and patients alike (Fig. 11.1). Maslow suggests that people strive from a basic level of physiologic needs toward a level of self-actualization. This highest level is characterized by confidence in who the person is and what the person's goals are in life. Essentially, each level of needs must be satisfied before one can proceed to the next level. Students often begin their education at approximately the third level, which relates to belonging or affection needs. Once instructors, classmates, and staff radiologic technologists have accepted the student, he or she must move toward the fourth level, which addresses self-esteem and respect needs. Many students achieve this level during the second year, once many of the required clinical skills have been mastered. As graduation and the certification examination are successfully completed, level seven, the self-actualization level, can begin in a professional context.

As jobs or roles change, moving up and down the various levels of the hierarchy and being at different levels in different roles would be normal. For example, a new husband may be at the fourth level at work but at the third level in marriage.

PATIENT NEEDS

To interact effectively with patients, understanding that patients may be in an altered state of consciousness is important. They are in an unfamiliar environment in which they are no longer in complete control. In addition, they often fear not knowing the exact state of their health. Preferring bad news to uncertainty—because at least plans can be made to cope with bad news—is not unusual for a patient, whereas uncertainty leaves

a person without the means to attempt to control the situation. Empathizing with these feelings is difficult until they have been experienced personally.

Most patients would prefer not to be in the care of health care professionals, including radiologic technologists. Even the kindest and most cooperative patients are simply making the best of a situation they would prefer to avoid. An injury or the potential for disease or illness exists; otherwise they would not be seeking medical care. In many instances, patients' fear of what the images may confirm or uncover causes them to be inconsiderate, arrogant, impatient, rude, overly talkative, or to exhibit other characteristics as they attempt to cope with their situation.

PATIENT DIGNITY

The patient may arrive for care at the first level of Maslow's hierarchy of needs, which is the physiologic or survival level. Illness or trauma may have altered many physiologic functions, which in turn may cause the patient to behave out of character.

A lack of satisfaction in level one needs can cause a patient to be unable to satisfy the other, higher needs. For example, if a female patient is very sick, she might lose sleep (level one) over how she will keep her job and maintain her home or belongings (level two). When a patient arrives with a nasogastric tube (Fig. 11.2), although normally very friendly and talkative, he or she may not want to be around other patients while the nasogastric tube is in place (level three).

As with most medical professionals, radiologic technologists have an awesome responsibility when interacting with patients because of the tremendous power that is held by health professionals over patients. This power is so great that it includes the most basic elements of a person's dignity and self-respect. Inconsiderate abuse of this power may seem to be difficult to avoid because of the nature of the examination procedures. Consequently, special attention is needed to ensure that the power is not abused. For example, when patients are required to wear flimsy patient gowns, when they are referred to as "the upper gastrointestinal series" or "the barium enema" instead of by name, or when they are placed in proximity to other patients who are more critically ill, patients can feel dehumanized. Maintaining self-respect is difficult while trying to get to a toilet before evacuating barium from the bowel, when vomiting, and in other uncomfortable situations.

Professional radiologic technologists should learn about different types of patients, along with various methods of communication that are effective with each. Two main classifications of patients can be considered—inpatients and outpatients. Each type has typical characteristics that require different approaches and interaction skills on the part of the technologist. Whether the patient is an inpatient or an outpatient, one of the initial patient communication skills is **patient assessment**. Initial patient assessment by the technologist usually comes in the form of chart or procedure request review, or both. Much information can be learned from reviewing these two sources concerning patient history and indications for or contraindications to the requested procedure. Second, patient assessment by the

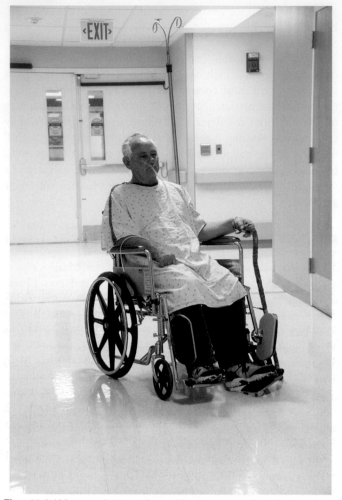

Fig. 11.2 When patients arrive with a nasogastric tube in place, although they may normally be friendly and outgoing, they may prefer to wait in a location where they do not have to face the public.

technologist usually comes in the form of verbal communication. All health care professionals should introduce themselves to their patients, explain the procedure to patients, and obtain a brief history. Many medical imaging departments have patient questionnaires requiring that the technologist ask patients pertinent questions regarding their history and medical status before a procedure can be performed. In other instances, if a patient is scheduled to have an invasive procedure or if the use of intravascular contrast media is required, obtaining informed consent is often the responsibility of the technologist. In either instance, good communication skills are a must.

Inpatients

An **inpatient** is someone who has been admitted to the hospital for diagnostic studies or treatment. In general, these persons occupy a hospital bed for longer than 24 hours. Inpatients often move up and down Maslow's hierarchy before arriving in the care of the radiologic technologist. Gaining the patient's confidence is important, even though he or she may be in a somewhat agitated or bewildered state of mind. Previous experiences in the hospital may have shaped the manner in which the patient responds to these initial interactions with the technologist. For

example, a patient with severe lower back pain who has been transferred from a bed to a cart by inexperienced nursing staff may be skeptical of a radiologic technologist's assurances of a smooth and careful transfer onto a medical imaging procedure table.

The inpatient may be transported to the radiology department by wheelchair or cart or may walk (ambulate). While in the waiting area of the department, the patient has an opportunity to hear and see many departmental activities. Technologists should always be aware that, although they are familiar with the department and may take waiting patients for granted, patients are listening and watching everything in anticipation of how they may be treated.

Outpatients

An **outpatient** is someone who has come to the hospital or outpatient center for diagnostic testing or treatment but does not usually occupy a bed overnight. Outpatients arrive in the radiology department with prior expectations. They often expect to be seen immediately on arriving in the department because they have a scheduled appointment. Maintaining a schedule in any medical setting is difficult because of unforeseen circumstances. For example, follow-up images on a previous patient may take longer than expected; a radiologist may require extra projections to be certain of a diagnosis; or patients may become ill, refuse examinations, or be unable to cooperate fully. Apologizing for delays and trying to keep waiting patients up to date on their status is certainly appropriate and important—for example, telling a patient that it will be 20 minutes before he or she can be seen is appropriate if no emergencies exist. If something unforeseen occurs, then little extra time is required to say, "I'll be with you as soon as I finish with one more patient," as you walk by 15 minutes later. Patients greatly appreciate the simple fact that you are aware they are waiting and you perceive their patience. More positive comments are received by hospitals from these types of interactions than for any other reason.

Because outpatients often have insurance or government benefits of some type, they may expect priority treatment. A professional should provide the same care and attention to all patients regardless of status. This care can be especially difficult when a patient is a famous personality, a correctional inmate, or public official or otherwise known.

INTERACTING WITH THE PATIENT'S FAMILY AND FRIENDS

The patient's family and friends who are visiting also must receive attention. Because they spend much time waiting, they tend to critique everything about the technologist, from appearance to tone of voice to smile (or lack thereof). Being courteous to visitors and relatives, as well as to the patient, is important. Relatives are justifiably concerned and may ask questions such as whether the technologist sees anything abnormal or whether a fracture is present. Thinking about how the family and friends feel or considering how concerned you would be about a member of your own family would help. But the technologist must also be aware and remember that he or she is prohibited from rendering a diagnosis at any time and of any sort.

The same needs function for family and friends as for the patient and technologist. Abnormal or rude behavior may be the result of anxiety, concern, or stress. Being asked for an interpretation of images is common for the technologist. An important point to remember is that family and friends often listen closely to everything a professional says (Fig. 11.3). Any statements in response to this type of question may be construed as diagnosing, which is practicing medicine without a license and is illegal. The best response is usually to indicate that the findings are available to the referring physician and that only he or she can provide the information.

The radiologic technologist has a responsibility to make patients, as well as their family and friends, feel confident that they are receiving the best possible care and that they are considered important and special. A smile and brief explanation of the procedure, with extra attention when delays occur, goes a long way in making everyone feel more relaxed and confident.

METHODS OF EFFECTIVE COMMUNICATION

Attention to the various forms of interaction and communication techniques that have proved effective in improving relationships with patients can produce dramatic results in clinical situations. Accurate and timely communication is essential to providing high-quality patient care. A coordinated, team approach is required, with the patient at the center. Developing patient–provider rapport paves the way for an interchange of information that makes the patient feel at ease, leading to better cooperation. Communication comes in many forms, and health care practitioners must be aware of them all; otherwise, although they may not verbally communicate an idea or thought, other forms of communication may be conveying the message, positive or negative.

Verbal Skills

Speech and Grammar. The methods of verbal communication that are used in establishing an open relationship between the health professional and the patient are basic to the quality of the interaction. Vocabulary, clarity of voice, and even the organization of sentences must be at a level appropriate for the patient. For example, a discussion of units of radiation dose is probably not of interest to a Protestant minister. Conversely, telling a physics teacher that a chest x-ray examination is similar in dose to a few minutes of sun tanning is equally inappropriate.

An important point to remember is that, whenever possible, verbal communication should occur face to face. This approach typically makes others believe that they have your undivided attention, that your concern is only for them, and that they are the only person about whom you care at this specific point in time. Be polite and focus attention on the listener's perception of the manner in which you are communicating. Remember that cultural, generational, and individual differences may affect a person's perception of what you are trying to convey. Be careful not to patronize or otherwise demean an individual.

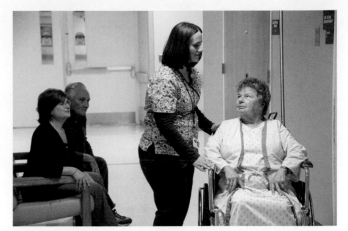

Fig. 11.3 Family members often listen closely to everything a professional says. The radiologic technologist should be careful not to attempt to interpret images because this is diagnosing, which is illegal.

Humor. The value of humor in medical settings is well documented. Using humor to relax and open up conversation is acceptable, but the technologist must be extremely careful to avoid cultural slurs and references to age, sex, diseases, and the abilities of other health professionals. The fact that many patients use self-deprecating humor about their disabilities or fears as an emotional release must not be construed as permission for the radiographer to joke in a similar manner. Laughter is good medicine, but when humor is used in an incorrect manner or wrong context or is perceived as unprofessional, it becomes a tool that may prohibit good communication. For example, if a patient asks about the specifics of a medical imaging procedure and the reply is, "I don't know; this is my first time performing this procedure," this response may be humorous to the technologist, but the patient may become apprehensive about having an inexperienced person performing the examination. This apprehension may lead to closure of all communication channels between the two parties.

Nonverbal Communication

Paralanguage. Paralanguage is the music of language; it is often considered a form of nonverbal communication. Patients receive signals about your attitude toward them from the pitch, stress, tone, pauses, speech rate, volume, accent, and quality of your voice. For example, because the mind works faster than the voice, thinking of a response when someone who is talking pauses is common. This knowledge can be used to structure productive questions. For example, asking a patient "Exactly where does it hurt most?" may not produce as much information as saying "You said it hurts a lot around your stomach. Now exactly where would you say the pain is usually greatest?" The second statement gives patient time to recall what he or she said and to think specifically about the statement before being asked to answer.

Body Language. Patients quickly perceive nonverbal communication such as the tone of voice, speed of speech, and position of the speaker's extremities and torso (body language). Radiographers must be cautious to avoid giving confusing signals to

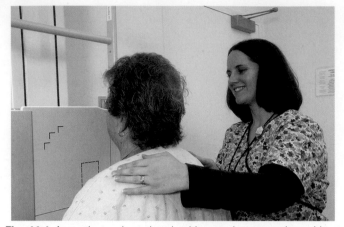

Fig. 11.4 A gentle touch at the shoulder can be reassuring without being offensive.

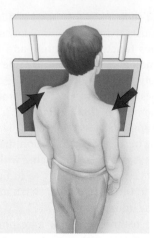

Fig. 11.5 Touching for emphasis to help a patient turn the left side toward a chest unit. A gentle touch at the posterior left shoulder accompanied by a similar touch at the anterior right shoulder accomplishes the movement quickly and efficiently.

patients by saying one thing and acting in a totally different manner. For example, asking a patient if he or she is comfortable but neglecting to offer a positioning sponge to hold an oblique position may call into question the sincerity, and consequently the trustworthiness, of the technologist. Positive nonverbal cues increase the quantity and quality of communication and improve the history. For example, the technologist should look at patients and show interest in their statements. Eye contact in many cultures, but not all, is seen as reassurance that the person is concentrating only on the individual with whom he or she is speaking. Smiling, responding candidly, and using a friendly tone of voice all work toward this end. Negative nonverbal cues can also be used to improve the history. For example, looking puzzled may prompt the patient to elaborate on exactly how an injury occurred and may provide the radiologist with details on the direction of the force that caused a fracture. While speaking with patients, the radiologic technologist, as well as the radiologist, should avoid standing away from them with the arms folded across the chest. This body language is generally perceived as someone who is on the defensive, has something to hide, or is repulsed by the patient. Rolling of the eyes, shrugging of the shoulders, and looks of disgust should never be exhibited.

Touch. The radiologic technologist commonly uses three types of touch: (1) touching for emotional support, (2) touching for emphasis, and (3) touching for palpation. Few things are more reassuring than a gentle pat on the hand or shoulder as a form of emotional support (Fig. 11.4). Many people respond extremely well to touch, and using this technique is acceptable, as long as proper social conventions are followed. The use of touch conveys to patients that the technologist is trying to understand, be empathetic, and care about them as people. Gentle support under the arm to assist patients to and from the imaging room and onto and off of the table often provides reassurance to the patient that he or she is being cared for by a professional practitioner.

Touching for emphasis involves using touch to highlight or to specify instructions or locations. For example, after a postero-anterior chest radiograph has been performed, patients can be instructed to turn their left side toward a chest unit by a gentle

touch at the posterior left shoulder accompanied by a similar touch at the anterior right shoulder (Fig. 11.5). Likewise, after a patient states, "My stomach hurts here," and places a hand on the upper abdomen, the technologist can elicit further information by asking, "Does it hurt more here or here?" while touching the duodenal and gastric regions.

Palpation is the application of light pressure with the fingers to the body. Palpating to locate various bony radiographic landmarks when positioning patients is advisable and helpful. In a similar fashion, using specific palpation is often useful to determine a more exact localization during history taking. Effective and precise palpation requires the *gentle* use of fingertips (Fig. 11.6). The use of the palm or several fingers is less precise than using fingertips and may in some instances be painful or even offensive to patients. For example, a 14-year-old girl is usually more comfortable if a male radiographer palpates for the iliac crest with the tip of a finger than if the entire hand is used to feel the hip region. Before touching a patient, his or her permission to do so should be obtained. Touching without consent can have legal ramifications.

Professional Appearance. Most programs in radiologic technology have a dress code for students. Although dressing according to a code does not produce better technologists, a professional appearance in the medical setting says as much about technologists as their technical abilities say about their competence. Professional dress helps the patient feel comfortable and confident in the technologist's abilities. Gaining the patient's confidence and trust is a considerable part of being a competent radiologic technologist.

Personal Hygiene. Personal hygiene is as important as professional appearance. Personal grooming sends a powerful message. Unkempt individuals may prompt patients to suspect that the person's professional behavior is similar to his or her appearance—neglected and disheveled. Hair, nails, and teeth should be neat and clean. Nails should be kept at a manageable length, without the use of acrylics, which have been banned in many health care institutions. Body odor emanating from anyone

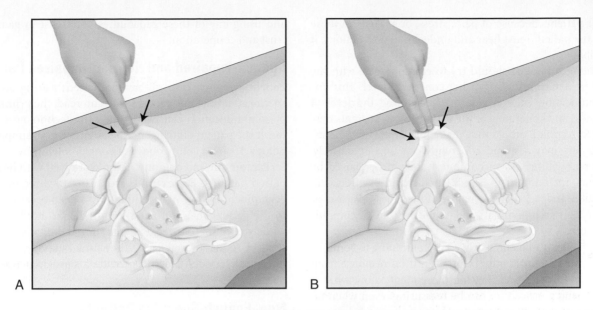

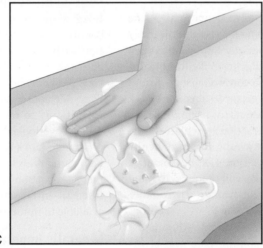

Fig. 11.6 Proper palpation is accomplished by using fingertips to provide precise and gentle localization information. (A) Proper use of a single fingertip. (B) Proper use of several fingers. (C) Improper use of the palm.

causes others to react negatively, suggesting that the person is unclean. Daily baths or showers, good oral hygiene, and the use of personal hygiene products may be eliminate this problem. The use of strong perfumes, colognes, and aftershaves should also be avoided. Patients may react to certain smells by becoming nauseated by any smell that may affect them negatively. A patient will not communicate with someone with whom they do not desire to be in close contact.

Physical Presence. Appearance and physical presence go together. Posture is important because it is perceived as relating to confidence and self-esteem. Facial expressions are vital nonverbal cues that give people information on the importance of instructions and questions, as well as both positive and negative reinforcement of their actions and statements. For example, confusion and frustration are easily communicated in this manner.

Visual Contact. As stated previously, eye contact may help ensure that questions, instructions, and other information have

been understood. Visual inspection of a patient's condition can be critical when changes such as blood pressure and allergic reactions produce symptoms.

UNDERSTANDING THE VARIOUS TYPES OF PATIENTS

Patients in radiology departments often have unusual conditions, in addition to the conditions for which they are undergoing examination. The medical population is as diverse as the general population and will continue to grow more diverse as time passes. An understanding of the most common special conditions can be valuable in meeting the needs of patients.

Seriously Ill and Traumatized Patients

Not all patients with whom the technologist comes into contact want to talk or are able to cooperate during their procedure. A seriously ill or traumatized patient may act differently from other patients because of pain, stress, or anxiety. In these instances, the patient must hear and understand instructions, if at all possible.

First, the technologist should try to communicate with the patient while determining his or her coherence level. This initial communication can provide cues regarding the level of consciousness and coherency of the patient. Some patients may be unable to respond, others may make incoherent statements, and still others may respond coherently but uncooperatively. Inability or unwillingness to communicate can be caused by many factors, including pain, shock, medication reaction, and disorientation. Indeed, the very nature of the illness, disease, or trauma can alter an individual's ability to cooperate or communicate, or both.

Working quickly and efficiently while continuing to communicate with the patient is important, even if no response from the patient is forthcoming. Letting the patient know what is going on during a procedure can be reassuring, even when no apparent sign of understanding is evident.

Because seriously ill and traumatized patients may not be able to communicate effectively, watching for visual indications of changes in vital signs becomes especially important. When patients cannot tell anyone they are having difficulty breathing, they must rely completely on the technologist to recognize potential problems promptly. For example, a patient's neck vasculature and musculature being distended, flaring nostrils, involvement of abdominal muscles (retraction) when breathing, or blueness of the skin (cyanosis) are all indicative of difficulty breathing and may require medical attention. Helping someone is a great feeling; however, when a seriously ill or injured patient must rely on you, the added responsibility can greatly enhance these feelings.

Radiologic technologists interact with patients who exhibit a wide variety of impairments. Combining common sense, empathy, and classroom knowledge will enable you to provide high-quality images for patients who would otherwise receive suboptimal examinations. Remember that the patient's cooperation is one of the main factors essential to producing high-quality images technologists can be proud of, and allow the interpreting physician to make definitive diagnoses.

Visually Impaired Patients

A blind patient, a patient who has decreased vision without glasses, or an optically injured patient needs special attention. The technologist should attempt to gain the patient's confidence as soon as possible by giving clear instructions before the examination, as well as informing him or her of what is occurring at all times. Reassuring the patient through a gentle touch establishes that someone is near if needed. Continued verbal communication assists persons who are blind and visually impaired with satisfying many of the basic needs attributed to Maslow. Many times, technologists may feel that talking loudly to a blind person may somehow make them able to see. These individuals are blind, not deaf, and talking loudly cannot make them see. The same goes for speaking loudly to a profoundly deaf person. Even if you scream at them, they will not hear you, but usually they can see and write and many also read lips. Inquiring about

and using any of these capabilities will assist in gaining their trust and cooperation.

Speech-Impaired and Hearing-Impaired Patients

Patients who are deaf or have impaired hearing also require special attention. For persons who can read, the primary means of communication can be writing. The technologist must not insult the patient's intelligence by attempting to simplify terminology. Hearing ability does not control intelligence.

Pantomime and demonstration work well with hearing-impaired patients. For example, counting to three on your fingers, pinching your nose, and taking a deep breath symbolizes to the patient that you need him or her to hold their breath while you count to three. Patients should demonstrate instructions in return to make sure they understand. Many facilities offer deaf services and will provide a sign language expert as necessary.

Non–English-Speaking Patients

Imagine the frustration you would feel if you were in a foreign country where no one understood English. Effective interaction with non–English-speaking patients is greatly enhanced by using touch, facial expressions, and pantomime. Nearly all such patients understand basic words such as *yes, no,* and *stop.* Everyone appreciates any attempt to speak his or her language, even if only to say *yes* and *no.* Pronunciation and accents are quickly overlooked when good intentions are shown. Most hospitals maintain a list of bilingual employees who are available to help patients and visitors. The use of telephonic translators has increased nationwide. In addition, many facilities have made essential instructions, consent forms, and other paperwork available in numerous languages.

Mentally Impaired Patients

Generally speaking, mental impairment means any mental or psychological disorder. These types of disorders include intellectual disability, organic brain syndromes, emotional or mental illnesses, and specific types of learning disabilities. Manifestations of such disorders range from mild to severe and cover a very broad spectrum, inclusive of all age groups. Although all health care workers cannot be expected to know the specific characteristics of each type of mental impairment, they must certainly be aware that a patient has one. They must also be aware that communicating with the mentally impaired may be difficult, although not impossible. Remember that exhibiting respect for every patient, including the mentally impaired, goes a long way in gaining their trust and cooperation. Communicating with gentle tones and smiles will often illicit a positive response, although sometimes other measures may be necessary.

Working with mentally impaired patients also requires a thorough knowledge of equipment and immobilization techniques. Although degrees of mental impairment vary, using a strong yet reassuring tone of voice with these patients is important. A continuous conversation while preparing the patient for the examination usually helps keep the patient calm and aware that the technologist is working with him or her.

Substance Abusers

Radiologic technologists who work weekends, holidays, and evenings are often involved with patients who are under the influence of drugs or alcohol. These patients may not be totally aware of where they are or what they are doing, and may need to be restrained from leaving the room or from playing with tubes, wires, or high-voltage cables.

The best mode of interaction with these patients often includes assessing their capabilities, attempting to establish a means of communication, using technical knowledge, and working efficiently to decrease the total examination time.

Patients who are under the influence of drugs or alcohol may be relaxed, or they may be hyperactive and irrational. The technologist must observe them closely and use immobilization techniques as necessary. If patients are hyperactive and loud, they obviously require close supervision. Calm, quiet patients are of increased concern because they may react without warning and fall or otherwise injure themselves.

Some substance abusers respond well to firm directions about what to do, whereas others are best handled by requesting that they return for examination at a later time when the effects have diminished considerably. The technologist will always encounter some patients who simply cannot be examined properly without assistance from other medical personnel. Waiting until the patient becomes cooperative is often best. Seriously injured patients are seldom uncooperative, especially when they believe their life may be in jeopardy.

Restraints may be needed when dealing with mentally ill and other patients. Remember that using restraints can lead to legal ramifications. Using restraints must occur only as prescribed in facility procedure and policy. Restraint without consent is termed unlawful restraint. Please see departmental protocol on the use of restraints.

MOBILE AND SURGICAL EXAMINATIONS

Many patients who require mobile examination are too sick or injured to be transported to the medical imaging department for their procedure. Patients may be unconscious and attached to an array of tubes, monitoring lines, ventilators, and other medical equipment. Except in surgery, during which the patient is normally incapable of interacting because of anesthesia, attempting to establish a line of communication with the patient is important. Begin by calling the patient's name, identifying yourself to the patient, and explaining the procedure. This approach permits assessment of the patient's condition and level of coherence.

Under no circumstances should the technologist assume that a patient does not comprehend comments that are made within the patient's range of hearing. Patients may be cognizant, although they appear to be comatose. Several studies have reported instances in which patients in deep anesthesia or even long-term comatose states were able to recall jokes and derogatory comments that were made about them. Both cognizant and incoherent patients will demonstrate increased cooperation if they hear a kind voice of explanation before being touched. Even if the words are not understood, a caring tone of voice and a gentle touch often have a positive effect.

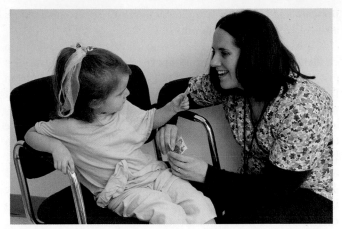

Fig. 11.7 "To stand tall in pediatrics, you have to get down on your knees." Entering the child's environment by squatting to the child's eye level can begin a rewarding relationship.

In interacting with the patient's family and friends, you should introduce yourself, explain the procedure briefly, and explain why they must leave the immediate area during the exposure. In most instances, no need exists to send visitors far, and explaining that the exposure is only a fraction of a second often encourages them to wait nearby while the equipment is removed. Remember that visitors sometimes arrive from distant places at considerable expense and that every moment may be precious with a dying parent or favorite aunt. Family members and visitors appreciate courtesy, empathy, and thoughtfulness.

AGE AS A FACTOR IN PATIENT INTERACTIONS

Age differences between the radiologic technologist and the patient should not be a barrier to effective communication. Nearly everyone has family members and friends of different ages, from grandparents to infants, and interactions with patients should be similar. Every patient deserves the best that all health care professionals can offer, but some require increased strategic care based on their age or condition.

Pediatric Patients

Pediatric patients always require special attention. The proper method for dealing with young children is summarized by the famous statement of Dr. Armand Brodeur, long-time chief radiologist at Cardinal Glennon Children's Hospital in St. Louis: "To stand tall in pediatrics, you have to get down on your knees." In other words, simply getting down to the child's level—physically, in language, and in spirit—establishes a positive relationship. For example, instead of picking a child up and setting him or her on an imaging table, which is the technologist's environment, the technologist should squat at the child's eye level, which is the child's environment, to begin the relationship (Fig. 11.7). The pediatric patient can provide valuable clinical information. For example, before a procedure, a 5-year-old girl may reveal that she has been battered if she is alone with a friendly and nonthreatening technologist whom she believes she can trust. Technologists need to be aware of their facility's policies and procedures on reporting suspected child abuse, also called nonaccidental trauma.

Children are special patients who are capable of presenting a challenge to the technologist's interpersonal skills. A technologist who can perform procedures effectively and competently on the pediatric patient is probably capable of handling any imaging procedure on any type of patient. Patience, technical knowledge, understanding of the pediatric patient, and the effective use of communication skills and immobilization devices can assist in obtaining a high-quality image.

Many hospitals provide soft toys such as stuffed animals for children, and stocking these items in the radiology department is a good idea. However, please make sure that such items are not contaminated with germs from previous patients. Never try to separate a child from a security object such as a blanket or toy unless absolutely necessary for image quality. Even then, the object should remain within the child's sight so that he or she is assured it will be returned momentarily. If the parents accompany the child, try to sit with the parents in the waiting room while you hold the child and explain the procedure to the parents. This additional time, 2 or 3 minutes, provides the child the opportunity to become familiar with you, your professional attire, and the department. Always remember that children must *never* be left alone, even if properly immobilized.

Another very important thing to remember when imaging pediatric patients is that radiation protection methods must be employed in order to limit the amount of radiation these children receive from medical imaging studies, especially those using ionizing radiation. Technical factors should be child-sized, as should doses of contrast media or other medications used in the medical imaging department. Remember to "Image Gently."

Infants (Birth to 1 Year). First communications are established using facial expressions, body movements and other nonverbal behaviors, and vocalizations. Very young infants like to be held in a familiar position. Observe how the parents are holding the child, or ask what the favorite position is—at the shoulder, lying on the right side, and so forth. In addition, most small infants respond well to being held closely with a tight blanket (called swaddling). A steady, soothing voice, male or female, also often helps. Simply repeating "It's all right; that's okay" usually works.

Mobile imaging of infants in the neonatal intensive care unit is especially tedious and requires expeditious and accurate use of the technologist's knowledge and skills. These infants are usually very premature or seriously ill. They are usually unclothed, with numerous tubes and wires attached to their small bodies. In addition, they may be housed in an incubator, or other structures that limit access for imaging purposes. The technologists must learn and implement facility procedure for accomplishing imaging of these infants.

At approximately 8 months of age, most infants express definite anxiety when removed from a familiar person. Permitting the parents to assist with the entire examination if possible is often helpful. If separation is necessary, it should be for the minimum amount of time.

At approximately 12 months of age, children are beginning to develop memories, ideas, and feelings. A child with previous experiences with hospital personnel may rebel at the sight of a laboratory coat or surgical scrub suit. The strength a 1-year-old child is capable of mustering is amazing when a vivid memory of an injection or being restrained for a previous imaging procedure is triggered.

Toddlers (1 to 3 Years). Although toddlers may understand simple abstractions, their thinking is basically related to tangible events. They usually cannot take the viewpoint of another (this is why statements such as "See, it doesn't hurt Mommy" are seldom effective), and they cannot understand more than one word for something. Asking a parent what word the child uses for urination is important if asking the child to urinate becomes necessary. Toddlers' concept of time is essentially now, and distance is whatever can be seen. Therefore speaking with simple words that are familiar to children is important, and expecting them to think about how they will feel in an hour should be avoided. Toddlers are often concerned only with what you are going to do to them at the moment.

Preschoolers (3 to 5 Years). Preschool children are not yet able to reason logically or understand cause and effect. Telling a 4-year-old boy that he needs a procedure to see if he is sick is meaningless. If his arm hurts, however, he will long remember that he broke it when he fell. Because preschoolers are very much involved with self-image, this is the age at which children may form an opinion that they are sick because they were bad. They may perceive relationships such as *big*, *little*, or *first* but may not understand *next in line*. They must see or hear something to understand and must be actively involved to maintain their short attention span. They will not hold still for long, although they can be remarkably cooperative if their trust has been won.

School-Aged Children (5 to 10 Years). At approximately 7 years of age, children begin to think logically and to analyze situations. At this point, children can reflect and develop deeper understandings. With these advancements, children often develop a special fear of bodily injury, disease, separation from loved ones, death, and punishment.

Remember that many diagnostic procedures may appear as punishment to children, and special attention is warranted to divert their attention from the negative aspects of various examinations. This task often can be accomplished by using the child's capacity for depth of understanding. For example, helping a child rationalize how an excretory urogram helps the physician find out why it hurts to urinate is appropriate as a method of diverting attention from the pain of the venipuncture.

Adolescents (10 to 25 Years). Adolescence is not a well-defined age group, although it begins earlier for girls than it does for boys. The primary consideration in early adolescence focuses on body awareness, and modesty becomes especially important. Persons in this age group usually require special consideration to avoid embarrassment when changing clothes and during examinations. Asking unnecessary personnel to leave a room is appropriate during these examinations. Same-sex peer groups have a dominant role at this age, and conversation that focuses on friends of the same sex often eases tensions during procedures.

Middle adolescents are often bridging the gap between peer group influence and early sexual relationships. Persons in this age group are often developing their first real independence and often appreciate being treated as adults in conversation, preferences, and consultation about procedures.

Late adolescents are often focusing on mature relationships with both sexes and may be financially independent. They easily relate to adult conversation and should essentially be treated as adults, although their experiences may be limited in some areas.

Young Adults (25 to 45 Years)

Young adults are usually entering new roles of responsibility at home and in their work. They often experience problems in handling their multitude of new roles and may neglect one area while they concentrate on another. For example, focusing on child rearing at home may result in neglect of work duties. Conversation and interaction should be on the same level as for other adults.

Middle-Aged Adults (45 to 65 Years)

In middle age, most people have found their place in life and tend to be relatively comfortable with their roles and success (or lack of it). When poor health or a threat of poor health occurs, considerable stress and special concern over how to maintain responsibilities, such as keeping a job and providing for a family, may outweigh personal health concerns. That is one of the reasons that they may delay seeking diagnosis and treatment for troubling symptoms.

Mature Adults (65 Years and Older)

Research shows that most persons 65 years old or older do not consider themselves old. They tend to consider themselves middle-aged. Because of this self-image, radiologic technologists should not attempt to interact with them as though they are geriatric patients. Senility is not a natural part of aging, and only approximately 10% of people in this age group demonstrate memory loss. They should be treated as middle-aged persons, with conversation centering on life activities. A much-reprinted saying, *I may be old and wrinkled on the outside but I'm young and vulnerable on the inside*, is well worth considering when phrasing statements to this age group. Remember, this is the age group that will continue to grow, because the first of the baby boomers have turned 60, as mentioned in Chapter 10. These individuals are well educated and health savvy. They watch shows such as *Dr. Oz*, and are provided a multitude of information via the American Association for Retired Persons and the like. It is certainly best not to patronize them and to respond to any questions or concerns with factual information.

Gerontology

Gerontology (geriatrics) is the study of aging and diseases of older adults. Studies show that the geriatric group will continue to increase in size and importance in American society for many years to come, primarily as a result of improvements in living standards, dietary practices, physical fitness, and medical care. At the end of the 20th century, more than 33 million Americans were over 65 years of age—more than 12% of the total population, compared with only 4% in 1900. In addition, the elderly population itself is aging. From 1960 to 1994, the US population grew by 45%, whereas the over-65 population grew by 100% and the over-85 population grew by almost 275%, to a total of 3 million persons. In addition, the 2000 census revealed a 49% increase in the 45- to 54-year-old category. According to census data, from 2000 to 2010, there was a 31.5% increase in people from age 45 to 64, and a 15.1% increase in the population aged 65 and above. This population group has now reached the *mature persons* category. These data have caused significant concern as young workers begin to realize that current retirement and medical care systems rely on active workers to fund care of older adults. Real concern exists that worldwide economies may not grow sufficiently to fund this increasing burden. As a result, current pressure on the medical system to find ways to decrease costs while increasing the efficiency of care for older adults is apparent.

Referring to all older patients as *geriatric* is inappropriate. American culture tends to be oriented toward youth, productivity, and a rapid pace. Automatically considering a person as *geriatric* results in feelings of alienation, which can be made worse by a lack of respect. One author points out that although everybody wants to live a long life, hardly anybody wants to be old because the word connotes frailty, narrow-mindedness, incompetence, and loss of attractiveness. Furthermore, the use of terms such as *senior citizens* or *golden agers* constitutes prejudice and discrimination and should be avoided. To minimize these feelings, technologists should treat geriatric patients as mature adults, with all the normal interaction that would be used with healthier or younger patients (Fig. 11.8). Talking loudly or using childish terms should be avoided when speaking with geriatric patients. At the same time, accommodating older adults by using gentle handling and extra time for movements and verbal responses is also important. This approach is identical to adjustments that must be made for other types of patients, such as a partially paralyzed patient.

Geriatric patients are now being classified as young-old, old-old, and oldest-old, in an attempt to differentiate between widely varying conditions that accompany the aging process. Although these classifications can be chronologic, classifying by functional age is equally appropriate. Both classifications are given in Table 11.1. The aging process itself is now divided into *primary aging* and *secondary aging*. Primary aging is the gradual and inevitable process of deterioration that begins in childhood and extends through old age. Secondary aging consists of disease, abuse, and disuse, which are often within control of the individual. Some of the changes that are especially important when patients are undergoing imaging procedures are provided in Table 11.2. The cardinal rules when dealing with geriatric patients are patience and respect.

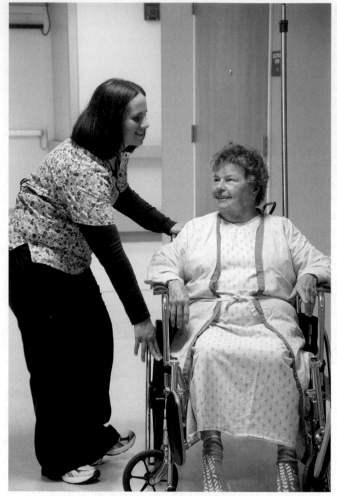

Fig. 11.8 To minimize feelings of alienation, the radiation technologist should treat geriatric patients as mature adults, with all the normal interaction that would be used with healthier or younger patients.

TABLE 11.1	Gerontologic Aging Categories	
Category	**Chronologic**	**Functional**
Young-old	Age 65–74 years	Healthy and active
Old-old	Age 75–84 years	Transitional
Oldest-old	Age 85 years and older	Frail and infirmed

INTERACTING WITH THE TERMINALLY ILL PATIENT

The general agreement asserts that the primary care of the dying patient falls on the nurse; however, this concept does not release the radiologic technologist from an obligation to understand the basics of current practices toward terminally ill patients. Because few new technologists have had experiences with this type of patient, being prepared personally is important.

Unexpected death is much more complicated than anticipated death, but it is guided by a principle of trying to meet as many of the patient's needs as possible. Many technologists eventually experience patient death during imaging procedures, often as a result of anaphylactic shock. Calling a "false alarm" emergency code is always better than waiting too long to save a patient. With this guideline followed, obtaining assistance may still become necessary when working through the personal aspects of having a patient die.

When death is expected because of age or disease, studies show that for most people the crisis is not death but where and how it will occur. For example, older patients who have adjusted to living at home often become anxious if they are removed from their home before death. However, by comparison, geriatric patients who have adjusted to living in an institution are much more willing to accept death in the same setting.

Patients who are kept in *closed awareness* are not told of their condition. Many of these patients deduce that they are terminally ill but lack assistance in working through the various stages of acceptance. Even heavily sedated patients may know more than the health care team suspects. Some patients develop *suspicious awareness* in that they watch for clues to their condition but attempt to keep the health care team from knowing exactly how much they understand. A state of *mutual pretense* exists when patient, staff, and family all know but are pretending not to know in hopes of avoiding interpersonal conflicts. A condition of *open awareness* is usually considered desirable because it permits everyone to work through the various stages that precede death.

The stages delineated by Elisabeth Kübler-Ross have been generally regarded as an acceptable sequence of events. *Denial* and *isolation* may be the initial reactions and should be supported by silence and acceptance of the person without discussing death. *Anger* may occur as a result of the realization that life will be interrupted before everything the person planned has been accomplished and feelings that the person will soon be forgotten. Anger is often expressed in terms of complaints about health care, which may include radiologic services. These complaints should be addressed, and special care should be taken to avoid situations such as long waits without attention that will increase the patient's anger.

Some patients experience a *bargaining* stage that focuses on hope and may be based in religion—for example, prayers for small extensions of life to perform good deeds and heal family wounds. Supporting the patient's beliefs at this time is important because the hope itself can reduce stress. This stage may be followed by *depression*, which often occurs when remission ends and additional treatments must begin. This reaction is normal and should be encouraged by giving realistic praise while letting the patient express his or her feelings.

Preparatory depression comes with the realization of the inevitability of death and is accompanied by a desire for death as a release from suffering. The most important thing at this time is to permit the behavior. Attempting to cheer the patient may meet the needs of the health care provider but not of the patient. Touch and silence are often construed as acceptance and are appropriate at this time. *Acceptance*, which is considered the final stage, can occur only if enough time is provided and if the patient is appropriately helped through the other stages. This stage is characterized by a near-total lack of feelings.

The radiologic technologist also needs to be sure that personal feelings do not override patient concerns when caring for the terminally ill patient. Most hospitals can offer assistance in

TABLE 11.2 Physical Changes of Functional Aging

Body System	Physical Change	Considerations for Radiologic Examinations
Nervous	Slowing of psychomotor responses	Give patient time to move.
	Slowing of information processing	Give patient time to think before expecting a response.
	Decreased visual ability	Stand directly in front of patient, hold items to be seen or read at an appropriate distance without moving for a short time, and provide extra time for visual adjustments after dramatic changes in light levels.
	Decreased hearing ability	Speak directly to the patient's ear, move closer, or (as a last resort) talk more loudly.
Respiratory	Decreased cough reflex	Avoid aspiration by giving patient time to swallow when drinking.
Musculoskeletal	Osteoporotic loss of bone mass	Increase sensitivity to patient paranoia about potential falls with potential for permanent loss of mobility.
	Arthritis	Expect decreased joint flexibility.
	Decreased muscle strength	Prepare to provide assistance in moving if needed.
	Atrophied muscle mass	Expect decreased tolerance of positioning requirements and discomfort in placement on hard imaging tabletops.
Cardiovascular	Decreased cardiac efficiency	Avoid orthostatic hypotension by allowing time for blood pressure adjustment when moving a patient from supine to sitting or from sitting to erect position.
	Arteriosclerosis	Avoid chilling discomfort by providing extra blankets and sheets.
Integumentary	Loss of texture and elasticity	Avoid skin lacerations (especially to the backs of hands) by not abrading skin with draw sheets during patient transfers or applying tape to sensitive areas.
Gastrointestinal	Decreased secretions	Expect difficulty when requiring a patient to drink quickly or from a recumbent position.
	Decreased gastrointestinal motility	Expect delays during completion of small bowel studies. (Prepare for long-term patient comfort via extra blankets, pillow under knees, communication of reasons for delays, and so on.)
	Decreased sphincter muscle tone	Prepare for potential loss of barium from rectum during lower gastrointestinal examinations. Expect more frequent requests for time or assistance with moving.

dealing with personal feelings about caring for terminally ill patients through their nursing departments. Students should consult with their program directors about assistance or appropriate courses. The technologist should not become hardened in dealing with dying and severely injured patients but learn to handle feelings appropriately during interactions with the patient, relatives, and friends.

Health care options now provide terminally ill patients with some control over their death. An **advance directive** provides an individual a means to direct health care if a situation occurs in which he or she is unable to make decisions. Such directives allow the will of the patient to be known regarding certain health care options. For instance, a person having an advance directive stating that he or she does not wish to be placed on a ventilator should there be injury or disease requiring its use to sustain life would probably not be placed on the device if it were required. Other health care advances have supported **patient autonomy** in much the same way as advance directives. In the past, patients with terminal illnesses were faced with few options regarding their death. The only options generally available to them were dying in pain or in a medically induced haze. Today, physicians and their terminally ill patients are making decisions together on how patient symptoms are controlled and how conscious and alert patients desire to be at life's end. Radiologic technologists and other health care professionals should be aware that some of their patients have made these choices and should abide by their patients' wishes.

SUMMARY

- The importance of interacting effectively with the patient is critical to the radiologic technologist, as well as to the patient. Maslow's hierarchy of needs provides insight into the behavior of professionals and patients alike. Maslow's hierarchy proceeds in seven levels of needs, from basic physiologic needs toward a level of self-actualization. The technologist holds significant power, including the most basic elements of a person's dignity and self-respect. Special attention is needed to ensure that the power is not abused.

- The inpatient is someone who has been admitted to the hospital for diagnostic studies or treatment. Previous experiences in the hospital may have shaped the manner in which such a patient responds. Outpatients arrive in the radiologic department or center with prior expectations. They often expect to be seen immediately on arriving in the department because they have a scheduled appointment. Apologizing for delays and keeping waiting patients up to date on their status are appropriate and important. Family and friends of patients who are visiting must also receive attention.

- Attention to the various forms of interaction and communication techniques that have proved effective in improving relationships with patients can produce dramatic results in clinical situations. These skills include verbal skills, including humor, and nonverbal communications, such as paralanguage, body language, and touch. Touching can be used for emotional support, emphasis, and palpation. Professional appearance, personal hygiene, physical presence, and visual contact are also important.

- Special consideration and techniques are necessary when dealing with seriously ill and traumatized patients, as well as impaired patients. Patients with vision, speech, hearing, and mental impairments; patients who do not speak English; and patients who are substance abusers require extra care. Mobile and surgical examinations also have special techniques for effective communication.

- Age is also a special factor in patient interactions. Knowledge of growth and development differences for infants, toddlers, preschoolers, school-aged children, adolescents, young adults, middle-aged persons, mature persons, and geriatric persons can be useful in clinical practice. The cardinal rules when dealing with geriatric patients are patience and respect. When death is expected because of age or disease, studies show that for most people the crisis is not death but where and how it will occur. Understanding the various stages that many terminally ill patients undergo once they have reached a condition of open awareness about their disease is helpful for the technologist. The Kübler-Ross sequence includes denial and isolation, anger, bargaining, depression, preparatory depression, and acceptance. Preparing personally for dealing with the death of a patient is important for the radiologic technologist.

BIBLIOGRAPHY

Bradberry T, Greaves J: *What emotional intelligence looks like: understanding the four skills. Emotional Intelligence 2.0*, San Diego, Calif, 2009, TalentSmart.

Ehrlich RA, Daly JA: *Patient care in radiography: with an introduction to medical imaging*, ed 8, St. Louis, 2013, Elsevier, p 23.

Faguy K: Emotional intelligence in health care, a directed reading, *Radiol Technol* 83:237, 2012.

Freiberg K: *Human development: a life-span approach*, ed 4, Boston, 1992, Jones & Bartlett.

Gurley LT, Callaway WJ: *Introduction to radiologic technology*, ed 7, St. Louis, 2010, Mosby.

Kübler-Ross E: *Death: the final stage of growth*, Englewood Cliffs, NJ, 1975, Prentice-Hall. Available at: https://hr.blr.com/HR-news/Discrimination/Disabilities-ADA/znt1-ADA-Regulations-What-is-a-Mental-Impairment#.

Papalia D, Olds SW: *Human development*, ed 11, New York, 2008, McGraw-Hill.

Purtilo R, Haddad A, Doherty R: *Health professionals and patient interaction*, ed 8, Philadelphia, 2013, Saunders.

Torres LS, Dutton AG, Linn-Watson T: *Patient care in imaging technology*, ed 8, Philadelphia, 2013, Lippincott Williams & Wilkins.

U.S Department of Commerce: *U.S. Bureau of the Census: Growth of America's oldest-old population (profiles of America's elderly no. 2)*, Washington, DC, 2010, U.S. Government Printing Office.

U.S Department of Commerce: *U.S. Census Bureau: Profile of general demographic characteristics for the United States: 2020*, Washington, DC, 2010, U.S. Government Printing Office.

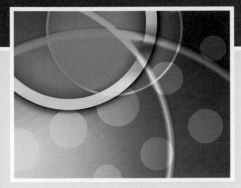

12

History Taking

Richard R. Carlton, MS, RT(R)(CV), FAEIRS,
Arlene M. Adler, MEd, RT(R), FAEIRS

When you talk with the patient, you should listen, first for what he wants to tell, secondly for what he does not want to tell, thirdly for what he cannot tell.

L. J. Henderson
Physician and Patient as Social Systems

OBJECTIVES

On completion of this chapter, the student will be able to:
- Describe the role of the radiologic technologist in taking a clinical history
- Describe the desirable qualities of a good patient interviewer
- Differentiate objective from subjective data
- Explain the value of each of the six categories of questions useful in obtaining clinical histories
- Describe the importance of clarifying the chief complaint
- Detail the important elements of each of the *sacred seven* elements of the clinical history

OUTLINE

KEYTERMS

Chief Complaint Primary medical problem as defined by the patient; important because it focuses the clinical history toward the single most important issue

Chronology Time element of the history, usually including the onset, duration, frequency, and course of the symptoms

Clinical History Information available regarding a patient's condition; traditionally comprises data on localization, quality, quantity, chronology, setting, aggravating or alleviating factors, and associated manifestations

Leading Questions Undesirable method of questioning; provides information that may direct answers toward a suggested symptom or complaint

Localization Determination of a precise area, usually through gentle palpation or careful wording of questions

Objective Perceptible to the external senses

Quality Description of the character of the symptoms—for example, the color, quantity, and consistency of blood or other body substances; size or number of lumps or lesions; frequency of urination or coughing; or character of pain

Subjective Pertaining to or perceived only by the affected individual; not perceptible to the senses

PATIENT INTERVIEW

The clinical history describes the information available regarding a patient's condition. To extract as much information as possible during a clinical history, the event must be viewed as an interview with the patient. Because the radiologic and imaging sciences professional's job often involves obtaining the **clinical history,** learning methods of accomplishing a valid patient interview is important.

Role of the Radiologic and Imaging Sciences Professional

Radiologists often do not have the opportunity to obtain a clinical history from the patient. Although more complex procedures such as angiography and radiation therapy permit extensive history taking by the radiologist or radiation oncologist, most patients scheduled for diagnostic imaging are never examined or interviewed by the radiologist. Because history taking is one of the most critical and valuable diagnostic tools, possessing good history-taking skills is an essential responsibility of the radiologic and imaging sciences professional.

Many radiologic and imaging sciences professionals fail to appreciate the importance of their roles as clinical historians. Unquestionably history taking is one of the most valuable opportunities to acquire clinical information that can contribute to the diagnostic process. A radiologist can be instructed to give special attention to the exact anatomic area where pain is focused. For example, stating that a patient has pain in the right hand is less focused than stating that the pain is over the anterior aspect of the distal portion of the second metacarpal.

In addition, the interaction with the patient plays an important role. A unique opportunity to become part of the healing process presents itself with each new patient. Eric Cassell, a physician noted for his teaching of the art of practicing medicine, tells about how, late one night, he felt powerless to help a patient with severe pulmonary edema. While waiting for equipment to arrive, he began to talk calmly with the patient, explaining how the water would begin to ease bit by bit, until, much to his amazement, that was precisely what happened. By reducing the patient's fear, he had reduced the hypertension and actually eased the pathologic process. Cassell refers to this action as the *art of healing,* and it is directly related to the role of the radiologic technologist in taking a history. Genuine interest in what the patient has to say, attentiveness, and an aura of professional competence can convey a real sense of caring.

Desirable Qualities of the Interviewer

Taking a history must be a cooperative event between the patient and the radiologic technologist. Because patients wish to have a medical problem resolved, most want to help with the history; however, sick people may be combative as a symptom of their frustration. In these instances, acknowledging the patient's anger as a method of overcoming it often helps. For example, a patient who complains about already having given a history to someone and who then rants about incompetent health professionals will often become an ally if the technologist agrees with the inconvenience and suggests that because the radiologist needs specialized information, the interview will be as short as possible and can be taken while the patient is getting ready for the x-ray examination.

Carl Rogers identified several qualities that appear to be important in establishing an open dialogue. These qualities include respect, genuineness, and empathy. When patients perceive any of these qualities to be missing, the interview may become increasingly difficult as the good faith between the two persons decreases. Patients need to believe that the information they are providing is important. When they lack these thoughts because of intimidation or lack of respect, they may withhold information as unimportant or unworthy of being mentioned. Because many patients often perceive physicians as being busy authority figures, radiologic technologists can serve a useful role in that they are usually seen as less threatening and easier to talk with than physicians.

The radiologic and imaging sciences professional should maintain a polite and professional demeanor during the interview, especially when introducing himself or herself to the patient, verifying the patient's name (by using *Mr.* or *Ms.* instead of first names), and explaining that a history is needed.

Notes should be added to the paperwork, usually the examination request or requisition. Most patients perceive note taking as positive because the technologist is making it clear that the information being given is important enough to be recorded. In addition, there is little point in acquiring the clinical history if it is not written on the paperwork that will be in front of the radiologist when the images are read.

Data Collection Process

Good history taking involves the collection of accurate objective and subjective data. **Objective** data are perceptible to the senses, such as signs that can be seen, heard, or felt and such things as laboratory reports. **Subjective** data pertain to or are perceived only by the affected individual. They include factors that involve the patient's emotions and experiences, such as pain and its severity, and are not perceptible to the senses. *Objective data are not necessarily more important than subjective data.* In fact, much has been written on the therapeutic value of the interview itself. Many patients come to see the physician with a personal agenda of finding a professional to listen to and empathize with a problem that may or may not have physical manifestations. The technologist must realize that conversation with the patient has great value by itself in addition to the diagnostic information that may be obtained. The art of radiologic technology includes this aspect of patient interaction.

An important point to realize is that an objective approach to the collection of subjective data is also necessary. For example, never disregard anything the patient says, *especially* if it does not fit with the opinion you are forming about the patient's symptoms. Disregarding some comments constitutes subjective collection of the data. Asking patients to define and clarify the words they use can considerably accelerate the diagnostic process. For example, the word *pain* can often provide significant additional information if the pain can be localized and a chronology established.

Questioning Skills

Adult patients are usually experienced in providing medical histories, especially if they have been hospitalized previously. The student can use this experience to advantage by simply letting patients tell their stories. Listening instead of asking more questions often provides the necessary information. Effective histories result when the following questioning techniques are used:

- Open-ended questions (nondirected, nonleading) let the patient tell the story.
- Facilitation (nod or say *yes, okay, go on …*) encourages elaboration.
- Silence (to give the patient time to remember) facilitates accuracy and elaboration.
- Probing questions (to focus the interview) provide more detail.
- Repetition (rewording) clarifies information.
- Summarization (condensing) verifies accuracy.

All histories should begin with open-ended questions to encourage the patient's spontaneous associations about the clinical problem. For example, "What type of chest problem are you having?" These questions should be followed by increasingly focused and directed probing questions based on what the patient has already said. For example, "When you breathe deeply, exactly where does it hurt—on the left side of your chest?" This technique permits the radiologic technologist to pick up where the patient had left off and provides medically specific information that might not occur to the patient otherwise.

The use of *precise and clear wording* cannot be overemphasized. Words do not always mean the same thing to patients as they do to radiologic technologists. For example, many patients refer to the entire abdomen as the *stomach*. Therefore recording *gastric pain* when a patient says the left side of the stomach hurts may be inaccurate. If this information is verified by asking the patient to point to the area, the technologist may discover that the complaint the patient is actually experiencing is left lower quadrant abdominal distress. The medical terms learned in radiologic technology are professional ones and will not be understood by all patients. On the other hand, some patients will understand medical terms, and they should not have their intelligence offended by the use of overly simplified words. For example, there is no need to tell a high school biology teacher that the esophagus is a tube leading to the stomach.

The ability to assess the patient's background can be a difficult skill to develop. Probably the most helpful technique is to begin with a question that provides an opportunity for the patient to respond in a manner that reflects his or her life experience and educational background. For example, a patient who responds to a question about the location of pain with a specific anatomic term such as *epigastric* clearly signals that medical terminology may be used. Conversely, a response using the word *belly* may indicate lack of knowledge about abdominal organs and should signal the use of simpler terms.

The use of **leading questions** should be avoided whenever possible because they introduce biases into the history. For example, "Does the pain travel down your leg?" may lead the patient to a description of sciatica. Asking the question, "Does the pain stay deep within your hip, or does it move?" provides a more reliable indication.

A useful tool is to *repeat information* obtained as a part of the history for two reasons: (1) to verify that the radiologic technologist has perceived the information correctly and (2) to ensure that the patient has not changed his or her mind.

ELEMENTS OF THE CLINICAL HISTORY

Determining the Chief Complaint

Physicians attempt to determine the patient's **chief complaint**. This effort is valuable because it focuses the history toward the single most important issue (Box 12.1). In many instances the chief

---

BOX 12.1 Sample Patient History Guide

Review the Chief Complaint
Indications for This Examination
Localization
Chronology
Quality
Severity
Onset
Aggravating or alleviating factors
Associated manifestations

Has There Been Any Trauma?

Has There Been Any Previous Surgery?

Depending on the Chief Complaint
Skeletal System
Pain location
Injury location
Injury chronology

Central Nervous System
Pain
Unconsciousness or lethargy
Bleeding location
Vision
Vertigo
Seizures

Respiratory System
Cough
Dyspnea
Hemoptysis

Infection
Pain location
Pain duration

Gastrointestinal and Genitourinary Systems
Pain location
Gastric
Nausea
Vomiting
Bowel
Constipation
Diarrhea
Stool description
Date of last bowel movement
Urinary
Known allergies and contrast media reactions
Blood pressure
Hematuria
Blood urea nitrates
Creatinine
Burning
Frequency

complaint is directly related to the first symptom that is discussed; however, there is a danger in becoming too focused on determining a single chief complaint. Permitting the patient to add more than a single complaint when multiple complaints are apparently valid is important. Ignoring all symptoms except the most predominant can obscure other important clinical information.

Sacred Seven

The radiologic and imaging sciences professional typically does not need to compile a complete medical history on patients. The physician or the nursing staff who first saw the patient will have completed this job. The interviewer's role is to collect a focused history specific to the procedure that is to be performed. Seven elements are recognized for a complete history. These elements are often referred to as the *sacred seven:*

- Localization
- Chronology
- Quality
- Severity
- Onset
- Aggravating or alleviating factors
- Associated manifestations

Localization. Localization is defining as exact and precise an area as possible for the patient's complaint. It requires the use of carefully worded questions accompanied by proper touching of the patient. By consenting to the procedure, the patient gives implied consent for the technologist to touch his or her body for both information and positioning. Remember that the patient can use verbal or nonverbal communication to withdraw this permission at any time. Two types of touch that the technologist commonly uses in gathering a clinical history are (1) touching for emphasis and (2) touching for palpation.

Touching for emphasis involves using touch to highlight or specify instructions or specify locations. A history can be clarified by a light touch to specify the region. For example, after a patient states, "My stomach hurts here" and places a hand on the upper abdomen, the radiologic technologist can add information by asking, "Does it hurt more here or here?" while touching the upper left side and then the upper middle region. *Palpation,* or applying the fingers with light pressure, can also be useful in history taking. For example, palpating the olecranon process of the elbow can help the patient to localize pain within that region.

Sometimes localization is not possible because of the nature of the problem. For example, a radiating pain may also be a deep pain that the patient cannot localize. When this confusion occurs, the radiologist should be informed that the pain is not localized. This description tells the radiologist that attempts were made to confine the complaint to a specific region. The term *nonlocalized* then becomes valuable clinical information.

Chronology. The chronology is the time element of the history. The *duration since onset, frequency,* and *course* of the symptoms should be established. This information should be described in seconds, minutes, hours, days, weeks, or months. For example,

the onset of a chest problem may have been several weeks before the examination, the duration of coughing may average 10 to 15 seconds, the frequency may be several times per hour, and the course may reveal that it is worse during the night and in the morning. The radiologist may derive important diagnostic clues from a good chronology. For example, a stress fracture may first be visualized 10 to 20 days after the onset of symptoms.

It helps to avoid giving dates or days as a chronology. For example, reporting that an injury occurred last Thursday or on July 14 requires that the physician find a calendar to determine how much time elapsed between the trauma and the examination.

Quality. The quality describes the character of the symptoms. Examples include the color and consistency of body fluids, the presence of clots or sores, the size of lumps or lesions, the type of cough, and the character of pain.

When pain is involved, it must be described carefully. This description should include either the word *acute,* meaning having a sudden onset, or the word *chronic,* meaning having a prolonged course. It should also include specific descriptors, such as *burning, throbbing, dull, sharp, cutting, aching, prickling, radiating, pressure,* and *crushing.* Again, the patient's understanding of medical terms is important. For example, a patient may describe acute pain as *sharp* or *recent.* Gaining this additional information often requires the use of focused, probing questions, such as, "When did the pain begin?"

Severity. The severity of a condition describes the intensity, quantity, or extent of the problem. Examples are the intensity of pain, the number of lesions or lumps, and the extent of a burn, as when a patient says that he or she is having a light burning sensation versus a very intense one.

Onset. Describing the onset of the complaint involves the patient explaining what he or she was doing when the illness or condition began. A review of the onset can help to determine whether predictable events preceded the recurrence of a symptom. For example, a patient might have had a series of mild headaches before a seizure.

Aggravating or Alleviating Factors. The circumstances that produce the problem or intensify it should be well defined, including anything that aggravates, alleviates, or otherwise modifies it. For example, heartburn may occur only after a full meal or a stressful day on the job and may be aggravated by certain foods and alleviated by assuming a right anterior oblique position with the head elevated slightly.

Associated Manifestations. It may be necessary to find out whether other symptoms accompany the chief complaint in order to determine whether all of the symptoms relate to the chief complaint or are related to a separate condition. For example, the patient may describe gastrointestinal symptoms as a part of, or separate from, a cardiac condition.

SUMMARY

- The radiologic and imaging sciences professional who sees himself or herself as a clinical historian realizes the value of this service. Understanding the fine art of accomplishing patient interviews can often assist in gaining increased insight and information, thus adding significantly to the radiologist's ability to diagnose.
- Good history taking involves the collection of accurate objective and subjective data. Objective data are perceptible to the senses. Subjective data pertain to or are perceived by the affected individual only.
- Thorough histories result from using such techniques as open-ended questions, facilitation, silence, probing questions, repetition, and summarization. Physicians need to determine the patient's chief complaint. This effort is valuable because it focuses the history toward the single most important issue. Seven elements are recognized as producing complete history. These elements, often referred to as the *sacred seven*, are localization, chronology, quality, severity, onset, aggravating or alleviating factors, and associated manifestations.

BIBLIOGRAPHY

Aldich CK: *The medical interview: gateway to the doctor-patient relationship*, ed 2, New York, 1999, Parthenon.

Bickley L: *Bates' guide to physical examination and history-taking*, ed 11, Philadelphia, 2012, Lippincott.

Carlton R: Radiographers as clinical historians, *RT Image* 4:16, 1991.

Carlton R, Adler AM: *Repeating radiographs: setting imaging standards: postgraduate advances in radiologic technology*, Berryville, Va, 1989, Forum Medicum.

Carnevali DL, Thomas MD: *Diagnostic reasoning and treatment decision making in nursing*, Philadelphia, 1993, Lippincott.

Cassell E: *The healer's art*, Boston, 1985, MIT Press.

Cassell E: *Talking with patients, vol. 1: theory of doctor-patient communication*, Cambridge, Mass, 1985, MIT Press.

Cassell E: *Talking with patients, vol. 2: clinical technique*, Cambridge, Mass, 1985, MIT Press.

Cassell E: *The nature of healing: the modern practice of medicine*, Oxford, UK, 2012, Oxford University Press.

Cole S, Bird J: *The medical interview: the three-function approach*, ed 2, St. Louis, 2000, Mosby.

Coulehan JL, Block MR: *The medical interview*, ed 5, Philadelphia, 2005, FA Davis.

Enelow A, Forde D, Brummel-Smith K: *Interviewing and patient care*, ed 4, New York, 1996, Oxford University Press.

Fortin A, Dwamena C, Frankel R, et al.: *Smith's patient centered interviewing: an evidence-based method*, ed 5, New York, 2012, McGraw-Hill.

Henderson M, Tierney Jr LM, Smetana GW: *The patient history: evidence-based approach to differential diagnosis*, ed 2, New York, 2012, McGraw-Hill.

Hillman R, Goodell BW, Grundy SM, et al.: *Clinical skills: interviewing, history taking, and physical diagnosis*, New York, 1981, McGraw-Hill.

Levinson D: *A guide to the clinical interview*, Philadelphia, 1987, Saunders.

McGee S: *Evidence-based physical diagnosis*, ed 4, St. Louis, 2017, Elsevier.

Park C, Morrell RW, Shifren K, editors: *Processing of medical information in aging patients: cognitive and human factors perspectives*, Mahwah, NJ, 1999, Lawrence Erlbaum.

Prior JA, Silberstein JS, Stang JM: *Physical diagnosis: the history and examination of the patient*, St. Louis, 1981, Mosby.

Purtilo R, Haddad A: *Health professionals and patient interaction*, ed 8, St. Louis, 2012, Elsevier.

Reiser D, Schroeder K: *Patient interviewing: the human dimension*, Philadelphia, 1989, Williams & Wilkins.

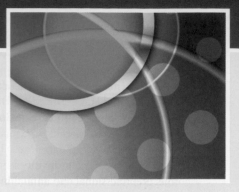

13

Safe Patient Movement and Handling Techniques

Jan Bruckner, PhD, PT, CLT-LANA

At no time in the day is the patient in more peril than when being transferred from bed to wheelchair. More injuries of consequence occur to patients, and health care personnel serving them, during transfer than at any other time.

Marilyn Rantz and Donald Courtail
Lifting, Moving, and Transferring Patients, 1981

OBJECTIVES

On completion of this chapter, the student will be able to:
- List four factors that account for the reduction of injuries that occur during handling and moving patients and explain the contribution of each factor.
- Define concepts of body mechanics used in moving and handling a patient.
- Describe the cause, signs, symptoms, and treatment of orthostatic hypotension.
- Describe the basic principles of proper lifting and transfer techniques.
- Explain or demonstrate four types of wheelchair-to-bed transfers.
- Explain or demonstrate a standard cart transfer procedure.
- Identify five standard patient positions.
- List three types of commonly attached medical equipment and explain how this may influence how to move or position a patient.

OUTLINE

KEYTERMS

Base of Support Foundation on which a body rests or stands; when people stand, their feet and the space between the feet define the base of support.

Biomechanics A component of physics, the laws of Newtonian mechanics, applied to living bodies at rest and in motion.

Center of Gravity Hypothetical point around which all mass appears to be concentrated.

Commonly Attached Medical Equipment Items clipped, fastened, or affixed to patients' bodies to deliver substances, such as oxygen, medications, hydration, or nutrition, or drain away substances, such as postsurgical fluids or urine. Care must be taken when moving or positioning patients with these attachments. Neither the patient nor the clinician should get injured during this activity. The equipment should also survive intact without damage or functional impairment.

Mobility Muscles Muscles that are found in the four extremities and designed for movement; examples include the biceps femoris, biceps brachii, and gastrocnemius. These muscles have long white tendons and are also called white muscles.

Orthostatic Hypotension A sudden drop in blood pressure in the brain when a person stands up quickly from a sitting or supine position, causing the oxygen in the brain to drop and the person to become dizzy and prone to falling.

Stability Muscles Muscles that support the torso and are designed to provide postural stability; examples include the latissimus dorsi, abdominal group, and erector spinae. These muscles tend to have thick red muscle bellies and are also called red muscles.

OVERVIEW OF SAFE HANDLING AND MOVING PATIENTS

The US Department of Labor Statistics cites sprains, strains, and other musculoskeletal problems as the leading causes of disability for people in health care, estimating the involvement of over 600,000 employees each year and a cost estimated of about $50 billion. Fortunately the incidence of injury has been decreasing. Analyses credit four factors in this declining morbidity: rigorous preprofessional and annual in-service training, improvements in equipment and technology, postinjury investigation into the causes, and the establishment of a "culture of safety" that sets institutional policies and procedures supporting health professions' decisions about the safety of any specific task. For example, if a radiologic technologist does not think that she can safely move a patient from a cart onto an exam table, the culture of safety supports her professional judgment not do the transfer without additional help. Ethical issues can arise if health professionals work in settings that do not have a culture of safety and the demands of their jobs require them to perform activities that risk injury to themselves and their patients.

Safe handling and moving people starts with applying the laws of physics to the human body. This application, called body mechanics, enables health professionals to transfer a patient safely from one place to another or move body parts into desired positions. Examples include patients transferred to and from examination tables, on and off toilet seats, and in and out of bathtubs.

Radiologic technologists position patients' arms and legs for diagnostic imaging. The patient's physical and cognitive abilities determine the amount of assistance required for each move. Some patients can perform the movement tasks independently or with verbal directions from the health professional. Other patients need manual assistance or the use of special equipment, such as lifts or transfer devices. To promote safety for patients and staff, health professionals involved with patient handling and movement must decide on the appropriate type of transfer. Special clinical skills are required to choose the appropriate method. Continuing educations classes and in-service training help clinicians stay abreast of new techniques as they develop.

BODY MECHANICS

Biomechanics is a branch of physics that applies the laws of mechanics to living creatures. Biomechanics examines the action of forces on bodies at rest or in motion and can be used to optimize exercise programs, promote greater athletic skills, and design safer work environments. Fundamental to good patient handling techniques are the concepts of the base of support, center of gravity, and mobility and stability muscles.

Base of Support

The base of support is the foundation on which a body rests. When a person is standing, the feet and the space between the feet constitute that person's base of support (Fig. 13.1A).

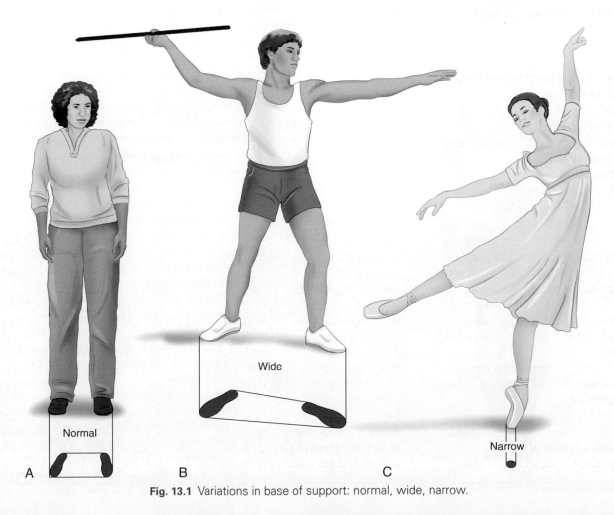

Fig. 13.1 Variations in base of support: normal, wide, narrow.

Standing with the feet far apart enlarges the base of support (see Fig. 13.1B). Standing on one foot or tiptoe provides the person with a small base of support (see Fig. 13.1C). Narrow bases of support characterize unstable and mobile systems. Wide bases of support characterize stable systems. In transferring a patient, the health professional must establish as stable a base of support as possible. Standing with feet farther apart to increase the base of support improves stability.

Center of Gravity

Center of gravity is a hypothetical point at which all the mass appears to be concentrated (Fig. 13.2); gravitational forces appear to act on the entire body from this specific point. In humans aligned in the anatomic position, the center of gravity is at approximately sacral level two, with slight variations between men and women. Moving heavy objects is relatively easy and safe if the object is held close to the mover's center of gravity. Stability can be achieved when a body's center of gravity is over its base of support (Fig. 13.3A). Instability results when the center of gravity moves beyond the boundaries of the base (see Fig. 13.3B). For safe, stable lifting, the center of gravity must always be over the base of support.

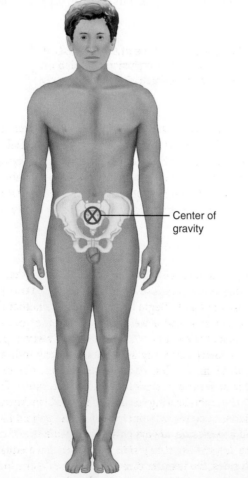

Fig. 13.2 The center of gravity for most people is located at approximately S-2.

Mobility and Stability Muscles

The body contains muscles that are designed for mobility and other muscles that are designed for stability. Mobility muscles are found in the limbs. Typically these muscles have long white tendons and cross two or more joints. Examples include the biceps muscles, which flex the elbow, and the hamstring muscles, which flex the knee (Fig. 13.4). Stability muscles are found in the torso. Typically stability muscles are large expanses of red muscle belly and provide postural support. Two examples are the latissimus dorsi, girthing the back, and the rectus abdominis, supporting the abdomen. For effective patient moving and handling, clinicians should use white mobility muscles for lifting and red postural muscles for support. Lifting should be done by bending and straightening the knees. The back should be kept straight or in a position of slightly increased lumbar lordosis.

PRINCIPLES OF LIFTING

In performing a transfer, let the patient do as much of the work as possible (Box 13.1). Before attempting a transfer, always ask the patient whether he or she can move independently. Patients can often transfer on their own or with minimal assistance. If assistance is required, let the patient help. This approach minimizes trauma to the patient and avoids stress on the clinician. In addition, this approach enhances rapport and mutual respect between patient and technologist.

Patients may be unsure whether they need assistance. Patients sometimes believe that they are capable of transferring themselves when they are not. Before executing the transfer, check the patient's chart and verify whether he or she has a restricted weight-bearing status. Be especially protective of patients with diagnoses such as lower extremity or pelvic girdle fracture; painful, inflamed, or unstable joints; or any weakened or debilitated condition. Patients with cognitive impairments, such as dementia, may overestimate their transfer abilities and require assistance. Offer assistance as required. Allow ample time and handle patients with a firm, gentle grasp. Identify yourself and give your title. Inform the patient of what you are going to do and how you intend to proceed. For example, tell the patient your name and that you are a radiologic technologist who is going to help him or her move from the wheelchair to the table. List the specific steps for doing this activity: scoot your pelvis to the front of the wheelchair, put your hands on the arms of the wheelchair, lean forward with your nose over your toes, stand up, reach for and hold the table with the hand closest to the table, pivot so you are standing with your pelvis against the table, and sit down gently on the table. Let the patient perform as much of the transfer as he or she can. Execute the transfer slowly, with grace and control, so that the patient will feel secure.

In lifting a patient, the technologist should stand with feet apart to increase the base of support. The patient's center of gravity (S-2) should be held close to the clinician's center of gravity (S-2). This positioning provides the best mechanical advantage for lifting. Some patients may be wearing bathrobes or hospital gowns. Loose clothing inhibits the clinician's ability to hold a patient securely. One solution is to place a transfer belt around

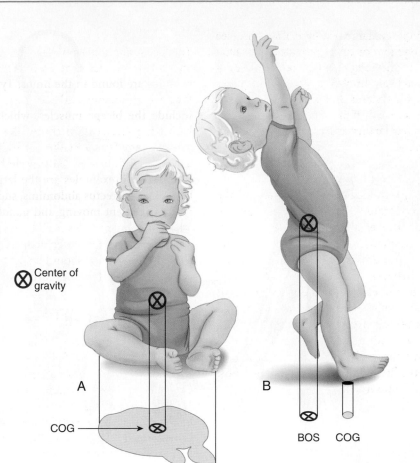

Fig. 13.3 (A) A body is stable when its center of gravity *(COG)* rests over its base of support *(BOS)*. (B) A body is unstable when its COG is not over its BOS. In the picture, the child is standing on his left heel. The right foot is off the ground, and the COG is just anterior to S-2, considerably posterior to the left heel. The child is unstable and likely to fall.

the patient's waist. Transfer belts are usually made of webbing or muslin and can provide a good grip with minimal trauma to the patient. Using a transfer belt is a good practice in planning to perform transfers. In lifting patients, *keep your back stationary and let your legs do all of the lifting;* also avoid any twisting.

Technologists should be aware of **orthostatic hypotension,** which is a drop in blood pressure that occurs when a person stands too quickly. A slight drop in blood pressure occurs normally when any person rises quickly from a recumbent to an upright position. This condition becomes increasingly serious when patients have been in bed for long periods and have a debilitated status. These weakened patients tend to have blood vessels with decreased vasomotor tone, compromised lymph vessels, and other circulatory problems. As a result, blood pressure may be affected. Rising too quickly can deprive patients of oxygen-rich blood to the brain. Symptoms of orthostatic hypotension include dizziness, fainting, blurred vision, and slurred speech.

To minimize the severity of orthostatic hypotension, have the patient stand slowly and talk during the transfer. Ask patients open questions. For example, "How are you feeling?" or "Where do you come from?" The questions do not matter, but the patient's answers do. Listen to the patient's speech. Slowing or slurring of words may indicate decreased blood flow to the

brain. If signs occur, slow the speed of the transfer and ask the patient to take slow, deep breaths. Provide additional verbal and physical assistance as needed. If a patient reports symptoms, let him or her pause and take deep breaths for a few moments until he or she feels better. *Do not send symptomatic patients on their way* and risk having them faint on the way to their rooms.

WHEELCHAIR TRANSFERS

Radiologic technologists use four types of wheelchair transfers: (1) standby assist, (2) assisted standing pivot, (3) two-person lift, and (4) hydraulic lift. Begin by determining whether the patient has a strong side and a weak side or whether both sides are equal. Look at the patient. A long-leg cast, a severe foot deformity, or a lower extremity amputation clearly indicates a unilateral problem. For less easily observed transfer precautions, check the patient's chart, ask the patient, or inquire of staff about restricted weight-bearing status, generalized weakness, arthritic conditions, or cognitive impairment. If the patient has a strong side and a weak side, *always position the patient so that he or she transfers toward the strong side.* If patients have equal strength on both sides, the transfer direction may be determined by convenience or space limitations. In all wheelchair transfers, be

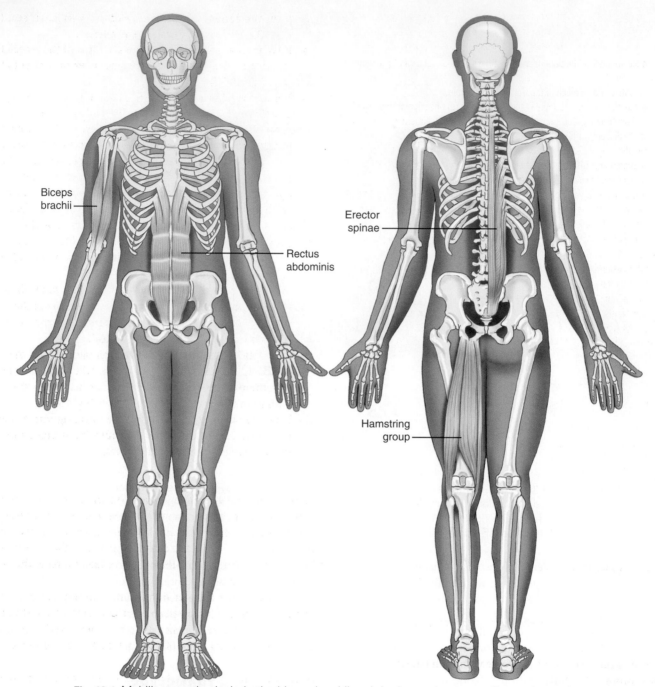

Fig. 13.4 Mobility muscles include the biceps brachii and the hamstring group. Postural muscles include the rectus abdominis and the erector spinae muscles.

sure that the wheelchair wheels are locked and that the footrests are removed or folded away so that they do not obstruct patient movement.

Standby Assist Transfer

Some patients have the ability to transfer from a wheelchair to a table on their own. Position the wheelchair at a 45-degree angle to the table (Fig. 13.5). Talk to the patient before he or she moves to determine how much, if any, assistance is required. Divide the transfer into single-step components, and talk the patient through each step. Perform the following tasks and give the following commands to the patient to provide assistance for a wheelchair-to-table transfer:

1. Task: Move the wheelchair footrests out of the way.
2. Task: Be sure that the wheelchair wheels are locked.
3. Command: "Sit on the edge of the wheelchair seat."
4. Command: "Push down on the arms of the chair" (to assist in rising).
5. Command: "Nose over toes and stand up slowly."
6. Command: "Reach out and hold onto the table with the hand closest to the table."
7. Command: "Turn slowly until you feel the table behind you."

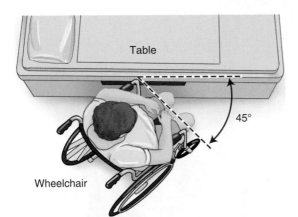

Fig. 13.5 Angle the wheelchair to be 45 degrees from the table.

8. Command: "Hold onto the table with both hands."
9. Command: "Sit down."

If the table is too high for the patient to sit comfortably, after step 6 give the patient a footstool. Provide assistance as needed for the patient to step up on the stool and sit on the table.

Assisted Standing Pivot Transfer

For patients who cannot transfer independently but can bear weight on their legs, a standing pivot technique is used. Position the wheelchair at a 45-degree angle to the table with the patient's stronger side closest to the table. If the patient is wearing loose-fitting clothes, place a transfer belt around the patient's waist (Fig. 13.6A). The transfer belt enables a secure grip on the patient without traumatizing any of the patient's joints. Execute the following steps one at a time:

1. Move the wheelchair footrests out of the way.
2. Be sure that the wheelchair wheels are locked.

3. Have the patient sit on the edge of the wheelchair seat (see Fig. 13.6B). Provide assistance as needed.
4. Have the patient push down on the arms of the wheelchair to assist in rising with patient's nose over the patient's toes (see Fig. 13.6C).
5. Bend at the knees, keep your back straight, and grasp the transfer belt with both hands. The patient's feet and knees must be blocked to provide stability, especially for paraparetic and hemiplegic patients who have muscle weakness and may not be able to move or feel sensation in lower extremities. The technologist must block the patient's knees and feet so the patient can bear enough weight to move safely. This task is accomplished by placing one foot outside the patient's foot while the knee is placed at the medial (inside) surface of the patient's knee (see Fig. 13.6D).
6. As the patient rises to a standing position, rise also by straightening your knees (see Fig. 13.6E).
7. When the patient is standing, ask, "How are you feeling?" If the patient reports or exhibits dizziness or any of the other signs of orthostatic hypotension, stand for a moment and take slow, deep breaths (see Fig. 13.6F).
8. When the patient is ready, both of you pivot toward the table until the patient can feel the table against the back of the thighs.
9. Ask the patient to support himself or herself on the table with both hands and to sit down (see Fig. 13.6G).
10. Help the patient to sit by gradually lowering him or her to the table. Be sure that your back remains straight and that the lowering occurs from the knees.

Two-Person Lift

Some patients cannot bear weight on their lower extremities and must be lifted onto the table. If the patient is lightweight, a two-person lift can be executed. The stronger person should lift the patient's torso while the second person lifts the patient's feet. The person lifting the patient's torso usually directs the other person's actions.

Prepare for the transfer by verbally planning out the procedure. This verbal planning enables a coordinated effort among the people doing the transfer and the patient. Verbal planning also allows for troubleshooting before the execution of the transfer.

Begin with the wheelchair. Lock the wheelchair wheels, remove the armrests, and swing away or remove the leg rests. Ask the patient to cross his or her arms over the chest. The stronger person stands behind the patient, reaches under the patient's axillae, and grasps the patient's crossed forearms. The second person should squat in front of the patient and cradle the patient's thighs in one hand and calves in the other hand (Fig. 13.7A). On command, the patient is lifted to clear the wheelchair and is moved as a unit to the desired place (see Fig. 13.7B).

Hydraulic Lift Techniques

Some patients are too heavy to lift manually and require a hydraulic lift. Lift transfers have multiple steps and require some skill. Health professionals should familiarize themselves with and practice using the equipment before attempting to lift a patient.

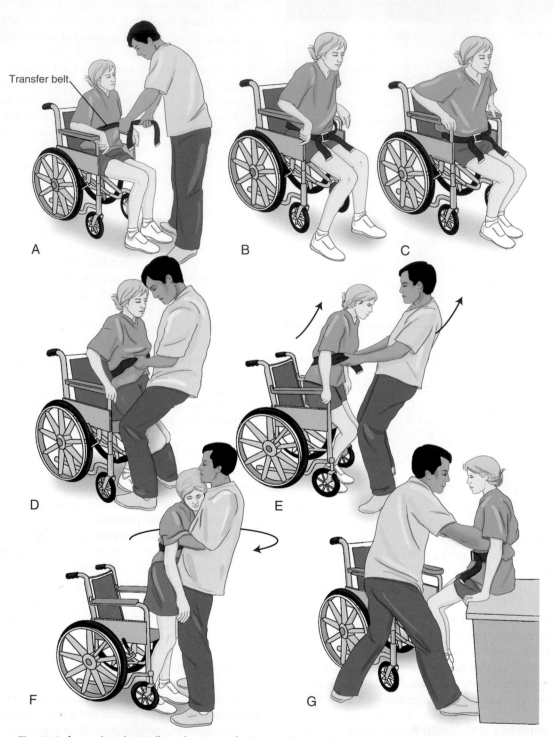

Transfer belt

A

B

C

D

E

F

G

Fig. 13.6 An assisted standing pivot transfer is used in transferring a patient from a wheelchair to a table. (A) Use a transfer belt to hold the patient securely. (B) Have the patient sit on the edge of the wheelchair seat. Provide assistance as needed. (C) Have the patient push down on the arms of the wheelchair to assist in rising. (D) Bend at the knees, keeping your back straight, and grasp the transfer belt with both hands. (E) As the patient rises to standing, rise also by straightening your knees. (F) When the patient is standing, ask, "How are you feeling?" If the patient reports or exhibits dizziness or any of the other signs of orthostatic hypotension, stand for a moment and take slow, deep breaths. (G) Ask the patient to hold onto the table with both hands and to slowly sit down.

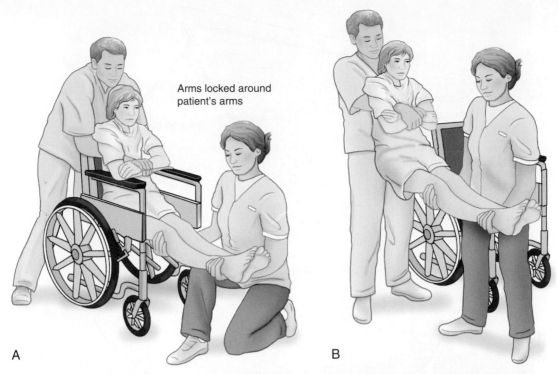

Arms locked around patient's arms

A   B

Fig. 13.7 Two-person lift. (A) The first person asks the patient to cross his or her arms over the chest. The person making the transfer stands behind the patient, reaches under the patient's axillae, and grasps the patient's crossed forearms. The assistant squats in front of the patient and cradles the patient's thighs in one hand and the patient's calves in the other. (B) At the command of the person supporting the patient's upper body, the patient is lifted to clear the wheelchair and moved as a unit to the desired place.

Most hydraulic lifts have several basic features. To facilitate moving, they often have four caster wheels but no wheel locks. The lift's base of support can be widened or narrowed by means of a lever. Most lifts have two handles for steering, a manual pump for raising the support arm, a release valve for lowering the support arm, and a spreader bar for the sling attachment (Fig. 13.8). Identify these features and learn their operation before attempting to lift a patient.

Prior arrangements should be made with the nursing staff to have patients needing hydraulic lift transfers arrive in the radiology department sitting on a transfer sling. If this patient arrives without a sling, call the nursing staff and discuss the need for a sling. One option is to send the patient back to the floor and have the patient return sitting on the sling. Avoid risking injury to patient or staff by using equipment correctly.

The sling attaches to the spreader bar by hooks and chains. The chains have a short segment for attachment to the sling back and a longer segment for attachment to the sling seat. Adjust the chain length according to the size of the patient. Hook the chains to the sling from the inside out (Fig. 13.9A). This precaution minimizes the risk of a patient being injured by the hooks.

Check that the release valve is closed and that the patient is positioned comfortably in the sling. Gently raise the patient (see Fig. 13.9B). When the patient has cleared the wheelchair seat, the wheelchair can be removed and the patient can be positioned on the table. Manual assistance may be required to position the patient appropriately.

To lower the patient, open the release valve and gently lower the patient. Guard the patient's head from contact with the spreader bar. Remove the chains with care; they have a tendency to swing and must be steadied to avoid patient injury. After the patient has achieved a safe, stable position, the lift can be removed. If possible, leave the sling under the patient in anticipation of the return transfer.

CART TRANSFERS

Many patients are transported by cart (also called a *stretcher* or *gurney*). To move a patient from a cart onto a radiographic table, position the cart alongside the table on the patient's strong or less affected side. The cart must be wheeled as close to the table as possible and then secured. Simply engaging wheel locks may not be sufficient to keep a cart from moving. Placing sandbags or other devices on the floor is often necessary to block the wheels satisfactorily.

If the patient can assist with the transfer, all that may be required is stabilization of the cart and support for the involved body part. For example, a patient with a plaster long leg cast may be able to move his or her body if the cast is supported

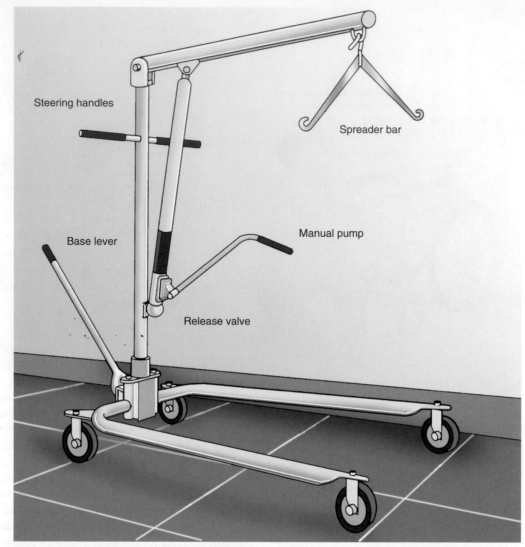

Fig. 13.8 Hydraulic lifts often have four caster wheels but no wheel locks. The lift's base of support can be widened or narrowed by means of a lever. The lift has two handles for steering, a manual pump for raising the support arm, a release valve for lowering the support arm, and a spreader bar for the sling attachment.

during the transfer. If the patient cannot assist, a moving device or draw sheet should be used. Three people usually perform a cart-to-table transfer.

Numerous commercially manufactured moving devices are available. Some devices are smooth, thin sheets of plastic, and others are composed of canvas or plastic over small rollers; all are designed to be used as aids during cart-to-table transfers. To do the transfer, begin by rolling the patient onto his or her side away from the direction of the transfer. Place the moving device in the midpoint of the patient's back. Roll the patient supine so that he or she is positioned on the moving device. The device slowly moves the patient onto the table (Fig. 13.10). If necessary, the patient can be rolled to remove the moving device.

A second type of moving device is a low-friction plastic sheet that enables health practitioners to slide rather than lift their patients during transfers. The Arjo Company manufactures such products under the names of MaxiSlide, MaxiTube, and MaxiTransfer. A patient must be placed on a double thickness of this fabric and then glided from one place to another. The top layer moves with the patient so that the patient's skin is protected from abrasions. Because the patient is pushed or pulled into position rather than lifted, each transfer requires less effort and fewer personnel.

To perform a lateral transfer from, for example, a gurney to a radiographic table with plastic transfer sheets, two sheets are needed. One sheet must be directly under the patient, and the second sheet must be under the first sheet to serve as a track on which the patient will slide. If the patient arrives without a transfer sheet, one can easily be placed under the patient. Roll the patient to one side, place a double thickness of the sheeting under the patient, and then roll the patient on top of the transfer sheets.

For the actual lateral transfer, both transfer surfaces must be side to side, as close to each other as possible, and at the same

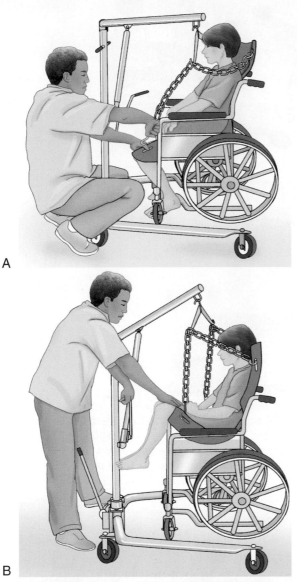

A

B

Fig. 13.9 Hydraulic lift transfer. (A) The chains have a short segment for attachment to the sling back and a longer segment for attachment to the sling seat. Adjust the chain length according to the patient's size. Hook the chains to the sling from the inside out. This precaution minimizes the risk that a patient will be injured by the hooks. (B) Check that the release valve is closed and that the patient is positioned comfortably in the sling. Gently begin to raise the patient.

height. The wheels of the gurney must be locked so the two surfaces cannot separate during the transfer. Two technologists, one at the patient's head and chest and a second at the patient's pelvis and legs, can grasp the top sheet and slide the patient laterally into the desired position.

To perform a cart-to-table transfer without a moving device, a draw sheet is needed. Begin by checking that the sheet is properly positioned for the transfer. Then roll up the draw sheet on both sides of the patient (Fig. 13.11A). The person directing the transfer should support the patient's head and upper body from the far side of the radiographic table. Another person should support the patient's pelvic girdle from the cart side. A third person should support the patient's legs from the table side. The

patient's arms should be crossed over the chest to avoid injury or interference with a smooth transfer (see Fig. 13.11B).

The person supporting the pelvic girdle stands on the opposite side of the cart and makes sure that the cart does not move away from the table during the transfer. The person in charge, at the patient's head, gives the commands and directs the transfer. On command, everyone grasps the rolled-up draw sheet and slowly pulls the patient to the edge of the cart. Depending on the length of their reach, the assistants may need to reposition themselves in anticipation of moving the patient from the cart onto the table. When everyone is ready, the person in charge again issues the command and the patient is slowly lifted and positioned onto the table.

The transfer without a moving device is difficult. Because of the potential for strain and injury to the persons performing the maneuver, it is generally not recommended for most patients, especially those who are heavy or who have serious injuries. The transfer personnel should never kneel or stand on the radiographic table to perform transfers.

POSITIONING *Pg. 151*

For the desired body part to be examined, patients need to be moved into a variety of different positions. In general, the patient must be transferred as a single unit, placed on the table in a safe and secure position, and then moved segmentally into the desired body position. Before executing the move, talk through the steps to prepare the patient and any assistants. Let the patient assist as much as possible. To minimize trauma and discomfort for the patient, take an extra moment to make sure that the patient is ready to make the move. In moving a patient, always roll the patient *toward* you. Provide positioning sponges to support the patient comfortably in the desired position. The proper terms for the most common positions are given in Fig. 13.12. All radiologic technologists should become familiar with both the positions and the appropriate methods to assist patients in achieving them.

COMMONLY ATTACHED MEDICAL EQUIPMENT

Patients may arrive in the radiology department with items clipped or affixed to their bodies designed to deliver or drain away fluids. Commonly attached medical equipment includes oxygen tubing, intravenous lines, central lines, postsurgical drains, and urine bags. Before moving or positioning a patient, clinicians should check for attached equipment. Items hanging above a patient may be easier to see than items hooked onto the wheelchair frame under the seat or secured inside patient clothes. The patient's chart and transport personnel can also provide information about commonly attached medical equipment. Clinicians must consider attached equipment when moving and positioning patients. Equipment must not hinder patient or clinician movement and the transfer should not damage or impair function of equipment. Training and in-service instruction assists clinicians in safely handling patients with attached equipment during transfers.

▲ *Draw string transfer has the greatest potential for back strain*

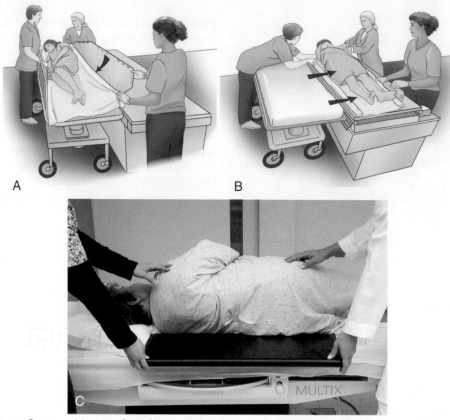

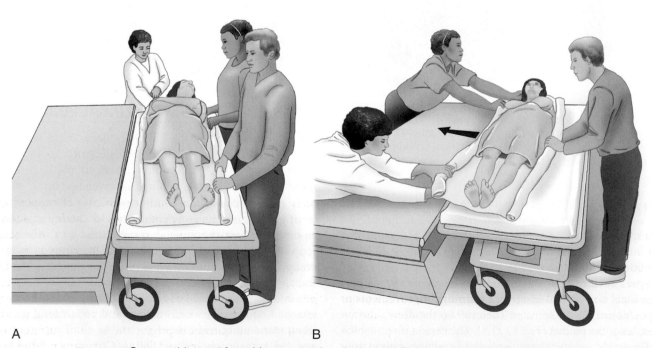

Fig. 13.10 Cart-to-table transfer with a moving device. The preferred method of moving a patient from a cart to a table is with a moving device. (A) The patient should be rolled away from the table while the device is placed halfway underneath both the patient and the draw sheet. The patient is then returned to a supine position, and the draw sheet is gently pulled to move the patient onto the table. If necessary, the patient may be rolled again to remove the moving device. (B) A plastic moving device in use. (C) A roller moving device in use.

Fig. 13.11 Cart-to-table transfer without a moving device. (A) Begin by rolling up the draw sheet on both sides of the patient. (B) The person directing the transfer supports the patient's head and upper body from the far side of the radiographic table. An assistant supports the patient's pelvic girdle from the cart side. A second assistant supports the patient's legs from the tableside. The patient's arms can be crossed over the chest to avoid injury or getting in the way.

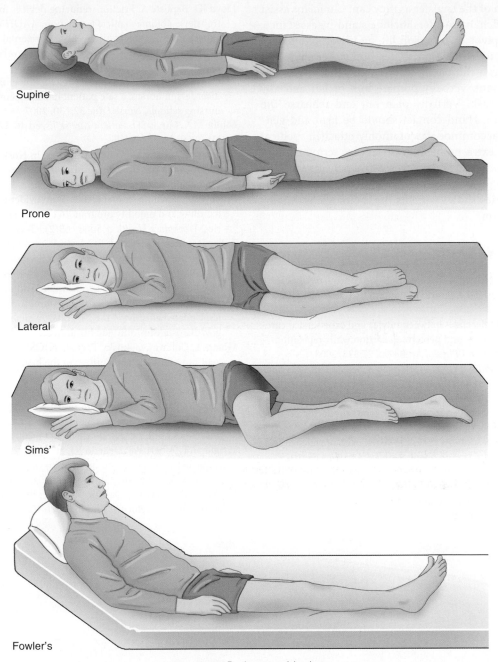

Supine

Prone

Lateral

Sims'

Fowler's

Fig. 13.12 Patient positioning.

SUMMARY

Sprains, strains, and other musculoskeletal injuries distinguish health care workers as having one of the most dangerous occupations in the United States. Fortunately the incidence of injury has been decreasing due to four factors: rigorous pre-professional and annual in-service training, improvements in equipment and technology, postinjury investigation into the causes, and the establishment of a "culture of safety," which establishes institutional policies and procedures supporting health professions' decisions about the safety of any specific task. The first factor requires the radiologic technologists to learn and use proper body mechanics. Basic principles of body mechanics include knowledge of base of support, center of gravity, and the body's mobility and stability muscles. In moving a patient, the clinician should maintain a wide base of support, hold the patient's center of gravity close to the technologist's center of gravity, avoid trunk twisting, keep the back stable, lift from the knees, and let the patient assist as much as possible. One danger in moving patients is orthostatic hypotension. Patients may suffer a sudden drop in blood pressure when standing quickly, depriving the brain of sufficient oxygen and causing fainting and falling. Clinicians need to know the cause, signs, symptoms, and treatment of orthostatic hypotension to avoid patient falls. When moving from one place to another or moving a body part into a specific position, patients should do as much of the transfer as they can. Clinicians assist as required. Wheelchair transfers include stand-by assistance, assisted standing pivot, two-person lift, and hydraulic lift. In initiating any activity with a patient, tell him or her name and identify yourself as a radiologic technologist. Before moving or handling a patient, verbally prepare him or her and any assistants for the task. Verbally plan out and rehearse the intended procedure. Hand contact should be firm and gentle. Take time to accommodate commonly attached medical equipment. These extra moments can prevent serious injury. Handle patients with care and respect. Move patients with the application of professional knowledge and skill. Demonstration of these abilities shows patients the radiologic technologist's professionalism.

BIBLIOGRAPHY

Baptiste A, Boda SV, Nelson AL, et al.: Friction-reducing devices for lateral patient transfers: a clinical evaluation, *AAOHN J* 54:173, 2006.

Daikoku R, Saito Y: Differences between novice and experienced caregivers in muscle activity and perceived exertion while repositioning bedridden patients, *J Physiol Anthropol* 27:333, 2008.

Ehrlich RA, Daly JA: *Patient care in radiography: with an introduction to medical imaging*, ed 8, St. Louis, 2012, Mosby.

Hubley-Kozey CL, Vezina MJ: Differentiating temporal electromyographic waveforms between those with chronic low back pain and healthy controls, *Clin Biomech (Bristol, Avon)* 17:631, 2002.

Karahan A, Kav S, Abbasoglu A, et al.: Low back pain: prevalence and associated risk factors among hospital staff, *J Adv Nurs* 65:516, 2009.

Kelsey JL, White 3rd AA, Pastides H, et al.: The impact of musculoskeletal disorders on the population of the United States, *J Bone Joint Surg Am* 61:959, 1979.

Lloyd JD, Baptiste A: Friction-reducing devices for lateral patient transfers: a biomechanical evaluation, *AAOHN J* 54:113, 2006.

McGill SM, Kavcic NS: Transfer of the horizontal patient: the effect of a friction reducing assistive device on low back mechanics, *Ergonomics* 48:915, 2005.

Menzel NN, Hughes NL, Waters T, et al.: Preventing musculoskeletal disorders in nurses: a safe patient handling curriculum module for nursing schools, *Nurse Educ* 32:130, 2007.

Minor MA, Minor SD: *Patient care skills*, ed 46, Upper Saddle River, NJ, 2009, Prentice Hall.

Norkin CC, Levangie PK: Biomechanics. In Norkin CC, Levangie PK, editors: *Joint structure and function: a comprehensive analysis*, ed 5, Philadelphia, 2011, FA Davis.

Przybysz L, Levin PF: Initial results of an evidence-based safe patient handling and mobility program to decrease hospital worker injuries, *Workplace Health & Safety* 65(2):83–88, 2017.

Tullar JM, Brewer S, Amick BC, Irvin E, et al.: Occupational safety and health interventions to reduce musculoskeletal symptoms in the health care sector, *J Occup Rehabil* 20:199–219, 2010.

U.S. Department of Labor: Back disorders and injuries. In *Occupational Health and Safety Technical Manual, Section VII: Ergonomics*. Updated effective, June 24, 2008. Available at http://www.osha.gov/dts/osta/otm/otm_toc.html. Accessed July 9, 2014.

Waters T, Collins J, Galinsky T, et al.: NIOSH research efforts to prevent musculoskeletal disorders in the healthcare industry, *Orthop Nurs* 25:380, 2006.

White Paper: Strategies to improve patient and health care provider safety in patient handling and moving tasks. Available at http://www.osha.gov/ergonomics/guidelines/nursinghomes/final_nh_guidelines.html. Accessed February 24, 2004.

Wrigley AT, Albert WJ, Deluzio KJ, et al.: Differentiating lifting technique between those who develop low back pain and those who do not, *Clin Biomech (Bristol, Avon)* 20:254, 2005.

Wrigley AT, Albert WJ, Deluzio KJ, et al.: Principal component analysis of lifting waveforms, *Clin Biomech (Bristol, Avon)* 21:567, 2006.

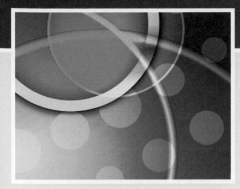

Immobilization Techniques

Melynie Durham, MS, RT(R)(MR)

> *Uncooperative behavior can be viewed as active resistance, a defensive action which serves to preserve self-esteem and ward off the invasiveness of intervention. … Resistance is therefore a sign of strength … the therapeutic solution is not to confront resistance, but to honor it.*
>
> *Helen Burr, 1987*

OBJECTIVES

On completion of this chapter, the student will be able to:

- Demonstrate a range of immobilization techniques.
- Explain the importance of high-quality communication with the patient.
- Describe reduction of patient radiation exposure by using proper immobilization methods.
- Apply immobilization techniques in routine situations.
- Use immobilization devices effectively.
- Describe trauma immobilization techniques as they pertain to specific anatomic involvement.
- Explain the importance of establishing rapport with pediatric patients.
- Use various methods of pediatric immobilization.
- Describe appropriate application of immobilization techniques pertinent to geriatric patients.

OUTLINE

KEY TERMS

Ambulatory Able to walk

Anteroposterior Direction of x-ray beam from front to back

Artifacts Substances or structures not naturally present but of which an authentic image appears on an image

Axial Projection Any projection not at right angles to the long axis of an anatomic structure

Empathy Recognition of and entering into the feelings of another person

Flexion Act of bending or condition of being bent

Geriatric Pertaining to the treatment of the aged

Immobilization Act of rendering immovable

Neonates Newborn infants

Pediatric Pertaining to the branch of medicine that treats children

Plantar Surface Sole of the foot

Rapport Relation of harmony and accord between two persons

Restraint Hindrance of an action (movement)

Trauma Wound or injury

SCOPE OF IMMOBILIZATION TECHNIQUES

When **immobilization** techniques are discussed, the effect of motion and positioning inaccuracy on the diagnostic quality of the procedure is important to understand. One of the many factors that affect diagnostic quality is motion. When one attempts to photograph a fast-moving object (e.g., a sprinter or a race car), a good possibility exists that the image will appear streaked or blurry because of the motion of the object photographed.

The same phenomenon occurs when radiographing a wiggly 3-year-old patient's chest or the shaking hand of a badly injured accident victim. The movement of the toddler or the shaking hand results in a blurred image and necessitates a repeat exposure, which increases patient dose. The important fact is that the motion of the subject does not have to be considerable or exaggerated to affect the procedure. Even the slightest movement can seriously compromise the image.

Another important factor affecting diagnostic information is inaccuracy when positioning the patient during an examination. Many positions for procedures require exact degrees of rotation of the patient or body part. Use of positioning aids such as sponges or supports enables the radiologic technologist to position the patient accurately. At the same time, this support of the patient significantly lessens the possibility of motion.

A thorough knowledge of the various methods that can be used to reduce the possibility of motion problems and positioning inaccuracies is therefore extremely important when studying the art and practice of radiologic technology.

Simple Versus Involved Immobilization Techniques

Although some forms of immobilization or restraint techniques can be intricate, understanding that immobilization techniques cover a wide range of applications, from minimal to highly sophisticated, is important. The simplest techniques involve the use of a positioning sponge to support the anatomic area of interest or gently laying a sandbag across a patient's forearm to minimize shaking caused by patient anxiety. More complex techniques might involve completely wrapping an infant or small child in a sheet (often referred to as a *mummy wrap* or *bunny method*) or securing a trauma patient to a backboard to facilitate transport of the patient to the emergency department and minimize the possibility of more severe complications, such as spinal cord damage, during the transport process. In the latter case, the radiologic technologist has not applied the immobilization device but must recognize the importance of the device and be able to use it to the best advantage.

Protection From Radiation

A conscientious, professional radiologic technologist strives to produce the most diagnostic image possible with the least amount of radiation to the patient and others. If the patient moves, either voluntarily or involuntarily, the images may be of less-than-optimal quality and therefore need to be repeated. When the projection is repeated, the patient receives an additional dose of radiation. Voluntary movement can be controlled by the patient and most often occurs as a result of inadequate communication by the technologist. Involuntary movement is the result of many contributing factors (e.g., examination room temperature, medication, movement disorders, posttraumatic shock) and cannot be controlled by the patient. To minimize the radiation dose to the patient, performing the procedure correctly the first time is important.

Communication

Various physical restraints can be used to reduce the possibility of motion, but perhaps one of the most effective means of reducing motion on the part of the patient is also one of the simplest and, unfortunately, one of the most overlooked. The method is *communication*.

Communication is a skill that is often used ineffectively. Ineffective or unskillful communication can occur at all levels—between radiologist and radiologic technologist, from one technologist to another, from clinical instructor to student, from department manager to secretary, from technologist to patient, and so forth. Keeping in mind the objective of reducing repeated procedures and exposure to radiation, the most important communication that occurs in a radiology department may take place between the technologist and patient.

The patient is often capable of cooperation and would be more than willing to facilitate the examination if he or she were simply informed of what was going to happen and apprised of the importance of cooperation in producing an accurate diagnosis. A key component to effective communication with the patient is the establishment of rapport.

Rapport is a relation of harmony and accord between two persons, as between patient and physician. This harmony and relationship building should begin as soon as the technologist introduces himself or herself to the patient and continue throughout the history-taking process. While obtaining the history, the technologist has the opportunity to display empathy, respect, and concern for the patient as a person, as well as to ascertain the clinical facts behind the examination. Once the radiologic technologist has established rapport with the patient, the patient becomes increasingly comfortable, a sense of trust and confidence is established, and the patient is able to focus on the explanation of what will occur during the examination.

Whereas a good explanation of the examination is important and will better enable the patient to cooperate, the explanation generally need not be highly technical or filled with professional jargon. A simple explanation, in lay terms, stressing the importance of cooperation on the part of the patient is usually all that is needed. Care must be taken, however, that in simplifying the explanation one does not make the patient feel insulted by underestimation of his or her intelligence. A proper assessment of the patient's replies and questions allows the technologist to explain the examination at a level appropriate to each patient. The explanation should emphasize that cooperation on the part of the patient will make the examination proceed quickly and result in the highest quality diagnostic information possible. Keeping the explanation simple is important, but make sure the patient understands that his or her cooperation is essential.

The radiologic technologist will not always be able to communicate effectively in a verbal sense, as in the case of a very young child or someone who is highly stressed because of the nature of his or her injury or condition. If the technologist is truly genuine in his or her empathy for the patient, communication of a subtle nature will occur. For example, a newborn infant often senses and responds positively to warmth, gentle holding, a soft calm voice, and a sense of security.

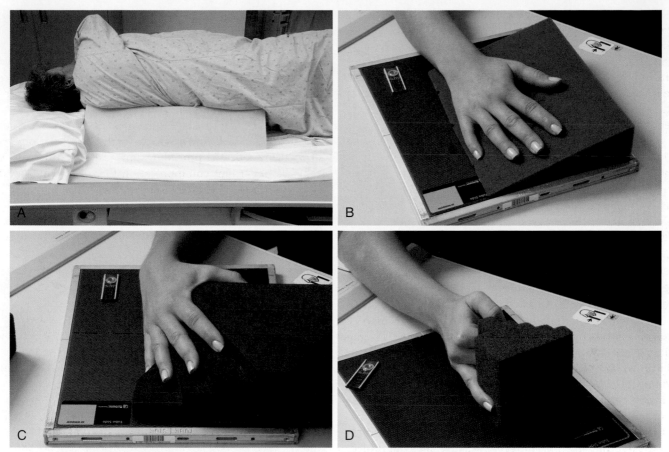

Fig. 14.1 (A) Patient positioned with sponge for oblique lumbar spine image. (B) Hand in oblique position on sponge. (C) Hand in fan lateral position on sponge. (D) Fourth finger in lateral position using sponge.

ROUTINE APPLICATIONS

Although some immobilization methods may seem mundane to the experienced technologist, their dedicated use results in fewer repeated procedures as a result of patient motion.

Positioning Sponges

One of the most common methods of reducing patient motion involves the use of positioning sponges. These sponges come in a variety of shapes and sizes and are designed to support the patient or the anatomic area of interest by reducing physical strain on the patient from having to hold a position that might otherwise be difficult to achieve (Fig. 14.1). Positioning sponges also allow for increased accuracy in positioning by supporting the patient or anatomic area of interest in the correct position (Fig. 14.2). The use of positioning sponges is limited only by the creativity of the technologist.

Stability Bar

Stability bars are located on most upright Bucky units (see Fig. 8.13)—originally created to assist patients when performing lateral chest examinations. The purpose is twofold: to move the patient's arms above their head and out of the area of interest as well as providing stability and steadiness. By eliminating patient swaying or movement, the need for repeats can be reduced and

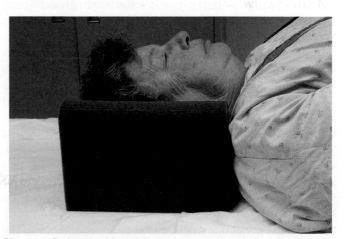

Fig. 14.2 Patient positioned for anteroposterior skull radiograph with head holder in place.

patient radiation exposure can be kept at a minimum. The stability bar is adjustable and can be used while the patient is standing or sitting as well as for standing lateral lumbar examinations.

Velcro Straps

Although often not considered a form of restraint, Velcro straps can be effective as restraining or positioning devices. A good example of the use of straps is provided by an upright lateral

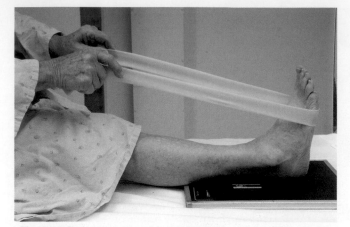

Fig. 14.3 Patient positioned for axial calcaneus image using strap.

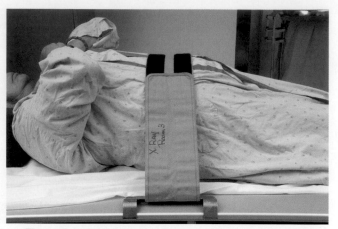

Fig. 14.4 Patient supine on table with Velcro straps in place.

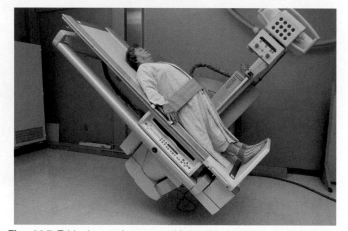

Fig. 14.5 Table in semi-erect position with compression band over patient. If more support is needed, then additional bands may be applied to the chest, hips, and knees.

chest position. The patient should be standing for a chest examination if at all possible. Although capable of standing, a patient who has not been regularly **ambulatory** for a time may be unsteady when standing at the upright cassette holder. Placing Velcro straps across the upper portion of the patient's chest can help the patient hold still and also provides a sense of security. Holding the arms up out of the way when positioning for a lateral chest radiograph raises the center of balance and can cause slight swaying even in the steadiest subject.

Velcro straps can also be used in immobilizing only the area of interest during the procedure. For example, an **axial projection** of the calcaneus requires extreme dorsiflexion of the ankle to produce an optimally diagnostic image (Fig. 14.3). The use of the strap beneath the **plantar surface** of the foot allows the patient to maintain the extreme **flexion** required and at the same time reduces the possibility of motion that may result from maintaining an uncomfortable position.

Velcro straps can serve as a safety precaution when performing a procedure on a patient who is not completely cognizant, such as those who are heavily medicated or intoxicated or who have diminished mental capacities. This type of patient should never be left unattended; the straps serve only to facilitate protection of the patient from injury. With straps in place, sudden or unexpected movement by the patient would not result in injury to the patient and would allow the attendant to respond to the situation.

Velcro Strap Restraints   *used for non-ambulatory pts*

Velcro strap restraints are designed to be attached easily to the radiography table. These types of restraints include two brackets that mount to each side of the table with a strap that is adjustable for any size patient. It can be adjusted to cover any part of the body, such as the chest, abdomen, or legs (Fig. 14.4). These restraints can also be used for compression. Tightening the strap a little further applies gentle pressure to the abdomen to enhance diagnostic information in certain procedures.

When performing gastrointestinal procedures—for example, placing the patient in the semi-erect position—may be desirable. In these circumstances, when a patient is too weak to stand unassisted, Velcro strap restraints can be applied across the patient's upper and lower abdomen to support the patient firmly during the procedure (Fig. 14.5). This precaution helps reassure the patient that he or she will not fall.

Sandbags

Sandbags are useful positioning and immobilization devices and can be used in a variety of ways. By themselves or in combination with positioning sponges, sandbags are extremely helpful in reducing voluntary motion (Figs. 14.6 and 14.7). Sandbags, unlike radiolucent positioning sponges, are radiopaque (i.e., radiation does not pass through easily). As a result, they cannot be placed in such a way that diagnostic information is obscured within the anatomic area of interest. They must be placed gently on or against the areas adjacent to the anatomic area of interest so as not to injure or cause further damage.

A common use of sandbags as positioning aids is in performing examination of a lateral cervical spine or of the acromioclavicular joints. Both examinations require that the shoulders lie in the same transverse plane and that the patient hold sandbags of equal weight. For the lateral cervical spine, the patient must depress the shoulders as much as possible to demonstrate the lower cervical vertebrae (Fig. 14.8).

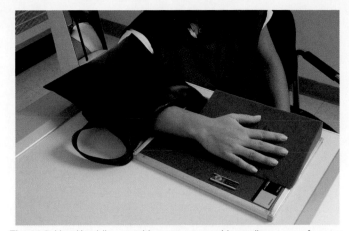

Fig. 14.6 Hand in oblique position on sponge with sandbag across forearm.

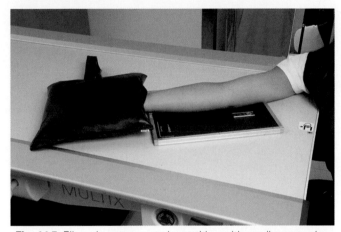

Fig. 14.7 Elbow in anteroposterior position with sandbag on palm.

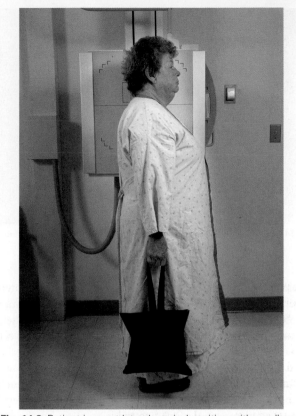

Fig. 14.8 Patient in erect lateral cervical position with sandbags.

Here again, as in the case of positioning sponges, the variety of uses for sandbags is limited only by the technologist's imagination.

Head Clamps

Head clamps can be attached to radiographic imaging devices (e.g., radiographic table, upright cassette holder) and are designed strictly for use in positioning various projections of the skull. When applied safely and appropriately, head clamps serve more as positioning aids than as immobilization devices. A patient so desiring can easily pull away from the head clamps. Head clamps serve as a reminder to the patient of the importance of remaining as still as possible, and they ensure the reduction of voluntary movement on the part of the patient.

SPECIAL APPLICATIONS

Immobilization techniques are often required for use with trauma, pediatric, and geriatric patients. Each type of patient provides unique opportunities to apply immobilization techniques.

Trauma Applications

Methods for safely and expeditiously performing examinations on badly traumatized patients involve entirely different concepts. Immobilization is one of the most critical considerations when working with seriously injured patients. In these instances, the technologist is faced with immobilization devices that already have been applied to the trauma patient by the emergency medical team to stabilize the area of injury and to facilitate safe transport to the trauma center. The technologist must be familiar with the various types of traction and immobilization techniques and devices used by emergency medical personnel. This familiarity must include knowledge of which devices are radiolucent, which must be left in place for initial examinations, and when these devices can safely be removed for more detailed procedures.

In many situations the technologist must consider performing the initial examination with immobilization devices left in place. In fact, more often than not, the technologist has no choice but to perform the procedure in this manner. Fortunately, manufacturers of emergency traction devices are designing equipment to use radiolucent materials whenever possible. This equipment permits initial studies to result in increased diagnostic information without endangering the trauma patient by necessitating the removal of immobilization devices.

In most instances, initial images can and should be produced without removing immobilization devices. Only after a radiologist or an attending physician has read the initial images and approval has been given should the technologist remove the immobilization device for a more complete examination.

Immobilization devices should be removed gently while maintaining patient comfort and safety by immobilizing the injured area above and below the device. Positioning sponges

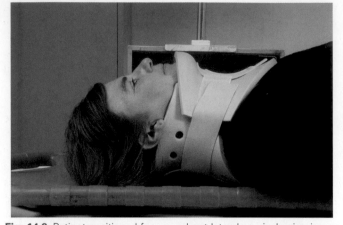

Fig. 14.9 Patient positioned for recumbent lateral cervical spine image with a cervical collar in place.

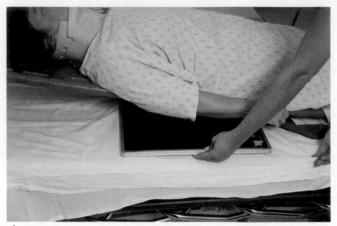

Fig. 14.10 Patient on backboard with grid cassette placed under backboard for anteroposterior lumbar spine image.

should be placed to support the anatomic area of interest. Depending on his or her condition, the patient may be moved or rolled slightly to facilitate removal of the device. If help is available, safety and comfort for the patient are enhanced if two people, working together, remove immobilization devices.

Spinal Trauma. The most common spinal trauma traction device encountered by a technologist is probably the cervical collar. This device is designed to place traction on the cervical spine to prevent further life-threatening movement in this vital area. The cross-table lateral, anteroposterior (AP), and AP open-mouth positions may be used to evaluate the cervical spine during a cervical trauma examination. After evaluating the images, the attending physician or neurosurgeon can determine the next step in treatment. All projections can be produced with the cervical collar in place (Fig. 14.9), and it will be removed only after the physician has reviewed the radiographic images and determined that it is safe to move the patient without the collar.

The backboard, or spineboard, is another spinal immobilization device often seen in trauma situations. Although the backboard is mentioned here under spinal trauma considerations, its uses are by no means limited to spinal injury. It is used to immobilize and support the victim's entire body. A backboard can be used if the thoracic or lumbar spine is involved. Additional trauma situations in which the backboard is used include injuries to the pelvis, hips, and lower extremities, and when multiple injuries in addition to spinal trauma are present.

Most backboards are made from radiolucent materials (e.g., wood, plastic), making radiography of patients relatively easy. With assistance, one end of the backboard can be lifted and a cassette placed under the area of interest beneath the board (Fig. 14.10). All AP projections from head to toe can be accomplished in this manner.

Another advantageous purpose for the backboard is to transport a stable trauma patient to the radiology department for the initial examination. Moving the patient onto the table by sliding the entire backboard onto the examination table is relatively easy for the movers and comfortable for the patient. Once the radiologist has evaluated the initial images, the backboard can be moved from

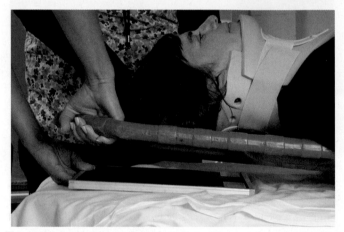

Fig. 14.11 Patient on backboard positioned for acanthoparietal projection with cervical collar in place.

under the patient for further projections. Conversely, if the findings indicate the presence of fracture or other traumatic involvement, the patient can be safely moved back onto a stretcher for transport to surgery, the emergency department, or the appropriate treatment area.

Head Trauma. The technologist will encounter trauma immobilization devices applied to other areas of interest besides the spine. In many instances, examining the skull of a patient wearing a cervical collar or similar immobilization device is necessary. Because of the presence of the cervical collar, a radiographer must become versatile in the production of skull images. Instead of being able to rotate and tilt the head or flex and extend the neck so as to position the patient correctly, the radiographer must be able to manipulate the radiographic equipment to compensate for the patient's lack of mobility (Fig. 14.11). Often, the cervical collar cannot be removed for more difficult skull projections until after approval by a physician.

Extremity Trauma. Other anatomic areas of interest that may involve the use of traction devices are the extremities, particularly the lower extremities. In these cases the traction devices are in the form of splints, most often inflation or traction splints.

An inflation or air splint is simply an inflatable plastic cuff that is slipped over the affected limb and inflated to provide stability for transport by the emergency team. These splints are readily radiolucent, and routine radiography can usually be achieved with little discomfort or danger to the patient. An exception would be when a patient has multiple injuries that complicate the procedures.

Traction splints are designed for use on the lower extremities. They exert a steady force on the affected limb by applying pressure against the pelvis and groin area. Although traction splints often contain radiopaque materials, satisfactory initial images can be obtained with the splint in place. Most splints designed for use on the upper extremities are made from radiolucent materials and do not present any great obstacles to the procurement of diagnostic images.

femur, lower leg

An antishock garment might also be occasionally encountered. The antishock garment is a pair of inflatable trousers applied to the trauma patient. This garment is used in instances in which the patient has sustained trauma to the abdomen, pelvis, or lower extremities and internal hemorrhage is suggested. Once the antishock garment is in place around the patient, the garment is inflated to slow the rate of hemorrhage. Performing radiography is sometimes necessary on these patients for pelvic or other fractures with the garment in place. Because the trousers are radiolucent, they can be left in place while the examination is being performed.

Pediatric Applications

Special problems are encountered when performing radiographic examinations on pediatric patients. Although many methods and devices are available to facilitate pediatric radiography, perhaps the most overlooked aspects of positioning and immobilizing children are communication and the establishment of rapport. In many instances, children as young as 3 or 4 years of age can be convinced to hold still without immobilization when communication is well done. This rapport is established with kindness, patience, honesty, and understanding. Although this communication may not be difficult to convey under normal circumstances, an entirely different situation arises within the context of a busy radiographic department with a child who is injured or sick. Kindness, patience, honesty, and understanding are best conveyed to children literally on their level by dropping to one knee to talk with the children face to face. To quote Armand Brodeur, former chief radiologist at Cardinal Glennon Children's Hospital in St Louis, "To stand tall in pediatric radiology, you have to get down on your knees." A diagnostic examination will be obtained relatively quickly if a little time is spent in establishing rapport with the child. Speak in a calm, soothing voice, perhaps while offering a toy to the child. Young children often respond well to making a game of having their *picture taken* or seeing how long they can hold still. Allow the child time to explore the new surroundings and ask questions. Threats and force must be avoided at all times, with restraints being applied gently.

Another preliminary consideration for pediatric radiography is how to manage parents while the examination is being performed. Some possibilities include having the parent accompany the child into the radiography room to assist the radiographer, having the parents wait outside the radiography room during the procedure, or having a parent accompany the child but observing only. With the use of department protocol and experience, the radiographer must decide what option will yield the best results.

As is often the case, when departmental policy or the situation calls for parents to be present during the examination, the radiographer absolutely must share the importance of cooperation and understanding with the parents. Being objective is difficult for parents when they observe their child being placed in a pediatric immobilization device. Although a child who is confined in an upright chest immobilization device or strapped to a restraint board may appear uncomfortable, the parent must be made to understand that the technique or device used for immobilization is the safest, surest way to produce optimal diagnostic images with a minimal amount of discomfort and radiation exposure for the child.

Pediatric positioning and immobilization are increasingly appropriate for neonates and small children. If well done and genuine, rapport and communication should be the only techniques necessary for older children. The radiographer must determine what methods are required according to the situation.

Sheet Restraints. One of the most effective, simple, inexpensive, and reliable methods of restraining or immobilizing a child is a mummy wrap. Although this method can be used on children 4 or 5 years of age, it is beneficial for children who are still too young to understand cooperation. Basically, the child is wrapped in a sheet, which effectively limits the movement of the extremities and gives the technique its name (Fig. 14.12). Sheets or blankets can be used in many ways for immobilizing infants and small children. Again, the technologist is limited only by imagination.

Commercial Restraints. Commercial restraints usually take one of two forms: upright restraint devices or restraint boards. Two common useful upright restraint devices are the Pigg-O-Stat and Pedia-Poser Pediatric Positioning Chair (Fig. 14.13). These devices are useful for upright chest and abdominal radiographic examinations. They can accommodate children up to approximately 3 to 4 years of age, depending on their size. Once secured, the patient can be rotated 360 degrees to demonstrate various oblique and lateral positions. The Pigg-O-Stat has a built-in, adjustable lead shield which provides gonadal protection, respiration phase indicators, and left and right markers. Because the Pigg-O-Stat is made of clear plastic, patient movement can be easily observed during exposures. The Pedia-Poser Pediatric Positioning Chair has an adjustable back and head tilt supports. It comes equipped with soft adjustable straps to help secure the child's arms and a chinstrap to bring the chin up out of the chest. Both devices hold children securely and safely and greatly reduce the need for repeated exposures or the necessity of having someone hold the patient. One disadvantage of the Pigg-O-Stat is possible artifacts caused by the plastic sides, which can overlap the anatomic area of interest.

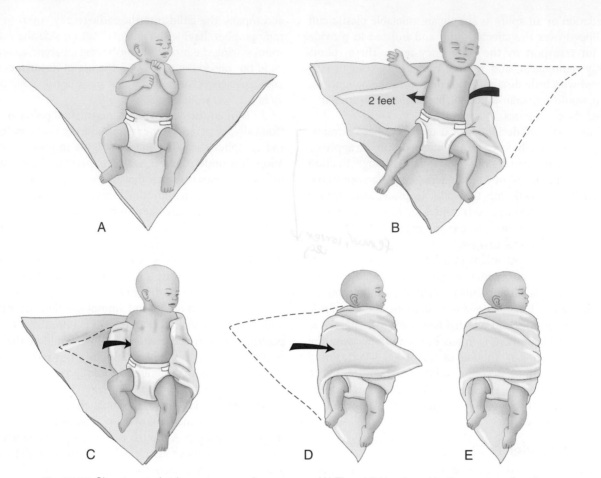

Fig. 14.12 Sheet restraint (mummy wrap) sequence. (A) The child is placed in the center of a triangular folded sheet as shown so that the shoulders are just above the top fold. (B) The left corner of the sheet is brought over the left arm and under the body so that approximately 2 feet of the sheet extends beyond the right side of the body. Make sure the child is not lying on the left arm. (C) Tuck the 2 feet of sheet over the right arm and under the body. Again, make sure the child is not lying on the arm. (D) Bring the remaining sheet over the body. (E) Tuck the sheet securely under the left side of the body. Remember that this technique restrains most movement but is not satisfactory as a complete immobilization procedure. Restraint bands are still required, and the child should not be left alone, even for the amount of time needed to make a radiographic exposure.

Another type of commercial restraint device occasionally used in radiology departments is the restraint board (infant immobilizer). Even though several variations of restraint boards exist, all of them consist basically of a contour-fitting pad, mold, or sponge with attached Velcro straps for securing the patient (Fig. 14.14). The restraint board is a good way to immobilize an infant or small child when radiographic studies of the abdomen are desirable. Similar to the upright restraint device, these restraint boards allow the child to be safely and securely immobilized while eliminating the need for someone to hold the child.

A modification of the Velcro strap restraint board is the Octostop board (Fig. 14.15). Octagonal frames are attached to the end of the board, and the child is restrained on the board with Velcro straps around the limbs and across the torso and head. The patient can be rotated 360 degrees into eight different positions (Fig. 14.16). The disadvantage of the regular restraint board and the octagonal framed version is size. Only infants

and small children up to 1 year of age should be immobilized with these devices.

Noncommercial Restraints. A clever means of immobilizing the hands, fingers, feet, and toes of young patients is the use of a radiolucent Plexiglas paddle (Fig. 14.17). Pediatric patients have a tendency to wiggle fingers and toes. Applying gentle pressure to the affected area of interest aids the child in holding still while at the same time allowing the production of a diagnostic image of the entire subject with one exposure. One other immobilization technique worthy of consideration is the use of Velcro straps and tape. Velcro straps can be used in pediatric situations in much the same way as for adult applications. Because children are curious, they tend to be easily distracted by the new surroundings of a radiographic room with all its new information. With their attention wandering from one new wonder to another, even the best rapport and communication may not be able to overcome entirely a slight bit of motion as the child

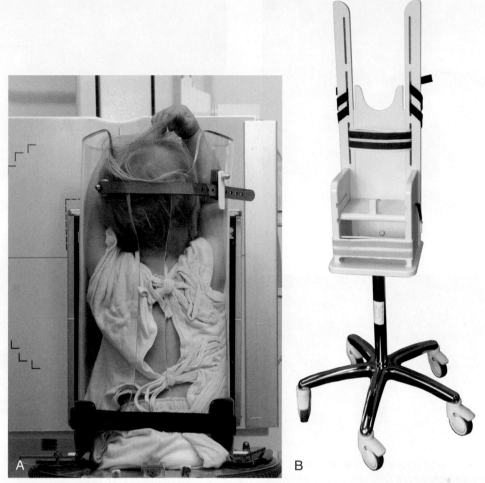

Fig. 14.13 (A) Patient positioned in Pigg-O-Stat for posteroanterior chest image. (B) Pedia-Poser Pediatric Positioning Chair for chest image.

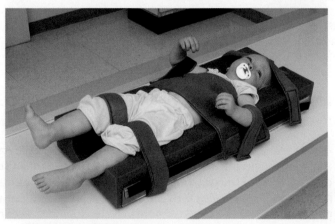

Fig. 14.14 Pediatric patient in a Velcro strap restraint board.

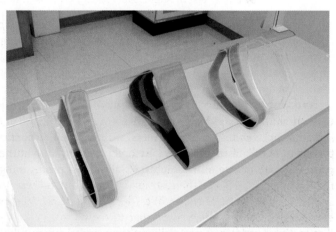

Fig. 14.15 Octostop restraint board.

continues to investigate the surroundings during the examination. Using Velcro straps for a 5- or 6-year-old child during an upright chest examination not only keeps the patient more still, but also serves as a reminder to the child that he or she should hold still.

Tape is also sometimes used when immobilizing pediatric patients. Tape should be used more as a reminder to the patient to hold still than as an absolute restraining device. The radiographer should keep in mind that the skin of infants and young

children is much more tender and sensitive than that of an adult. Caution should be exercised when using tape to restrain so as not to abrade the skin of the child. When tape is used, it should be twisted where it comes in contact with the skin so that the nonadhesive side is in contact with the skin (Fig. 14.18A). Another technique to protect the skin is to place a gauze pad between the skin and the tape (see Fig. 14.18B).

A stockinette is also an invaluable pediatric immobilization device. A stockinette is stretchable cotton fabric in the shape of

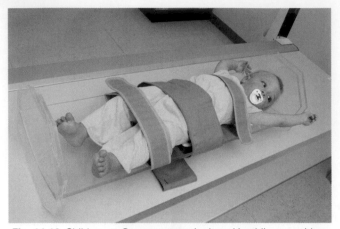

Fig. 14.16 Child on an Octostop restraint board in oblique position.

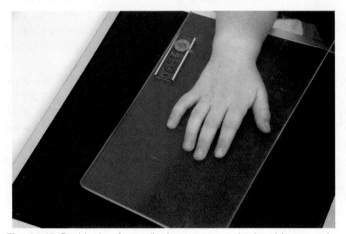

Fig. 14.17 Positioning for pediatric posteroanterior hand image using Plexiglas paddle.

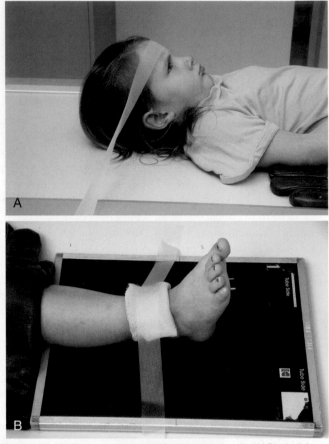

Fig. 14.18 (A) Patient positioned for anteroposterior (AP) skull image with tape twisted across the forehead. (B) Gauze pad between the skin and tape for an AP ankle image.

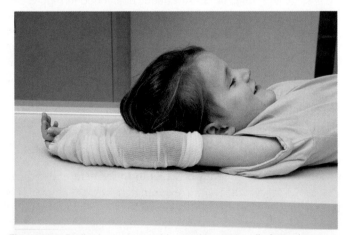

Fig. 14.19 Pediatric patient with stockinette applied to the upper extremities.

a sleeve that is pulled over a fractured extremity before a plaster cast is applied. Its purpose is to prevent chafing and irritation of the skin while the limb is in the cast. It comes in a roll and can be cut to any length. A stockinette is effective as a restraint when pulled over the upper or lower extremities of a child and secured with tape. This technique is good for immobilizing the upper limbs above and behind the child's head (Fig. 14.19).

Pediatric radiography is an art, and it is a special radiographer who is its master. Radiography of a patient who is at the other extreme of age also requires a skillful and professional radiographer.

Geriatric Applications

Radiographic studies of **geriatric** patients can be difficult, but the radiographer can make the examination go smoothly if a few considerations are kept in mind. The first of these considerations is security.

In many instances, one of the greatest concerns of an older person is fear of falling. A natural part of the aging process is loss of mobility, agility, and sense of balance. What would be considered a minor fall for a younger person often has catastrophic results for an older adult. Therefore in addition to communication and rapport, the radiographer must take extra care to make a geriatric patient feel secure. This measure always includes patience in allowing for extra time during the examination so that the geriatric patient does not feel rushed or hurried. Using an extra assistant or two to help move the older patient onto the radiographic table can increase the patient's feeling of security. Always take extra care not to make the geriatric patient feel disoriented by rushing through the examination or by quickly moving from one radiographic position to another. This precaution will allow the geriatric patient to feel more relaxed and better able to concentrate on holding still, thus reducing the need for repeated exposures.

An often overlooked consideration of geriatric radiography that goes along with security is keeping the patient warm. Older persons tend to become chilled easily. This fact, along with the necessity of wearing thin hospital gowns and robes, can add to the difficulty of a geriatric radiographic examination. If the patient is cold and concentrating on trying to keep warm, he or she will be less likely to be able to cooperate by maintaining a radiographic position. If the older patient is going to be in the department for a long time or is undergoing a lengthy examination such as a barium enema, which requires an extended time on the radiographic table, the radiographer should cover the patient or offer extra blankets during the procedure.

A third factor that can interfere with an older patient's ability to cooperate and maintain position is comfort, and this factor too must be considered during the radiographic examination. Just as security and warmth are part of patient comfort, consideration must be given to how long the geriatric patient must lie on the radiographic table. Radiographic tables are hard and cold. Many older patients are thin and are therefore conscious of the hardness of the table. To enable the geriatric patient to cooperate easily and fully, a radiolucent pad should be placed on the table before the examination (Fig. 14.20). A radiographic examination that might take 20 to 30 minutes can seem to take an eternity on an unpadded radiographic table. In addition, a sponge or radiolucent pad beneath the patient's knees can greatly reduce strain on the patient's back and increase the patient's ability to cooperate during the examination. A disadvantage of using a pad is the possibility of slight artifact production or loss of radiographic detail because of increased object to image receptor distance. In some instances, a pad might be objectionable to a radiologist.

Although the previously mentioned aspects of security, warmth, and comfort should be considered for all patients, these elements are of extra importance for geriatric patients and can greatly reduce the amount of stress to the patient and radiographer during a radiographic examination if extra emphasis is placed on them.

SUMMARY

- Although patient immobilization is only one of many factors in the production of a successful radiographic study, awareness of the various elements to be considered in immobilization techniques must be a part of the radiographer's professional repertoire.
- Before learning the various methods of immobilization and restraint pertinent to radiographic studies, the radiographer must first understand that immobilization techniques are used to eliminate or minimize movement by the patient and

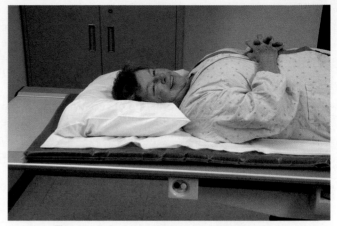

Fig. 14.20 Geriatric patient on a radiolucent pad.

to enhance the proper positioning of the anatomic area of interest. Appropriate use of immobilization or restraint techniques can greatly reduce the negative effects of movement or improper positioning on the diagnostic quality of the finished image.

- The skill that may be the single most important technique in patient immobilization and the one that must be developed by all radiographers is high-quality communication. High-quality communication allows the patient to become an active participant and assistant in the radiographic examination, thus accelerating the examination and reducing the need for repeated exposures. Two key essentials for effective communication are explanation of the procedure and establishment of rapport with the patient.
- The range of immobilization techniques runs from simple involvement, such as the use of a positioning sponge or sandbag to reduce patient motion, to rather involved techniques, such as using sheet restraints in pediatric radiographic studies or making decisions about removal of traction splints in trauma situations. Within this range are a significant number of different immobilization techniques and considerations for their use. The radiographer should be familiar with all these applications and be able to adapt them to fit each radiographic situation and each patient's condition.
- Some of the commonly used routine immobilization methods are positioning sponges, Velcro straps, Velcro strap restraints, sandbags, and head clamps. Many ways exist to use these methods of immobilization, and their use is limited only by the creativity of the radiographer.
- Because immobilization is one of the most critical aspects of trauma radiography, the radiographer should be familiar with numerous trauma immobilization devices, methods for producing diagnostic images with these devices in place, and when removing these devices for further radiographic studies is appropriate. Some of these trauma immobilization devices are cervical collars, backboards, air splints, and traction splints.
- One area of radiography that often requires the use of immobilization methods is pediatric radiography. Perhaps

the most effective method of immobilization is establishing rapport with the young patient. Methods for pediatric immobilization with which the radiographer should be acquainted are sheet restraints, upright and board restraint devices, radiolucent paddles, stockinettes, and the correct use of tape.

- Although radiographic examination of geriatric patients can be difficult, certain considerations can greatly facilitate these studies. In addition to communication, rapport, and respect, key considerations for successful geriatric radiography are security, warmth, and comfort.

- Familiarity with various immobilization techniques is one aspect of the art of radiography that enables the radiographer to attain the highest levels of professional standards—that is, the production of optimal diagnostic quality images with the least amount of radiation exposure to patient, radiographer, and ancillary personnel.

BIBLIOGRAPHY

Bontrager K, Lampignana J: *Textbook of radiographic positioning and related anatomy*, ed 9, St. Louis, 2017, Mosby.

Campbell J: *Basic trauma life support for advanced providers*, ed 5, Englewood Cliffs, NJ, 2003, Prentice-Hall.

Ehrlich RA, Coakes DM: *Patient care in radiography with an introduction to medical imaging*, ed 9, St. Louis, 2016, Mosby.

Frank E, Long B, Smith B: *Merrill's atlas of radiographic positions and radiologic procedures*, ed 13, St. Louis, 2015, Mosby.

Godderidge C: *Pediatric imaging*, Philadelphia, 1995, Saunders.

Gurley LT, Callaway WJ: *Introduction to radiologic technology*, ed 7, St. Louis, 2010, Mosby.

M.D. McCauley Co., Inc.: Positioning Foam Blocks and Positioning Aids. Available at: http://www.xraymdm.com/positioning_blocks.htm Accessed September 15, 2017.

Torres LS, Dutton AG, Linn-Watson TA: *Patient care in imaging technology*, ed 8, Philadelphia, 2012, Lippincott Williams & Wilkins.

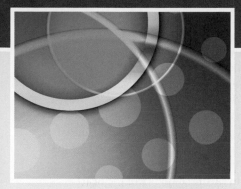

Vital Signs, Oxygen, Chest Tubes, and Lines

Julie Gill, PhD, RT(R)(QM)

> *Life is only known as the complex of many functions, and health as the integrity of these functions, each in itself and in harmony.*
>
> **Peter Latham**
> **General Remarks on the Practice of Medicine**

OBJECTIVES

On completion of this chapter, the student will be able to:

- Discuss the significance of homeostasis.
- Explain the mechanisms that adapt and maintain homeostasis.
- Discuss the significance of each of the four vital signs: temperature, respiration, pulse, and blood pressure.
- Identify the normal range for each of the vital signs.
- Explain the implications of abnormal vital signs.
- Describe how vital signs are assessed.
- Explain the indications for administering oxygen therapy.
- Differentiate high-flow and low-flow oxygen-delivery devices.
- Explain why caution must be used when performing radiographic procedures on patients receiving oxygen therapy.
- Describe the uses of, or indications for, the following thoracic tubes and lines to manage compromised patients: endotracheal tubes, thoracostomy tubes, and central venous lines.
- Describe the radiographic appearance and proper placement of endotracheal tubes, thoracostomy tubes, and central venous lines.
- Differentiate various types of central venous lines.
- Recognize the clinical complications associated with use and placement of tubes and lines used in the thorax.

OUTLINE

KEY TERMS

Apnea Cessation of spontaneous ventilation

Atelectasis Absence of gas from part or the whole of the lungs as a result of failure of expansion or reabsorption of gas from the alveoli

Auscultation Listening to sounds of the body, typically through the use of a stethoscope

Body Temperature Measurement of the degree of heat of the deep tissues of the human body

Bradycardia Slowness of the heartbeat as evidenced by slowing of the pulse rate to less than 60 beats per minute (BPM)

Bradypnea Abnormal slowness of breathing

Diaphoresis　Profuse sweating

Diastolic　Pertaining to dilation, or a period of relaxation of the heart, especially of the ventricles

Dyspnea　Difficult or labored breathing

Febrile　Pertaining to or characterized by fever

Homeostasis　Constancy in the internal environment of the body, naturally maintained by adaptive responses that promote healthy survival

Hypertension　Persistently high arterial blood pressure

Hyperthermia　Abnormally high body temperature, especially that induced for therapeutic purposes

Hypotension　Abnormally low blood pressure; seen in shock but not necessarily indicative of shock

Hypothermia　Low body temperature

Hypoxemia　Decreased oxygen tension (concentration) in the blood

Hypoxia　Reduction of oxygen supply to the tissue

Intubation　Insertion of a tubular device into a canal, hollow organ, or cavity

Orthopnea　Difficulty breathing except when sitting up or standing erect

Pleural Effusion　Increased amounts of fluid within the pleural cavity, usually the result of inflammation

Pneumothorax　Presence of air or gas in the pleural cavity

Pulse Oximeter　Photoelectric device used for determining the oxygen saturation of the blood

Respiration　Action of inhaling oxygen and exhaling carbon dioxide during breathing

Sphygmomanometer　Instrument for measuring blood pressure

Systolic　Pertaining to tightening, or a period of contraction of the heart (myocardium), especially that of the ventricles

Tachycardia　Rapidity of the heart action, usually defined as a heart rate greater than 100 BPM

Tachypnea　Abnormal rapidity of breathing

Tidal Volume　Volume of air inhaled and exhaled during one respiratory cycle

Ventilation　Mechanical movement of air into and out of the lungs

VITAL SIGNS AS INDICATORS OF HOMEOSTASIS STATUS

Homeostasis is a relative constancy in the internal environment of the body that is naturally maintained by adaptive responses that promote healthy survival. The primary mechanisms that maintain homeostasis are the heartbeat, blood pressure, body temperature, respiratory rate, and electrolyte balance. These adaptive response mechanisms identified as homeostasis are continuously interacting with and adjusting to changes originating inside or outside the body to maintain the constant internal environment. Every health care professional should have a fundamental comprehension of the mechanisms that maintain homeostasis. For example, *vital signs* are primary mechanisms that adapt to responses, inside or outside the body, to maintain homeostasis. Collectively, the vital signs are body temperature, pulse rate, blood pressure, and respiratory rate. In addition, assessment of the patient's mental alertness (*sensorium*) is often reported along with the vital signs.

Vital signs can be assessed quickly in the clinical setting and serve as objective, noninvasive evidence of the patient's immediate condition; similarly, vital sign measures are physiologic indicators of a patient's response to therapy. Most notably, vital signs provide important information because they often reveal the first clue of adverse reactions associated with treatments and diagnostic procedures. Improvement in a patient's vital signs is strong evidence that a treatment is having a positive effect. For example, a decrease toward normal in the patient's heart rate and respiratory rate after oxygen therapy suggests a beneficial effect. In addition, records of vital sign measurements obtained at the onset of diagnostic procedures serve as important benchmarks indicating the patient's initial status should the patient experience adverse reactions during such procedures.

BODY TEMPERATURE

Description

Body temperature reflects the degree of heat of the deep tissues of the human body. The normal mean body temperature is approximately 98.6°F (37°C), with a daily variation of 1°F to 2°F (0.5°C to 1.0°C). Because humans are warm-blooded animals, the cells of the human body function best within a narrow range of temperature variations. Body temperature must maintain a relatively constant level despite extremes in environmental temperatures. *Thermoregulation* is the term used to describe the body's maintenance of heat production and heat loss. The hypothalamus plays an important role in regulating heat loss and can initiate peripheral vasodilation and sweating (**diaphoresis**) to dissipate body heat. Similarly, the respiratory system plays an important role by removing excess heat through ventilation. The hypothalamus also plays an important role in the preservation of heat by initiating shivering (to generate heat) and vasoconstriction (to conserve heat).

Measurement

Historically, mercury-filled glass bulbs were used to assess core body temperature. However, today, electronic thermometers are most commonly used and are recommended. Many electronic thermometers are also digital, meaning that the temperature reading is digitally displayed as a number. Depending on the type of thermometer used, electronic or glass bulb, the thermometer stays in place for 20 seconds to 3 minutes, until a stable reading has been obtained. When a mercury-filled bulb is used, it is important to note differences in bulb shape for oral and rectal measures. The rectal thermometer has a rounded bulb, whereas the oral type has a slender, more pointed tip. Because of risk for toxic exposure, mercury-filled bulbs are seldom used in a health care facility; however, they continue to be sold and used in the private sector. If a mercury spill should occur, the local health department should be notified and proper clean-up procedures followed.

Five routes are commonly used to measure and extrapolate core body temperature: (1) oral, (2) axillary, (3) tympanic, (4) temporal, and (5) rectal. Oral measurements are obtained by placing a thermometer under the patient's tongue (Fig. 15.1).

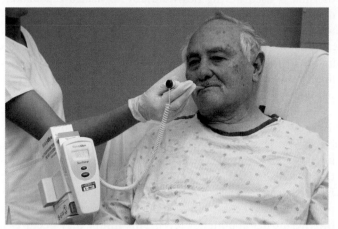

Fig. 15.1 A common method for measuring body temperature is the oral route; the thermometer is placed under the tongue.

Axillary temperatures are obtained by placing the thermometer high between the upper arm and the torso. This method, used for children and infants, is notoriously inaccurate and time consuming. The thermometer must remain in place 5 to 10 minutes to obtain a stable reading. Its shortcomings make this technique almost useless. For rectal temperatures to be measured, the bulb of a rectal thermometer is lubricated, inserted into the anal opening, and held in place in the rectum of the patient for 2½ to 5 minutes. Tympanic temperatures are obtained by placing a tympanic membrane thermometer in the ear (Fig. 15.2A). A stable reading is displayed within 3 seconds. In any case, for infection control reasons, the thermometer is covered with a disposable protective sheath, and proper hand washing before and after patient contact is also essential.

In the past, tympanic and rectal temperatures were the preferred assessments for all infants, as well as for adults, when oral measures were not feasible. Even today, rectal thermometry is believed to be the most accurate reflection of core body temperature; however, *temporal artery (TA) thermometers* have been introduced (see Fig. 15.2B). The TA lies superficial in the temporal region of the skull. A noninvasive swipe of the thermometer along the forehead and across the temporal region

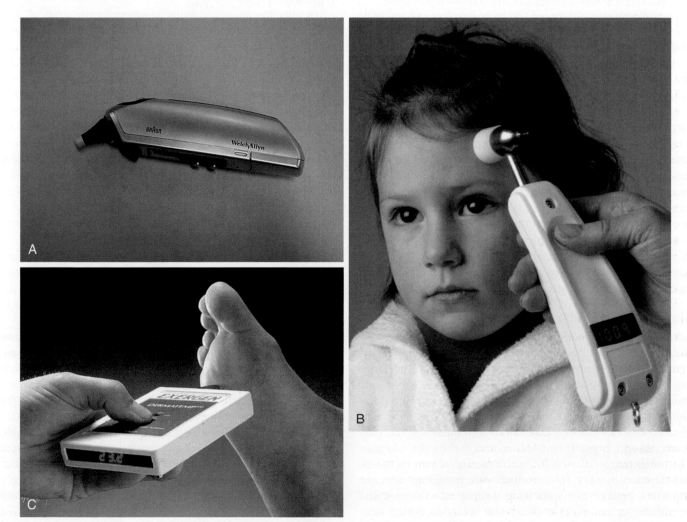

Fig. 15.2 (A) Tympanic thermometer. (B) Temporal thermometer. (C) Infrared digital thermometer.

TABLE 15.1 Normal Vital Signs

Sign	Range
Temperature (Varies With Meter Type)	97.6°F–100°F (36.5°C–37.8°C) (method of measurement is also charted as follows)
Average oral	98.6°O
Average tympanic	97.6°T
Average temporal artery	100°TA
Average rectal	99.6°R
Average axillary	97.6°A
Respirations	
Adult	12–20 breaths/min
Child	20–30 breaths/min
Pulse	
Adult	60–100 beats/min
Child	70–120 beats/min
Blood Pressure	
Systolic	<120 mm Hg
Diastolic	<80 mm Hg

provides immediate, accurate measures closely correlating to core body temperature. Today, TA thermometry is popular.

In addition, infrared digital thermometers have gained popularity for identifying subtle skin temperature variations associated with vascular diseases (see Fig. 15.2C). The thermographic unit conveniently scans and measures skin temperatures and is especially useful in wound management and with patients' potential for diabetic foot neuropathies producing diminished blood supplies. It is important to recognize that infrared digital thermometers are not useful for measuring core body temperature and are strictly used to detect superficial skin temperature variations.

Body temperature readings may be measured in either degrees Fahrenheit (°F) or degrees Celsius (°C). Oral temperature readings in healthy adults and children are within the narrow range of 97.7°F to 99.5°F (36.5°C to 37.5°C) (Table 15.1). Tympanic measurements range from 95.9°F to 99.5°F (35.5°C to 37.5°C). Axillary temperatures register slightly lower, and rectal and TA temperatures register approximately 1°F higher than oral readings.

Significance of Abnormalities

When the oral temperature is higher than 99.5°F, a fever exists (hyperthermia). A patient with a fever is said to be febrile. When the body temperature falls outside the normal range (e.g., with an illness or a head injury), the metabolic rate changes accordingly, and the demands on the cardiopulmonary system also change. For example, when the body temperature increases, the metabolic rate also increases, resulting in increased oxygen consumption and carbon dioxide production at the cellular level. As the metabolic rate increases, the cardiopulmonary system must work harder to meet the additional cellular demands by providing more oxygen and eliminating carbon dioxide. As a result of increased body temperature, an increase in cellular metabolism occurs; therefore

any event that increases cellular metabolism also increases body temperature.

Conversely, when the patient's temperature falls below the normal range, hypothermia is said to be present. Although not common, hypothermia may be present in patients exposed to cold environmental temperatures and in those with trauma to the hypothalamus. In addition, medically induced hypothermia is used during heart surgery to decrease metabolic demands, thereby decreasing the demand on the cardiopulmonary system.

Fevers are common with viral and bacterial infections as a natural response of the human body to increase cellular activity to combat the invading organism. Similarly, a patient may become febrile for a day or two after a surgical procedure as the body responds to initiate healing. Prolonged fever in these patients is evidence of postoperative infection. The culprit is often an infection in the wound, lungs, or urinary tract. Patients having a myocardial infarction might be febrile because of increased cellular activity. Hyperthermia may also result from injury to the temperature-regulating center of the hypothalamus, causing it to set the thermostat at a higher level. This injury may occur as a result of a cerebrovascular accident, cerebral edema (swelling), or tumor.

Despite the increased body temperature in some disease states, cellular function is optimal within only a narrow temperature range. Prolonged hyperthermia can lead to serious complications and resultant cellular damage. Patients with hyperthermia may become confused, dizzy, and even comatose. Conversely, hypothermia may be medically induced or the consequence of accidental exposure. Medically induced hypothermia is performed to therapeutically decrease the body's need for oxygen. Because temperature is an easily measured indicator of the presence of disease, it is routinely followed as a yardstick of response to therapy for many conditions.

RESPIRATORY RATE

Description

Adequate breathing (minute ventilation) is predicated on respiratory rate and depth of the breath. The depth of breath determines tidal volume. At rest, minute ventilation will generally be adequate provided the respiratory rates are at least 10 to 12 breaths/min.

While assessing a patient's respiratory rate, the health care professional obtains a general impression of the functional status of the respiratory system. The respiratory system is responsible for delivering oxygen (O_2) from the environment to the tissues and eliminating carbon dioxide from the tissues to the environment. This action of inhaling oxygen and exhaling carbon dioxide while breathing is called respiration. The cells of the body require a constant supply of oxygen for cellular metabolism. As a result of cellular metabolism, the waste product carbon dioxide is produced. Unless oxygen is continually supplied and carbon dioxide is continually eliminated, death will occur. Consequently, failure of the respiratory system is a life-threatening event.

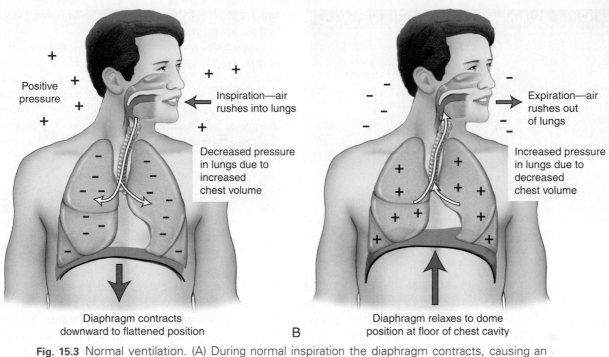

Fig. 15.3 Normal ventilation. (A) During normal inspiration the diaphragm contracts, causing an expansion of the chest cavity. This expansion decreases the pressure in the lungs to below the atmospheric pressure; consequently, air rushes into the lungs. (B) During normal expiration the diaphragm relaxes, returning to its original position at the floor of the chest cavity and causing a decrease in the volume of the chest cavity. The decrease in chest cavity volume increases the pressure of air in the lungs to above atmospheric pressure so that air flows out of the lungs.

Measurement

The major muscle of **ventilation** is the diaphragm. During inspiration the diaphragm contracts, moving downward in the abdominal cavity and pushing the abdominal contents outward. The downward movement of the diaphragm causes an expansion of the chest cavity, along with a decrease in chest cavity pressure. With decreased internal pressure, air moves into the lungs. Expiration is achieved by simple relaxation of the diaphragm. As the diaphragm relaxes, it returns to its original position at the floor of the chest cavity. This action causes an increase of pressure, and subsequently air flows out of the lungs to the environment (Fig. 15.3).

In a healthy adult, a single respiration consists of an inspiratory phase and an expiratory phase. Because the diaphragm is responsible for the movement of air in and out of the lungs, respirations are often counted by observing the movement of the abdomen. A respiratory rate is also assessed by observing the rise (*inspiration*) and fall (*expiration*) of the chest; however, abdominal and chest wall movement may be difficult to detect by observation alone, particularly in patients who are breathing shallowly. In these cases the hand of the health care professional may be placed on the patient's abdomen or chest to assist in assessing each ventilation. However, obtaining a patient's respiratory rate without the patient's knowledge is best because, when aware, patients often alter their breathing rate and pattern. Therefore, after obtaining a pulse rate, many health care professionals leave their hand on the patient's wrist and count the respiratory rate; the patient assumes that a pulse rate is still being assessed.

In the healthy adult, normal respirations are silent and effortless, automatically occurring at regular intervals. Respiratory rates are measured as the number of breaths per minute; normal range at rest is 12 to 20 breaths/min (see Table 15.1). Children under the age of 10 years have slightly increased rates, averaging 20 to 30 breaths/min. Newborns' respiratory rates average 30 to 60 breaths/min. Because respiratory rates are higher in children than in adults, counting respirations for a minimum of 1 minute is important to obtain an accurate measurement. In addition, while counting respirations, the health care professional assesses the depth (shallow, normal, or deep) and pattern (regular or irregular) of ventilation. Therefore, by assessing the rate, depth, and pattern, an overall impression of the respiratory system can be obtained.

Significance of Abnormalities

Any deviation from normal indicates a change in the status of the respiratory system. If cellular metabolism increases, then the demand for oxygen increases, as does the production of carbon dioxide. The respiratory system responds by increasing the respiratory rate to deliver additional oxygen to the blood. Similarly, with increasing respiratory rates, more carbon dioxide will be exhaled by the lungs. **Tachypnea** is the term used to describe respiratory rates greater than 20 breaths/min in the case of an adult patient. Common causes of tachypnea include exercise, fever, anxiety, pain, infection, heart failure, chest trauma, decreased oxygen in the blood, and central nervous system disease.

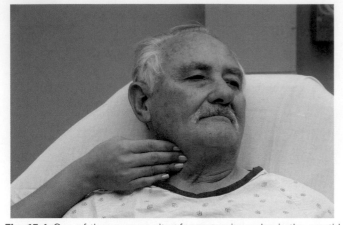

Fig. 15.4 One of the common sites for measuring pulse is the carotid artery in the neck.

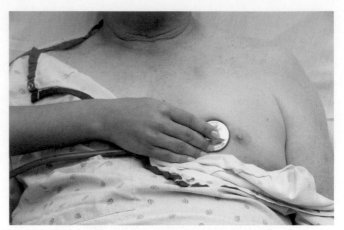

Fig. 15.5 Apical pulses can be counted by listening to the chest with a stethoscope.

Bradypnea is the term used to describe a decrease in the respiratory rate. Bradypnea occurs much less frequently than tachypnea. Bradypnea results from depression of the respiratory center of the brain—common with drug overdoses, head trauma, and hypothermia. **Dyspnea** is a common term used to describe difficult breathing. **Orthopnea** refers to difficulty breathing (dyspnea) unless sitting up or standing erect. **Apnea** is the term used to identify the absence of spontaneous ventilation; it is an ominous sign.

PULSE

Description

The cardiovascular system is a closed fluid system composed of a pump (the heart) and many blood vessels. When the left ventricle of the heart contracts, blood is pumped out of the heart into the aorta and throughout the arteries of the body. The function of the cardiovascular system is to transport oxygenated blood from the lungs to the cells of the body and to return deoxygenated blood back to the heart and lungs to become reoxygenated. In addition, the cardiovascular system transports carbon dioxide from the cells to the lungs for removal.

As previously stated, the cells of the human body require a constant supply of oxygen to effectively function, and any impairment to the cardiovascular system will result in decreased oxygen to the cells and injury; furthermore, if the heart stops beating, death is imminent.

Measurement

Under normal conditions, the pulse can be palpated at superficially located arteries. Three common sites are used for measuring pulse rate: (1) the radial artery on the thumb side of the wrist, (2) the brachial artery in the antecubital fossa of adults and the upper arm of infants, and (3) the carotid artery in the neck (Fig. 15.4). In addition, listening to the chest with a stethoscope placed over the heart (**auscultation**) and counting each heartbeat can be used to measure the pulse rate. Pulses obtained in this manner are called *apical* pulses (Fig. 15.5). When measuring the pulse rate, the second and third digits are placed over the pulse point; the pulse should be counted for 60 seconds

for the most accurate assessment. In addition to the rate, the strength and regularity of the beat should be assessed.

During cardiopulmonary resuscitation, the pulse is routinely assessed at the carotid artery; however, peripheral pulse points—the femoral, pedal, and radial arteries—may also be assessed to verify the effectiveness of chest compressions. Presence of a peripheral pulse indicates a systolic blood pressure of at least 80 mm Hg and verifies effective chest compressions.

Pulse rates reflect the rapidity of each heart contraction and are recorded as the number of beats per minute (BPM). Counting the pulse rate for 1 minute is important for an accurate measurement. Resting pulse rates in the normal adult vary from 60 to 100 BPM (see Table 15.1). A normal pulse range for children younger than 10 years is 70 to 120 BPM.

In critical care settings, patients' arterial oxygen saturation (Sao_2 and Spo_2), respiratory rate, and pulse rate are monitored. Arterial oxygen saturation (Sao_2) levels are measured through periodically performed blood gas analyses. However, some devices may be used for continuous vital sign monitoring, including electrocardiographs, arterial lines, and pulse oximeters. Electrocardiographs, discussed in more detail in the next chapter, continually monitor the patient's heart rate and rhythm. Electrodes placed on the patient's chest monitor the electrical activity of the heart and transform this electrical activity to rate values and waveforms visible on a monitor (Fig. 15.6).

An arterial line is a catheter that is inserted into an artery. The catheter is connected to a pressure transducer that is attached to a monitor. A continual measurement of the patient's heart rate and blood pressure is visible on the monitor.

A **pulse oximeter** is a noninvasive device used to provide ongoing assessment of the hemoglobin oxygen saturation of arterial blood, as well as the patient's pulse rate. A light-emitting probe is placed on the finger, foot, toe, earlobe, temple, nose, or forehead of the patient. Hemoglobin oxygen saturation (Spo_2) and pulse rate are determined by measuring absorption of selected wavelengths of light by the circulating blood. When the heart pulses, the oximeter converts the light intensity information into hemoglobin oxygen saturation and pulse rate values (Fig. 15.7). Normal pulse oximeter (Spo_2) values for a healthy person would be 95% to 100%.

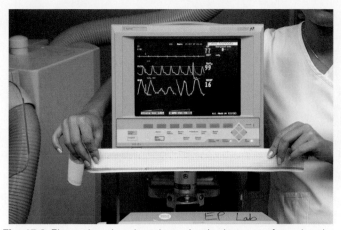

Fig. 15.6 Electrodes placed on the patient's chest transform the electrical activity into pulse rate values and waveforms visible on a monitor.

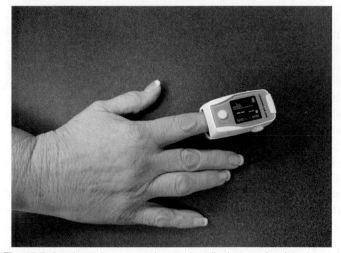

Fig. 15.7 A pulse oximeter can be used to display a patient's pulse and oxygen saturation.

Several factors can affect the accuracy of electronic devices used to monitor pulse rates. For example, patient movement can give rise to inaccurate readings. In addition, misplaced or loose electrodes, lines, or probes also yield inaccurate values. Poor peripheral perfusion caused by low blood pressure, nail polish, and acrylic nails are common causes of pulse oximetry inaccuracies. However, when the factors or situations that limit the device's precision are corrected, these monitoring instruments provide reliable, continual, and rapid assessment of patients.

Significance of Abnormalities

Because the cardiovascular system is responsible for delivering oxygenated blood to the cells, when cellular demand for oxygen increases, the heart responds by sending more blood to the tissues. The heart accomplishes this task by increasing the number or force of each myocardial contraction. When heart contractions, and therefore pulse rates, increase by more than 20 BPM in the resting adult or reach a rate greater than 100 BPM, the patient is said to be experiencing **tachycardia.** Exercise, fever, anemia, respiratory disorders, congestive heart failure, hypoxemia, and shock can cause a patient to become tachycardic because of the increased cellular demands for oxygen. Pain,

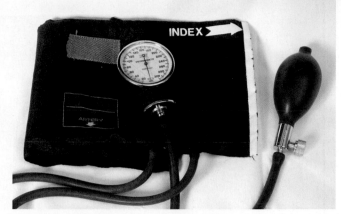

Fig. 15.8 Aneroid-style sphygmomanometer consisting of an air bladder (cuff), a bulb and valve to control airflow in and out of the cuff, and a calibrated pressure gauge or dial.

anger, fear, anxiety, and medications may also induce tachycardia, but the stimulus is through the nervous system, not through an increased demand for oxygen.

Bradycardia refers to a decrease in heart rate. Although initially pain can cause tachycardia, unrelieved, severe pain can in fact lead to bradycardia, subsequent heart problems, and even heart failure. Bradycardia may also be seen in hypothermia and in physically fit athletes.

If no pulse can be felt at the wrist, or if cardiac arrest is thought to occur, the pulse should be assessed at the carotid artery for a full 5 seconds while emergency help is summoned. If pulse irregularities are accompanied by patient reports of palpitations, dizziness, or faintness, a physician should be notified because these irregularities can be life threatening.

BLOOD PRESSURE

Description

Blood pressure is a measure of the force exerted by blood on the arterial walls during contraction and relaxation of the heart. An analogy can be made to water being pumped through a hose. A constant pressure is exerted on the inner surface of the hose by the water. When pumping occurs, the pressure increases as more water is added to the system, causing the water to flow. A similar situation exists in the human body. The pump is the heart, arterial blood vessels are analogous to the hose, and the fluid component is blood instead of water. A constant pressure is exerted on the arterial vessels by the blood when the heart is relaxed. This pressure is called the **diastolic** pressure. During a contraction of the heart, blood is ejected from the ventricles into the arterial blood vessels, creating an increase in pressure. The peak pressure present during contraction of the heart is known as the **systolic** pressure.

Measurement

Blood pressure readings are obtained with the use of a **sphygmomanometer** and stethoscope. The sphygmomanometer consists of a cuff, tubing, a valve, a bulb, and a manometer attached to the cuff (Fig. 15.8). The two commonly used types of sphygmomanometers are mercury and aneroid (more common). Regardless

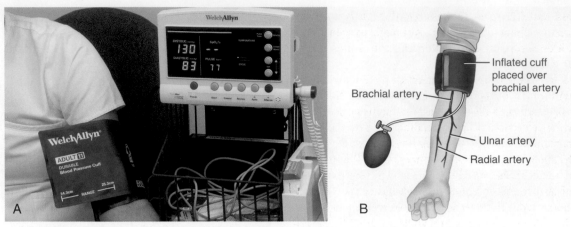

Fig. 15.9 Blood pressure may be monitored through an electronic, digital readout vital signs manometer. (A) The cuff is directly connected to the manometer. (B) The cuff of the sphygmomanometer is placed on the upper arm midway between the elbow and shoulder and is then inflated.

of which type is used, the cuff of the sphygmomanometer is typically placed on the upper arm midway between the elbow and shoulder. It is important that the proper size cuff, depending on the size of the arm, be used. The bulb is used to inflate the cuff with air. Inflation of the cuff above the patient's systolic pressure stops blood flow to the arm by collapsing the brachial artery. With the stethoscope placed over the brachial artery in the antecubital fossa of the elbow, opening the valve slowly deflates the cuff of the sphygmomanometer. When cuff pressure no longer exceeds the internal pressure of blood in the brachial artery, blood flow returns and can be heard through the stethoscope. The first sound of blood flow (turbulence of blood flow through the artery) corresponds to the values (numbers) observed on the manometer and indicates the systolic pressure. When the sound of blood flowing through the arm can no longer be heard, the corresponding values on the manometer indicate that the diastolic pressure is reached. The turbulent sound of blood flow through the arteries during blood pressure measurement is called *Korotkoff sounds*, named for the Russian physician who first described them. Blood pressures are recorded in millimeters of mercury (mm Hg) read from the manometer, with systolic measurements recorded over diastolic measurements (systolic/diastolic).

Blood pressure may also be measured and displayed through a cardiac or vital signs monitor. The cuff is placed around the patient's arm and may be inflated manually by a health care professional or through an automatic, timed sequence controlled through the monitor. Once the cuff inflates and deflates, blood pressure values electronically display on the monitor (Fig. 15.9).

Normal blood pressure in the healthy adult includes a systolic pressure of less than 120 mm Hg and diastolic pressure of less than 80 mm Hg (see Table 15.1). Pressures are most often recorded with the patient in a sitting position and the arm at approximately the level of the heart. Variations in these conditions can cause some difference in blood pressure readings.

Significance of Abnormalities

The persistent elevation of blood pressure greater than 140/90 mm Hg is known as **hypertension.** Hypertension is further categorized. Prehypertension involves consistent systolic pressure of 120 to 139 mm Hg or when consistent diastolic pressures measure between 80 and 89 mm Hg. Stage 1 hypertension is diagnosed when the systolic pressure is consistently recorded at 140 to 149 mm Hg or when diastolic pressure is consistently between 90 and 99 mm Hg. Stage 2 hypertension involves consistent systolic pressures of 160 mm Hg or greater or when diastolic pressures fall to 100 mm Hg or greater.

Hypertension is common, but patients are usually unaware of its presence because no symptoms exist. Hypertension causes a significant increase on the workload of the heart. Extreme elevations in the blood pressure can damage the brain within minutes. Moderate degrees of hypertension can cause damage to the heart, brain, kidneys, lungs, and other organ systems. In addition to various disease states, stress, medications, obesity, and smoking can contribute to hypertension. The incidence of hypertension is higher in men than in women, and it is more common in African Americans than in whites.

Hypotension is defined as low blood pressure and may be identified by a blood pressure of less than 95/60 mm Hg. Low blood pressure is generally desirable and is usually not problematic unless it produces symptoms (e.g., syncope). In other words, in a healthy adult without any accompanying symptoms, hypotension presents no cause for alarm. A hypotensive patient reporting dizziness, confusion, or blurred vision may have an inadequate circulating blood volume, and further evaluation needs to be initiated immediately. A patient in shock from severe bleeding, burns, vomiting, diarrhea, trauma, or heat exhaustion is hypotensive as a result of a decrease in total blood volume. These persons require immediate care.

OXYGEN THERAPY

The moment-to-moment sustenance of human life depends on a single external substance. This substance is so important that its absence in the environment causes irreversible damage to the brain in approximately 6 minutes. In its absence, production of cellular metabolism is grossly inadequate and death ultimately occurs. This substance is, of course, oxygen, which is essential to each of the billions of cells making up the human body. Oxygen is a colorless, tasteless, and odorless gas that plays a critical role in efficient cellular metabolism. Although oxygen is not flammable, it does support combustion and constitutes 21% of atmospheric gases.

The need for oxygen becomes critical to patients when the internal environment of the body is not consistent. Normally, the 21% of oxygen supplied in room air maintains homeostasis; however, when oxygenation levels become low, the metabolic rate is compromised and the patient's homeostasis is altered. Accordingly, the patient's cardiopulmonary system has to adapt to maintain homeostasis caused by **hypoxemia.** Approximately one-third of all patients in acute care settings receive oxygen therapy of some type. The overall goal of oxygen therapy is to maintain adequate tissue oxygenation while minimizing cardiopulmonary work.

Indications for Oxygen Therapy

The primary clinical indications for oxygen administration are to correct hypoxemia or possible tissue hypoxia and prevent or minimize the increased cardiopulmonary workload (increased heart rate, blood pressure, and respiratory rate). Tissue **hypoxia** is a term used to describe an inadequate amount of oxygen at the cellular (tissue) level. The tissues most sensitive to hypoxia are the brain, heart, lungs, and liver. When hypoxia is present, the metabolic rate of the body is compromised, resulting in altered homeostasis.

To compensate for hypoxia, respiratory rates, depth of breathing, blood pressure, and heart rates increase. A patient with hypoxia feels short of breath and has to work harder to breathe, thereby allowing the body's adaptive response mechanisms to maintain homeostasis. During this event, oxygen therapy is administered to alleviate the cardiopulmonary work. As a result, blood pressure, heart rate, and respiratory rate and depth may return toward normal.

Oxygen as a Drug

Oxygen is listed in the *US Pharmacopeia* and is defined as a drug in the *Federal Food, Drug, and Cosmetic Act* of 1962. Like any drug, oxygen has both good and bad biologic effects; the minimum dose should always be given to obtain the desired result, and no more. Therefore a physician must prescribe oxygen. In terms of dosage, and depending on equipment, oxygen is usually ordered either in liters per minute (LPM) or as a concentration. When a concentration is prescribed, it may be either a percentage, such as 24%, or a fractional concentration of oxygen (Fio_2), such as 0.24. Once the desired result has been achieved, the dosage is maintained and the patient's response is continually monitored.

OXYGEN DEVICES

The radiologic technologist will encounter a variety of devices used to deliver oxygen. Oxygen therapy may be accomplished using a pressurized gas or liquid oxygen systems. Liquid oxygen delivery systems provide a convenient method for home use and during the patient's normal daily activities. At very low temperatures, oxygen, as a gas, converts to a liquid state.

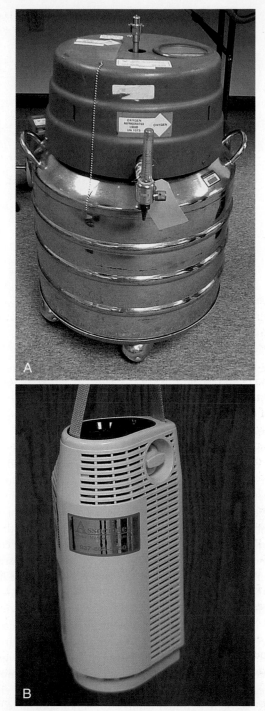

Fig. 15.10 (A) Large stationary liquid oxygen supply. (B) Small portable liquid oxygen canister.

A large stationary tank for liquid oxygen is available to serve in the home as the supply source for a smaller, portable oxygen canister (Fig. 15.10).

Regardless of the type of system used, these devices in no way hamper the technologist's ability to perform radiologic procedures, although sometimes repositioning the devices is necessary to avoid artifacts on the image. If the oxygen device must be repositioned, the responsibility of the technologist is to ascertain that any tubing leading to the device is not kinked or disconnected and that the device is properly repositioned on

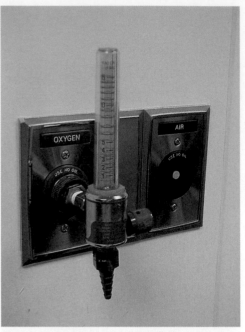

Fig. 15.11 Flowmeter for a wall supply of oxygen.

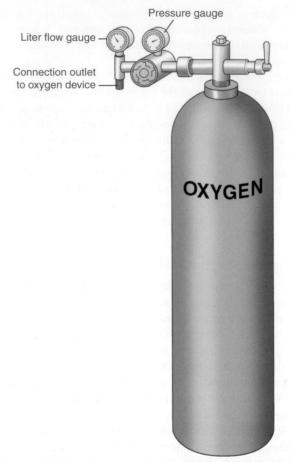

Fig. 15.12 Typical portable oxygen cylinder—small size (E-tank).

the patient at the conclusion of the radiologic procedure. *Under no circumstances should an oxygen device be completely removed from the patient for the purpose of taking a radiograph without the consent or supervision of a physician, respiratory care practitioner, or attending nurse.*

Supplemental oxygen administration for patients requires an oxygen-delivery device, a gas source, and a means by which the two can be connected. Oxygen devices may be continuous flow or conserving device systems.

Oxygen-delivery devices are designed to operate at a certain LPM value. An oxygen flowmeter is a reducing valve that permits flows (LPM) safe for patient use and serves as the connection between the oxygen-delivery device and the gas source. The oxygen flowmeter is green (or has green labeling) and has the word *OXYGEN* on it (Fig. 15.11).

In the patient's hospital room, these oxygen devices are usually attached to a wall outlet through which a continuous oxygen supply is piped. However, patients receiving oxygen frequently need to be transported to the radiographic examination room for procedures. This task is accomplished by attaching the tubing from the oxygen device to either a portable oxygen cylinder (tank) or small, portable liquid oxygen canister. Portable systems include a regulator consisting of a flowmeter and pressure manometer (Fig. 15.12). The pressure manometer indicates pressure or the volume of oxygen inside the cylinder or canister, and the flowmeter control operates the rate of oxygen flow in LPM to the patient. Although various configurations of flowmeters may be seen on the regulator, all serve as a means of setting the LPM flow of oxygen required (Fig. 15.13). It is important to check the portable oxygen system before transporting a patient to ensure that an adequate oxygen supply is available throughout the patient transport period and duration of the radiographic procedure. On the patient's arrival in the radiographic suite, the oxygen supply is usually transferred from the portable oxygen system back to a wall outlet during

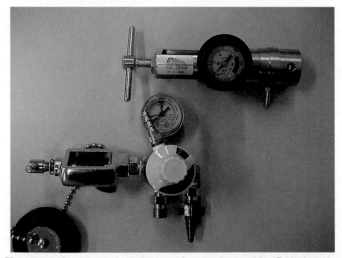

Fig. 15.13 Oxygen tank regulators for small portable (E-size) tanks. Each regulator has a flowmeter (dial and knob styles). Also note the small-bore connectors for hooking up oxygen tubing.

the examination. If this is the case, the technologist should ensure correct transfer of the LPM settings and turn off the portable supply of oxygen. Although portable oxygen systems and regulators are extremely durable, they should be secured during transport to prevent them falling and possibly developing cracks or leaks. It is important to note that when magnetic resonance imaging studies are performed, aluminum tanks or cylinders must be used.

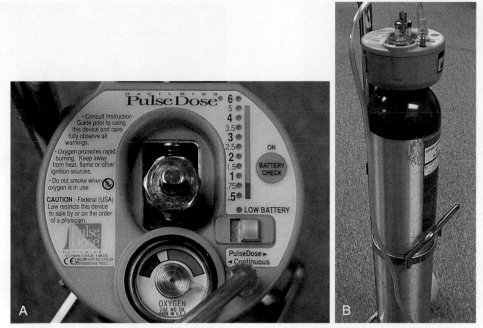

Fig. 15.14 (A) Pulse dose regulator. (B) Pulse dose regulator on an E-tank.

Primarily for home use, oxygen-conserving devices have gained popularity. An outpatient requiring oxygen therapy may need a medical imaging procedure using conserving systems of liquid or pressurized gas. There are two categories of oxygen-conserving devices that deliver a specifically measured dose to the patient: pulse dose and demand devices. A pulsed dose device delivers a fixed volume of oxygen supply during breathing. Based on the patient's rate of breathing, a special electronic circuit opens a valve in the device, delivering a fixed oxygen supply to the patient during the inspiratory phase of breathing. By delivering oxygen only during inspiration, oxygen supply is conserved, whereas conventional regulators provide a continuous flow of oxygen regardless of the patient's phase of breathing. A demand device delivers a variable-volume oxygen dose. The dose supplied with a demand device is dependent on the length of the patient's inspiration. In both these systems, oxygen pressure is continually adjusted to provide an accurate flow of oxygen (Fig. 15.14).

Oxygen devices are divided into low-flow and high-flow delivery systems. A low-flow, or *variable-oxygen concentration*, device does not meet the entire inspiratory needs of the patient. An unknown amount of room air is entrained through the nose or mouth of the patient and mixes with the constant amount of 100% oxygen delivered. The exact oxygen concentration or FiO_2 the patient receives is unknown and can vary as the patient's breathing pattern changes. As the patient takes in more air (either by deeper breaths and a normal respiratory rate or by normal-volume breaths and a faster respiratory rate), the oxygen concentration decreases as more room air dilutes the 100% oxygen source. Oxygen concentration increases if the patient takes in less air (either by smaller volume breaths and a normal respiratory rate or by normal-volume breaths and a decreased, slower respiratory rate) because less room air is entrained to dilute the 100% oxygen coming from the flowmeter. Consequently, in the low-flow delivery systems, the percentage of

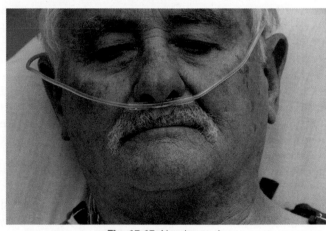

Fig. 15.15 Nasal cannula.

oxygen that a patient receives may fluctuate with a change in depth of respiration, respiratory rate, or breathing pattern when a low-flow device is used.

A *high-flow* device, sometimes referred to as a *fixed* or *precise oxygen concentration* device, does meet or exceed the inspiratory needs of the patient when the device is functioning properly. The inspired concentration of oxygen does not change with altered breathing patterns because high-flow systems function on an air-entrainment principle. In this case, room air gases are precisely mixed with 100% oxygen before reaching the patient. The constant ratios used in the mixing of the gases (oxygen and room air) will provide the patient a precise oxygen percentage or FiO_2 regardless of the breathing pattern.

Nasal Cannula

The most common device used to deliver low concentrations of oxygen is the nasal cannula (Fig. 15.15). The nasal cannula delivers oxygen through short prongs inserted into the nares. Because the patient inhales oxygen from the cannula, as well as

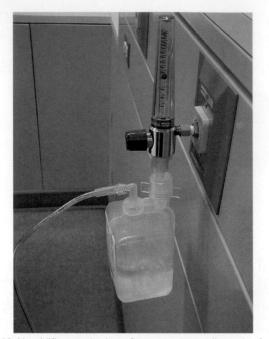

Fig. 15.16 Humidifier attached to a flowmeter in a wall supply of oxygen.

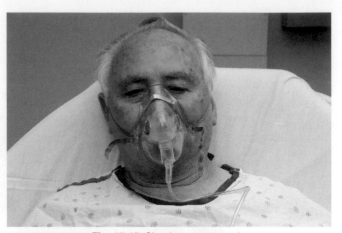

Fig. 15.17 Simple oxygen mask.

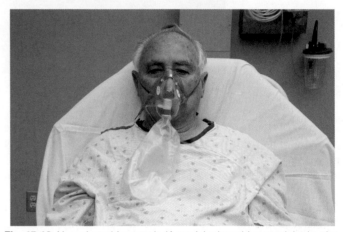

Fig. 15.18 Nonrebreathing mask. (A partial rebreathing mask looks similar to this.)

room air, this device is classified as a low-flow device. Although flow rates up to 6 LPM may be administered through the cannula, usually oxygen flow rates of 1 to 4 LPM are used, delivering approximately 24% to 36%. Humidity is added to the nasal cannula delivery system when flows greater than 4 LPM are used, because the higher flows can dry the nasal mucosa and cause patient discomfort (Fig. 15.16). The nasal cannula is well tolerated by the patient because talking, eating, and sleeping are not hindered.

Masks

Various kinds of masks, including simple, nonrebreathing, partial rebreathing, aerosol, and air-entrainment masks, are used for oxygen therapy. A mask is generally not tolerated as well as a nasal cannula. Masks can be hot and because they are made of plastic tend to stick to the patient's face. Masks need to be removed for eating. They muffle speech, and frequently the head strap does not fit well around the patient's head. Therefore masks often become dislodged during sleep. Masks also increase the risk for aspiration in the patient who vomits. Despite these disadvantages, masks provide an effective way to deliver accurate as well as high concentrations of oxygen and are effective when a nasal cannula cannot be used.

Simple oxygen masks, low-flow devices, cover the patient's nose and mouth (Fig. 15.17). They require oxygen flow rates greater than 6 LPM to prevent an accumulation of carbon dioxide. Simple oxygen masks are capable of delivering 35% to 50% oxygen, depending on the oxygen flow rate and the respiratory pattern of the patient. Although not commonly used, simple masks are convenient for short-term oxygen therapy.

A nonrebreathing mask can deliver a higher percentage of oxygen than the nasal cannula or simple mask. These masks have bags attached to them known as *reservoirs* that fill with oxygen (Fig. 15.18). As disposable units, these nonrebreathing

masks are constructed with one-way valves at the opening of the reservoir bag, preventing exhaled air from being rebreathed and ensuring that only oxygen from the device is inhaled. A partial rebreathing mask is similar to a nonrebreathing mask, but it does not contain the valve. Because of the small volume of the reservoir, the partial rebreathing mask and nonrebreathing mask might not necessarily meet the total inspiratory demands of a patient exhibiting variable respiratory rates or variable inspiratory volumes. The masks should always be maintained with a liter flow high enough to keep the reservoir bag inflated. Theoretically, a high liter flow and a tight seal against the face should provide 100% oxygen; however, clinically, these devices may deliver as little as 60% or as much as 80% oxygen, depending on how tightly the mask is affixed to the face.

Nebulizers (high-flow devices) generate an aerosol mist with precise oxygen concentrations; they can be connected via corrugated tubing to an aerosol face mask, tracheostomy mask or collar, or T-piece adapter for endotracheal tubes (Fig. 15.19). An aerosol mist is desired when the patient's inspired gases bypass the normal humidification function of the nasal passages and upper airways, which occurs through the insertion of an artificial airway after intubation or tracheostomy. The nebulizer is connected to an oxygen flowmeter at a flow rate of at least 8 LPM (and/or according to manufacturer's guidelines) to provide

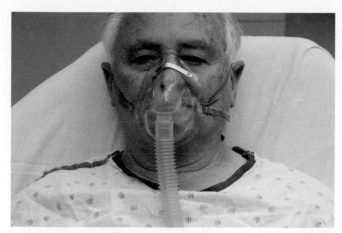

Fig. 15.19 Aerosol mask.

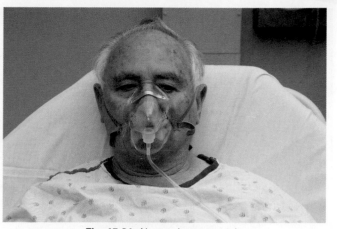

Fig. 15.21 Air-entrainment mask.

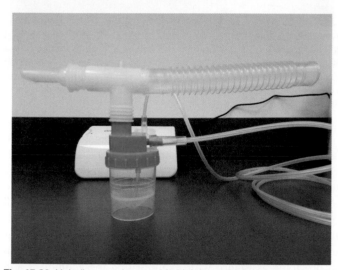

Fig. 15.20 Nebulizer used to provide high humidity in the form of a mist.

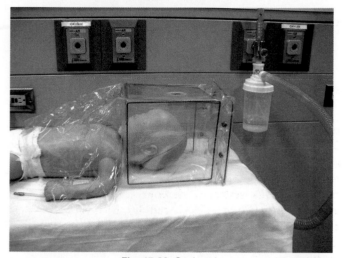

Fig. 15.22 Oxyhood.

precise ratios of oxygen to room air entrainment through the oxygen concentration (28% to 100%) dialed or set on the nebulizer device. The nebulizer is filled with 0.45 saline, 0.9 normal saline, or sterile water (Fig. 15.20). Because the aerosol mist condensates in the corrugated tubing on its way to the patient, caution must be used as the tubing, delivery device, and patient are manipulated or moved. Failure to do so may inadvertently flush the patient's airway with the fluid accumulated within the corrugated tubing. Nebulizers are also used to administer medications in the form of an extremely fine mist that patients inhale.

The air-entrainment mask, a high-flow device, is constructed to provide an accurate concentration of oxygen to the patient by propelling a high-velocity of source oxygen through a narrowed opening near the mask (Fig. 15.21). This method results in room air being drawn into the mask. The source oxygen, along with the entrained room air, provides a flow of gas that is capable of meeting the total need of the inspiratory capacity of the patient. Therefore the set liter flow must not be altered for the purpose of maintaining accurate oxygen concentrations. Air-entrainment masks provide consistent concentrations of oxygen, even though the patient's respiratory pattern may change. Depending on the manufacturer, air-entrainment masks generally can provide consistent oxygen concentration values at 24%, 28%, 35%, 40%, and 50%.

Tent and Oxyhood

Pediatric patients requiring oxygen therapy and additional humidity can be placed either in oxygen tents or oxyhoods. An oxygen tent covers the child's bed. Controlling the oxygen concentration is difficult in a tent because the frequent openings necessary for childcare allow oxygen to escape. Because oxygen supports combustion, care should be exercised and machines that are likely to produce sparks should not be used in the vicinity of oxygen tents or free-flowing oxygen. Therefore the technologist is responsible for ascertaining that the mobile x-ray unit is safe for use in situations in which combustibility is a risk.

Oxyhoods are generally used on infants. These consist of a disposable or permanent plastic box that fits over the infant's head (Fig. 15.22). Oxygen concentrations of 21% to 100% can be delivered using these devices.

Table 15.2 provides a summation of low-flow and high-flow oxygen therapy systems. The flow rates and FiO_2 ranges described in Table 15.2 are the generally accepted values; however, patient-specific physician prescription is to be followed.

Ventilators

When the cardiopulmonary system is unable to supply adequate oxygen to the tissues, a patient may have an artificial

TABLE 15.2 Summary of Oxygen Devices

Category	Device	Liters per Minute	Fio$_2$ (%)
Low flow	Nasal cannula—adult	0.25–8	24–40
	Nasal cannula—infant	<2	22–45
	Nasal catheter	0.25–8	22–45
	Transtracheal catheter	0.25–4	22–35
	Simple mask	5–10	35–50
	Partial rebreathing mask	No less than 10	40–70
	Nonrebreathing mask	No less than 10	60–80
High flow	Air-entrainment mask	Varies; should provide ≥60	24–50
	Air-entrainment nebulizer	10–15; should provide ≥60	28–100
Enclosure	Oxyhood	≥7	21–100
	Isolette	8–15	40–50
	Tent	12–15	40–50

Fio$_2$, Fractional concentration of oxygen.
Kacmarek R, Stoller J, Heuer A. *Egan's Fundamentals of Respiratory Care*. 11th ed. St. Louis: Elsevier; 2017.

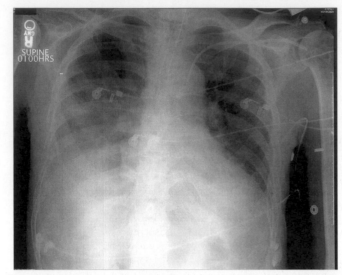

Fig. 15.24 Anteroposterior projection of the chest with endotracheal tube in normal position. Note that the patient is slightly rotated to the left, underscoring the importance of proper patient positioning during imaging. Also note the left subclavian central venous line with catheter tip in the hemiazygous vein and overlying cardiac monitor wires and leads.

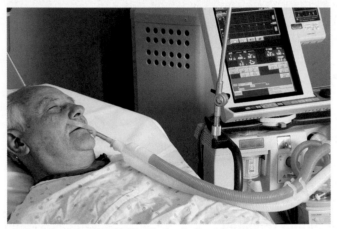

Fig. 15.23 Mechanical ventilator.

airway inserted in the trachea, which is then connected to a mechanical ventilator (Fig. 15.23). The ventilator delivers a minimum set respiratory rate, preset inspiratory volume, and consistent Fio$_2$. A radiograph of the patient's chest is frequently required to determine whether the artificial airway is in the proper place (Fig. 15.24). The attending nurse or respiratory care practitioner must be informed before the initiation of any radiologic procedure because care must be taken not to dislodge the artificial airway when positioning the patient or when adjusting the ventilator tubing. Care must also be exercised when moving the corrugated tubing, because moisture collects inside the tubing and may be passed into the patient's lungs, as previously discussed. The radiographer must also be aware that proper head position is critical because flexing or extending the neck can adversely influence artificial airway placement, particularly in neonatal patients. Audio and visual alarms on the ventilator monitor the patient's response. Occasionally, the alarms sound when the patient is repositioned. *These alarms on the ventilator should not be silenced or altered by the radiologic technologist.*

The nursing staff or respiratory care practitioners should assist the technologist in positioning the patient, thereby preventing accidental disconnection and patient endangerment. If a mobile procedure is to be performed on a mechanically ventilated patient, the radiographer must carefully observe the rise and fall of the patient's chest to determine full inspiration or full expiration. Ideally, the technologist should collaborate with the respiratory therapist before initiating the mobile procedure. In addition to providing assistance with manipulating the equipment and patient, the therapist can control the ventilator to yield an effective inspiratory volume to produce a high-quality chest image.

CHEST TUBES AND LINES

Provided they are well informed, radiographers can play an important role in the early detection of problems associated with malpositioned lines. As experts in radiographic quality, radiographers have a clear responsibility in this area that is separate from the issue of interpretation of images. Without any expectation of the radiographer to interpret the image from a pathologic diagnostic standpoint, when malpositioning is thought to occur, alerting the appropriate authority (e.g., radiologist, attending physician) is both appropriate and beneficial to the patient.

Endotracheal Tubes

Endotracheal tubes are used to manage a variety of respiratory complications (Fig. 15.25). Indications for use include (1) a need for mechanical ventilation or oxygen delivery because of inadequate ventilation (breathing), inadequate arterial oxygenation, severe airway obstruction, shock, and parenchymal diseases that impair gas exchange; (2) upper airway obstruction; (3) impending gastric acid reflux or aspiration; and (4) provisions for tracheobronchial lavage.

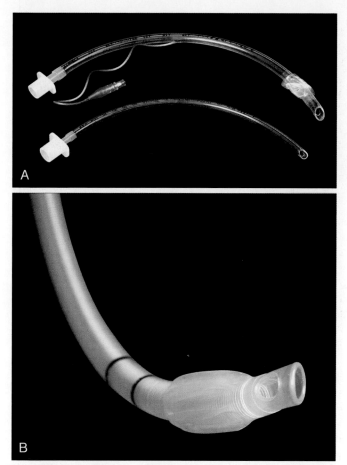

Fig. 15.25 (A) Adult endotracheal tube *(top)* and pediatric endotracheal tube *(bottom)*. Note the absence of cuff. (B) Distal end of endotracheal tube with cuff deflated.

Tracheal **intubation** is accomplished most often using a translaryngeal approach via the mouth or nose, but in certain cases the use of a tracheostomy is necessary (Fig. 15.26). The nasal tracheal approach is preferred except during emergency situations or when anesthesia is administered. Historically, the cuff's structure and pressure often damaged the tracheal mucosa, especially during long-term care; thus in extended-care settings or when intubation was required for prolonged periods of time, tracheostomies were often substituted. Today, endotracheal cuffs are softer and exert lower pressure on tracheal tissues and therefore are more compatible with long-term use.

Once an endotracheal tube has been inserted, placement of the tube is confirmed by chest radiography and is assessed periodically thereafter. Properly positioned tubes will show the distal tip 1 to 2 inches (3 to 5 cm) superior to the tracheal bifurcation (Fig. 15.27). The cuff is inflated with air and is positioned at midtrachea; however, the cuff is not radiographically apparent. The most common example of malpositioning involves intubation of the right main-stem bronchus because it originates at the trachea at less of an angle compared with the left main bronchus. Complications may include overventilation of the right lung and potential airway obstruction of the left. When the tip of the tube slides into the right main bronchus, its shaft may occlude the left main bronchus, causing severe **atelectasis** of the left lung (Fig. 15.28).

Collapsed lung ←

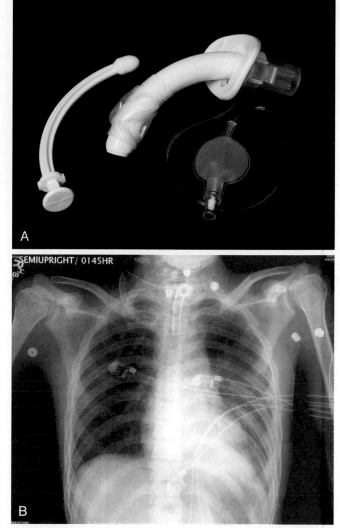

Fig. 15.26 (A) Tracheostomy tube with obturator. The obturator is used only to guide the insertion and is removed once the insertion is complete. (B) Anteroposterior chest projection with tracheostomy tube in normal position.

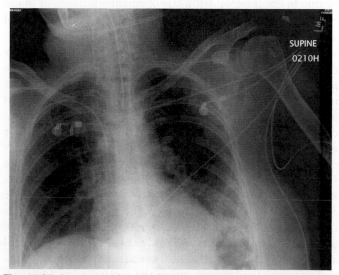

Fig. 15.27 Anteroposterior mobile chest projection showing endotracheal tube properly positioned with right peripherally inserted central catheter line tip in the superior vena cava overlying cardiac monitor leads.

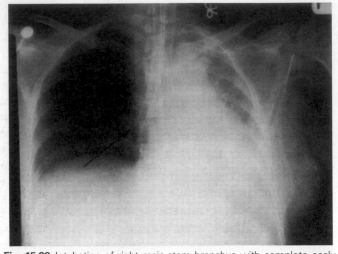

Fig. 15.28 Intubation of right main-stem bronchus with complete occlusion of the left bronchus causing left lung atelectasis. (From Moore DE. ET, CV, VAD, PA, Swan: what's it all about? *Semin Radiol Technol.* 1997;5:49.)

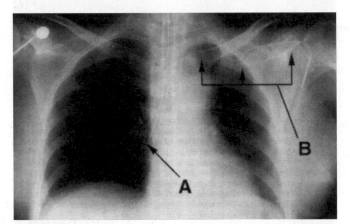

Fig. 15.29 (A) Distal tip of endotracheal tube in right main bronchus. (B) Central venous catheter in the left subclavian vein. (From Moore DE. ET, CV, VAD, PA, Swan: what's it all about? *Semin Radiol Technol.* 1997;5:49.)

Occasionally, endobronchial tubes are used to provide ventilation to one lung, as in the case of pneumonectomy, or to use two mechanical ventilators, one for each lung. Endobronchial tubes are designed so that the tip is inserted in one of the main-stem bronchi. In such cases, the tip will be located in either the right or the left system. Once inserted properly, two cuffs are inflated to anchor the endobronchial tube in position, one at the bronchial end and one in the trachea. When dual ventilation is used, a side hole in the endobronchial tube is positioned adjacent to the nonintubated bronchus to facilitate ventilation to the contralateral lung.

Radiographic demonstration of complications associated with tracheal intubation and mechanical ventilation includes the following:

1. Bronchial intubation, most often involving the right main-stem bronchus (Fig. 15.29)
2. Intubation not far enough, so cuff inflation damages vocal folds and inadequately provides ventilation
3. Erosion of the tracheal mucosa as a result of cuff trauma, causing subcutaneous or mediastinal emphysema
4. Pneumothorax

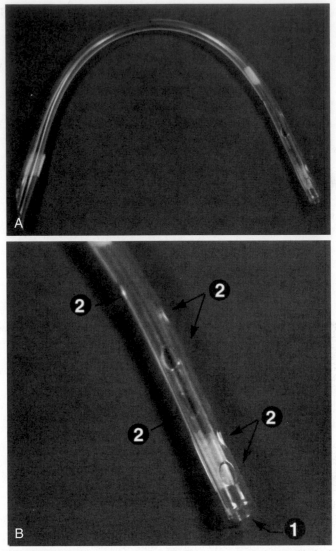

Fig. 15.30 (A) Thoracostomy tube. (B) Thoracostomy tube: end hole *(1)* and side holes *(2)*. (From Moore DE. ET, CV, VAD, PA, Swan: what's it all about? *Semin Radiol Technol.* 1997;5:49.)

Thoracostomy Tubes

Thoracostomy (intrapleural) tubes, more commonly called *chest tubes* (Fig. 15.30), are used to drain the intrapleural space and the mediastinum. Fluid or air accumulation, or both, in either space will have deleterious effects and may be life threatening, depending on volume.

The pleural cavity is a potential space where parietal and visceral pleurae meet. A minimal amount of serous fluid exists to provide a lubricant for ease of movement between the two pleural layers during breathing. Negative pressure in the intrapleural space provides a suction-type mechanism between the lung and thorax that facilitates lung expansion. When fluids or air accumulate in the space, negative pressure is lowered or lost and the lung fails to fully expand. If pressure falls too low, then the lung will collapse.

Thoracostomy tubes are inserted through the chest wall to reestablish negative intrapleural pressure in cases of **pneumothorax,** hemothorax, **pleural effusion,** and empyema. In addition to chest tubes, mediastinal drains (usually small chest tubes) are used after cardiac surgery to drain residual blood

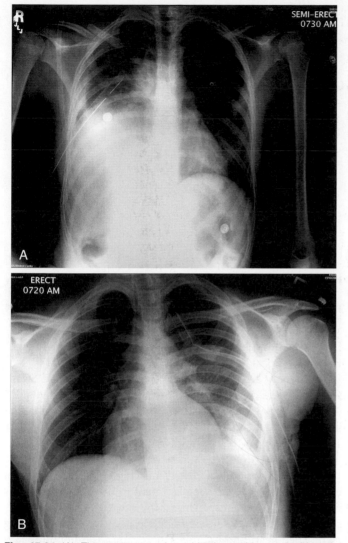

Fig. 15.31 (A) Thoracostomy tube with tip positioned at fifth and sixth intercostal spaces to treat pleural effusion of right lung. (B) Left upper lobe pneumothorax with thoracostomy tube in place to evacuate extrapleural air and reexpand lung.

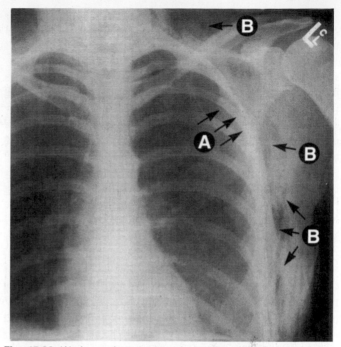

Fig. 15.32 (A) An expiratory, anteroposterior projection showing an approximate 10% pneumothorax on the left. (B) Also note moderate subcutaneous emphysema in the left chest wall extending up to the neck. (From Moore DE. ET, CV, VAD, PA, Swan: what's it all about? *Semin Radiol Technol.* 1997;5:49.)

from the mediastinum. Postoperative blood accumulation around the pericardium can cause cardiac tamponade, which is a life-threatening event.

Insertion sites for thoracostomy tubes vary with the intrapleural substances to be removed. In the case of hemothorax and pleural effusions, fluids flow with gravity and tend to accumulate near the lung base (Fig. 15.31A). Typical insertion sites in these instances are the fifth to sixth intercostal spaces and laterally at the midaxillary line. Tubes can also be inserted as high as the fourth and as low as the eighth rib. In cases of pneumothoraces, air will rise to the upper pleural spaces, requiring higher insertion sites in the apical region. In general, the second to third intercostal space at the midclavicular line is preferred.

Pleural fluid accumulation becomes apparent radiographically when enough fluid is present to show costophrenic blunting. Once radiographically apparent, the angles typically show medial displacement. Costophrenic fluids may approach 300 mL or more before becoming radiographically evident on posteroanterior or anteroposterior chest projections, but as little as

150 mL of fluid may be visible on lateral decubitus views. Supine imaging may obscure visualization of pleural fluids and should be avoided when possible.

Causes of pneumothorax include a break in the continuity of the visceral pleura (rupture of an emphysematous bleb, fractured rib, central venous [CV] line insertion error), penetration of the external chest wall seen in trauma, or in rare instances a gas-producing microorganism *(empyema)*. When air accumulates in the intrapleural space, creating a loss of negative pressure, the lungs cannot fully expand, creating a space between the lung edge and the costal border.

Radiographically, pneumothoraces are shown when the increased density of the collapsed lung is contrasted with a lateral radiolucency that is absent of lung markings (see Fig. 15.31B). During inspiration, the lung expands laterally and meets the lateral rib edge, rendering small pneumothoraces that are difficult to detect. Therefore pneumothoraces are best shown by expiratory posteroanterior or anteroposterior projections of the chest. Lateral decubitus filming with the ipsilateral side up may also be useful.

After thoracostomy, sutures are applied to anchor the tube so that patients can move with caution. Radiographic studies require erect or semi-erect imaging whenever possible, and care must be exercised to avoid dislodging the tube. Partially dislodged tubes, leaks at the insertion site, and extracostal insertions may lead to subcutaneous emphysema (Fig. 15.32).

Various degrees of pneumothoraces exist. Small pneumothoraces are typically classified as *simple* and *spontaneous*, usually caused by a ruptured bleb, and may resorb naturally. *Secondary* pneumothoraces are complications of parenchymal disease, or they may be caused iatrogenically during CV catheter insertion.

Because of coexisting conditions and the fact that these patients are already in a compromised state, secondary pneumothoraces require chest tube evacuation of the pleural cavity.

Tension pneumothorax is a dramatic event that requires aggressive care. In these cases, air continues to enter the pleural cavity through either a valvelike opening in the external chest wall (trauma) or a similar opening in the visceral pleura whereby air continues to enter the pleural space but cannot escape. Pressure increases on the ipsilateral side, causing a shift of the mediastinum toward the opposite side and producing a life-threatening event.

Tension pneumothorax may occur during mechanical ventilation. Rupture of the visceral pleura allows air to enter the pleural space without escape. Immediate aspiration of the intrapleural air relieves pressures and is standard treatment for tension pneumothorax.

Central Venous Lines

CV lines are catheters that are inserted into a large vein. They have a multitude of uses and descriptive terms. Initially, CV lines were developed to administer chemotherapeutic drugs and parenteral nutrition. Today, they may also be used to administer a variety of drugs, manage fluid volume, serve as a conduit for blood analysis and transfusions, and monitor cardiac pressures.

Commonly known as *central venous catheters* and *venous access devices*, venous lines are also named for their developers. One of the first modern CV lines was developed by Broviac and later enlarged by Hickman. Leonard and Groshong catheters are also widely used. Groshong catheters have a unique rounded, closed-end tip with a three-way valve mechanism that reduces the risk for blood loss and air embolism during withdrawals and infusions.

Catheters generally vary by size and composition and are available in single, double, and multiple lumens for short-term and long-term use. They are available as percutaneous catheters (subclavian insertion catheter), totally implanted access ports (Infusa Port, Port-a-Cath, Mediport), peripherally inserted central catheters (PICCs) (Fig. 15.33), and externally tunneled catheters (Broviac, Hickman, Groshong) (Fig. 15.34). In cases of chronic illness, implantable ports are desired when access is required intermittently over a long period; however, PICC insertion into the basilic or cephalic veins near the antecubital area also allows for long-term intravenous treatments, especially for patients receiving intravenous therapy home care.

Regardless of the style used, the goal is to position the catheter tip in a central vein. The preferred location is the superior vena cava, approximately 2 to 3 cm above the right atrial junction. Superior vena caval placement is preferred because of the size of this vein. Infusions of intravenous fluids are much less caustic in central veins than in smaller, peripheral veins.

The most common insertion site for CV catheters is the subclavian vein (Fig. 15.35). Other common sites include the internal jugular and femoral veins. Recent technologic advancements in catheters and safer insertion techniques now provide the opportunity to access the subclavian vein from a peripheral approach. When percutaneous subclavian and internal jugular approaches are contraindicated, the antecubital area may be accessed for line insertion, as is the case with PICC line insertions. Ports used in conjunction with PICCs are smaller than

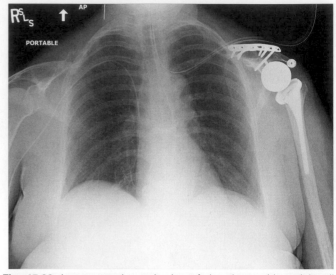

Fig. 15.33 Anteroposterior projection of the chest with peripherally inserted central catheter (right arm) tip properly positioned in the superior vena cava. Also note the nasogastric tube and that the patient has no clavicles.

those used in a subcutaneous pocket in the thorax but are functionally identical.

Pulmonary arterial (PA) lines are commonly called Swan-Ganz catheters, so named for the developers of the catheter. PA lines are specialized single-lumen or multilumen CV lines that incorporate at the distal end a small electrode used to monitor PA pressures (Fig. 15.36).

PA lines are used to estimate left ventricular end-diastolic pressure. Access to the left ventricle requires an arterial approach. Because catheter placement in the left ventricle has major physiologic consequences, the safest way to assess left-sided heart pressure is to extrapolate its value by monitoring right-sided heart and pulmonary pressures. Cardiopulmonary circulation is a continuous network of vascular structures interconnected by valves. Some valves are open, whereas others are simultaneously closed. When atrioventricular (AV) valves (tricuspid and bicuspid) are open, semilunar valves (pulmonary and aortic) are closed; when the semilunar valves open, the AV valves close.

PA catheters have a balloon located at the distal end. During pressure monitoring, this balloon is inflated, allowing the catheter tip to float and wedge in a small pulmonary artery. During this interval, the electrode, at the most distal end of the catheter, measures PA (wedged capillary) pressures. PA-wedged pressure is indicative of left atrial pressure, which in turn is indicative of left ventricular pressure. PA lines are routinely used to monitor venous oxygenation discretely or continuously.

Other than PA lines, no central catheter should appear beyond the superior vena cava. In the case of PA lines, the distal tip will be located in one of the two pulmonary arteries (Fig. 15.37). During pressure recordings, the balloon floats and wedges in a small arterial branch. Balloon wedging is synchronized with the cardiac monitor and lasts momentarily to avoid potential ischemia and infarction of the lung. The cardiac monitor generates pressure tracings during the wedge procedure.

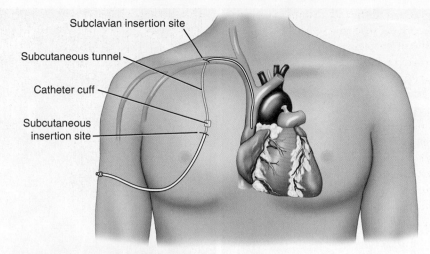

Fig. 15.34 Tunneled catheter.

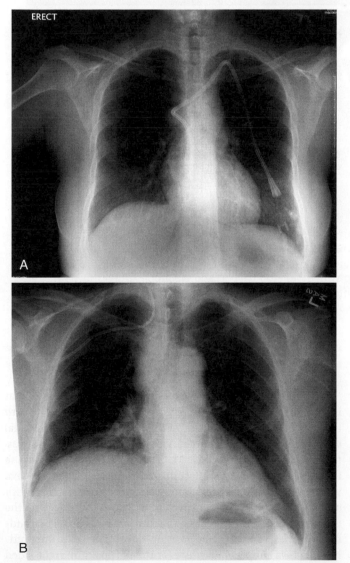

Fig. 15.35 (A) Posteroanterior projection of the chest shows double-lumen tunnel catheter in left subclavian vein with the tip in the superior vena cava at the right atrium. (B) Posteroanterior projection of the chest with right side peripherally inserted central catheter (PICC) line passing through right subclavian vein with tip up the internal jugular vein, and left side PICC line passing through left subclavian vein into the superior vena cava.

Once the measurement is complete, the balloon is deflated and blood flow beyond the catheter tip is resumed (Fig. 15.38).

CV access devices can improve and extend quality of life for many patients, but the potential for complications demands the attention of all members of the health care team. Reported incidence of CV complications varies, but those related to the management of CV lines by health care workers is significant. Examples of complications include catheter dislodgment and occlusions resulting from the accumulation of blood clots or drug precipitates. Catheter flushing procedures conducted by nursing staff help to prevent occlusive problems. One of the most critical concerns of radiographers is catheter dislodgment, which can be prevented only with increased awareness of the catheter's presence. Care must be exercised when handling patients with CV lines. Assessing the patient before performing radiographic procedures is essential to avert the possibility of line displacement (Fig. 15.39).

Regarding insertion problems, as many as one-third of CV catheters are placed incorrectly at insertion time. Malpositioning, pinching, and kinking also occur with significant frequency. Pneumothorax and hemothorax are potential complications associated with catheter insertions (Fig. 15.40).

Radiographic confirmation of line placement is essential at the time of insertion and thereafter as needed. Aberrant tip location is one of the most common complications associated with CV catheters. Additional medical imaging modalities may also prove useful when catheter placement is difficult or complications occur. For example, complications involving catheter fracture and subsequent migration can be resolved using angiography and fluoroscopy.

Recognition of catheter malposition requires thorough knowledge of CV structures and their branches. Typically, CV lines inserted from a right-sided approach will follow the course of the subclavian vein in a lateromedial direction and then descend through the right brachiocephalic vein. From the right brachiocephalic vein, the catheter passes into the superior vena cava, where it should terminate above the right atrium. Because of the right-sided position of the superior

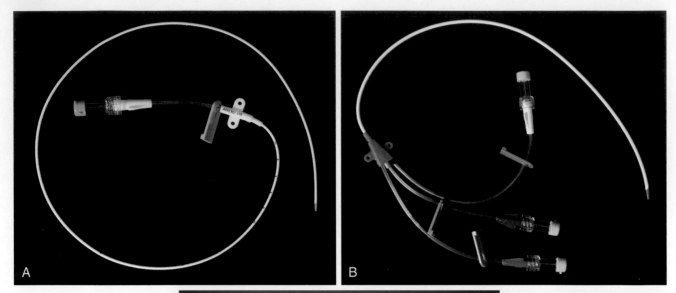

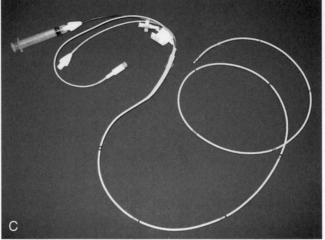

Fig. 15.36 (A) Single-lumen central venous catheter. (B) Triple-lumen central venous catheter. (C) Pulmonary arterial catheter. Note the distal tip with a deflated balloon and electrode. During pressure measurement, the balloon is inflated, drifting the catheter into a small pulmonary artery, where it wedges. The electrode at the tip of the catheter measures pulmonary pressure.

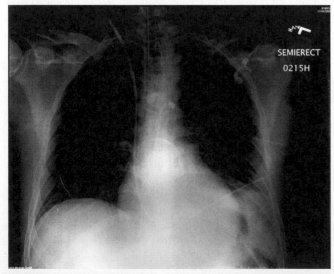

Fig. 15.37 Anteroposterior chest projection showing pulmonary arterial line through an internal jugular vein approach. The catheter tip is located in the right pulmonary artery.

vena cava, as the catheter advances, its image should remain to the right of the vertebral column and should not cross midline (see Fig. 15.33).

A left-sided approach involves a slightly longer catheter that is advanced lateromedially through the left subclavian vein to the left brachiocephalic vein. Because the left brachiocephalic vein courses in a relatively horizontal fashion as it crosses to the right of midline (see Fig. 15.35A), the catheter will traverse from left to right, where it terminates in the superior vena cava with a short descending pattern. One problem associated with a left-sided approach is placement of the catheter tip in the thoracic duct. In this instance, the catheter does not cross midline. Checking for catheter position in orientation to the midline can be a simple way to assess catheter position; right-sided approaches never cross midline, whereas a left-sided approach should always cross midline.

Although recognition of problems related to tubes and line use is not specifically identified in the radiographer's scope of practice, an implied responsibility certainly exists. As

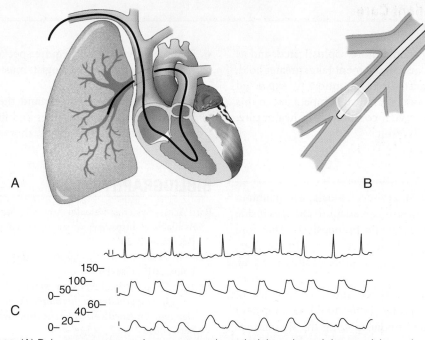
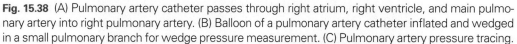

A

B

C

Fig. 15.38 (A) Pulmonary artery catheter passes through right atrium, right ventricle, and main pulmonary artery into right pulmonary artery. (B) Balloon of a pulmonary artery catheter inflated and wedged in a small pulmonary branch for wedge pressure measurement. (C) Pulmonary artery pressure tracing.

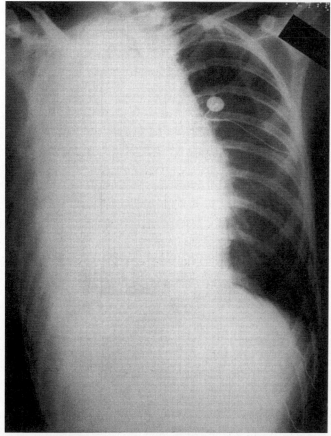

Fig. 15.39 Right hydrothorax caused by displacement of a central venous line during dressing change; 1300 mL of intravenous fluids were evacuated via thoracentesis. (From Moore DE. ET, CV, VAD, PA, Swan: what's it all about? *Semin Radiol Technol.* 1997;5:49.)

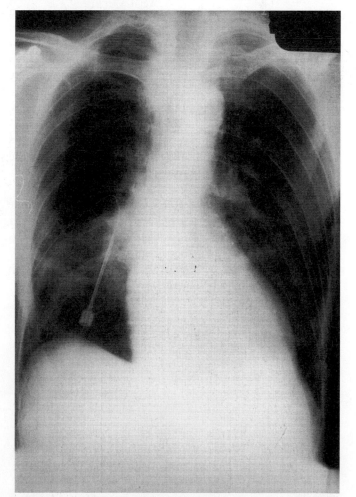

Fig. 15.40 Pneumothorax on the right resulting from complications associated with central venous line insertion. Note the small angiographic catheter inserted to evacuate the pleural cavity and the oxygen tube across the lower field, creating an artifactual distraction. (From Moore DE. ET, CV, VAD, PA, Swan: what's it all about? *Semin Radiol Technol.* 1997;5:49.)

techniques for patient care become more sophisticated, and as the team concept of health care management takes greater hold, practicing radiographers must direct attention to expanded learning opportunities to maintain clinical competency. In this regard, radiography remains a vital component of health care, and improved patient care will result.

SUMMARY

- Vital signs represent the primary mechanisms that maintain homeostasis. These mechanisms can adapt to changes inside or outside of the body to maintain homeostasis. Therefore the vital functions provide a relative constancy in the internal environment of the body to promote healthy survival. Assessment of vital signs is an objective, noninvasive evaluation of the patient's immediate condition or response to therapy. Every health care professional should be competent in obtaining vital signs and understanding the significance of any abnormalities. Because the primary mechanisms that maintain homeostasis are represented by vital signs, accuracy in obtaining and recording the data is crucial. The need for oxygen becomes critical to patients when the internal environment of the body is not consistent. Normally, room air gases containing 21% oxygen are sufficient to maintain homeostasis; however, when vital signs are abnormal, supplemental oxygen therapy is necessary. Supplemental oxygen therapy relieves the increased stress on the cardiopulmonary system.
- Oxygen therapy can be administered by high-flow devices, such as air-entrainment masks, which deliver consistent concentrations of oxygen and supply entire inspiratory volumes as required by the patient. Low-flow devices, such as nasal cannulas, simple masks, aerosol masks, and partial rebreathing and nonrebreathing masks, can also deliver oxygen therapy. Because of the variance of the patient's respiratory rate or change in breathing pattern, these devices provide neither consistent concentrations of oxygen nor the entire inspiratory volumes required by the patient.
- Oxygen tents and oxyhoods are used to deliver oxygen to children requiring supplemental oxygen or humidity.

- Patients on ventilators require special care in handling, and the radiographic technologist must never alter ventilator alarms and settings.
- Radiographers must understand the use and radiographic appearance of common tubes and lines used in the thorax, including endotracheal tubes, thoracostomy tubes, and CV lines.

BIBLIOGRAPHY

Bard Access Systems: *Vascular Access Devices*, Salt Lake City, Utah. Available at: https://www.bardaccess.com/index.php. Accessed December 7, 2017.

Cairo JM, Pilbeam SP: *Mosby's Respiratory Care Equipment*, ed 8, St. Louis, 2010, Elsevier.

Exergen Corp Medical Division, Medical Education Center: *Technology, temporal artery thermometry*. Available at: http://www.exergen.com/medical/eductr/technology.htm. Accessed December 7, 2017.

Exergen Corp Medical Division, Medical Products: *Derma Temp Infrared Surface Skin Scanners*. Available at: http://www.exergen.com//medical/product/DermaTemp.html. Accessed December 7, 2017.

Foto J, Brasseaux D, Birke JA, et al.: Essential features of a handheld infrared thermometer used to guide the treatment of neuropathic feet, *J Am Podiatr Med Assoc* 97:360, 2007.

Jardins Des TR: *Cardiopulmonary Anatomy and Physiology: Essentials of Respiratory Care*, ed 6, Albany, NY, 2012, Thomson Delmar Learning.

Kacmarek R, Stoller J, Heuer A: *Egan's Fundamentals of Respiratory Care*, ed 11, Philadelphia, 2017, Elsevier.

Kozier B, Erb G, Berman A, et al.: *Fundamentals of Nursing*, ed 10, Upper Saddle River, NJ, 2016, Pearson Education.

LifeART: *CD-ROM Collections*, Cleveland, Ohio, 1994, TechPool Studios.

Longo D, Fauci A, Kasper D, et al.: *Harrison's Principles of Internal Medicine*, ed 19, New York, 2015, McGraw-Hill.

Morgan Jr GE, Mikhail MS, Murray MJ: Patient monitors. In Morgan Jr GE, Mikhail MS, Murray MJ, editors: *Clinical anesthesiology*, ed 5, New York, 2013, Lange.

Sapna P: *Vascular Access, Central Catheter, Tunneled*, 2013. Available at: http://emedicine.medscape.com/article/1375734-overview. Accessed December 7, 2017.

Wilkins R, Dexter A, Heuer A: *Clinical Assessment in Respiratory Care*, ed 6, Philadelphia, 2010, Mosby.

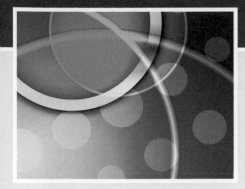

Basic Cardiac Monitoring: The Electrocardiogram

Julie Gill, PhD, RT(R)(QM)

> *In this current turmoil of the world, we are expected to use our resources. Because our two main resources are people and things, we must clarify the value of using people and loving things, versus using things and loving people.*
>
> **Bishop Ernest A. Fitzgerald**

OBJECTIVES

On completion of this chapter, the student will be able to:

- Describe the structural and physiologic mechanisms involved in a complete cardiac cycle.
- Explain the ordered sequence of events in a normal cardiac neural conduction process.
- Discuss the significance of electrical membrane potentials as they function in depolarization, repolarization, and the action potential sequence.
- Describe the electroconduction system of the heart in correlation with normal and abnormal electrocardiographic findings.
- List the steps useful in the analysis of an electrocardiographic tracing.
- Differentiate common arrhythmias and the cardiac structures involved.
- Recognize common treatments associated with cardiac arrhythmias.

OUTLINE

KEYTERMS

Action Potential Processes of depolarization and repolarization of the cardiac membrane.

Arrhythmia Irregularity of cardiac actions associated with physiologic or pathologic interruption of the neuroconductive tissues of the heart (also synonymous with dysrhythmia).

Asystole There is no evidence of any cardiac neuroconductive activity (full cardiac arrest).

Automaticity Process whereby cardiac cell membranes spontaneously depolarize at recurrent periods.

Bradycardia Slowness of the heartbeat, as evidenced by slowing of the pulse rate to less than 60 beats/min.

Cardiac cycle Events that occur from the beginning of one ventricular contraction (systole) until the beginning of another.

Cardiac Output Amount of blood ejected from the ventricles each minute; calculated as the product of stroke volume times heart rate.

Depolarization Myocardial cells are stimulated to contract.

Fibrillation Quivering contraction of cardiac muscle fibers.

Repolarization Myocardial muscle cells relax.

Tachycardia Heart rate above 100 beats/min.

BASIC CARDIAC MONITORING: THE ELECTROCARDIOGRAM

Cardiac output is the product of heart rate and stroke volume and is the vital event necessary to maintain blood flow throughout the cardiovascular system. To accomplish adequate cardiac output, there must be adequate blood volume and a regular cycle of muscular relaxation and contraction. Assessment of the heart's ability to perform its vital function is possible using a device called an electrocardiograph, which produces an electrocardiogram (EKG or ECG). Historically, EKG was the abbreviated term commonly used to describe the electrocardiogram, based on the Greek term *kardia* for heart; however, based on English versions of medical terminology, the word *cardia* is used to refer to the heart. Today, both abbreviations (EKG and ECG) are used synonymously. For the purposes of this text, ECG is used.

PRINCIPLES OF CARDIAC FUNCTION

Although the heart is a complex organ, its purpose is simple: to pump blood through vessels to vital organs and tissues. Through the pumping of blood through the vascular system, a pressure (systolic blood pressure) is created that can easily be assessed using a stethoscope and sphygmomanometer. Systolic pressures greater than 90 mm Hg generally ensure adequate perfusion of tissues. For systolic pressure to be sustained, the sequence of cardiac events must remain normal. This sequence of events is known as the *cardiac cycle.*

In practice, the term cardiac cycle refers to events that occur from the beginning of one ventricular contraction (systole) until the beginning of another. The ventricles fill with blood during rest (diastole) and eject blood into the pulmonary artery and aorta during systole; however, a cardiac cycle includes many complex events that specifically occur to maintain normal cardiac output.

Classic events required for a normal cardiac cycle are the rhythmic contraction and relaxation of the chambers of the heart, the atria, and the ventricles. The heart is composed of two principal cell types, working cardiac cells, and specialized neural conductive cells. Working cells are the cardiac muscle or myocardium of the atria and ventricles. Specialized cells include the sinoatrial (SA) node, atrioventricular (AV) node, bundle of His, and Purkinje fibers (Fig. 16.1). These cells originate in and transmit electrical impulses across the myocardium and regulate the rhythm of a cardiac cycle.

To initiate the neural conduction process throughout the myocardium, the specialized neural cells possess the ability to spontaneously originate electrical impulses. This action is independent of any nerves or hormones; however, actual firing rates can be influenced by the autonomic nervous system. The autonomic nerves include sympathetic and parasympathetic fibers. Sympathetic nerves can increase activity or rate of cardiac impulses, whereas parasympathetic nerves slow their rate. Each cardiac cycle begins with a spontaneous neural impulse generated by the SA node. Subsequently this impulse spreads throughout the remainder of the cardiac neural conductive tissues, stimulating the muscle (myocardial) cells to contract. Abnormalities within the neural conduction system will adversely affect cardiac output. These abnormalities are called arrhythmias or *dysrhythmias;* the terms are used synonymously.

ELECTRICAL MEMBRANE POTENTIALS

To comprehend the electrical impulses and the information provided by an ECG, one must understand the basic concepts regarding electrical membrane potentials. All cell membranes are positively charged on their outer surface owing to the relative distribution of cations. This resting membrane potential is maintained by an active transport mechanism called the *sodium-potassium ion pump.* When the cell is stimulated, movement of ions in and out of the membrane alters its charge, reversing the resting potential. This period is referred to as depolarization. When depolarization occurs, myocardial cells are stimulated to contract. The depolarization period is short. Reversal of ion flow reestablishes a positive charge to the outside of the membrane, a process called repolarization, which returns the membrane to its resting potential. During repolarization, myocardial muscle cells relax. The processes of depolarization and repolarization are collectively referred to as an action potential. This event perpetuates itself as an "impulse" along the entire surface of a cell and from one cell to another, provided cell membranes are connected to one another. The following steps summarize the action potential sequence:

1. The resting cell membrane is charged positively on the outside and negatively on the inside.
2. After stimulation, positive ions enter the cell, reversing this polarity.
3. This process continues until the entire cell membrane is depolarized.
4. Ions return to their normal location, and the cell repolarizes to its normal resting potential.

Unique to the tissue of the cardiac neural conduction system is a process called automaticity, which allows cell membranes to spontaneously depolarize at recurrent periods. Another unique feature of this specialized tissue is that cell membranes are in direct contact with cardiac muscle, and their action potential directly initiates depolarization of the cardiac muscle cells. Cardiac muscle cells are fused to one another, which allows the cells to function as a continuous sheet of cells (a syncytium). The sheet of cells of the atria is separated from that of the ventricles by a layer of connective tissue that acts as an insulator. The SA node initiates depolarization of the atrial muscle, but the insulation prevents transmission into the ventricles. The AV node delays and finally relays the impulse along the common bundle of His, which penetrates the connective tissue to enter the ventricles. The impulse continues along the common bundle of His and its branches until it finally reaches the Purkinje fibers, stimulating the ventricular muscular sheet.

Action potentials that spread throughout the muscle sheets of the heart may be detected by surface electrodes to record and produce a tracing known as an electrocardiogram. What is observed in an ECG tracing is the action potentials of the atrial and ventricular muscle cells. However, other events can be deduced from the tracing.

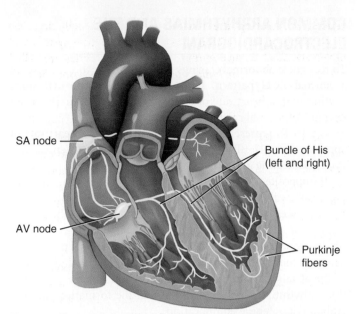

Fig. 16.1 Electroconduction tissues of the heart. *AV*, Atrioventricular; *SA*, sinoatrial.

ELECTROCARDIOGRAPHIC TRACING

The electrical sequence of a cardiac cycle is initiated by the SA node, known as the *pacemaker* of the heart. This is because the SA node has a faster rate of spontaneous firing than the remaining specialized tissues (see Fig. 16.1).

The baseline of an ECG is called the isoelectric line and signifies resting membrane potentials. Deflections are the positive or negative changes in the tracing relative to the isocenter over the time of the cycle. These deflections are lettered in alphabetic order, and after each the tracing normally returns to the isoelectric point.

P wave. The first deflection, the P wave, represents depolarization of atrial muscle cells. It does not represent contraction of this muscle, nor does it represent firing of the SA node. These events are deduced, based on the shape and consistency of the P waves. The assumption is that the SA node fires at the start of the P wave and atrial contraction begins at the peak of the P wave. Although atrial repolarization follows depolarization, the ECG provides no evidence of this event because atrial repolarization is too minor in amplitude to be recorded by surface electrodes.

QRS complex, T, and U waves. The QRS complex represents depolarization of ventricular muscle cells. The Q portion is the initial downward deflection, the R portion is the initial upward deflection, and the S portion is the return to the baseline (isoelectric point). Often the Q portion is not evident, and the depolarization manifests as only an RS complex. In any case the complex does not represent ventricular contraction. The assumption is that contraction will commence at the peak of the R portion of the complex. After depolarization, ventricular muscle repolarizes, and this event is significant enough in amplitude to generate the T wave on the ECG tracing. Although not always seen, the U wave is typically small and, when evident, follows the T wave. The U wave is theorized to represent repolarization of the papillary muscles and Purkinje fibers.

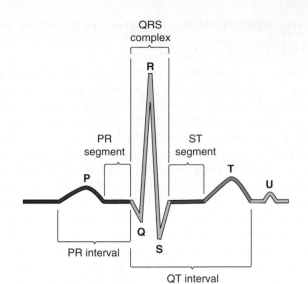

Fig. 16.2 A typical electrocardiographic tracing with labeled waves.

PR interval. The PR interval is measured from the beginning of the P wave to the beginning of the R portion of the QRS complex. (This is conventional practice because the Q portion of the complex is so frequently indiscernible.) Because the PR interval commences with atrial muscle depolarization and ends with the start of ventricular depolarization, it can be assumed that the electrical impulse passes through the AV node into the ventricle during this interval. If the PR interval is prolonged, it can be deduced that AV block is present.

The electrical events of an ECG are illustrated and summarized in Fig. 16.2.

SUMMARY OF EVENTS OF A CARDIAC CYCLE

Of the following eight physiologic events listed for a cardiac cycle, only three are actually observed on an ECG tracing.

1. SA node initiates impulse (fires 60 to 80 times per minute): not visible on ECG tracing
2. Depolarization of atrial muscle: P wave
3. Atrial contraction: not visible on ECG tracing
4. Depolarization of AV node (fires 60 to 80 times per minute) and common bundle: not visible on ECG tracing
5. Repolarization of atrial muscle: not visible on ECG tracing
6. Depolarization of ventricular muscle: QRS complex
7. Contraction of ventricular muscle: not visible on ECG tracing
8. Repolarization of ventricular muscle: T wave

ANALYSIS OF THE ELECTROCARDIOGRAM

How one chooses to analyze an ECG rhythm strip is arbitrary. Each clinician must adopt a sequence of analysis that accommodates personal methods of reasoning. Always keep in mind that events during the PR interval pertain to supraventricular activity. When abnormalities are detected, try to establish the event as either ventricular or supraventricular in origin. The following sequence represents one suggestion for analysis of an

ECG tracing, described for convenience as a five-step analysis. Refer to Fig. 16.3 during the following explanation.

Step 1: Is the rhythm regular or irregular?

If the intervals between QRS complexes (RR intervals) are consistent, ventricular rhythm is regular. In Fig. 16.3, note the four large labeled time boxes and note that the recurrence of the QRS complexes is consistent. If intervals between P waves (PP intervals) are consistent, the atrial rhythm is regular. In Fig. 16.3 the rhythm is regular.

Step 2: Are all QRS complexes similar, and are they narrow?

The duration of the QRS complex should not exceed 0.12 seconds (three small squares). A widened complex indicates ventricular enlargement (hypertrophy) or that ventricular depolarization is being initiated by pacemaker tissue below the AV node—for example, ventricular-paced rhythm. In this example, one ventricle depolarizes first and the current must spread into the second ventricle. This takes more time than when the current spreads down the bundle of His into both ventricles simultaneously. If QRS complexes are narrow, the rhythm is being initiated by a pacemaker at the AV node or higher and is described as a *supraventricular rhythm*. If the complexes are wide, the pacemaker is in the ventricles and is described as a *ventricular rhythm*. Should complexes vary in appearance, more than one pacemaker is generating impulses. This is referred to as *ectopic pacemakers,* and the rhythm is described as *ectopy.*

Step 3: Are all P waves similar, and are PR intervals normal?

If P waves are all similar, and normal in shape, one can assume that the SA node is the primary pacemaker. In this case the rhythm is sinus. If P waves vary in shape or are absent, other tissue(s) are functioning as pacers.

The PR interval is normally 0.12 to 0.20 seconds (three to five small squares). Longer intervals indicate that the impulse is being delayed from entering the ventricles, and the condition is designated *AV block*.

Step 4: Is the rate normal?

Provided rhythm is regular, count the number of large squares between QRS complexes and divide this number into 300. However, if the rhythm is irregular, count the number of QRS complexes in a 6-second segment and multiply by 10. Rates below 60 indicate bradycardia; those above 100 indicate tachycardia. In Fig. 16.3 there are approximately four large boxes between QRS complexes, so the rate is approximately 75 beats/min (BPM).

Step 5: Do waves and complexes proceed in normal sequence?

Each P wave should be followed by a QRS complex, which is followed by a T wave. This ensures a normal sequence for each cardiac cycle.

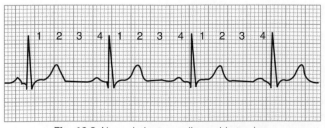

Fig. 16.3 Normal electrocardiographic tracing.

COMMON ARRHYTHMIAS AND THE ELECTROCARDIOGRAM

To recognize abnormal tracings, it is important to first observe a normal ECG pattern. Fig.16.4A represents normal sinus rhythm with a heart rate of approximately 79 BPM. This is an example of normal cardiac neural conduction.

Fig. 16.4B represents sinus bradycardia with a heart rate of approximately 47 BPM. Note the wide space between cardiac cycles, indicating a slow heart rate.

The opposite of sinus bradycardia is sinus tachycardia, as seen in Fig. 16.4C, with an estimated heart rate of 140 BPM. Note that the space between cardiac cycles is narrow, indicating a fast heart rate.

One of the most common cardiac arrhythmias is atrial **fibrillation,** as seen in Fig. 16.4D. Additional ectopic pacemaker firings in the atria exceed those of the SA node, creating a quiver of the atria syncytium instead of a full contraction. Although this arrhythmia is not life-threatening, the formation of atrial emboli is a potential complication.

Most cycles contain narrow QRS complexes, but occasionally a wide QRS complex may appear interposed between cardiac cycles. Occasionally an extra impulse is fired from within the ventricle and creates a wide QRS complex. These complexes are called *premature ventricular contractions* (PVCs). Fig. 16.4E shows normal sinus rhythm with PVCs.

Ventricular tachycardia ("V-tach"), seen in Fig. 16.4F, involves an abnormally high heart rate that exceeds 100 BPM and can be as high as 240 BPM. Ventricular tachycardia is a heart rhythm that abnormally originates in the ventricles; when the event lasts for a prolonged period of time (>30 seconds), it is called *sustained V-tach* and requires treatment. In some cases this abnormal heart rhythm can lead to ventricular fibrillation, as seen in the next illustration.

Ventricular fibrillation ("V-fib") is a serious arrhythmia that is life-threatening (Fig. 16.4G). Instead of competent myocardial contraction, the muscle fibers twitch or quiver. As a result, little to no blood is pumped and cardiac output is virtually zero. This is a case of cardiac arrest, and unless it is reversed, death will occur.

Fig. 16.4H is an example of **asystole** (straight-line tracing). There is no evidence of any neuroconductive activity. The patient is in full cardiac arrest, and, as in the case of fibrillation, unless this condition is resolved, death is imminent.

COMMON TREATMENTS OF CARDIAC ARRHYTHMIA

Cardiac arrhythmia is caused by abnormalities of the heart that negatively interfere with its neural conduction system and consequently affect cardiac output. Arrhythmias are typically classified by the origin of the abnormality (atrial or ventricular) or are classed by the speed of the resulting heart rate. Tachycardias may involve the atria or ventricles, whereas bradycardia typically involves either SA or AV node abnormalities.

Depending on the cause and the severity of the arrhythmia, treatment may be as simple as administering antiarrhythmic medications, but it may also require more physical and invasive forms of therapy, including cardiac surgery.

Cardioversion therapy is useful for treating atrial-related causes of arrhythmias, including atrial fibrillation. It involves external shock therapy to the chest to restore normal cardiac rhythm. In severe cases of ventricular tachycardia or fibrillation, electric shock defibrillation therapy is administered.

Ablation therapies involve either heating or freezing tissues within a chamber of the heart that is considered to be the cause of the arrhythmia. Catheters are advanced through the vascular system into the involved chamber of the heart. Most frequently, radiofrequency ablation (RFA) is performed. RFA involves the use of electrodes at the tip of catheter wires; these are heated with radiofrequency energy (high-frequency AC current). Whether heating or freezing, the involved tissue is ablated and the arrhythmia is resolved.

Arrhythmias may also be treated with an implantable device such as a cardiac pacemaker or an implantable cardioverter-defibrillator (ICD). A pacemaker is used most often to treat bradycardia. It consists of a small battery-powered generator to which one to three wires tipped with electrodes are attached. The battery

and generator are implanted in a subcutaneous pocket near the clavicular region of the thorax. The wires are inserted and advanced through veins leading into the right cardiac chambers of the heart. In a single-wire unit, the electrode is placed in the right ventricle. In a dual-wired unit, the electrodes are positioned in the right atrium and right ventricle. In a three-wired pacemaker, wires are positioned with electrodes in the right atrium and right and left ventricles. The battery and generator stimulate myocardial pacing of the heart.

ICDs are typically used to treat tachycardia and irregular cardiac contraction disorders involving the ventricles of the heart, although ICDs treat bradycardia as well. Similarly to the pacemaker, the battery and generator are implanted in a subcutaneous pocket near the clavicle. Wires with electrodes are inserted and positioned in the ventricles of the heart, and the ICD monitors cardiac rhythm. In a case of bradycardia, the ICD sends a signal to pace the heart at normal rates. In cases of ventricular tachycardia or fibrillation, the ICD send shocks to reset normal pacing. Fig. 16.5 demonstrates both an ICD *(A)* and a dual chamber pacemaker *(B)*.

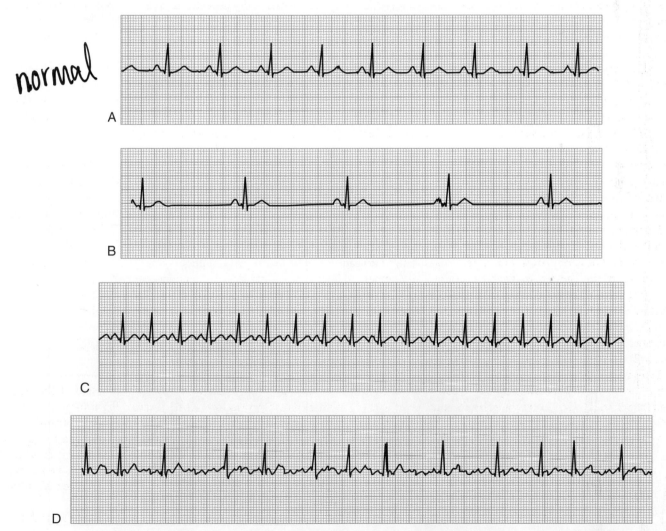

normal

Fig. 16.4 (A) Normal electrocardiogram pattern. (B) Sinus bradycardia. (C) Sinus tachycardia. (D) Atrial fibrillation. (E) Normal sinus rhythm with premature ventricular contractions. (F) Ventricular tachycardia. (G) Ventricular fibrillation. (H) Asystole.

Continued

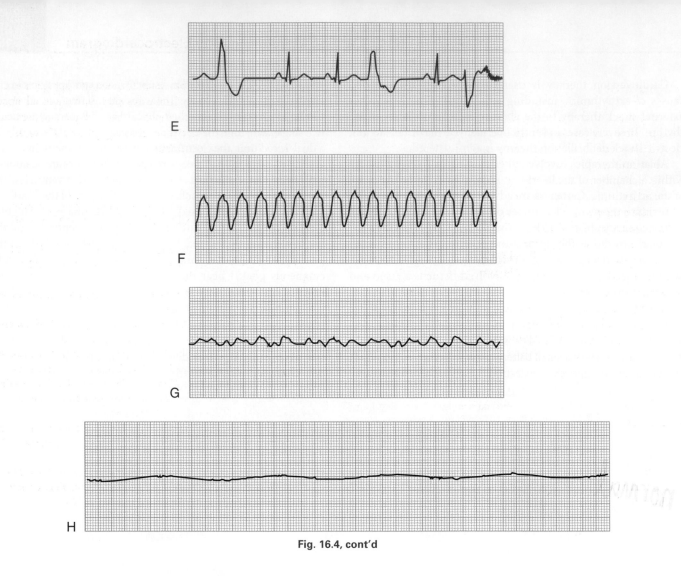

E

F

G

H

Fig. 16.4, cont'd

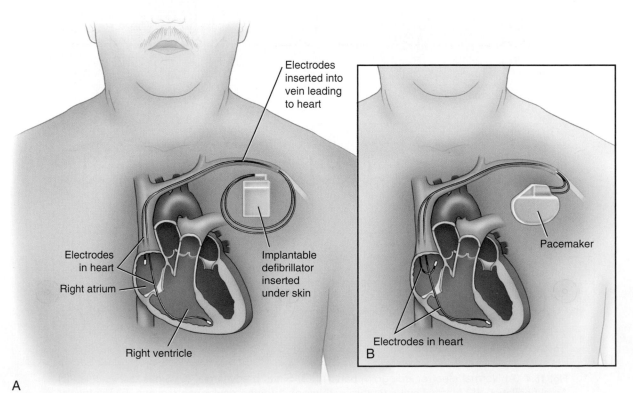

Electrodes
inserted into
vein leading
to heart

Electrodes
in heart

Right atrium

Right ventricle

Implantable
defibrillator
inserted
under skin

Pacemaker

Electrodes in heart

A

B

Fig. 16.5 Implantable defibrillator device with electrodes in place (A); implanted cardiac pacemaker with electrodes in place (B). (Courtesy National Institute of Health National Heart Lung and Blood Institute.)

SUMMARY

- Assessment of the heart's ability to perform its vital function is possible using a device called an *electrocardiograph*. Systolic and diastolic actions of the heart pump blood through the heart and out to the lungs and body. Specialized neural cells possess the ability to spontaneously originate and transmit electrical impulses across myocardial cell sheets that generate cardiac muscle contraction. The SA node initiates spontaneous neural impulses across atrial muscle. The AV node relays the impulse along the bundle of His, which penetrates to enter the ventricles. The impulse continues along the bundle of His and its branches until it finally reaches the Purkinje fibers, stimulating the ventricular muscular sheet. Action potentials that spread throughout the muscle sheets of the heart may be detected by electrodes to record and produce a tracing known as an *electrocardiogram*.

- The ECG tracing consists of a P wave, representing depolarization of the atria; the QRS complex, representing depolarization of the ventricles; a T wave, representing repolarization of the ventricles; and—sometimes visible—a U wave, believed to represent repolarization of the papillary muscles and Purkinje fibers. Various abnormalities involving the electrical system of the heart can be detected through the ECG. These abnormalities are referred to as *arrhythmias* or *dysrhythmias*.

- Abnormalities of the heart that interfere with its neural conduction system cause cardiac arrhythmias. Treatments of arrhythmia are varied based on the severity and location of the disorder. Antiarrhythmic drug therapy, external shock therapy, and implanted devices such as pacemakers and ICDs have proved effective in the management of a variety of cardiac rhythm abnormalities.

BIBLIOGRAPHY

Des Jardin TR: *Cardiopulmonary anatomy and physiology: essentials of respiratory care,* ed 6, Clifton Park, NY, 2013, Delmar Cengage.

Ganong WF: Dynamics of Blood and Lymph Flow. In Ganong WF, editor: *Review of medical physiology,* ed 24, New York, 2012, McGraw-Hill.

Goldberger AL: *Clinical electrocardiography: a simplified approach,* ed 8, Philadelphia, 2013, Elsevier.

Guyton AC, Hall JE: *Textbook of medical physiology,* ed 13, Philadelphia, 2016, Elsevier.

Holmes Jr DR: Cardiogenic Shock. In Goldman L, Ausiello D, editors: *Cecil textbook of medicine,* ed 23, Philadelphia, 2008, Saunders.

LifeART: *CD-ROM Collections,* Cleveland, Ohio, 1994, TechPool Studios.

Longo D, Fauci A, Kasper D, et al.: *Harrison's principles of internal medicine,* ed 19, New York, 2015, McGraw-Hill.

Morgan Jr GE, Mikhail MS, Murray Jr MJ: Patient Monitors. In Morgan GE, Mikhail MS, Murray MJ, editors: *Clinical anesthesiology,* ed 5, New York, 2013, Lange.

U.S. Department of Health & Human Services: Implantable cardioverter defibrillator. Available at: http://www.nhlbi.nih.gov/health/health-topics/topics/icd/. Accessed December 7, 2017.

Infection Control

Kristi Moore, PhD, RT(R)(CT)

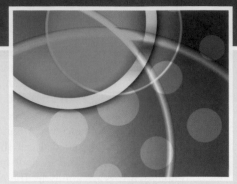

What man does not avoid contact with the sick, fearing lest he contract a disease so near?

Ovid, 43 BC–17 AD

OBJECTIVES

On completion of this chapter, the student will be able to:
- Define the terminology related to infection control
- Categorize the four basic infectious agents along with their unique characteristics
- Explain the steps involved in the establishment of an infectious disease
- Discuss the four factors involved in the spread of disease and the chain of infection
- Describe the various sources of health care–associated infection
- Explain the constituents of microbial control within the host
- Contrast medical and surgical asepsis
- List the chemical and physical methods of asepsis
- Demonstrate the medically aseptic hand-washing technique
- Describe the basic premises of standard precautions
- Relate types of transmission-based precautions with appropriate clinical situations
- Demonstrate the contact precautions technique

OUTLINE

KEY TERMS

Asepsis Freedom from infection

Bacteria Prokaryotic, ubiquitous single-celled organisms

Bloodborne Pathogens Disease-causing microorganisms that may be present in human blood

Chemotherapy Treatment of disease by chemical agents

Cyst Stage in the life cycle of certain parasites during which they are enclosed in a protective wall

Dimorphic Occurring in two distinct forms

Diseases Deviations from or interruptions of the normal structure or function of any part, organ, or

system (or combination thereof) of the body that are exhibited by a characteristic set of symptoms and signs and whose cause, pathologic mechanism, and prognosis may be known or unknown

Disinfectants Chemicals used to free an environment from pathogenic organisms or to render such organisms inert, especially as applied to the treatment of inanimate materials to reduce or eliminate infectious organisms

Eukaryotes Organisms whose cells have a true nucleus

Flora Microbial community found on or in a healthy person

Fomite An object such as a book, wooden object, or article of clothing that is not in itself harmful but is able to harbor pathogenic microorganisms and thus may serve as an agent of transmission of an infection

Fungi General term used to denote a group of eukaryotic protists—including mushrooms, yeasts, rusts, molds, and smuts—that are characterized by the absence of chlorophyll and by the presence of a rigid cell wall

Health Care–Associated Infection (HAI) Infection that patients acquire while they are receiving treatment for another health care issue

Host An animal or plant that harbors or nourishes another organism

Iatrogenic Resulting from the activities of physicians

Immunity Security against a particular disease

Infection Invasion and multiplication of microorganisms in body tissues that may be clinically inapparent or may result in local cellular injury as a result of competitive metabolism,

toxins, intracellular replication, or antigen–antibody response

Medical Asepsis Reduction in numbers of infectious agents, which, in turn, decreases the probability of infection but does not necessarily reduce it to zero

Microorganisms Microscopic organisms—those of medical interest including bacteria, viruses, fungi, and protozoa

Nosocomial Pertaining to or originating in the hospital; said of an infection not present or incubating before admittance to the hospital but generally developing 72 hours after admittance

Pathogens Disease-producing microorganisms

Prokaryotes Cellular organisms that lack a true nucleus

Protozoa A subkingdom comprising the simplest organisms of the animal kingdom, consisting of unicellular organisms ranging in size from submicroscopic to macroscopic; most being free-living but some having commensalistic, mutualistic, or parasitic existences

Reservoir Alternative or passive host or carrier that harbors pathogenic organisms, without injury to itself, and serves as a source from which other individuals can be infected

Standard Precautions Precautions to prevent the transmission of disease by body fluids and substances

Sterilization Complete destruction or elimination of all living microorganisms accomplished by physical methods (dry or moist heat), chemical agents (ethylene oxide, formaldehyde, alcohol), radiation (ultraviolet, cathode), or mechanical methods (filtration)

Surgical Asepsis Procedure used to prevent contamination by microbes and endospores before, during, or after surgery using sterile technique *eliminate*

Vaccine Suspension of attenuated or killed microorganisms (bacteria, viruses, or rickettsiae) administered for the prevention, improvement, or treatment of infectious disease

Vector A carrier, especially an animal (usually an arthropod), that transfers an infective agent from one host to another *misquito*

Virion Complete viral particle found extracellularly and capable of surviving in crystalline form and infecting a living cell; comprises the nucleoid (genetic material) and the capsid; also called a viral particle

Viruses Any of a group of minute infectious agents not resolved in the light microscope, with certain exceptions (e.g., poxvirus), and characterized by a lack of independent metabolism as well as the ability to replicate only within living host cells

MICROBIAL WORLD

Well over 300 years have passed since Anton van Leeuwenhoek first observed what he called *wee animalcules* under his crude microscope. At the time, he reported his findings to the Royal Society of London; the fact that these tiny creatures, known as *microbes,* could be anything more than a mere curiosity was beyond anyone's imagination.

At the beginning of the twentieth century, the major causes of death in the United States were microbial infectious diseases. These **diseases** included pneumonia, tuberculosis, gastroenteritis, and diphtheria. Although today most microbial infections are under control, microbes still present a major threat to survival for the immunosuppressed person. Furthermore, microbial disease in less developed countries still constitutes the

major causes of death. Millions of people still die annually of illnesses such as malaria, cholera, and dysentery.

The last century saw an explosion in knowledge of the sciences. The tiny amusing creatures of Leeuwenhoek's time have proved to be literally a matter of life or death. Microbes are essential to life through their ability to recycle organic and inorganic matter and are devastating through their ability to produce disease. Most important, by studying these microbes at the molecular level, scientists have learned to identify them and determine their capabilities. Through use of this knowledge, many microbial functions can be controlled, making them beneficial or preventing potential harm.

The health care practitioner must have an understanding of what infectious diseases are, how they are spread, and how they are controlled. Health care providers have been granted responsibility not only to the patients entrusted to their care but also to the entire public sector.

Many microorganisms can grow in or on a host organism and cause disease. These diseases are known as *infections*. Infection refers to the establishment and growth of a microorganism on or in a host. Only when the infection results in injury to the host is the host said to have a disease. Pathogenic microorganisms cause *infectious diseases*. Most often, pathogens have the ability to do one of three functions extremely well: (1) they can multiply in large numbers and cause an obstruction, (2) they can cause tissue damage, and (3) they can secrete organic substances called *exotoxins*. These exotoxins can produce certain side effects, such as an extremely high body temperature, nausea, vomiting, or shock. Pathogens are divided into four basic infectious agents: bacteria, viruses, fungi, and protozoan parasites.

Bacteria

Bacteria are microscopic single-celled organisms with a simple internal organization (Fig. 17.1). Bacteria are prokaryotic rather than eukaryotic organisms. Prokaryotes lack a nucleus and membrane-bound organelles, whereas eukaryotes have a true nucleus. Most of the cellular metabolic activities take place on the cytoplasmic membrane. Prokaryotes do not have the capacity to ingest particulates or liquid droplets. Although bacteria are single-celled, they may reside in the host in a group or cluster called a *colony*.

Bacteria are identified and classified according to their morphology, biochemistry, and genetic constitution. Morphology is considered a major criterion for classification. *Morphology* is the size or shape of the bacterium and is routinely determined by a simple staining technique called *Gram staining*. The medically important bacteria are classified into three general morphologies: cocci or spheres, bacilli or rods, and spirals.

Some bacteria have the ability to produce a highly resistant resting form known as an *endospore*. This structure is internal, as reflected in its name. Endospores are metabolically

dormant structures that are highly resistant to the external environment. Spores possess extreme resistance to chemical and physical agents. They can remain viable for many years and then germinate in response to specific requirements. The endospore is a survival form of the bacterium that is most often produced in response to nutritional deprivation. Of all the bacteria able to produce endospores, only two genera, *Bacillus* and *Clostridium,* are of medical importance. Among the common bacterial infections encountered today are streptococcal pharyngitis ("strep throat"), *Klebsiella pneumoniae* infection (bacterial pneumonia), and *Clostridium botulinum* infection (food poisoning).

Viruses

Viruses are much simpler in form than bacteria or animal cells (Fig. 17.2). Viruses are neither prokaryotic nor eukaryotic; they are considered obligate intracellular parasites. Viruses cannot live outside a living cell. They lack the components necessary for their own survival because of their inability to synthesize specific required proteins. Viruses depend on the host cell to provide these missing factors. A virus carries its own genetic information in the form of deoxyribonucleic acid (DNA) or ribonucleic acid (RNA), but never both. A protein coat called a *capsid* surrounds the viral DNA or RNA.

Viruses are generally characterized by the chemical nature of their nucleic acid, their size, and their symmetry. Nucleic acids within a virus are, as stated earlier, either DNA or RNA, but these nucleic acids may be double or single, positively or negatively stranded. Nucleic acids of differing viruses also possess varying weights. The size of a virus may vary from 20 to 250 nm. A *nanometer* is equal to 10^{-9} m; therefore direct observation of a virus is possible only through an electron microscope.

Viral infection is the result of a viral particle, also called a virion, which attaches to a host cell and inserts its genome or genetic information into the host. The viral genome then redirects the host cell. The virus uses the organelles and metabolic functions of the host cell to produce new viruses. Once this process is completed, the new viral particles are released from the host cell, sometimes resulting in destruction of the cell. Some viruses have the ability to travel within the nervous

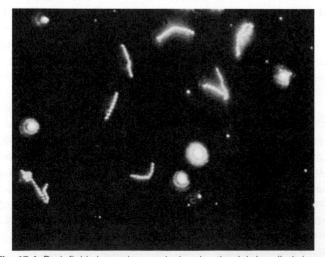

Fig. 17.1 Dark-field photomicrograph showing the tightly coiled characteristics of the spirochete *Treponema pallidum.* (From Forbes BA, Sahm DF, Weissfeld AS. Bailey and Scott's diagnostic microbiology. 12th ed. St Louis: Mosby; 2007.)

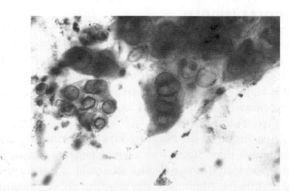

Fig. 17.2 Papanicolaou (Pap)-stained smear showing multinucleated giant cells typical of herpes simplex or varicella zoster viruses. (From Forbes BA, Sahm DF, Weissfeld AS. Bailey and Scott's diagnostic microbiology. 12th ed. St Louis: Mosby; 2007.)

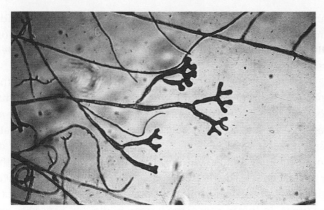

Fig. 17.3 Antler hyphae showing swollen hyphal tips resembling antlers, with lateral and terminal branching (favic chandeliers) (×500). (From Forbes BA, Sahm DF, Weissfeld AS. Bailey and Scott's diagnostic microbiology. 12th ed. St Louis: Mosby; 2007.)

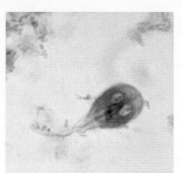

Fig. 17.4 *Giardia lamblia* trophozoite. (From Forbes BA, Sahm DF, Weissfeld AS. Bailey and Scott's diagnostic microbiology. 12th ed. St Louis: Mosby; 2007.)

system. They reappear sporadically and emerge at the nerve ending, causing various symptoms. They then leave the site and travel up the nerve again. This pattern can be repeated several times and is known as a *latent* or *dormant* infection. A cold sore caused by herpes simplex virus is an example of a latent viral infection. Common viral diseases in humans include the common cold (caused by the rhinovirus), infectious mononucleosis (caused by the Epstein-Barr virus), and warts (caused by the papillomavirus).

Fungi

Fungi (singular, *fungus*) can be macroscopic, as in the case of mushrooms and puffballs, or microscopic, such as yeasts and molds (Fig. 17.3). They are eukaryotic organisms with a nucleus and membrane-bound organelles. Fungi can be distinguished from bacteria by the fact that intracellular organelles can be visualized within the fungal cell. Fungal cells differ from animal cells in the type of sterol present in the cell membrane; the sterol present in animal cells is cholesterol. Fungi are also much larger than bacteria. Medically important pathogenic fungi are **dimorphic**—that is, they have the ability to grow in two distinct forms, either as a single-celled yeast or as filamentous hyphae. A filamentous hypha is better known as a *mold*. Whether the organism is present in either form depends on the growth conditions. Fungi are classified according to the type and method of sexual reproduction.

A photomicrograph of a typical mold would reveal a structure similar to that of a plant or small tree. The molds produce tiny branches that extend into the air. It is at these branches that spores are formed. These spores are called *conidia*; they are lightweight and resistant to drying, and they are easily dispersed to new habitats. Diseases caused by fungi can be of four different classifications. The first is a *superficial* infection, which usually causes discoloration of the skin. *Tinea nigra* is a fungal infection that results in a painless black or brown discoloration of the palmar surface of the hand and the plantar surface of the foot. Second are the *cutaneous* infections, which involve the keratinized tissues of the hair, nails, and skin. The most common clinical infection in this group is *tinea pedis,* or *athlete's foot.* The growth pattern of this fungus forms a ring

and is also known as *ringworm.* The third type is a *subcutaneous fungal* infection that enters the human host as a result of trauma to the skin. The fourth type is characterized by a *systemic* infection that enters the circulatory and lymphatic systems and may be fatal.

Protozoan Parasites

Protozoa are unicellular organisms that are neither plants nor animals (Fig. 17.4). They are distinguished from bacteria by their greater size and by the fact that they do not possess a cell wall. Protozoa are generally motile organisms and are eukaryotic. They are able to ingest food particles, and some species are equipped with rudimentary digestive systems.

Protozoa are classified according to their motility. The first group is classified by its slow cellular flowing, called *ameboid locomotion.* Few amebae are pathogenic. The motility of the second group is facilitated by a long *flagellum,* or protein tail. The third group moves by the action of numerous short protein tails called *cilia.* Sporozoans constitute the fourth group. This group is unique in that its members are nonmotile and, despite their name, do not form spores as do bacteria and fungi.

Some protozoa are able to form a **cyst,** which permits them to survive while they are not within a host. Cysts are resistant to chemical and physical changes.

Typical protozoan infections include *Trichomonas vaginalis* infection, a sexually transmitted disease that infects both male and female hosts, and *Plasmodium vivax* infection (malaria).

ESTABLISHMENT OF INFECTIOUS DISEASE

From the time the infectious agent comes in contact with the host until the devastation of a disease is apparent, several complicated processes must be completed. These can be categorized into the following six steps: (1) encounter, (2) entry, (3) spread, (4) multiplication, (5) damage, and (6) outcome (Fig. 17.5). Remember, all six steps require breaching of the host.

Encounter

The encounter involves the infectious organism coming in contact with the host. Each encounter varies according to the host and microorganism. Every individual and every microbe

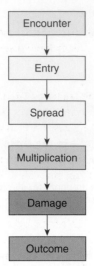

Fig. 17.5 The establishment of an infectious disease as a six-step process.

will respond differently. Some organisms can infect an unborn child, although this is difficult because the mother's womb is, microbially speaking, a sterile environment due to the selective passage allowed by the placenta. Still, some microorganisms are able to pass through the placenta to create what are called *congenital* infections. Examples of these infections are rubella and syphilis.

The initial encounter with infectious microorganisms takes place during the normal birthing process. The child comes in contact with the microbial world that is present in the mother's vaginal canal. Fortunately the newborn is born with antibodies obtained from the mother. These antibodies, plus those acquired through the mother's breast milk, provide the newborn with a sufficient immunologic base to cope with infection until its own immune system has matured.

During the entire human life span, the body comes in contact with new organisms; some are quickly eliminated and others are efficient colonizers. The colonizers either become part of the microbes normally found in the body or cause disease.

Entry

Much of the body is in contact with the external environment. The digestive, biliary, urinary, and respiratory systems are directly connected with the exterior. In women, the peritoneal cavity is also exposed via the fallopian tubes. An infectious microbe can gain entrance into the human body by either ingression or penetration.

Ingression does not involve deep-tissue penetration. Instead, these microorganisms adhere to the surface of the cell and excrete toxins that cause a distressed state within the system. Through the digestive system, infectious agents are ingested, most commonly through contaminated food or water. If the organism has the ability to survive the lower pH of the stomach and the small intestine, then it may become anchored on the colon and cause a diseased state. The most common example of a symptom caused by an ingressive organism is diarrhea. Ingression can also take place in the respiratory system. Inhalation of contaminated aerosols or

dust particles that are able to evade the powerful retrograde movement of the ciliary epithelium can lead to colonization within the lower respiratory tract. Pneumonia is contracted in this manner.

Penetration involves the microorganism invading past the epithelial barrier. This action can take place in various forms. Some microbes are equipped with a special apparatus, such as flagella. The bacteria that cause syphilis are able to penetrate using this mechanical device. Other microbes use vectors, as do mosquitoes or fleas, to penetrate into the tissue. Still others gain entry through tissue cuts and wounds. A *phagocyte*, which engulfs a foreign microbe, can transport it deeper into the tissue. In this instance, the human body itself is used to aid in penetration.

Spread

Spread, the propagation of the infectious organism, can take place before or after multiplication. In either case, the most important barrier for the microbe to overcome in this step is the host's immune defenses. Dissemination is dictated by the logistics of both the host and the microbe. In other words, the site of microbial entry, or the site where the microbe has taken up residence and the human anatomy at that site, determine the spread of the microbe. For example, the viruses that cause the common cold are easily spread as aerosols through coughing and sneezing.

Multiplication

The number of microbes that gain entrance into the host is usually much too small to cause the symptoms of a disease. Most infectious agents must first multiply for their impact to be recognized. The time frame applied to this phenomenon is termed the *incubation period,* and its parameters are defined from the time the host's defenses have been overcome until the time a substantial population has been achieved.

Damage

Virtually uncountable ways exist in which an infectious agent can cause damage to a host. Damage can be either direct or indirect. Cell death caused by destruction of the host cells or by toxins or poisons secreted by the infectious agent are examples of direct damage. The growth phase of a microbe is characterized by exponential growth; in a matter of hours, enough organisms may be present to cause complete obstruction of a major organ system.

Infectious microbes can also damage a host indirectly by altering the metabolism of the host. These infections are represented by some of the most life-threatening diseases. Once a person has ingested the toxins secreted by the organism that causes botulism, death can result in only a matter of hours.

A microbe can also induce host responses. Indirectly, the host's inflammatory and immune responses can cause further cell destruction than that already achieved by the microbe. This destruction is usually minimal compared with the overall devastation that an infectious agent can induce. The sacrificing of a few cells is justified when the integrity of the entire human body is at stake.

Outcome

An encounter with an infectious agent can result in one of three outcomes: (1) the host gains control of the infectious agent and eliminates it, (2) the infectious agent overcomes the host's immunities to cause disease, or (3) the host and the infectious agent compromise and live in a somewhat anxious state of symbiosis.

CHAIN OF INFECTION

In 1876, Robert Koch, a physician, introduced the germ theory of disease. Before this point the assumption had been that something was transmitted from an ill person to a well person. Up until the sixteenth century, evil spirits were a popular explanation for illness. In the sixteenth century, however, diseases were assumed to be spread by an unknown entity called a *contagion*, and the disease was said to be *contagious*, a term still in use today. Through scientific experimentation, Koch was able to prove that specific organisms caused specific diseases. He was able to prove that a precise series of events must occur for microorganisms from an infected person to be transmitted to an uninfected person. His postulates forever changed the relationship between microorganisms and humans.

According to the postulates of Koch, four factors are involved in the spread of diseases. Each factor is considered a link in the chain, and each link is connected to the next to form a ring. If at any point in the infection the chain is broken, the cycle cannot continue, and infection will cease. For infections to be transmitted, the following must exist: (1) a host, (2) an infectious microorganism, (3) a mode of transportation, and (4) a reservoir (Fig. 17.6).

Human Host

Humans provide a favorable **host** environment for the growth of many microbes because of the abundance of organic nutrients and metabolites found within the human body. Each region or organ of the body offers a different temperature, pH, or body fluid for microbial growth to occur. This diversity is optimal for the microbe with limited metabolic or aerobic requirements.

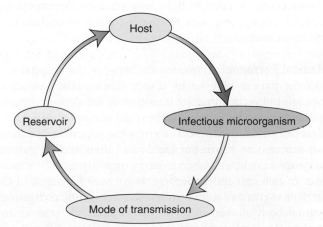

Fig. 17.6 The chain of infection. For infections to be transmitted there must be (1) a host, (2) an infectious microorganism, (3) a mode of transmission, and (4) a reservoir.

Infectious Microorganisms

Microorganisms include bacteria, viruses, fungi, and protozoa. These organisms have already been discussed.

Mode of Transmission

Microorganisms can be transmitted either *exogenously,* from outside the body, or *endogenously,* from inside the body. Exogenously acquired diseases are those that result from an encounter with a microbe in the environment. This transmission can occur by either direct or indirect host-to-host contact. Indirect transmission may also occur through a vector or a fomite.

Direct host-to-host transmission occurs when an infected individual transmits an infection by any number of methods, such as handholding, coughing, or sexual contact, just to name a few. Most important, direct contact involves touching of some sort. Sexually transmitted diseases use this route. Skin pathogens are also spread by the direct route. Staphylococcal infections can be spread by direct contact with the infected area, as demonstrated in impetigo infections.

Infective microbes are usually transported in a liquid medium. Secretions and excretions pick up organisms from infected areas and remove them during normal body functions. Body secretions such as phlegm and aerosols from sneezes and coughs are common transportation media.

Respiratory pathogens transmitted in the aerosols do not remain airborne and viable for long. Transmission is therefore considered to be of the direct route. Excretions, including urine and feces, are also pertinent carriers of microorganisms.

Some microorganisms require a **vector** to enter and exit the human host. A vector is usually an arthropod (mosquito, flea, tick, and so forth). When it consumes its blood meal from its human host, it can ingest an infectious microbe from the blood. When the vector goes on to obtain its next meal from a different individual, it can transmit the infection to that individual. The deer tick is a vector that transmits Lyme disease.

A **fomite** is an inanimate object that has been in contact with an infectious organism. Food and water, radiographic equipment, and latex gloves can all serve as fomites.

Endogenous transmission is the result of encounters with organisms already present in or on the body, the normal flora. This transmission usually happens when the normal flora of a specific area is transported to a different area. Staphylococci on the surface of the skin can invade deeper tissue through a laceration. In this case, the initial encounter with staphylococci may have been years earlier, but the infection was initiated as a result of the trauma. The primary encounter is termed the *colonization* and denotes the presence of a microbe. Do not assume, however, that because colonization exists, disease is present. *Disease* implies tissue damage and related symptoms.

Reservoir

A **reservoir** is the site where an infectious organism can remain alive and from which transmission can occur. People, animals, and inanimate objects can all serve as reservoirs.

A person who serves as a reservoir is called a *carrier.* A carrier is an infected person who does not display the disease symptoms; typhoid Mary is a classic example. Mary Mallon was a chronic carrier of *Salmonella typhi,* the organism that causes typhoid fever. She was employed in numerous households and institutions as a cook. Daily she exposed other people to the pathogen, which led to an epidemic. After extensive investigations of numerous outbreaks, she was revealed as the source of each one. When she was tested, her bacteria count for this specific species was incredibly high. She continued to shed the organism for many years. The assumption is that her infected gallbladder supplied a continuous wave of organisms to her colon. Public health officials offered to remove her gallbladder, an operation she refused. Their only recourse was to imprison Mary to prevent further epidemics. After 3 years in prison, Mary was released on the promise that she would cease to handle food and that she would continue to be monitored on a regular basis. Mary never appeared for her checkups; she changed her name and continued to cook. For 5 more years, she caused another epidemic of typhoid fever. After another epidemiologic investigation, the source of infection was, once again, traced to her. She was imprisoned and remained in prison for 23 years until her death in 1938.

Animals can also serve as reservoirs; a common animal reservoir is the cow. Some diseases can be passed from the cow to a human host through the ingestion of milk. Pasteurization has helped to obliterate most of these pathogens.

Insects are another common reservoir. After an insect ingests a blood meal infected with pathogens, protozoa may complete their life cycles within the insect and are introduced into the host in a different stage of life. Such is the case for malaria, which is spread primarily by a mosquito vector.

A dusty corner, contaminated linen, and food can serve as inanimate reservoirs.

HEALTH CARE–ASSOCIATED INFECTIONS

Health care–associated infections (HAIs) are infections that people acquire while they are receiving treatment in a health care setting for another condition. These infections can be acquired anywhere health care is delivered. This includes both outpatient and inpatient facilities. Outpatient facilities include ambulatory and long-term-care facilities such as outpatient urgent care clinics, nursing homes, and rehabilitation centers. Hospitals are inpatient acute care facilities. Specifically, hospital-acquired conditions are known as nosocomial infections (*nosocomium* is the Latin word for *hospital*). The statement that the hospital is a place where sick people can go to get better is a general concept, and for the most part this statement is true. However, approximately 5% of all inpatients acquire an additional condition while in the hospital. These HAI pathogens follow the chain of infection, but the links are limited to persons who are in contact with the microenvironment we know as the health care facility. In the United States, billions of dollars are spent annually on HAI management. HAIs are a significant cause of morbidity and mortality. The majority of HAIs include urinary tract infections, surgical site infections, bloodstream infections, and pneumonia. The US Department of Health and Human Services estimates that tens of thousands of lives are lost to HAIs, and such infections are the eighth leading cause of death.

Within the health care field, yet another microenvironment can be found: between patient and physician. An infection that is the result of intervention with a physician is an iatrogenic infection. This type of infection is strictly limited to the physician, whether he or she is in the hospital or not. For example, a patient may develop pneumonia after the performance of a lung biopsy by a physician.

The same organisms that cause HAIs, including nosocomial and iatrogenic infections, may be found elsewhere in the community, but the healthy population can usually combat these pathogens. HAI pathogens are opportunistic. Given the right conditions—a patient with an impaired immune system; the ability to bypass anatomic barriers through burns, wounds, or surgery; and introduction through a catheter, syringe, or respirator—these pathogens thrive and exert their maximum biologic effects. Health care facilities and their patients provide this optimal environment.

Compromised Patients

Hospital patients have a greater sensitivity to infection. Many patients have weakened resistance to infectious organisms because of their admitting illness. These patients are said to be *compromised* or *immunosuppressed.* For example, organ transplant patients are intentionally given drugs to suppress their immune systems. This action is taken to prevent rejection of the transplanted organ, but it provides the opportunistic pathogen with a suitable host at the same time. The severity of the admitting condition corresponds to the risk for acquiring an HAI and vice versa. An outpatient having a mole removed has an extremely small chance of acquiring an infection compared with a patient having emergency open-heart surgery.

Sources

Cross-infection within the hospital can come from a multitude of sources. The complexity of the hospital environment provides innumerable opportunities for the encounter of patients with infectious microbes.

Medical Personnel. Transmission between the hospital staff and the patient may be by direct skin-to-skin contact or through indirect contact by ingestion or inhalation. Unusual epidemics have been traced to hospital personnel. Food handlers can contaminate food eaten by the patient, and a nurse can sneeze onto his or her hands and then touch a patient. Surgeons have been known to carry organisms in their facial hair. In one epidemic, the organisms were harbored in the carrier's vagina and were presumed to be aerosolized through normal body movement. The possibilities for transfer are endless. Medical personnel can continually serve as active colonizers or transient carriers, or they, themselves, can become infected.

Patient Flora. Microorganisms are almost always found in regions of the body that are exposed to the external environment, such as the skin, gastrointestinal system, genitourinary system, and respiratory system. Potentially harmful bacteria such as staphylococci and streptococci are harbored in the nasopharynx of almost every healthy person. When a person is healthy, the relationship between the host and the microbe is either beneficial or neutral; but when this person is compromised, the microbe is harmful and seizes the opportunity to flourish.

Contaminated Health Care Environment. Many microorganisms are endemic to the health care environment. An example would be fungal infections acquired from the mildew that grows on moist walls. Infection can also be acquired through improperly sterilized surgical equipment or contaminated intravenous solutions. Contamination through the health care environment is often through fomites, such as instruments, fluids, food, air, and medications. Common fomites in the health care setting include indwelling medical devices such as bloodstream, urinary, and endotracheal catheters.

Blood-Borne Pathogens. Blood-borne pathogens are disease-causing microorganisms that may be present in human blood. They may be transmitted with any exposure to blood or other potentially infectious material. For this reason, these pathogens are considered HAIs.

Two blood-borne pathogens are of concern within the hospital setting: hepatitis B virus (HBV) and human immunodeficiency virus (HIV). Numerous other blood-borne pathogens exist, such as those that cause hepatitis C, hepatitis D, and syphilis, but they are not as prevalent as HBV and HIV.

HBV causes illness that primarily affects the liver. This infection results in swelling, soreness, and loss of normal function in the liver. HBV is a major cause of viral hepatitis.

The symptoms of hepatitis B include weakness, fatigue, anorexia, nausea, abdominal pain, fever, and headache. As the illness progresses, a yellow discoloration of the skin, called *jaundice,* may develop. In some patients, the disease may be asymptomatic and therefore may not be diagnosed.

A person's blood will test positive for the HBV surface antigen 2 to 6 weeks after symptoms of the illness develop. Approximately 85% of persons infected will recover in 6 to 8 weeks, and yet a blood test will always reveal that they have been exposed to the virus because of the presence of the HBV surface antigen.

A major source of HBV is the chronic active carrier of the virus. The carrier has the surface antigen present at all times. This presence may be the consequence of a problem with his or her immune system that prevents complete destruction of virus-infected liver cells. Estimates suggest that 1.25 million persons in the United States have chronic HBV and are potentially infectious to others. The carrier can unknowingly transmit the disease to a susceptible host through a contaminated needle or other penetrating injury and through intimate contact. Each year, 5000 people die as a result of liver disease caused by HBV.

HIV is a virus that specifically infects the immune system's CD4+ T cells in a human host. The presence of the virus renders the cells decreasingly effective in preventing disease. HIV is responsible for acquired immunodeficiency syndrome.

Symptoms of HIV infection may include weight loss, fatigue, glandular pain and swelling, muscle and joint pain, and night sweats. People with HIV infection may feel fine and not be aware of their previous exposure to HIV for as long as 10 years. As long as 1 year may be required for the results of a blood test to become positive for HIV antibodies; therefore more than one test over a specified period may be required to determine infection after exposure to HIV.

Invasive Procedures. Invasive diagnostic or therapeutic interventions allow a microbe to gain entrance into an area of the body where it may not normally be able to overcome that person's defenses. These procedures give the microbe a free ride. The most common nosocomial infection, a urinary tract infection, is introduced by a Foley urinary catheter. Other invasive procedures include any surgery and the insertion of such devices as needles, vascular catheters, endotracheal tubes, and endoscopes.

MICROBIAL CONTROL WITHIN THE HOST

Microbes can be controlled within the host by different mechanisms. Some of these defenses are part of the normal anatomic and physiologic mechanisms of the host. Others are introduced into the host, and microbes themselves control yet others.

Constitutive Defenses of the Body

The human body has defense mechanisms with which a host can protect itself from microbial invasion. These defenses are categorized as mechanical, chemical, or cellular. The intact skin and mucous membranes provide a mechanical and chemical barrier through which a microorganism must first pass. The sebaceous and sweat glands secrete moisture and fatty acids onto the skin, which kill many bacteria and fungi. In addition, the mechanical process of the shedding of cells caused by friction from rubbing the hands together during washing also provides a strong defensive system. Trauma—such as a burn, abrasion, or other type of wound—provides an obvious breach of this barrier.

The mucous membranes of the respiratory, gastrointestinal, and genitourinary tracts and conjunctiva of the eye secrete a gel-like substance called *mucus* that traps foreign particles and prevents them from invading the adjacent tissue. Some epithelial cells are ciliated. The beating action of the cilia on the mucous membranes provides for the continuous movement of the fluid mucus to the exterior.

Tears continually bathe the eyes, and urine cleanses the urinary tract. Both tears and urine are rich in *lysosome,* an enzyme that destroys the bacterial cell wall. The acidity of the stomach and vagina also provides a competent barrier to invasion.

Despite these efficient chemical and mechanical barriers, microbes penetrate the bloodstream and connective tissue daily. They gain entrance through everyday activity such as eating, brushing the teeth, scratching, and bowel movements. These daily attacks are survived through the cellular mechanism of defense, the *phagocytic cell*. The phagocyte is responsible for removing foreign particles—engulfing and destroying them through a process called *phagocytosis*. Phagocytosis is part of the inflammatory response.

Normal Microbial Flora

The human body contains thousands of species of microorganisms. Each of us is unique in that the types and amounts of each organism vary. Normal **flora** is defined as the microbial community found on or in a healthy person. The normal flora of one person may be completely different from that of the next. Because of this microbial uniqueness, pathogenicity is not a *black-and-white* issue. What constitutes the normal flora of one person may be life threatening to another. Although the normal flora may serve as the source of many opportunistic infections, the normal flora in many areas of the body inhibits the attachment and colonization of many pathogens. The old saying that *possession is nine-tenths of the law* also applies to microbes. Invaders that have found their niche are reluctant to concede their occupancy to other organisms, maintaining their physical advantage. Others secrete toxins that are inhibitory to other microbes.

Chemotherapy

Killing a microorganism outside the human body is a fairly simple task. To kill a microbe within the host requires the selective toxicity of a drug, also called selective **chemotherapy**. Most antimicrobial drugs have a single primary target, which most often are specific proteins, nucleic acids, and, in bacteria, the cell wall. Clinically useful antimicrobials must have the ability to inhibit reactions within the microbe but not interfere with the human cell with which the microbe is associated. Some chemotherapeutic drugs are termed *-static* because they inhibit growth but do not kill. Tetracyclines are examples of bacteriostatic drugs. Others are termed *-cidal* because of their ability to kill susceptible microbes. Penicillins are examples of bactericidal drugs.

Immunization

The awareness that persons who survived an epidemic did not contract that disease again has been evident in history for many centuries. As early as the tenth century, the Turks were inoculating their infant daughters with extracts from the pustules of smallpox patients. If they survived, their value on the market as concubines for harems was increased because their bodies were not pocked or scarred from the disease.

Modern immunology began with the experiments of Louis Pasteur, who developed vaccines for diseases, including anthrax and rabies. A **vaccine** is a mixture used to induce active **immunity** (the production of antibody). The importance of immunization is reflected in the marked drop in incidence of a specific disease after vaccination. The degree of immunity varies according to the patient and the quality and quantity of the vaccine. An important point to remember is that immunization rarely lasts throughout life. In many cases, booster vaccines must be administered.

ENVIRONMENTAL CONTROL

Up to this point, the primary concern has been with the intimate relationship between the infectious microbe and the host. The constituents of the body, other microbes, medicines, and immunizations all contribute their defenses in the constant battle against infection. Each of these factors is important in ensuring the integrity of the host, but another important step not yet considered exists. In a world populated by millions and millions of people, each with his or her own millions of microbes, focusing attention on the larger picture of environmental control is important. When the number of microbes is considered, the problem of environmental control seems overwhelming, and yet it is one of the easiest methods of control.

Within the United States, recommendations and guidelines for environmental control of infectious diseases are issued by the US Department of Health and Human Services (HHS) and the Centers for Disease Control and Prevention (CDC). The US Department of Labor's Occupational Safety and Health Administration (OSHA) enforces the established policies. All rules and regulations are strictly enforced at both the state and the federal levels. At the international level, the World Health Organization issues recommendations for infection control.

Asepsis

As radiologic technologists, we have the ability and the responsibility to prevent the spread of infectious organisms. Knowledge of the principles of sterilization and disinfection is fundamental. **Asepsis** means freedom from infection and can be divided into two categories: *surgical* asepsis and *medical* asepsis. **Surgical asepsis** is the procedure used to prevent contamination of microbes and endospores before, during, and after surgery using sterile technique. The absolute killing of all life forms is termed **sterilization.** If proper sterilization techniques are used, the probability of infection is theoretically zero. **Medical asepsis** involves a reduction in numbers of infectious agents, which in turn decreases the probability of infection but does not necessarily reduce it to zero. The microbes are not eliminated, however. Instead, their environment is altered so that it is not conducive to growth and reproduction.

Each microbial species has an optimal temperature range for growth. Any variation above or below this range results in a blockage of growth. Most organisms that infect humans survive best at 37°C (98.6°F). An increase in metabolic activity within the range results in an increase in growth. Once the temperature is above this range, the proteins or enzymes cannot perform their normal functions. A decrease within the range results in a slowing of growth; once the temperature is below the range, the protein loses its flexibility. This factor is one of the reasons why the operating room is kept so cold.

Another important environmental effect on microbial growth is pH. Most human infectious microbes grow best at a neutral or slightly alkaline pH (7.0 to 7.4). Some microbes prefer acidic or alkaline conditions and seek parts of the body that provide these conditions. Microbes are also sensitive to the presence or subsequent absence of oxygen. Consequently environmental microbial control can be achieved through both chemical and physical means.

Chemical Methods. Chemicals that alter the environment available to the microbe are called disinfectants. This term is ambiguous as it can refer to either the inactivation or inhibition of microbial growth. Disinfection may or may not entail the removal of bacterial endospores. If the disinfectant is applied topically, it is termed an *antiseptic*. Disinfectants can be classified not only according to whether they can be used on a living body but also by whether they kill or do not kill microbes. A *bacteriostatic* agent stops bacterial growth, and a *bactericidal* agent kills cells.

Chemical disinfectants common to the radiology department include the halogens chlorine and iodine, which are bactericidal. Chlorine is found in bleach. Because it is such a strong oxidizing agent, bleach is ordinarily used on inanimate objects. Iodine is used as the antiseptic in Betadine and Surgidine and is used in conjunction with alcohol swabbing. This antiseptic method is commonly used with invasive procedures. Alcohol cannot be used independently; although it is lethal to all vegetative cells, it cannot destroy endospores. Also common to the radiology department is hydrogen peroxide. This substance is used in a 3% solution as an antiseptic and is most effective in deep wounds. Ammonium-containing detergents are used as surface-active disinfectants throughout the hospital, and ethylene oxide is used for sterilization in the gas phase. Gas sterilization is used for electronic and plastic equipment that may be damaged by heat.

The effectiveness of chemical disinfectants is subject to concentration, temperature, time of exposure, types and numbers of microbes, and the nature of the object or person being treated. Reading all manufacturers' labels carefully is important to ensure maximal effectiveness.

Physical Methods. Heat is the most frequently used method of sterilization. Moist heat is much more effective and rapid at killing than dry heat. Moist heat involves using steam under pressure. This task is accomplished in a device known as an *autoclave*. Effective killing of vegetative cells and endospores is accomplished at 121°C (250°F) at a pressure of 15 lb/inch^2 for 15 minutes. Sterilization by dry heat is achieved in an oven. Compared with wet heat, dry heat requires a higher temperature for a longer time (160°C [320°F] for 120 minutes). *Pasteurization* involves moderate heating followed by rapid cooling. This process is used to kill heat-sensitive organisms in milk, beer, and wine. Pasteurization does not sterilize the liquid involved. Freezing can also kill certain organisms but is not a reliable form of sterilization. Ultraviolet (UV) light at 260 nm can produce maximal killing of microbes. UV light is used in germicidal lamps for control of airborne contaminants. UV light is restricted in its usage by its inability to penetrate glass, paper, body fluids, and thin layers of cells.

A host need not be a patient. The health care provider can also serve as a host. One of the simplest physical methods of microbial control, for the health care provider or the patient, is the use of barriers. Gloves, gowns, masks, protective eyewear, and face shields all serve as barriers and defend against invasion by infectious microbes.

Hand Washing

The discovery, in 1846, of the importance of hand washing in preventing the spread of infection is credited to Dr. Semmelweis of Vienna. He noted that when the medical students of the hospital went directly from class, in this case autopsies, to rounds in the hospital, the incidence of infection rose. What drew his attention to this practice was that when the students were on vacation, the incidence of infection dropped significantly. He noted that the nurses attending the patients were not permitted in the autopsy room. He established a policy that no medical students would be allowed to examine patients until they had cleansed their hands with a solution of chloride of lime.

Hand washing is a routine practice in all patient care settings. It is the single most important means of preventing the spread of infection. Washing or scrubbing the hands involves the removal of contaminants (transients) as well as resident microorganisms. Hand washing is both a chemical and a physical process. Many soaps and detergents are bactericidal, but their application during hand washing is usually too brief to kill microbes. Depending on the condition of the skin and the numbers of microbes present, as long as 7 to 8 minutes of washing may be required to remove the transients; resident microbes are even harder to remove because they are so firmly embedded. Soaps are effective at removing some fragile bacteria, such as pneumococci and meningococci. An important and effective portion of hand washing appears to be the mechanical action of rubbing the hands together.

Because a radiologic technologist comes in contact with myriad patients on a daily basis, hand washing absolutely must be performed *before and after tending to each patient*. This practice provides the simplest method of environmental control. The following specific protocol, which is accepted as medically aseptic, should be followed (Fig. 17.7):

1. Approach the sink. Consider it to be contaminated. Avoid contact with your clothing. Use foot or knee levers when available. If unavailable, use toweling to handle all controls. Adjust water flow to avoid splashing. Adjust water temperature to comfort.
2. Wet hands thoroughly with water. During the entire procedure, keep the hands lower than the elbow. This advantageous use of gravity allows organisms to flow down the arm and off the fingertips.
3. Apply soap. Soap should be available in liquid form and can be applied by using foot or knee levers. Soap can also be dispensed from a pump.
4. Use a firm, vigorous, rotary motion. Begin at the wrist and work toward the fingertips. Rub palms, back of hands, between fingers, and under the nails.
5. Rinse and allow water to run down over hands.
6. Repeat the entire process to cleanse from the elbow to the fingertips.
7. Turn off the water. Use toweling on handles if foot or knee levers are not available.
8. Dry from the elbow to the fingertips, never returning to an area.

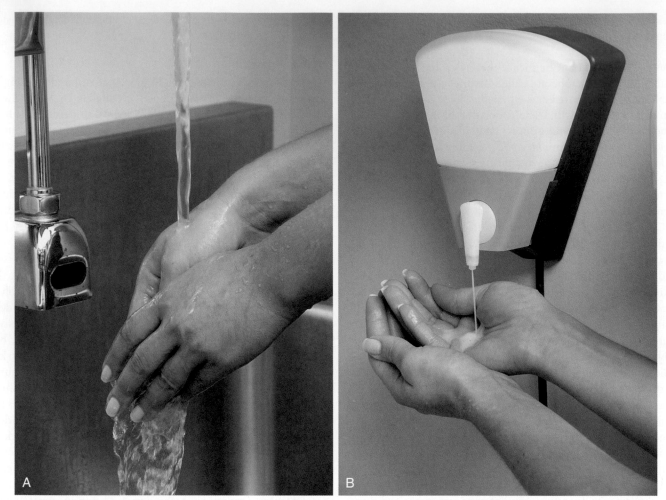

Fig. 17.7 Proper hand washing. (A) Wet hands thoroughly with water. (B) Apply soap.

Standard Precautions

The CDC and the Hospital Infection Control Practices Advisory Committee (HICPAC) recently revised the isolation precautions for hospitals and other health care facilities. To clarify the confusion regarding such terms as *universal precautions, body substance isolation precautions,* and the old disease-specific *isolation precautions,* the CDC and HICPAC reclassified infections, standardized terminology, and simplified precautions.

Standard precautions incorporate the features of both body fluid precautions and body substance isolation. Standard precautions should be used when performing procedures that may require contact with blood, body fluids, secretions, excretions, mucous membranes, and nonintact skin. Also included in this category are items soiled or contaminated with any of these substances. Because most patients in the radiology department have an unknown serostatus, all patients should be regarded as potentially infectious. Apply standard precautions to all patients regardless of diagnosis and infection status. Biosafety in the radiology department using standard precautions includes but is not limited to the following guidelines:

Hand Washing. Hands must be washed before and after performing invasive procedures and after touching body fluids,

blood, secretions, excretions, and contaminated items, regardless of whether gloves are worn. Gloves may have undetectable defects and may also be torn or damaged during use.

Gloving. Gloves must be worn during procedures that may involve contact with any patient's body fluids, blood, secretions, excretions, mucous membranes, nonintact skin, and contaminated items. Gloves must be worn during all vascular access procedures. Gloves must be promptly removed after use, before touching noncontaminated surfaces, and, of course, between patients.

Personal Protective Equipment. Personal protective equipment is provided by the hospital at no cost to the health care worker. This equipment provides a barrier between the patient and the health care provider to prevent exposure to the skin and mucous membranes. This equipment includes gloves, fluid-repellent gowns, face masks, protective eyewear, and resuscitation masks and bags. Personal protective equipment must be used when contact with body fluids, blood, secretions, and excretions is possible.

Needle Recapping. An estimated 800,000 needlestick injuries and other injuries from sharp objects occur to health care

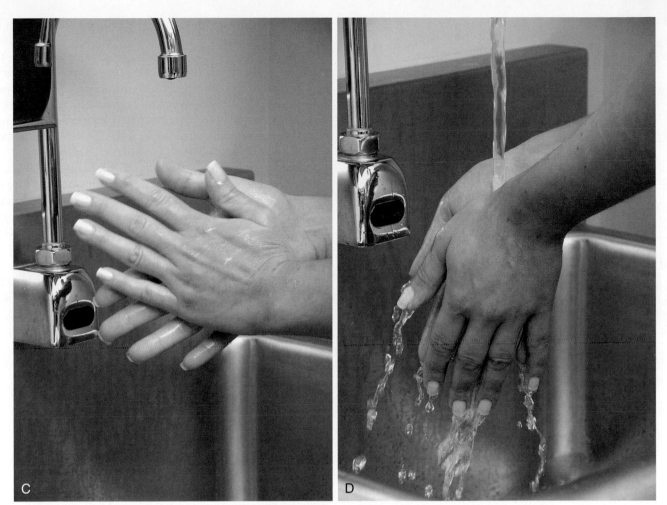

Fig. 17.7, cont'd (C) Rub hands using a firm, vigorous rotary motion. (D) Rinse, allowing the water to run down over the hands.

workers annually in the United States. Recapping used needles should be avoided. If recapping is necessary, the one-handed *scoop* technique or a needle-recapping device that holds the needle sheath can be used. All used sharps must be placed in a designated puncture-resistant container, commonly called a *sharps container*.

Biospills. For cleaning biospills, gloves and the appropriate personal protective equipment must be worn. Paper towels can be used to blot the spill and are then discarded into a designated medical waste container. The contaminated area can be cleaned with a bleach solution or a hospital-grade disinfectant.

Transmission-Based Precautions

Transmission-based precautions are applied whenever a patient is infected with a pathogenic organism or a communicable disease. Transmission-based precautions must also be applied when a patient is at risk for becoming infected, such as a patient who is immunosuppressed.

Transmission-based precautions are used along with standard precautions, serving as a double protection, protecting both the patient and the health care practitioner. The transmission-based precautions have replaced the old category of specific isolation precautions, such as contact and respiratory isolation.

Isolation techniques have been revised and combined into three sets of guidelines. An important point to keep in mind is that, under these guidelines, some infections and conditions fall into two categories.

Airborne Precautions. Pathogenic organisms that remain suspended in air for long periods on aerosol droplets or dust include tuberculosis, varicella (chickenpox), and rubeola (measles). Patients infected with pathogens that disseminate through the air are to be placed in a negative-pressure isolation room with the door closed. Health care practitioners should wear respiratory protection when entering the room. This type of respiratory protection should filter inspired air. An infected patient leaving his or her room should wear a surgical mask, which filters expired air.

Droplet Precautions. When caring for patients who are infected with such pathogenic organisms as rubella, mumps, influenza, and adenovirus, droplet precautions should be used. These pathogens disseminate through large particulate droplets expelled from the patient during coughing, sneezing, or even talking. The pathogens infect another person through contact with the mouth, nasal mucosa, or conjunctiva.

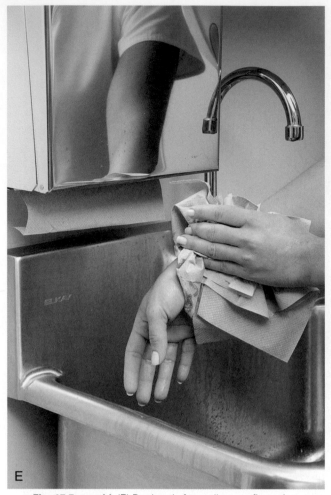

Fig. 17.7, cont'd (E) Dry hands from elbow to fingertips.

Patients infected with these pathogens are placed in private rooms or with another patient who is infected with the same disease. The door can remain open because large droplets typically travel 3 feet before dropping to the ground. Health care practitioners should protect themselves by wearing surgical masks when within 3 feet of the patient. Special ventilation precautions are not necessary. The patient should wear a surgical mask when leaving the room.

Contact Precautions. Contact precautions must be used when caring for a patient infected with a virulent pathogen that spreads by direct contact with the patient or by indirect contact with a contaminated object, such as patient's dressings or bed rails. Conditions that require using contact precautions include methicillin-resistant *Staphylococcus aureus,* hepatitis A, impetigo, varicella, and varicella zoster.

This patient will be housed in a private room or with another patient who is infected with the same disease. The health care practitioner should properly don gloves before entering the room. The gloves are removed and hands washed before the practitioner leaves the room. A gown should be worn if the practitioner anticipates contact with the patient or his or her environment; the gown is removed before the practitioner leaves the room. All radiographic equipment placed

in the contaminated environment should be cleaned with an antiseptic solution.

When a patient requiring contact precautions is sent to the radiology department, the patient must wear appropriate barriers. In many cases the patient will wear a mask and an impervious gown. Staff in the department should be notified before receiving the patient. All radiographic equipment should be decontaminated with an antiseptic after the radiographic procedure is completed.

Contact Precautions Technique. In many instances, a radiologic technologist is required to examine patients who are on contact precautions. Maintaining contact precautions usually requires teamwork. Acquiring the assistance of another health care provider is important. Contact precautions are maintained by the following steps (Fig. 17.8):

1. Determine the correct number of cassettes needed for the examination. Place each cassette into a protective bag, which may be either a plastic or cloth isolation bag. These bags should be available in the radiology department.
2. Move the portable machine to the isolation room.
3. Locate the isolation supplies for the room.
4. Remove all ornamentation (including watch, rings, earrings) and place them in a pocket.
5. Put on a lead apron.
6. Wash your hands as described previously.
7. Put on a clean gown, making sure it is sufficiently long to cover most of the uniform. Pick up the gown from the inside near the armhole openings and gently shake it open. Put one arm in and then the other. First tie the neck strings and then tie the waist strings.
8. Put on a mask, tying it securely, and then a cap. Goggles may also be worn if available.
9. Put on the gloves, which should be clean but need not be sterile. (See Chapter 18 if sterile gloving is required.)
10. Have the assistant put on a gown, gloves, and cap.
11. Enter the isolated area and explain to the patient who you are and what you are doing. You will appear intimidating. A gentle word will go a long way at this point.
12. Position the patient and the cassette.
13. Have your assistant manipulate the machine and make the exposure.
14. Remove the cassette from behind the patient. Fold the edge of the protective bag back, never touching the inside. Have your assistant remove the cassette, never touching the outside. Place the covering into an appropriate container. Have your assistant remove the portable equipment from the room.
15. Untie the waist ties of the gown.
16. Untie the neck strings of the gown and pull the gown forward and down from the shoulders. Pull the gown off so that the sleeves are inside out and the front of the gown is folded inward. Avoid touching the front of the gown. Discard it into an appropriate container.
17. Remove your gloves. Remove the first glove with the other gloved hand, never touching the inside of the glove. Grasp the top of the glove and pull it inside out. Remove the other glove with the exposed hand, touching the inside only. Discard into an appropriate container.

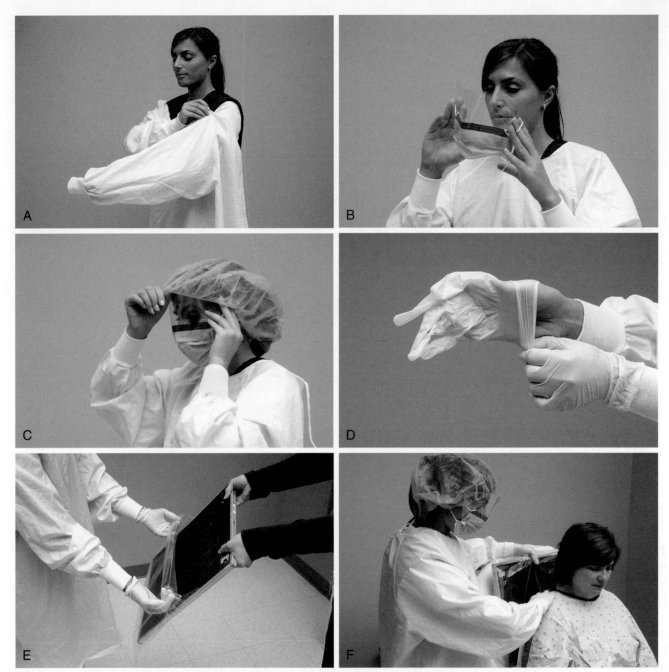

Fig. 17.8 An appropriate contact precautions technique. (A) Put on a lead apron and then gown, never touching the outside of the gown with your hands. (B) Put on a mask with eye shield if recommended. (C) Put on a cap. (D) Put on nonsterile gloves. (E) Place each cassette in a protective bag. (F) Position the bagged cassette beneath the patient.

18. Remove the cap and the mask and discard them in an appropriate container.
19. Wash your hands.
20. Have your assistant follow the same protocol. Clean the portable equipment with an antiseptic.
21. Wash your hands one last time.

SUMMARY

- Infection involves the establishment and dissemination of a microorganism on or in a host. Disease results when an infection causes physiologic damage to the host. Infectious diseases are caused by pathogenic microorganisms, which are divided into four basic types of infectious agents: bacteria, viruses, fungi, and protozoan parasites.
- For an infectious agent to become established in a host, a breach of the host's defenses must occur. The establishment of infectious disease involves six steps: encounter, entry, spread, multiplication, damage, and outcome.
- Four factors are involved in the spread of infectious diseases: the microorganism, the host, the mode of transmission, and the reservoir. Each factor is considered a link in the chain

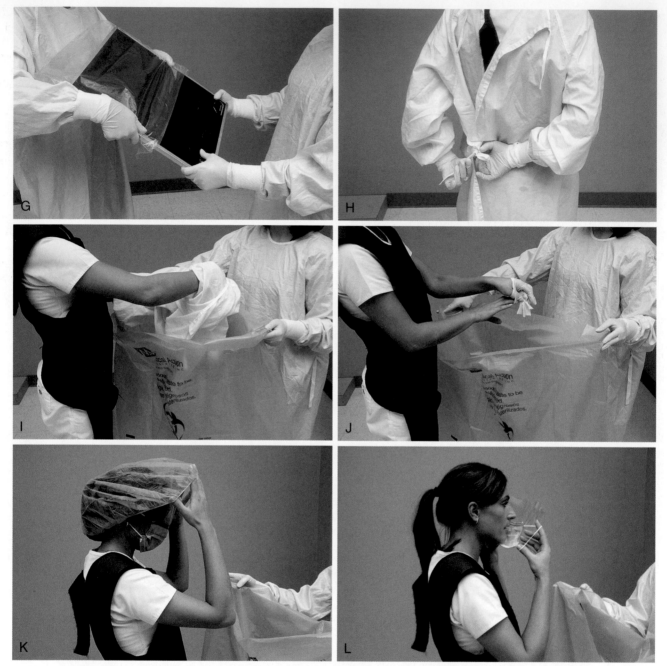

Fig. 17.8, cont'd (G) Remove the protective bag, never touching the inside, while an assistant removes the cassette without touching the outside of the bag. (H) Untie the gown at the waist. (I) Turn the gown inside out without touching the outside of the gown, and place the gown in the appropriate receptacle. (J) Remove the gloves, turning them inside out. (K) Remove the cap. (L) Remove the mask.

of infection. A break at any point in the chain results in the infectious disease's losing its ability to spread.

- HAIs are those acquired while in the health care setting. Hospitals and compromised patients provide the optimal environment for HAIs. Sources of this specific type of infection include the hospital proper and the medical personnel within, contaminated invasive diagnostic and therapeutic devices, and opportunistic microorganisms that are constituents of the normal flora.

- The human body has mechanical, cellular, and chemical mechanisms that it uses to fight infection. The presence of the microorganisms included in the normal flora inhibits the attachment and colonization of new microbes. Chemotherapy and immunization have aided in the reduction and eradication of many infectious diseases.

- Through asepsis, environmental control of infection is simple. Various chemical and physical methods can be used to achieve surgical or medical asepsis. The use of the medically aseptic hand-washing technique, standard precautions, and transmission-based precautions has contributed significantly in reducing the probability of spreading infectious diseases.

- Recommendations and guidelines are issued by HHS and the CDC. In turn, these guidelines are enforced by OSHA, part of the US Department of Labor. All rules and regulations are strictly enforced and reviewed to ensure the safety of every patient and health care provider within the clinical setting.

- Students and practicing technologists are continuously challenged both physically and mentally by the microbial world. In this world of newly found, life-threatening diseases, education has become the key to survival. Each health care provider must make a personal commitment to infection control so that, by collective effort, diseases can be conquered.

BIBLIOGRAPHY

Balows A: *Manual of clinical microbiology*, ed 5, Washington, DE, 1991, American Society for Microbiology.

Borton D: Isolation precautions: clearing up the confusion, *Nursing* 27:49, 1997.

Brown A: *Benson's microbiological applications: a laboratory manual in general microbiology*, ed 12, Blacklick, Ohio, 2011, McGraw Hill Science.

Engleberg NC, DiRita V, Dermody TS: *Schaechter's mechanisms of microbial disease*, ed 5, Baltimore, 2013, Lippincott Williams & Wilkins.

Gorbach SL, Bartlett JG, Blacklow NR: *Infectious diseases*, ed 3, Philadelphia, 2003, Saunders.

Jerome K: *Lennette's laboratory diagnosis of viral infections*, ed 4, vol 50. New York, 2010, Informa Healthcare.

Madigan MT, Martinko JM, Dunlap PV, et al.: *Brock biology of microorganisms*, ed 12, Upper Saddle River, NJ, 2009, Benjamin Cummings.

National Safety Council: *Bloodborne pathogens training manual*, Boston, 1992, Jones & Bartlett.

Pendergraph GE, Pendergraph CB: *Handbook of phlebotomy and patient service techniques*, ed 4, Philadelphia, 1998, Lea & Febiger.

Tille PM: *Bailey and Scott's diagnostic microbiology*, ed 14, St. Louis, 2017, Elsevier.

Turgeon ML: *Linne and Ringsrud's clinical laboratory science: concepts, procedures, and clinical applications*, ed 7, St. Louis, 2016, Mosby.

Volk WA, Bryan M, Gebhardt ML, et al.: *Essentials of medical microbiology*, ed 5, Philadelphia, 1996, JB Lippincott.

Walter JB: *An introduction to the principles of disease*, ed 3, Philadelphia, 1998, Saunders.

Aseptic Techniques

Lynn Carlton, MSRS, RDMS, RT(R)(M)

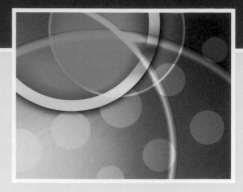

I would much prefer to suffer from the clean incision of an honest lancet than from a sweetened poison.

Mark Twain (1835–1910)

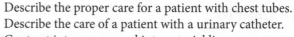

OBJECTIVES

On completion of this chapter, the student will be able to:
- Describe the use of a sterile drape to establish a sterile field.
- List the steps in a surgical scrub.
- Describe the procedures for gowning and gloving.
- List the basic principles of sterile technique.
- Describe the procedure for changing a dressing.
- Classify proper techniques for the safe removal of potential hazardous waste materials.

- Describe proper care for a patient with a tracheostomy.
- Describe the proper care for a patient with chest tubes.
- Describe the care of a patient with a urinary catheter.
- Contrast intravenous and intraarterial lines.
- Describe the use of fluoroscopy for guidance in the insertion of pacemakers.
- Identify common sterile techniques that are used during surgery using the C-arm.

OUTLINE

KEY TERMS

Angiography Radiographic procedure used to visualize blood vessels after the introduction of contrast material; used as a diagnostic aid in conditions such as cerebrovascular attacks (strokes) and myocardial infarctions

Arrhythmia Any change from the normal sequence of electrical impulses of the heart, such as bradycardia (slow), tachycardia (fast), atrial/ventricular fibrillation, or rhythm disorders

Arthrography Examination of a joint using x-rays after the injection of opaque contrast material

Aseptic Describes a product or method that is free of microbiological organisms

Atelectasis Medical condition in which the lungs are not fully inflated

Auscultation Technical term for listening to the internal sounds of the body, usually using a stethoscope; based on the Latin verb auscultare ("to listen"); performed for the purposes of examining the circulatory system and respiratory system (heart sounds and breath sounds), as well as the

gastrointestinal system (bowel sounds)

Benign Prostatic Hypertrophy Benign prostatic hypertrophy is a noncancerous enlargement of the prostate gland, commonly found in men over the age of 50

C-arm X-ray image intensifier, sometimes referred to as a fluoroscope in medical settings; a highly complex piece of equipment that uses x-rays and produces a live image feed that is displayed on a television screen

Central Venous Pressure (CVP) Pressure of blood in the thoracic vena cava, near the right atrium of the heart; reflects the amount of blood returning to the heart and the ability of the heart to pump the blood into the arterial system

Contaminated Presence or the reasonably anticipated presence of blood or other potentially infectious materials on an item or surface

Foley Catheter Indwelling catheter retained in the bladder by a balloon inflated with air or fluid

Isolette Used as an incubator for premature infants; provides controlled temperature and humidity and an oxygen supply

Lithotomy Position Common position for surgical procedures and medical examinations involving the pelvis and lower abdomen; patient is in the dorsal decubitus position with the hips and knees flexed and the thighs abducted and externally rotated; also called dorsosacral position

Manual Resuscitator (Proprietary name Ambu bag) is a hand-held device commonly used to provide positive pressure ventilation to patients who are not breathing or not breathing adequately

Microorganisms Microscopic organisms; those of medical interest include bacteria, viruses, fungi, and protozoa

Myelography X-ray examination of the spinal canal; a contrast agent is injected through a needle into the space around the spinal cord to display the spinal cord, spinal canal, and nerve roots on an x-ray; purpose of a myelogram is to evaluate the spinal cord and/or nerve roots for suspected compression

Pneumothorax Accumulation of air or gas in the pleural space, which may occur spontaneously or as a result of trauma or a pathologic process or which may be introduced deliberately

Purulent Consisting of or containing pus. The term purulent is often used with regard to drainage

Serous Resembling serum, having a thin watery constitution; various bodily fluids that are typically pale yellow and transparent and of a benign nature that fill the inside of body cavities

Sterile Aseptic; free of living microorganisms

Subungual Beneath a fingernail or toenail

Swan-Ganz Catheter The flow-directed balloon-tipped pulmonary artery catheter (also known as the Swan-Ganz or right heart catheter) has been in clinical use for more than 30 years. Initially developed for the management of acute myocardial infarction, the Swan-Ganz catheter provides right heart diagnostic information to rapidly determine hemodynamic pressures, cardiac output, and mixed venous blood sampling.

Tracheostomy Surgical creation of an opening into the trachea through the neck; also used to refer to the creation of an opening in the anterior trachea for insertion of a tube to relieve upper airway obstruction and to facilitate ventilation

Trendelenburg Position Position in which the patient is supine on the table or bed, the head of which is tilted downward 30 to 40 degrees, with the feet higher than the head; also, supine position with the patient inclined at an angle of 45 degrees so that the pelvis is higher than the head

Urinary Meatus External urethral orifice; the opening of the urethra on the body surface through which urine is discharged

Voiding Cystourethrogram Radiographic procedure obtained by the use of fluoroscopy and a contrast agent introduced through a catheter in the bladder; radiographic images are obtained before, during, and after voiding of the bladder, urethra, and kidneys

---

Aseptic technique can be applied in any clinical setting. Pathogens may introduce infection to the patient through contact with the environment, personnel, or equipment. All patients and the health care worker are potentially vulnerable to infection, although certain situations further increase vulnerability, such as extensive burns or immune disorders that disturb the body's natural defenses. Typical situations that call for aseptic measures include surgery and the insertion of intravenous lines, urinary catheters, and drains.

In health care settings, hand washing can prevent potentially fatal infections from spreading from patient to patient and from patient to health care worker and vice versa. The basic rule in the hospital is to cleanse hands before and after each patient contact by either washing hands or using an alcohol-based hand rub. Remember: If soap and water are not available, use alcohol-based gel to clean hands. When using an alcohol-based hand sanitizer, use the following procedure:

1. Apply product to the palm of one hand.
2. Rub hands together.
3. Rub the product over all surfaces of hands and fingers until hands are dry.

The goals of aseptic technique are to protect the patient from infection and prevent the spread of pathogens and harmful **microorganisms**. Often, practices that clean (remove dirt and other impurities), sanitize (reduce the number of microorganisms to safe levels), or disinfect (remove most microorganisms but not highly resistant ones) are not sufficient to prevent infection. Surgical asepsis is protection against infection before, during, and after surgery by using **sterile** technique. Medical asepsis is the removal or destruction of infected material. Practices performed are aimed at destroying pathological organisms after they leave the body in the care of patients. Included in these practices is to avoid reinfection and the spread of infection from one person to another. It is the responsibility of the radiologic and imaging sciences professional to be knowledgeable and practice these techniques daily.

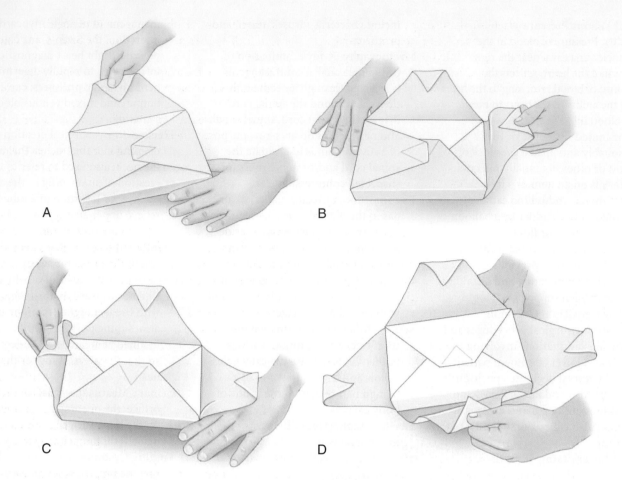

Fig. 18.1 Opening a sterile package. (A) Opening the first flap. (B and C) Opening the side flaps. (D) Pulling the last flap by grasping the corner.

Among the numerous imaging procedures that require sterile technique are angiography, arthrography, hysterosalpingography, myelography, and biopsies in the surgical environment. Other procedures described here require aseptic technique on the part of the radiologic and imaging sciences professional or an understanding of how aseptic technique is to be used for the specific procedure to improve care for patients.

STERILE DRAPING

A sterile field is a specified area (such as within a tray or on a sterile towel) that is considered free of viable microorganisms. In most instances a sterile field is established using a sterile drape. The first step in using a sterile drape is confirming that the package is sterile. If a package is not clean and dry, it is considered unsterile. If it appears to have been previously opened or if the expiration date has passed, it is also considered unsterile. The procedure for opening a sterile package (e.g., one prepared in the hospital) containing a sterile drape on a surface such as a table is as follows (Fig. 18.1):

1. Place the package on the center of the surface with the top flap of the wrapper set to open away from the person opening the package.
2. Pinch the first flap on the outside of the wrapper between the thumb and index finger by reaching around (not over) the package. Some packages require that the uppermost flap at

each corner be grasped. The flap should be pulled open and laid flat on the far surface.
3. Use the right hand to open the right flap and the left hand to open the left flap.
4. Grasping the turned-down corner, pull the fourth and final flap. If the inner surface of any of the package touches an unsterile object, such as a sleeve, the entire pack and contents are considered unsterile and must be replaced.

Note: The outer 1-inch edge of the sterile margin is not sterile.

A sterile package may also be opened as follows:

1. Hold the package in one hand with the top flap opening away from the person opening the package.
2. Pull the top flap well back and hold it away from both the contents of the package and the sterile field. Using the free hand to hold the flap against the wrist of the hand holding the package is an effective technique.
3. Drop the contents gently onto the sterile field from approximately 6 inches above the field and at a slight angle.

These techniques help ensure that the package wrapping does not touch the sterile field at any time.

Commercial packages usually have specific directions written on the package for opening. In general, available packages include those with partially sealed *corners*, in which the container is held in one hand and the flap is pulled back with the other, and those with partially sealed *edges*, in which both sides of the edge are grasped, one with each hand, and gently pulled apart (Fig. 18.2).

For a sterile field to be established, the drape is plucked with one hand by the corner and opened. This corner is used to fold back the top. Then the drape is lifted out of the cover and allowed to open freely without touching anything. Another corner of the drape then is picked up carefully and laid on a clean, dry surface with the bottom farthest from the person establishing the field (Fig. 18.3).

Adding Sterile Supplies to an Established Sterile Field

Necessary sterile supplies can be added to the field using the proper package-opening techniques. Remember the following:
1. Do not reach across a sterile field.

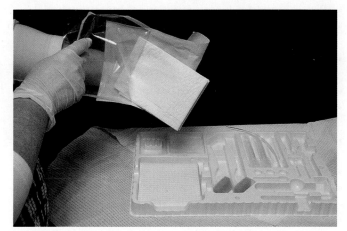

Fig. 18.2 Opening commercially prepared sterile packs to drop sponges onto a sterile field.

2. Do not flip or toss objects on the sterile field.
3. A 1-inch border around the sterile field is *not* considered sterile.
4. Discard the outer wrapper from each sterile item.
5. Repeat this process for adding additional items to the sterile field.
6. Any opened sterile item or sterile area is considered **contaminated** if left unattended.
7. Sterile items that are located at or below waist level are considered contaminated because they are not within critical view.

Pouring a Sterile Solution

Sterile solutions are frequently poured into a metal or other container within the sterile field. Bottles containing sterile solutions are usually considered sterile on the inside but contaminated on the outside; thus, special care is needed in pouring these solutions.

Begin with verifying the contents and expiration date on the solution. When possible, show the name to another health care person for verification.

Always try to use the exact amount of solution. Once opened, the solution can be considered sterile only if it is used immediately. Once the container has been set down, it is no longer considered sterile and a new container must be opened. The procedure for pouring sterile solutions is as follows:
1. Remove the lid or cap from the bottle; place it on an unsterile surface with the topside down immediately to ensure the sterility of the inner surface.
2. Hold the bottle with the label uppermost so that poured solution cannot stain and obscure the label.

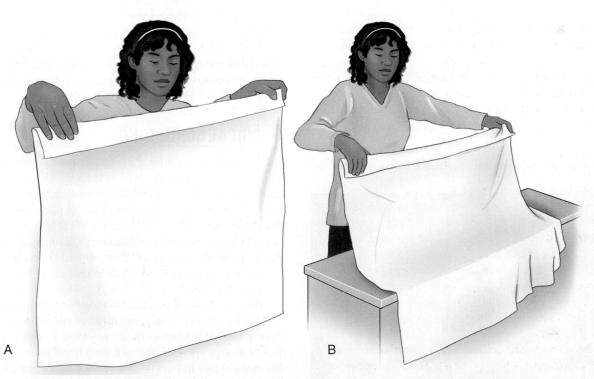

A   B

Fig. 18.3 Establishing a sterile field. (A) Holding the drape with one hand by the corner. (B) Folding back the top to lift the cover and laying the drape on a clean, dry surface with the bottom farthest from the person establishing the field.

3. Sterile basins into which sterile liquids will be poured are generally placed at the end of the table to avoid splashing over the entire sterile field.

4. With as little of the bottle as possible over the field, hold it at a height of approximately 1 to 2 inches over the bowl (Fig. 18.4). Gently pour the solution so that no splashing occurs. Splashing of liquids can destroy a sterile field by allowing microorganisms to move from the unsterile tabletop through the wet drape that forms the bottom of the sterile field.

5. Close the bottle with the cap if appropriate. Some institutions require marking on the label of the bottle with the date and time that the bottle was opened along with the initials of the person who opened the bottle.

STERILE PACKS

Commonly used sterile packs include myelography, minor procedures, and various special procedure packs used for exams such as venograms and angiograms. Items in the typical myelography pack are shown in Fig. 18.5 and often include the following:

- Injectable local anesthetic

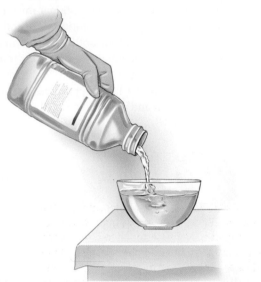

Fig. 18.4 Pouring a sterile solution into a sterile bowl on a sterile field.

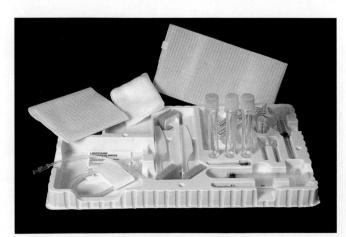

Fig. 18.5 A typical myelography pack.

- Syringes and needles of various sizes
- Sterile drape (fenestrated sheet or towel)
- Collection tubes (for spinal fluid)

A minor procedure pack, used for **arthrography** and biopsies (tissue and/or fluid samples), usually contains all of the preceding items, as well as a sterile gown. Although commercially prepared **angiography** packs are available, many hospitals prefer to make up their own trays. Typical supplies for angiography procedures and biopsies include the following:

- Needles, including three 18-gauge, one 20-gauge, one 22-gauge, and one 25-gauge (the larger-gauge needles are used to inject local anesthetic)
- Sterile containers for biopsy specimens
- Plastic connector for test injections of contrast material
- One manifold (three stopcocks) for the contrast test, heparin drip, or saline flush
- Scalpel handle and no. 10 scalpel blade, used for arterial cut-down techniques and superficial structures
- Large number of gauze pads or topper sponges
- Up to five 10-, 20-, or 30-mL Luer-Lok syringes for saline flush
- Three 10-mL Luer-Lok syringes: Two for contrast tests, one for local anesthetic
- Forceps for sponges
- Six sponges for preparation of the puncture site with anesthetic
- Three stainless steel basins—one for saline solution, one for antiseptic, and one used as a waste basin—and one emesis basin
- Straight and curved clamps for arterial cut-down techniques
- Clamp to keep guidewire wrapped

Several biopsies are performed under ultrasound guidance (thyroid, breast, kidney, and liver). These are done in real-time and utilize many of the same items in the sterile tray.

There are various items that may be different, depending on the procedure and/or the provider preference.

SURGICAL SCRUBBING

Although persons performing aseptic procedures wear gloves, the skin of their hands and forearms should be cleaned routinely to reduce the number of microorganisms in case a glove tears. A surgical scrub is required before participation in many interventional studies. The purpose of the surgical hand scrub is (1) to remove debris and transient microorganisms from the hands, nails, and forearms; (2) to reduce the resident microbial count to a minimum; and (3) to inhibit rapid rebound growth of microorganisms.

The sterile scrub consists of scrubbing with an antimicrobial agent. Surgical scrubbing involves two basic methods: (1) the numbered stroke method, in which a certain number of brush strokes are used for each finger, the palms, the backs of the hands, and the arms; and (2) the timed scrub. Although exact procedures and times for the scrub vary among different settings and institutions, the following can serve as guidelines for the timed scrub (currently a surgical scrub with 2%

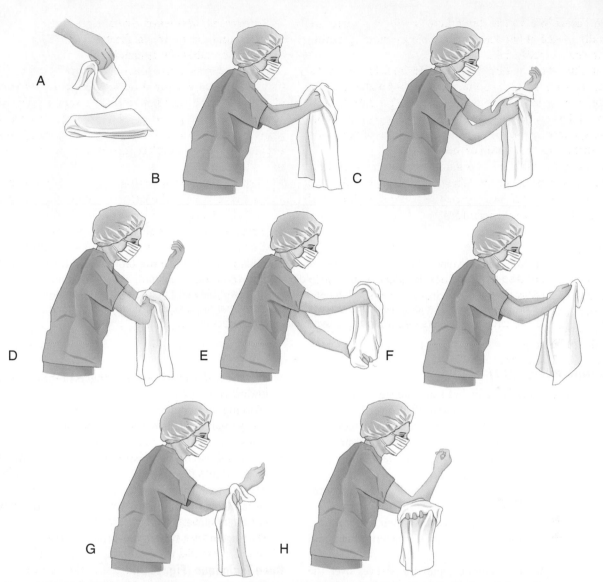

Fig. 18.6 Drying the hands and arms after a surgical scrub. (A) Pick up a sterile towel from the table, being careful not to drip water on the gown beneath it. (B) Fold the towel lengthwise. (C) Use one end of the towel only to dry one hand. (D) Rotate the arm as you proceed to dry it, working from the wrist to the elbow. Do not allow the towel to contact the scrub suit. (E and F) After the arm is dried, bring the dry hand to the opposite end of the towel and begin drying the other hand. (G) Dry the arm using the blotting rotating motion. (H) Proceed to the elbow. The towel must be discarded in the linen hamper or kick bucket.

chlorhexidine gluconate or 7.5% povidone-iodine is performed before each procedure):

1. Be sure that scrub brushes, antiseptic soap, and nail cleaners are available.
2. Remove all jewelry, including watches.
3. Wash hands and arms with antiseptic soap.
4. Clean subungual areas with nail file.
5. Scrub the sides of each finger, between the fingers, and the back and front of the hand for 3 minutes.
6. Scrub the arm with the hands higher than the elbows. Each side of the arm is washed to 3 inches above the elbow for 1 minute.
7. Repeat the process for the other hand and arm. The hands remain above the elbows at all times.
8. Dry the hands as shown in Fig. 18.6.

STERILE GOWNING AND GLOVING

Gowns and gloves are put on after the surgical scrub. Gowning can be done in two ways: (1) self-gowning and (2) gowning by another person. Sterile gowning differs from gowning for isolation in that the focus is on surgical rather than medical asepsis. Gloving can also be done in two ways: (1) self-gloving and (2) gloving by another person. A sterile surface is always required for sterile gloving. Gloves have two surfaces: an inside and an outside. Before the gloves are touched, the entire glove is sterile; however, once gloving has started, the inside surface of the cuff is considered nonsterile. Gloves are packaged in a paper wrapper with the palms of the gloves facing upward and the top of the glove folded over to form a 2- to 3-inch cuff. The exposed cuff is part of the inside of the glove and is therefore part of the nonsterile side.

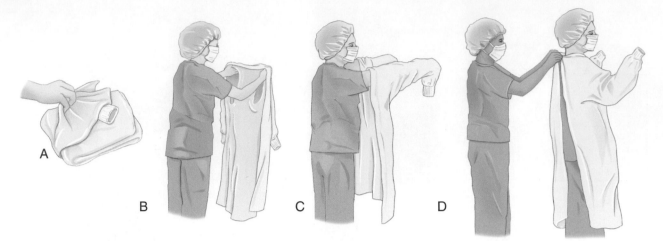

Fig. 18.7 Self-gowning. (A) Grasp the gown firmly and bring it away from the table. It has been folded so that the outside faces away. (B) Holding the gown at the shoulders, allow it to unfold gently. Do not shake the gown. (C) Place hands inside the armholes and guide each arm through the sleeves by raising and spreading the arms. Do not allow hands to slide outside cuff of gown. (D) The circulator assists by pulling the gown over the shoulders and tying it.

Self-Gowning (Fig. 18.7)

1. Standing approximately 12 inches from the sterile area, pick up the gown by the folded edges and lift it directly up from the package. The gown is folded so that the outside faces away.
2. Stepping back from the table, make sure no objects are near the gown. Holding the gown at the shoulders, allow it to unfold gently. Do not shake the gown.
3. Place the hands inside the armholes and guide each arm through the sleeves by raising and spreading the arms.
4. An unsterile assistant can adjust the gown by standing behind and reaching inside the sleeves, grasping them, and pulling gently.
5. For the open gloving technique, pull the sleeves over the hands. For the closed gloving technique, keep the hands and fingers covered by the sterile gown.
6. An assistant fastens the back and waistband of the gown.

After the gown is on, only the sleeves and front of the gown down to the waist are considered sterile. To maintain sterile technique once in sterile gown and gloves, persons must pass each other back to back.

Self-Gloving

Self-gloving can be done using a closed or an open gloving technique. It is performed after gowning or, in the case of the open gloving technique, may be used during sterile procedures that do not require donning a sterile gown. All jewelry should have been removed. Select the appropriate size and type then check to make sure that the package is intact and dry and no tears or water stains are seen. Hands must be washed and dried before opening and putting on the gloves.

The glove package should be opened facing the person who is going to wear the gloves with the right glove on the right side.

Closed Technique (Fig. 18.8).

1. After donning a sterile gown with the fingers still inside the cuff of the gown, pick up the glove and lay it palm-down

over the cuff of the gown. The fingers of the glove should face toward you.
2. Working through the gown sleeve, grasp the cuff of the glove and bring it over the open cuff of the sleeve.
3. Unroll the glove cuff so that it covers the sleeve cuff.
4. Pull the glove on by grasping the glove cuff and advancing the hand into the glove.
5. Proceed with the opposite hand, using the same technique. Never allow the bare hand to contact the gown cuff edge or outside of glove.
6. The fingers are adjusted until comfortable.

Open Technique (Fig. 18.9).

1. Pick up the glove by its inside cuff with one hand. Do not touch the outside surface of the glove or the glove wrapper.
2. Slide the glove onto the opposite bare hand, leaving the cuff down.
3. With the gloved (and now sterile) hand, pick up the other glove by reaching under the cuff. Touch only the outside surface of the glove with the sterile gloved hand.
4. The glove is then pulled onto the hand without touching the inside surface of the glove, which is actually the outside surface of the folded cuff.
5. Interlock your hands and remember to keep them at or above waist level.

Removal of Your Gloves.

1. At the completion of the procedure, grasp the cuff of one glove and pull it inside out and place it in the gloved hand.
2. Now reach inside the cuff of the gloved hand and pull the glove inside out and over the glove that you are holding and discard.
3. Wash and dry hands.

Gowning Another Person (Fig. 18.10)

1. The sterile person picks up the gown by the neckband, holds it at arm's length, and allows it to unfold.

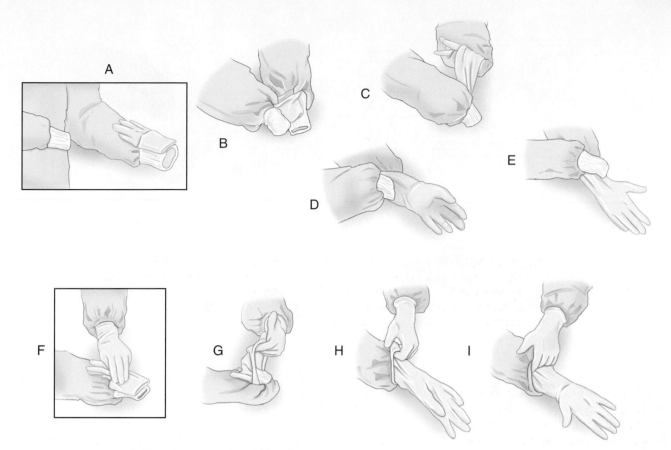

Fig. 18.8 Self-gloving, closed technique. (A) Lay the glove palm-down over the cuff of the gown. The fingers of the glove face toward you. (B and C) Working through the gown sleeve, grasp the cuff of the glove and bring it over the open cuff of the sleeve. (D and E) Unroll the glove cuff so that it covers the sleeve cuff. (F–I) Proceed with the opposite hand, using the same technique. Never allow the bare hand to contact the gown cuff edge or outside of glove.

2. The gown is held by the shoulder seams with the outside facing the sterile person.
3. The sterile gloves are protected by placing both hands under the back panel of the gown's shoulder.
4. The arms are slipped into the sleeves in a downward motion, sliding the gown up to the mid-upper arms.
5. A nonsterile circulator pulls the gown up and fastens the back and waistband of the gown.
6. Gently pull the cuff back over the person's hands, being careful that your gloved hands do not touch the bare hands.

Gloving Another Person (Fig. 18.11)

1. The sterile person opens the package, picks up the right glove, and places the palm away from himself or herself. Slide the fingers under the glove cuff and spread them so that a wide opening is created. Keep the thumbs under the cuff.
2. The person thrusts his or her hand into the glove. Having an extremely good grasp on the cuff is important because considerable force is exerted when the hand is pushed down into the tight glove.
3. Gently release the cuff while rolling it over the wrist.
4. Proceed with the left glove using the same technique.

The procedure for removing gloves aseptically is also important to avoid contamination. The procedure to avoid touching the outside portion of the glove is shown in Fig. 18.12.

STERILE PROCEDURES

Box 18.1 lists the basic principles of sterile technique. The field includes the patient, the table, and other furniture covered with sterile drapes, and the personnel wearing sterile attire.

Dressing Changes

Dressings are best changed in a team setting with another radiologic and imaging sciences professional or health care worker. The physician is responsible for ordering dressing changes and reapplication. Be sure to secure privacy for the patient, explain the procedure to the patient, and secure consent before beginning the procedure. The equipment needed is as follows:

STERILE
  Disposable gloves
  Pack containing scissors, forceps, sterile towel, dressings, cotton-tipped swabs, and solution cup
  Antiseptic solution and sterile saline

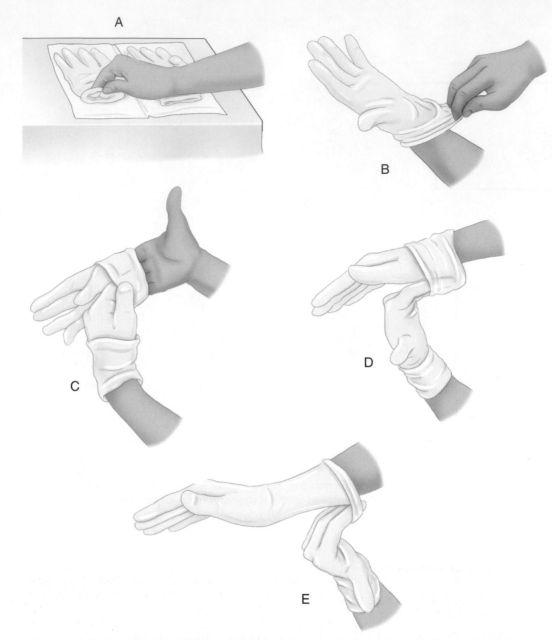

Fig. 18.9 Self-gloving, open technique. (A) Pick up the glove by its inside cuff with one hand. Do not touch the glove wrapper with the bare hand. (B) Slide the glove onto the opposite hand. Leave the cuff down. (C) Using the partially gloved hand, slide the fingers into the outer side of the opposite glove cuff. (D) Slide the hand into the glove and unroll the cuff. (E) With the gloved hand, slide the fingers under the outer edge of the opposite cuff and unroll it gently, using the same technique.

UNSTERILE

   Plastic bag for discarded dressings

   Properly sized adhesive

   Pads to protect surrounding area from secretions

   If the wound is draining (**purulent** or serous) material, to maintain a standard precautions environment, gowns are required at all times.

   All dressings are treated as though they are infected. Do not touch a dressing with bare hands. The procedure for changing a dressing is as follows:

1. The hands are washed, and patient privacy and consent are obtained. The adhesive tape surrounding the dressing must be removed. This procedure is often painful, and a solvent such as baby oil might be needed to loosen the tape. The amount of solvent should be limited to avoid contaminating the wound.

2. The dressing is removed with forceps or gloved hands, wrapped, and placed in the plastic bag. If the dressing does not come off easily, an appropriate person (e.g., department nurse, department supervisor, physician) should be contacted for additional instructions or to remove the dressing.

3. For reapplication, sterile technique is followed. The hands are washed, and the sterile towel is opened to use as a sterile field on which to place sterile dressings. The dressings are opened and placed on the sterile towel.

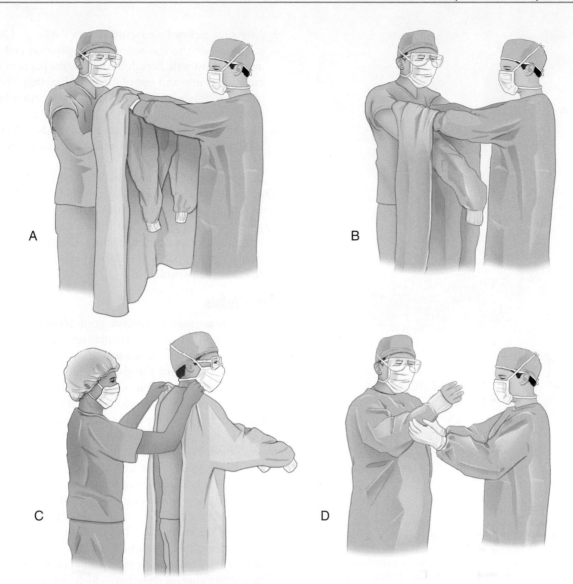

Fig. 18.10 Gowning another person. (A) Grasp the gown so that the outside faces toward you. Holding the gown at the shoulders, cuff your hands under the gown's shoulders. (B) The person steps forward and places his or her arms in the sleeves. Slide the gown up to the mid-upper arms. (C) The circulator assists in pulling the gown up and tying it. (D) Gently pull the cuffs back over the person's hands. Be careful that your gloved hands do not touch his or her bare hands.

4. The tape is cut into the lengths that will be needed. Because the tape is not sterile, it is placed near but not on the sterile field.
5. Gloves are put on, and the dressing is applied. The gloves are removed, and the dressing is secured with the adhesive tape. The hands are washed again, the patient is covered again, and the waste is discarded according to the institutional policy.

Tracheostomies

A **tracheostomy** is an operation performed under sterile technique that involves incising the skin over the trachea and then making a surgical incision in the trachea. This procedure provides for an airway during upper airway obstruction. It is used in emergency situations and to replace the airway provided by an endotracheal tube that has been in place for several weeks.

To prevent skin breakdown, tracheostomies are always covered with a dressing.

If at all possible, the first task in providing care to a patient with a tracheostomy is to establish communication. This provision usually consists of yes-or-no questions, hand signals, and simple sign language. Written communication methods are used less often than verbal methods. Because these patients are often extremely ill, they have difficulty in using written communication and little need for complicated messages. In some cases, after a few days, the tracheostomy may be changed to the talking type, which will allow for speech.

The technologist caring for the tracheostomy patient must also be sensitive to unmet and inexpressible needs and the need to keep the patient's anxiety level low. Thus, these patients often have a great need to have procedures explained and the explanations repeated.

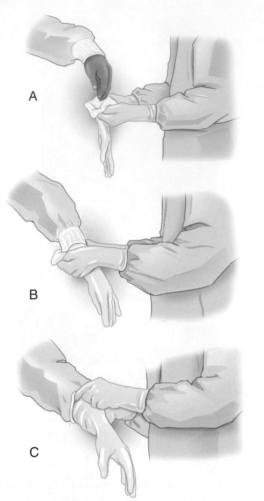

Fig. 18.11 Gloving another person. (A) Pick up the right glove and place the palm away from you. Slide the fingers under the glove cuff and spread them so a wide opening is created. Keep thumbs under the cuff. (B) The person thrusts his or her hands into the glove. Do not release the glove yet. (C) Gently release the cuff (do not let the cuff snap sharply) while unrolling it over the wrist. Proceed with the left glove, using the same technique.

To minimize the possibility of infection, the technologist should not touch a tracheostomy except under conditions of sterile technique. A tracheostomy must be suctioned often to remove secretions. This task is usually the responsibility of the respiratory therapist or nurse taking care of the patient, although in certain situations (i.e., emergencies), this responsibility may become the technologist's. It is recommended that only properly trained personnel suction the tracheostomy patient. The patient must be well aerated with 5 to 10 breaths of oxygen before suctioning, which can be accomplished using a **manual resuscitator** (Ambu bag) hooked to an oxygen source. In addition, before suctioning, the patency of the suction catheter must be tested by aspirating normal saline through the catheter. The procedure for suctioning is as follows:

1. Insert the catheter in the stoma without suction until the patient coughs or until resistance is met. Then withdraw the catheter approximately 1 cm before beginning suctioning.
2. Apply suction intermittently and withdraw the catheter in a rotating motion. Activate suctioning by placing the thumb over the hole in the suction line to cause the suction to pull from the end of the tube where it is placed in the patient's body.

3. Assess the airway by **auscultation** of the lungs. Use a stethoscope to listen to the sounds of inspiration and expiration over the chest wall. Breath sounds are the result of free movement of air into and out of the bronchial tree. The duration, pitch, and intensity of sounds indicate whether breathing is normal or abnormal.
4. Repeat the procedure until the airway is clear. Never suction for longer than 15 seconds, and allow the patient to rest in between.

In some patients the distance between the skin and trachea is too great to be safely bridged by the standard tracheostomy tube (e.g., obese patients). In such instances, an extra-long tube may be used. It is a single-lumen tube and does not have an inner cannula to remove for cleaning. Given that the tube is of a variable length, its position may be checked radiographically to avoid main-stem ventilation.

Chest Tubes

Chest tubes are used to remove fluid, blood, and air from the pleural cavity. They assist in reinflating collapsed lungs (**atelectasis**), alleviating **pneumothorax** (i.e., air in the thoracic cavity), and bleeding into the chest (hemothorax). They are also used in cases of thoracotomy and open-heart surgery. Normally the pleural cavity contains no air or blood, containing instead a thin layer of lubricant that allows the pleurae to slide and move over one another without friction. Chest drainage systems have three compartments to which chest tubes are attached (Fig. 18.13). The first compartment is the collection chamber, which collects any fluid leaving the lung. The second compartment is the water seal chamber, which contains water and prevents air from the atmosphere entering the cavity through the chest tube. The concept is similar to that of a drinking straw, through which air can be blown (e.g., into a glass of water) but none can return. The third compartment is the suction control chamber, which also contains water, the amount of which regulates the amount of suction. This suction removes unwanted air or fluid from the pleural cavity. Some units have an additional fourth chamber, a water seal vented to the atmosphere to prevent potential pressure buildup.

Radiographers often perform chest radiography, especially portable procedures, before and after the insertion of chest tubes to ensure proper placement. Fig. 18.14 shows proper placement of chest tubes on a portable chest radiograph. Radiographers also produce chest images to confirm that the tubes can be removed; these are sometimes taken in the radiology department. An initial radiograph confirms full lung expansion; a second is performed approximately 2 hours after clamping to verify continued expansion. A third image is often obtained after removal of chest tubes, again to confirm full lung expansion.

Radiologic and imaging science professionals must be careful when entering and leaving the patient's room after the tubes have been inserted; the tubes can be pulled from the body if caught by a mobile x-ray unit or tugged roughly during handling of the patient or cassette. Patients may also come to the radiology department by stretcher or wheelchair if they have had the chest tubes in place for a long time. The exterior assembly of the chest tubes must always remain lower than the patient's

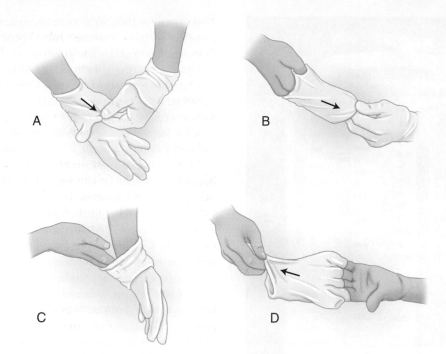

Fig. 18.12 Removing contaminated gloves aseptically. (A) Grasp the edge of the glove. (B) Unroll the glove over the hand. Discard the glove (not shown). (C) With the bare hand, grasp the opposite glove cuff on its inside surface. (D) Remove the glove by inverting it over the hand. Discard the glove (not shown).

BOX 18.1 Basic Principles of Sterile Technique

Only sterile items are used in sterile fields.

If in doubt about the sterility of an object, consider it unsterile.

An unsterile object should be removed, covered, or replaced.

A sterile field must be continually monitored to be considered sterile.

Create sterile fields as close to the time of use as possible.

Sterile persons should avoid unsterile areas.

Anything below the level of the table or the level of the waist, as well as the undersurface of the drape, is considered unsterile. Any item that falls below this level is considered contaminated.

Gowns are considered sterile on the sleeves and the front from the waist up. The back of the gown and the area below the waist are considered unsterile.

Persons in sterile gown and gloves must pass each other back to back.

A sterile person may touch only what is sterile.

Unsterile persons cannot reach above or over a sterile field.

Sterile materials must be kept dry. Moisture permits contamination. Packages that become wet must be resterilized or discarded.

If a solution soaks through a sterile field to a nonsterile field, the wet area may be redraped.

Sterile gloves must be kept in sight and above waist level.

---

chest. Caution is necessary when moving and positioning the patient to prevent compromising the integrity of the tubes. In addition, if the patient is in the department for a longer period (longer than 1 hour), drainage in excess in 100 mL/h should be reported, as well as any change from a serous fluid to a darker red color.

Urinary Catheters

Urinary catheterization is the insertion of a tube into the bladder using aseptic technique. The two main types of urinary catheters are the **Foley catheter** (a retention balloon type) and the straight-type catheter (Fig. 18.15). On insertion of the Foley catheter, the balloon is filled with sterile water to hold the catheter in place. Any catheter that remains in place is also called an indwelling catheter. Urinary catheters can be used to do the following:

- Empty the bladder (e.g., before surgery, radiologic or other examinations, or childbirth)
- Relieve retention of urine or bypass obstruction
- Irrigate the bladder or introduce drugs
- Permit accurate measuring of urine output
- Relieve incontinence
- Fill bladder with a contrast agent to assess the urinary system for structure and function, known as a **voiding cystourethrogram.** When the flow of the contrast is identified as traveling in reverse (bladder to kidney), vesicoureteral reflux is diagnosed.
- In addition, urinary catheters can be used in sonography to do the following:
- Fill the bladder to assess the wall thickness and/or pathology
- Fill bladder to assess the pelvic structures in the female patient (uterus, ovaries)
- Fill bladder and assess the volume of the prostate gland

The relative size of a Foley catheter is described using French units (F). The most common sizes are 8/F to 20/F. 1/F is equivalent to 0.33/mm = 0.013 inch = 1/77 inch of diameter.

This system indicates the outer diameter of the catheter. Thus, catheters range in diameter from approximately 2.6 to 5.9 mm. Choose a larger size when possible.

Because a urinary catheter can interrupt the body's defense mechanism against disease, a variety of catheters are available. Plastic catheters, for example, are suitable for short-term use only. Latex catheters can be used for 2 to 3 weeks and polyvinyl chloride catheters for 4 to 6 weeks, whereas the expensive pure silicone catheters are used only for long-term catheterization of 2 to 3 months.

There are also intraurethral catheters. These self-retaining devices are totally contained within the urethra and placed into position via a cystoscope. This type of catheter can provide continued relief of urinary retention in high-risk patients with **benign prostatic hypertrophy**. Early reports suggest low incidences of bacteriuria and symptomatic infection over weeks and months of use. An extension of this concept is the more recent use of temporary biodegradable and permanent intraurethral stents in men with benign prostatic hypertrophy, and in women with acontractile bladders and chronic urinary retention. Studies suggest that these stents are an attractive and simple alternative to conventional catheterization. These types of catheters will typically have a bag for drainage that will attach to the individual's leg and may not be readily identified as an indwelling catheter that continues into the bladder.

The urine collection bag should be kept low (below the level of the bladder) to prevent reflux of urine back into the bladder. Failure to do so can lead to infection. Keeping the collection bag low also facilitates drainage from the bladder by gravity. Bags should never drag on the floor. During the transfer of patients by wheelchair or stretcher, ensure that the drainage bag and tubing do not become entangled in wheels or caught on passing objects.

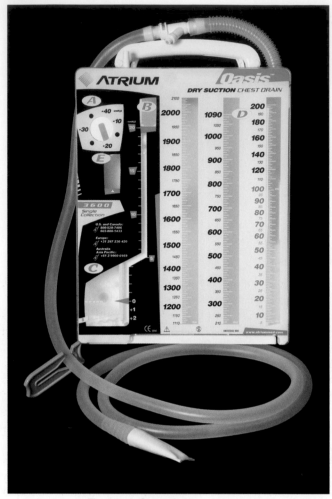

Fig. 18.13 Chest drainage system.

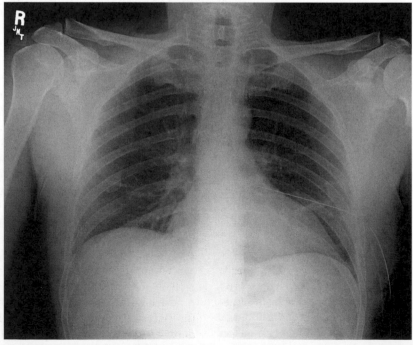

Fig. 18.14 Radiograph verifying proper placement of chest tube in the left lung.

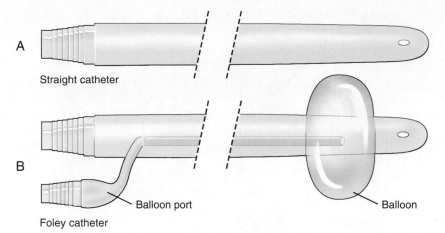

A

Straight catheter

B

Balloon port

Balloon

Foley catheter

Fig. 18.15 The two main types of urinary catheters: straight (A) and Foley (B).

If the radiographer empties the urine collection bag, then output must be measured and recorded, unless otherwise noted. Do not forget to reclamp the stopcock after the bag has been emptied. In many cases, the patient's intake of fluids is also being recorded; if the patient is given a drink of water or any other fluid, it should be recorded in the patient chart along with the recorded output. Always check with the nursing unit whenever a question of recording intake and output exists.

In most instances, radiologic and imaging sciences professionals do not catheterize patients, although this practice varies depending on the setting. In some institutions, they may be responsible for catheterizing a patient undergoing a voiding cystogram as an outpatient. The equipment needed to perform urinary catheterization consists of a sterile catheter, a sterile collecting bag, a syringe with sterile water or saline, and a catheterization kit or the following supplies:

- Sterile gloves
- Antiseptic solution
- Sterile cotton balls and sterile forceps
- Lubricant (water-soluble jelly)
- Container to receive urine
- Sterile drape for sterile field

The procedure for performing urinary catheterization is as follows:

1. Wash hands, provide for patient privacy, explain the procedure, and secure consent.
2. Place female patients in the **lithotomy position**; position male patients supine and expose the genitalia.
3. Open the kit and put on the gloves, which will remain sterile during the entire procedure.
4. Place the sterile drape around the penis for a male patient or under the buttocks for a female patient.
5. If a Foley catheter is being used, test-inflate the balloon by injecting a small amount (approximately 1 mL) of sterile water into the balloon port of the catheter. If the balloon holds, deflate it. If it fails to hold, obtain a new Foley catheter.
6. Pour antiseptic over the cotton balls.
7. Coat the catheter tip with sterile lubricant.

8. Expose the **urinary meatus** using the non-dominant hand. This hand is no longer considered sterile.
9. With female patients, separate the labia majora and minora. For male patients, hold the penis with the foreskin retracted.
10. Clean the urinary meatus with a cotton ball held by forceps. For men, circle the urinary meatus once and repeat. For women, wipe the labia minora from top to bottom, discard the cotton, and then clean the urinary meatus from top to bottom. The labia or foreskin must not contaminate the meatus before or after cleansing.
11. Insert the catheter slowly with the dominant hand until urine flows. For women, this distance is approximately 0.5 inch (Fig. 18.16); for men, it is approximately 8 inches (Fig. 18.17). Always apply gentle pressure, and never force a catheter.
12. Reattach the syringe to the balloon port and fill the balloon. A light tug on the catheter ensures that the balloon is holding the catheter in place.

The radiologic technologist and imaging science professionals are often responsible for removing a urinary catheter after procedures such as a voiding cystourethrogram and sonographic procedures. The materials needed to remove an indwelling catheter are a basin, such as an emesis basin, scissors, and several paper towels. The procedure is as follows:

1. Wash hands, provide for privacy, explain the procedure to the patient, and secure consent.
2. Uncover the patient and place the basin under the catheter valve. Cut the tip of the balloon valve with the scissors and allow the water from the balloon to drain into the basin.
3. Once the flow of water has ceased, place the towels under the catheter and pull gently. Stop and notify a physician or nurse if any resistance is noted.
4. When the catheter has been completely removed, wrap it in the towels, cover the patient, and discard the catheter.

Another type of urinary catheter is the suprapubic catheter, a closed drainage system inserted approximately 1 inch above the symphysis pubis into the distended bladder. The procedure is performed with the patient under general anesthesia. If the catheter is to be retained in place, it is sutured to the skin

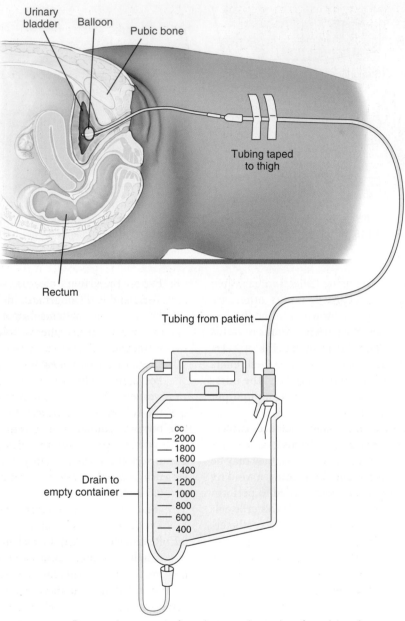

Urinary bladder

Balloon

Pubic bone

Tubing taped to thigh

Rectum

Tubing from patient

cc
— 2000
— 1800
— 1600
— 1400
— 1200
— 1000
— 800
— 600
— 400

Drain to empty container

Fig. 18.16 Proper placement of a urinary catheter in a female patient.

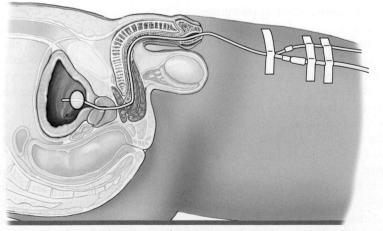

Fig. 18.17 Proper placement of a urinary catheter in a male patient.

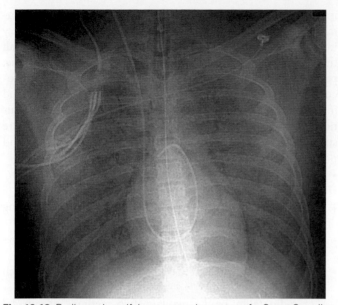

Fig. 18.18 Radiograph verifying proper placement of a Swan-Ganz line.

of the abdomen. Reasons for inserting a suprapubic catheter include the need for long-term catheterization, urethral injury or obstruction, and the period after some gynecologic surgeries.

Male patients may also have a condom catheter, a specially designed condom with a catheter at the end attached to a collecting bag. This device allows an incontinent male patient the use of a catheter without the permanence or inconvenience of a Foley or straight catheter. This type of catheter is associated with an increased susceptibility to infection at the tip of the penis and requires regular cleaning, care, and changing of the condom sleeve.

Intravenous and Intraarterial Lines

Sterile technique is required for the insertion of lines (catheters) into veins and arteries. These lines are also called central venous and arterial lines. Intravenous lines are inserted for a variety of reasons, including the introduction of medications and intravenous fluids and the measurement of **central venous pressure**. The **Swan-Ganz catheter**, a specific type of intravenous catheter, is used to measure the pumping ability of the heart and other heart parameters. Other types of venous lines include the Intracath, Hickman, Broviac, and Arrow-Howes triple lumen. Arterial lines include the radial arterial and femoral arterial lines. These lines are typically used for drawing blood and measuring blood pressure.

When performing special radiologic procedures, the radiologic technologist may encounter patients with arterial and venous lines in place. In addition, fluoroscopy and portable chest radiography are often used to verify placement of the lines. The portable chest radiograph is also used to assess for pneumothorax. Gloves, masks, and gowns are typically worn. The patient is usually in the **Trendelenburg position** when the line is placed. Fig. 18.18 demonstrates correct placement of a Swan-Ganz catheter.

Pacemakers

Permanent pacemakers are electromechanical devices inserted under the patient's skin and leads (wires) that are placed in the right atrium and/or the right ventricle to regulate the heart rhythm and normal speed. Single- or dual-chamber pacemakers may be utilized, depending on the correction needed. Patients with an **arrhythmia**, such as symptomatic bradycardia (a slow heart rate), are the most likely candidates for permanent pacemakers. A pacemaker can prevent bradycardia by sensing the heartbeats of a patient and pacing the heart when it does not initiate a heartbeat on its own.

Pacemaker units are approximately 1 inch wide in diameter and thickness, weighing just a little over 1 ounce. The unit consists of a pulse generator and accompanying circuitry and is connected to a lead. The tip of the lead contains a metal electrode that is put into contact with the heart. The electrode senses heartbeats and can also produce an electrical impulse to make the heart contract.

Using aseptic technique, the surgeon makes an incision at the level of the pectoral fascia, secures percutaneous access to a vein, and forms a pocket for the pulse generator. Before insertion of the pacing lead, a needle and syringe are inserted into the subclavian vein for verification. Then a guidewire is inserted through the needle to establish a pathway through the vein. The role of the radiographer is to operate the fluoroscopy unit, which will allow the physician to place the guidewire correctly. After the guidewire is determined to be in the correct position, an introducer sheath is used to place the pacing lead into the subclavian vein. Under fluoroscopy, the lead is advanced into the right atrium, the introducer sheath is withdrawn, and the lead is positioned in the apex of the right ventricle.

Temporary pacemakers are also usually connected to a transvenous pacing electrode, but the pacemaker is external to the patient's body. The fluoroscopic technique is similar to that for permanent pacemaker insertion.

A new magnetic resonance–conditional pacemaker system has been designed, tested, and approved for safe use in magnetic resonance imaging (MRI). This represents a major milestone in the evolution of implantable cardioverter-defibrillators. For the first time, patients with this new pacing system will be able to undergo MRI scans under certain conditions. Currently, most patients with implanted pacemakers are restricted from receiving MRI examinations.

Special care is also needed for the patient with a pacemaker undergoing radiation therapy; the pacemaker must be shielded from the radiation field, or damage to the circuit may occur.

Surgical and Portable Radiography

Radiography in the surgical environment requires strict attention to sterile technique. Specific guidelines are difficult to give because procedures vary greatly among surgeons and facilities. The one constant is the existence of a sterile corridor, the area between the patient drape and the instrument table. Radiographic cassettes are sometimes positioned under the table through a tunnel device; in other cases, they are enclosed in sterile covers and positioned by the physician.

In most cases, especially at first, the radiography student observes procedures performed in surgery. In some cases, the machinery is left outside the room until right before the procedure; in other cases, the surgeon or procedure demands that setup occur before the operation begins.

Use of the C-Arm in Surgery. A C-arm is an x-ray image intensifier. The name derives from the C-shaped arm used to connect the x-ray source and x-ray detector to one another. They are used primarily for fluoroscopic intraoperative imaging during surgical, orthopedic, and emergency procedures.

The use of the C-arm fluoroscopy in surgery requires increased attention to maintaining a sterile field. The surgical draping of the C-arm and the patient is performed by the surgical team. Basically, three approaches can be used to maintain a sterile field. The most common approach is draping the image intensifier and C-arm with what is known as a *snap cover*. A tension band is *snapped* in place when the image intensifier and C-arm are covered with a sterile cloth or bags. This approach allows the physician to manipulate the C-arm while maintaining a sterile field.

Hip pinning or femur rodding may use an approach known as the shower curtain approach. On the patient's affected side, a sterile clear plastic sheet is suspended from a long horizontal metal bar attached to two vertical suspending rods. An opening is located in the middle of the sheet, which is attached using a special adhesive to the patient, allowing access to the surgical site.

A third but less common approach is to drape the site with an additional sterile cloth. The C-arm then is brought over the anatomic area of interest. When the C-arm is no longer needed, it is removed, as is the cloth. This approach is a stop-gap measure in many cases and is useful only when the physician does not need to manipulate the C-arm. Care is needed when removing the cover. Gloves should be worn to protect the individual from any debris that may have been collected from the procedure.

Surgical and Portable Sonography

The same holds true for sterile technique in the surgical environment while utilizing sonography. The probe (transducer) may be used directly on a kidney in surgery to check the blood flow or on the brain that is open. All sterile draping of the probe must be performed and the machine must be cleaned prior to entering and exiting the surgical suite.

The same techniques are applied when working in the intensive care, neonatal units, and in neurointensive care units.

Ultrasound-guided procedures should be performed in accordance with the facility's infection control guidelines. The patient's skin should be cleansed with an antiseptic cleanser. The ultrasound probes represent a potential source of contamination. Probes should be disinfected between each procedure according to manufacturer recommendations and practice-specific infection control guidelines. The use of sterile drapes, sterile probe covers, and sterile ultrasound gel may provide the best method to reduce the risk of contamination and infection.

Neonatal Portable Radiography. Neonatal infant patients require many therapeutic interventions to support them, which may lead to frequent invasive procedures and long exposure to the hospital environment. Sepsis and nosocomial infections are recognized as major threats that result in significant morbidity and mortality each year in the neonatal unit. Thus, in neonatal radiography, maintaining asepsis as much as possible is important. The task of obtaining images of the infant and maintaining a safe environment without cross-infection are very important, and the radiographer must pay close attention to all that he or she is in contact with, including the x-ray machine, patient, bed and bedding, and protective lead shielding. Protocol for neonatal units should be outlined by the institution and implemented by the health care worker. Although some institutions may not be specific regarding protocol, the following are suggestions that may be helpful in reducing contaminants and possible infection in an already compromised patient:

- Hand washing (before and after each patient)
- Wiping down the machine (before and after use)
- Keeping multiple pieces of lead in the units and sterilizing after use
- Covering the lead with a pillowcase or other protective covering
- Assigning a piece of lead to each crib and cleaning after each use

For radiography of the neonate, two methods of gonadal shielding are accepted: (1) contact, which places lead directly on the infant's gonads, and (2) shadow, which hangs a piece of lead in the beam (or places a piece of lead on the isolette), casting a shadow in the collimator light. Each method has advantages and disadvantages. Shadow shielding, for example, requires low levels of ambient lighting for proper use. Contact shielding has the greatest potential for cross-infection.

Emergency Department, Patient Room, and Intensive Care Unit Portables. Some patients located in the emergency department, patient rooms, or intensive care unit may be unable to travel to the radiology department owing to the severity of their condition. This requires the radiographer to go to their rooms to obtain images. All precautions for the safety of the patient and health care worker must be considered.

The emergency department provides initial treatment to patients with a broad spectrum of illnesses and injuries, some of which may be life-threatening and require immediate attention. The patient undergoes a brief triage (sorting) interview to help determine the nature and severity of the illness or injury. After assessment, imaging studies may be ordered. These patients may require portable imaging to assist in appropriate treatment. Unfortunately, movement is necessary to obtain images, and this can cause additional injury to the patient if he or she is not moved correctly. In addition, with this movement comes increased exposure to possible infectious agents owing to contact with blood and other body fluids from a severely injured patient. It is very important to implement proper protection protocols. Care must be taken with the patient and all devices that are being used (e.g., respirators, central lines).

Recommended Good Practices for Removal of Hazardous Waste

Thick, leak-proof plastic bags, colored differently from other hospital trash bags, should be used for routine collection of discarded gloves, gowns, tubing, and other disposable material and labeled as Hazardous Drug-Related Wastes.

Hazardous Waste Disposal and Containers

The *Occupational Safety and Health Administration (OSHA) Technical Manual Part IV* (section c) requires the labeling of needle containers and breakable items of hazardous waste as hazardous drug waste only. It also mandates the use of properly labeled, sealed, and covered disposal containers, handled by trained and protected personnel, as required under the Bloodborne Pathogens Standard if such items are contaminated with blood or other potentially infectious materials.

SUMMARY

- The purpose of aseptic technique is to reduce the number of harmful microorganisms. Surgical asepsis is protection against infection before, during, and after surgery by using sterile technique. Medical asepsis is the removal or destruction of infected material. A variety of radiologic and other imaging procedures require sterile technique.
- A sterile field is a microorganism-free area that can receive sterile supplies. The patient is the center of the sterile field. The field includes the patient, the table and other furniture covered with sterile drapes, and the personnel wearing sterile attire.
- Commonly used sterile packs include myelography, minor procedure, and special procedure packs. Minor procedure packs are used for arthrography and biopsies.
- The purpose of the surgical hand scrub is to remove debris and transient microorganisms from the hands, nails, and forearms; to reduce the resident microbial count to a minimum; and to inhibit rapid rebound growth of microorganisms.
- Gowns and gloves are put on after the surgical scrub. Gowning can be done in two ways: self-gowning and gowning performed by another person. Sterile gowning differs from gowning for isolation in that the focus is on surgical rather than medical asepsis. Gloving can also be done in two ways: self-gloving and gloving performed by another person.
- All dressings are treated as though they are infected and are not touched with bare hands. Dressings are best changed with an assistant.
- A tracheostomy involves incising the skin over the trachea and then making a surgical wound in the trachea. This procedure provides for an airway during tracheal obstruction. If at all possible, the first task in providing care to a patient with a tracheostomy is to establish communication.
- Chest tubes are used to remove fluid, blood, and air from the pleural cavity. Special caution is needed when dealing with a patient with chest tubes to keep the drainage system below the chest and to maintain the integrity of the tube.
- Urinary catheterization is the insertion of a tube into the bladder using aseptic technique. The two main types of catheters are the Foley catheter (a retention balloon type) and the straight-type catheter.
- Intravenous and intraarterial lines are inserted for a variety of reasons, including the introduction of medications and pressure measurements. The radiographer may assist the physician in determining the placement of the line with fluoroscopy or a portable chest radiograph.
- Pacemakers are electromechanical devices inserted under the patient's skin to regulate the heart rate. They are further subdivided into permanent pacemakers, which are inserted in a pocket of skin, and temporary pacemakers, which are placed outside the patient's body. Both types use a transvenous pacing electrode that is monitored with fluoroscopy for proper placement.
- Surgical radiography procedures vary greatly among surgeons and institutions. The one consistency is the existence of a sterile corridor, the area between the patient drape and the instrument table. Portable radiography and other imaging equipment is a very important service for the critically ill patient who cannot be transported, and special care must be taken with all the equipment that may be associated with the patient. Special precautions must be taken for personal safety regarding patient body fluids and secretions, which includes the proper disposal of all potential hazardous waste. It is your professional responsibility to take care of yourself and your patients.

BIBLIOGRAPHY

American Thoracic Society: tracheostomy, 2009. Available at: http://www.thoracic.org.

AIUM practice parameter for the performance of selected ultrasound guided procedures, 2014. Available at: http://www.aium.org/resources/guidelines/usguidedprocedures.pdf. Retrieved 10/19/2017.

Askin DF: Bacterial and fungal infections in the neonate, *J Obstet Gynecol Neonatal Nurs* 24:635, 1995.

Berman A, Snyder S, Frandsen G: *Kozier and Erb's fundamentals of nursing: concepts, process, and practice*, ed 10, New York, 2015, Pearson.

Bontrager K, Lampignano JP: *Textbook of radiographic positioning and related anatomy*, ed 8, St. Louis, 2013, Elsevier.

Blasi M, Ferrai V: *Medical assisting, administrative & clinical competencies*, ed 8, Boston, 2017, Cengage Learning.

Chan D, Downing D, Keough CE, et al.: STANDARDS OF PRACTICE joint practice guideline for sterile technique during vascular and interventional radiology procedures: from the society of interventional radiology, association of periOperative registered nurses, and association for radiologic and imaging nursing, for the society of interventional radiology (Wael Saad, MD, Chair), standards of practice committee, and endorsed by the cardiovascular interventional radiological society of europe and the canadian interventional radiology association, *J Vasc Interv Radiol* 23:1603–1612, 2012.

Cheng SM, Garcia M, Espin S, et al.: Literature review and survey comparing surgical scrub techniques, *AORN J* A74:218, 2001.

Craig M: *Essentials to sonography and patient care*, ed 3, Philadelphia, 2013, Elsevier.

Donowitz LG: Nosocomial infection in neonatal intensive care units, *Am J Infect Control* 17:250, 1989.

Dugan L: What you need to know about permanent pacemakers, *Nursing* 21:46, 1991.

Ehrlich RA, Coakes DM: *Patient care in radiography*, ed 9, St. Louis, 2016, Mosby.

Frank ED, Long B, Smith B: *Merrill's atlas of radiographic positions and radiologic procedures* (vol 1), ed 13, St. Louis, 2015, Elsevier.

Fuller JR: *Surgical technology: principles and practice*, ed 6, Philadelphia, 2012, Saunders.

Goodman LR, Putnam CE, editors: *Intensive care radiology: imaging of the critically ill*, St. Louis, 1978, Mosby.

Greenspon A, Patel J, Lau E, et al.: Trends in permanent pacemaker implantation in the United States from 1993 to 2009 increasing complexity of patients and procedures, *J Am Coll Cardiol* 60:1540, 2012.

Kirkwood P: Ask the experts, *Crit Care Nurse* 22:70, 2002.

Levitsky MG, Cairo JM, Hall SM: *Introduction to respiratory care*, Philadelphia, 1995, Mosby.

Newby J: Nosocomial infections in neonates: inevitable or preventable, *J Perinat Neonatal Nurs* 22:221, 2008.

Polin R, Denson S, Brady M: Strategies for prevention of health care–associated infections in the NICU, *Pediatrics* 129(4):e1085, 2012. https://doi.org/10.1542/peds.2012-0145. Retrieved 7/11/2014. http://pediatrics.aappublications.org/content/129/4/e1085.full.

Ramakrishnan K, Mold J: Urinary catheters: a review, *Internet J Fam Pract* 3:2, 2004.

Snopek AM: *Fundamentals of special radiographic procedures*, ed 5, Philadelphia, 2006, Elsevier.

Strodtbeck F: Viral infections of the newborn, *J Obstet Gynecol Neonatal Nurs* 24:659, 1995.

Torres LS, Guillen Dutton A, Watson T: *Basic medical techniques and patient care for radiologic technologists*, ed 8, Philadelphia, 2013, Lippincott Williams & Wilkins.

United States Department of Labor: *OSHA technical manual (otm) section vi: chapter 2*, 2012.

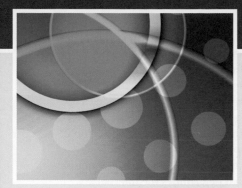

Nonaseptic Techniques

Lynn Carlton, MSRS, RDMS, RT(R)(M)

As it takes two to make a quarrel, so it takes two to make a disease, the microbe and its host.
Charles Chapin
The Principles of Epidemiology

OBJECTIVES

On completion of this chapter, the student will be able to:
- Describe the insertion, care, and removal of nasogastric tubes.
- Assist a patient with the use of the male urinal.
- Assist a patient with the use of a bedpan.
- Describe the common types of enemas.
- State the need for patient teaching regarding the barium enema—preparation, procedural, and postprocedural.
- Differentiate between the single-contrast and double-contrast barium enemas.
- Describe the procedure for a colostomy barium enema.
- State the needs of a colostomy patient undergoing a barium enema.

OUTLINE

KEY TERMS

Auscultation Is listening to the internal sounds of the body, usually using a stethoscope, such as heart, lungs, and the gastrointestinal system

Barium Bulky, fine white powder, without odor or taste and free from grittiness; used as a contrast medium in radiography of the digestive tract

Bedpan Vessel for receiving the urinary and fecal discharges of a patient unable to leave his or her bed

Colitis Inflammation of the lining of the colon

Colonoscopy Endoscopic examination of the large bowel and the distal part of the small bowel with a charge-coupled device camera or a fiberoptic camera on a flexible tube passed through the

anus. Biopsies can be performed during the procedure. Excellent method to identify small polyps or masses

Colostomy Surgical creation of an opening between the colon and the surface of the body; also used to refer to the opening, or stoma, that is created

Defecation Evacuation of fecal material from the intestines

Emesis Basin Kidney-shaped vessel for the collection of vomitus

Enema Liquid injected or to be injected into the rectum

Enterostomal Therapist Health professional (usually a nurse) with special training and certification in the care of ostomies and related concerns

Flatus Gas or air evacuated through the anus

Fowler Position Position in which the patient's head is raised 18 or 20 inches above the flat position; the knees are also raised

Hydration Term used to indicate that a liquid substance contains water

Loopogram The radiographic evaluation of the small and large bowel that has been connected to the skin surface as a substitute for the urinary bladder with an ostomy

Low-Residue Diet Diet that gives the least possible fecal residue, such as gelatin, sucrose, dextrose, broth, and rice

Lumen Cavity or channel within a tube or tubular organ (plural, lumina)

Nasogastric (NG) Tubes Tubes of soft rubber or plastic inserted through a nostril and into the stomach; for instilling liquid foods or other substances or for withdrawing gastric contents

Ostomate One who has undergone enterostomy or ureterostomy

Perineum Region between the thighs, bound in the male by the scrotum and anus and in the female by the vulva and anus

Purgation Catharsis; relief of fecal matter affected by a cathartic

Sigmoidoscopy Procedure used to see inside the sigmoid colon and rectum with a flexible tube that has a camera on the end (sigmoidoscope) and is placed through the anus

Sims' Position Position in which the patient lies on the left side with the right knee and thigh flexed and the left arm parallel along the back

Stoma Opening established in the abdominal wall by colostomy, ileostomy, and so forth

Urinal Vessel or other receptacle for urine (male and female types)

Virtual Colonoscopy It is performed on a multislice computed tomography scanner that takes up to 600 two-dimensional and three-dimensional images of the colon in approximately 30 seconds

Viscosity Physical property of liquids that determines the internal resistance to shear forces

---

In a health care environment that often seems impersonal and more concerned with the technical aspects of procedures than with the patients undergoing them, radiologic technologists must develop abilities of compassion, caring, and competency to be the excellent practitioners that we should all strive to be. Technical skill, experience, and understanding of nonaseptic techniques, including the use of nasogastric tubes, male urinals, bedpans, enemas, and colostomies, are imperative to providing the compassionate care that each patient deserves. Most of these nonaseptic techniques are often performed with patients who are very ill, have sustained major trauma, or are in great discomfort. Diana, Princess of Wales, once said, "If I am to care for people in the hospital, I really must know every aspect of their treatment and to understand their suffering." Students need to develop exceptional patient care skills to become competent in nonaseptic techniques, as well as understanding and sensitivity to patient needs to provide excellent care.

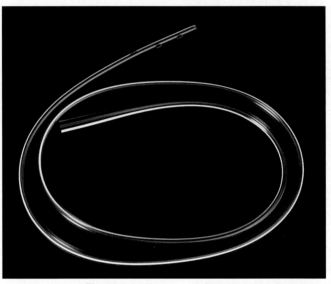

Fig. 19.1 Levin nasogastric tube.

NASOGASTRIC TUBES

Nasogastric (NG) tubes are plastic or rubber tubes inserted through the nasopharynx into the stomach. The primary use of an NG tube is for administration of medications and gastric decompression or removal of flatus and fluids from the stomach after intestinal obstruction or major trauma. NG tubes are increasingly used in the management of patients who typically require short-term enteral feeding. In these cases, the tube is often connected to an electronic pump that can control and measure the beneficiary's intake and signal any interruption in the feeding.

The most common NG tube used for gastric decompression is the Levin tube (Fig. 19.1). The Levin tube is a gastroduodenal catheter (tube) of sufficiently small caliber to allow transnasal passage. This catheter has a single lumen with several holes near its tip.

Other types of NG tubes include the Cantor, Keofeed, Miller-Abbott, and Sengstaken-Blakemore.

A patient with an NG tube in place usually experiences some discomfort. The discomfort of an NG tube often exceeds that of the surgical procedure that accompanies it. The use of topical anesthetics can provide some pain relief during the procedure. Educating patients about the procedure and reassuring them throughout the process are of utmost importance in ensuring

that the procedure is therapeutic as well as securing patient cooperation. Care must be taken to prevent accidental withdrawal of the tube after it has been inserted.

Insertion

In most cases, a physician or nurse is responsible for inserting an NG tube. The following materials are needed for the insertion of an NG tube:

- Rubber or plastic tube, usually a 14- to 18-F (4.7- to 5.3-mm) lumen for the average adult patient
- A basin of ice to make the rubber tube more rigid, facilitating passage
- Emesis basin
- Clean disposable gloves
- Towel
- Glass of water with a drinking straw
- 20- to 50-mL aspirating or bulb syringe
- Water-soluble lubricating jelly
- Tape to hold the tube in place at the nose (butterfly tape or 1-inch hypoallergenic tape)
- Stethoscope

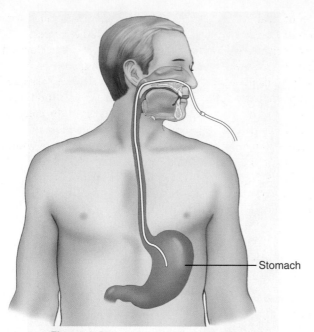

Fig. 19.2 Proper nasogastric tube position.

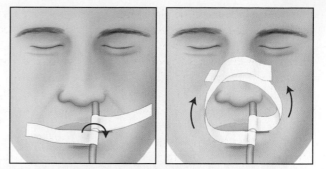

Fig. 19.3 Taping nasogastric tube properly with 1 inch of hypoallergenic tape.

- Clamp, drainage bag, or suction equipment if suction is to be used
- Facial tissues

The procedure for inserting an NG tube is as follows:

1. Identify the patient and explain the procedure. Verify that consent for the procedure has been obtained.
2. Place the patient in a high Fowlers position with pillows supporting the head and shoulders. Place the tissues and the emesis basin close for patient use. The procedure begins by externally measuring the distance from the nose to the stomach. Levin tubes have black markings on them that indicate how far the tube has been inserted.
3. Lubricate the tube at the distal end with the water-soluble lubricating jelly just before insertion. Instruct the patient to begin drinking water through the straw as the procedure begins. If the patient is unable to take fluids, air can be swallowed through the straw. The tube should go down easily with little force. The patient should be encouraged to continue swallowing as the tube is advanced. The proper position is shown in Fig. 19.2.

Verification of tube placement can be obtained through a variety of methods, including fluoroscopy. In most instances, a syringe is attached to the end of the tube, and the diaphragm of the stethoscope is placed over the upper left quadrant of the abdomen just below the costal margin. Air (10 to 20 mL) is injected while auscultation of the abdomen is performed. A *whooshing* sound indicates that the tube is properly placed in the stomach. As a further check, the syringe can be gently aspirated back to obtain gastric contents, which should appear greenish.

The tube is typically secured using the butterfly method, as follows (Fig. 19.3):

1. Cut two pieces of tape approximately 2 inches long and tear one lengthwise. Leave the other piece intact.
2. Wrap the intact piece of tape around the tubing.
3. Crisscross the two pieces of tape at the front of the tubing and place them over the bridge of the nose. A second piece of tape may be placed over the first two to hold them in place.

Levin tubes must be secured so they are not accidentally withdrawn. No pulling pressure should be present on the tube. Consumption of food or drink after the insertion of a gastric tube is not permitted unless specifically ordered by the physician. Occasionally patients are allowed to chew gum or suck on small ice chips to increase irrigation and to alleviate dryness of the mouth and throat.

Removal

Items needed to remove an NG tube are as follows:

- Emesis basin
- Tissues and several thicknesses of paper toweling
- Impermeable bag for disposal
- Clean disposable gloves

The procedure for removing an NG tube is as follows:

1. Identify the patient and explain the procedure. Verify that consent for the procedure has been obtained.
2. Wash hands, and then turn off and disconnect the suction equipment if in place.
3. Gently remove the tape from the patient's nose and ensure that the tubing is free from the patient's facial skin.
4. Put on clean gloves and instruct the patient to take in a deep breath as the tube is gently withdrawn. Wrap the tube in the paper toweling and place it in the disposal bag. If any resistance occurs, stop the procedure and seek assistance with the tube withdrawal from an appropriate individual, usually a supervisor or the department nurse.

Transferring a Patient With a Nasogastric Tube

When NG tubes are used for gastric decompression, they are typically connected to an intermittent gastric suctioning device. If a patient is to be transferred, the radiologic technologist must first confirm that the physician has given an order allowing the transfer and interruption of suctioning. The length of time that suction can be interrupted safely must also be known. Suction must be reestablished in the radiology department if the patient is allowed to be disconnected for a short amount of time. This task can be accomplished either by taking the patient's portable suction machine to the radiology department or by using suction equipment available in the department (Fig. 19.4). The level of suction pressure required must be determined before

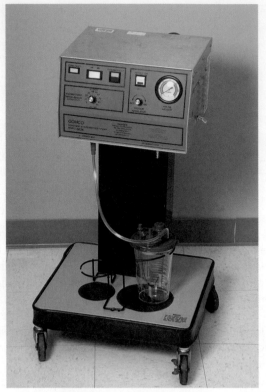

Fig. 19.4 Portable suction unit.

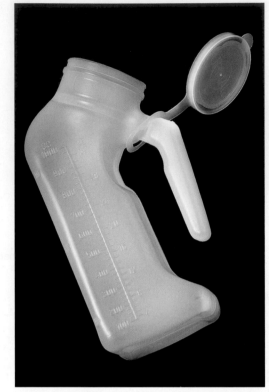

Fig. 19.5 Male urinal.

the patient is transferred. The amount of pressure ordered varies from patient to patient, and the correct level can be determined by reviewing the physician's orders or by asking the nurse in charge of the patient.

Items needed for discontinuing suction on a single-lumen tube are as follows:
- Clean disposable gloves
- Clamping device
- Package of sterile gauze sponges
- Two rubber bands

The procedure for discontinuing suction is as follows:
1. Identify the patient and explain the procedure. Verify that consent for the procedure has been obtained.
2. Wash hands, and then turn off the suction.
3. Open the package of sponges and put on the gloves.
4. Clamp or plug the gastric tube with the clamp or stopper. Cover the end of the tube with one gauze sponge and secure it with a rubber band.
5. Cover the connecting end of the suction tubing or the adapter with another gauze sponge and secure it with a rubber band. The gauze coverings will keep both ends of the tubing clean while not in use.
6. Secure the suction tubing to the suction machine to ensure that it will not fall onto the floor and ensure that the NG tube will not be dislocated during the transfer process.

If reestablishing suction is required on arrival in the radiology department, set the suction pressure gauge, turn on the suction, and reattach the tubing. This procedure is repeated when transferring the patient to the nursing unit.

A double-lumen tube must never be clamped closed with a hemostat or regular clamping device because to do so might cause the lumina to adhere to each other and destroy the double-lumen effect. To prevent leakage from this type of tube, the barrel of a piston-like syringe may be inserted into the suction-drainage lumen, and it is then pinned to the patient's gown with the barrel upward.

URINALS

The male **urinal** (Fig. 19.5) is made of plastic or metal and is shaped so that it can be used by a patient who is supine, lying on his right or left side, or in Fowler position. The urinal may be offered to the male patient who is not ambulatory—that is, one who is confined to a stretcher or wheelchair or is unable to walk.

If the patient is able to help himself, the imaging professional simply hands him an aseptic urinal and allows him to use it, providing privacy whenever possible. When he has finished, the radiologic technologist should put on clean disposable gloves, remove the urinal, empty it, and rinse it with cold water. If the patient's urinary output needs to be documented, note the level of urine indicated by the measurement scale on the side of the urinal and record it in the patient's chart. The urinal is then placed with the soiled supplies to be resterilized. Disposable urinals should be placed in the proper receptacle. The patient should be offered a wet washcloth with which to wash his hands. The imaging professional should then remove the gloves and wash his or her hands.

If the patient requires assistance in using a urinal, the radiographer would proceed as follows:
1. Put on clean disposable gloves and raise the cover sheet sufficiently to permit adequate visibility while being careful not to expose the patient excessively.
2. Spread the patient's legs and place the urinal between them. Place the penis adequately into the urinal so that it does not

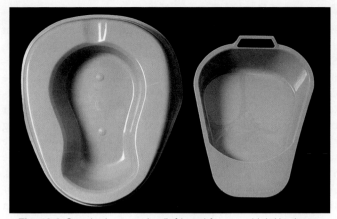

Fig. 19.6 Standard, or regular *(left)*, and fracture *(right)* bedpans.

slip out and hold the urinal in place by the handle until the patient finishes voiding. Remove the urinal, empty it, remove the gloves, and wash your hands.

A female urination device, female urination aid, or stand-to-pee device is a device that aids a female to urinate while standing upright. Female urination devices have increased in popularity since the 1990s. They are used for sanitary and medical reasons and outdoor pursuits.

BEDPANS

The patient who is not ambulatory must be offered a **bedpan** for **defecation**; a nonambulatory female patient requires a bedpan for both defecation and urination. Clean bedpans are stored in a specific area of the radiology department. If not disposable, bedpans must be sterilized between uses.

Bedpans are available in two types (Fig. 19.6). In the past, the standard bedpan was made of metal, but more often today, because of concerns over infectious diseases, most are made of plastic. A standard bedpan is approximately 2 inches high. If a patient has a fracture or another disability that makes using a pan of this height impossible, then a fracture pan is used. This type of bedpan may be used for those who cannot raise their hips high enough or to roll over onto a regular-size bedpan. Fracture pans are shallower and are contoured for patient comfort. The tapered end improves comfort and ease of placement with immobile patients. The built-in handle allows for easier placement and removal, and the plastic guard prevents spills. To reduce the spread of infectious diseases, proper hand washing is extremely important and should be performed both before and after assisting the patient with a bedpan. If the pan is cold, run warm water over it and then dry it before offering it to the patient. Patient privacy must be secured and respected. Always place a sheet over the patient.

The procedure for assisting a patient with a bedpan is as follows (Fig. 19.7):

1. Remove the bedpan cover and place it at the end of the table. In some instances, having a chair nearby on which to place the pan is best.
2. If the patient is able to move, place one hand under the lower back, asking the patient to raise his or her hips. Place the pan under the hips and position properly. Be sure the patient is covered with a sheet.

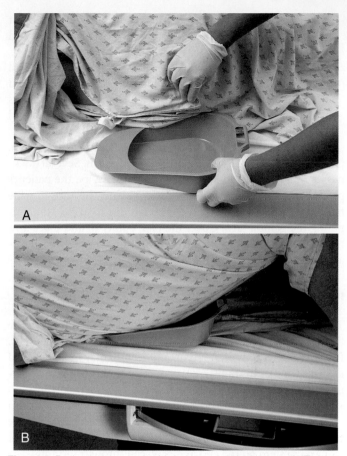

Fig. 19.7 Bedpan placement with helper wearing gloves. (A) Turn the patient onto side and position bedpan. (B) Turn the patient onto back.

3. If the patient is able to sit up, then this position is ideal. If possible, the patient's head should be elevated approximately 60 degrees.
4. Because a patient's balance is poor while on a bedpan, do not leave the patient alone for long. In most instances, leaving the patient alone is necessary, but be sure to indicate how assistance may be summoned.
5. When the patient has finished using the bedpan, offer tissues/washcloths for cleaning. When the patient is finished, put on clean disposable gloves. Have the patient lie back, place one hand under the lumbar area, and instruct the patient to raise the hips.
6. Then remove the pan, cover it, and empty it in the designated area. Plastic bedpans are discarded, and metallic ones are rinsed with cold water and returned to the area where used equipment is placed. Offer the patient a wet paper towel or washcloth to wash hands and a paper towel to dry them. Remove the gloves and wash your hands.

The aid of an assistant becomes necessary when a patient requires more assistance with a bedpan than can be provided by one person. The procedure is as follows:

1. Both persons put on nonsterile gloves.
2. The assistant should stand at the opposite side of the table.
3. Assist the patient to a lateral position.
4. Place the pan against the patient's hips, and then turn the patient back to a supine position while holding the pan in

proper position. Ensure that the hips are in proper alignment on the pan. Place pillows under the patient's shoulders and head and remain nearby if assistance is required.

5. When the patient has finished, put on clean gloves and reverse the procedure to remove the pan. The assistant should hold the pan as level as possible to avoid spilling the contents while the other person assists the patient to turn to a lateral position for the removal of the pan.

The patient may require assistance in cleaning the **perineum**. Clean disposable, nonsterile gloves must be worn. Several thicknesses of tissue should be folded into a pad. Wipe the patient's perineum clean and dry. For female patients, be sure to wipe from the mons pubis toward the rectal area to avoid contaminating the genital area. Cover the pan, empty it, and place it in the soiled equipment area for resterilization. Remove the gloves and wash your hands.

IMAGING THE COLON

The colon can be imaged in several ways. All methods require the colon to be free of fecal material to best visualize the walls. Imaging procedures of the colon and rectum may include any of the following or in some circumstances, a combination of imaging studies:

- **Colonoscopy:** Performed by a gastroenterologist or surgeon and takes about 30 minutes. It is a procedure used to see inside the entire colon and rectum with a flexible tube that has a camera on the end and is placed through the anus.
- **Virtual colonoscopy:** Performed in computed tomography (CT) and takes approximately 5 minutes.

Virtual colonoscopy is a minimally invasive alternative to conventional colonoscopy (endoscopy) that screens the colon and rectum for polyps and early cancer before symptoms occur. Virtual colonoscopy involves no scopes, sedation, recovery time, or referral from your doctor or insurance plan. It is performed on a multislice CT scanner that takes up to 600 two-dimensional (2D) and three-dimensional (3D) images of the colon in just 30 seconds. The combination of 2D and 3D images increases the radiologist's ability to detect and analyze areas of concern. The 3D images allow the radiologist to reconstruct the colon and do a "fly-through" of its entire length, simulating the views of conventional colonoscopy.

- **Sigmoidoscopy:** Performed by a gastroenterologist or surgeon; is a procedure used to see inside the sigmoid colon and rectum with a flexible tube that has a camera on the end (sigmoidoscope) and is placed through the anus.
- **Barium** enema: Performed by a radiologist, radiologist assistant, or physician assistant. Barium is inserted through a tip in the rectum and fills the colon in a retrograde fashion. Barium enema procedures are ordered less frequently these days since the availability of other examinations like colonoscopy, CT imaging, and magnetic resonance imaging have become increasingly available and affordable.

Oil retention: This method uses an oil-based solution and permits administration of a small volume (120 to 140 mL) to be absorbed by the stool. For best results the solution should be retained for 1 hour if possible. The absorption of oil softens stool for easier evacuation.

Aspects of Bowel Preparation

Bowel preparation is the least standardized aspect of barium enema examinations, but it is also one of the most important. Slight variations in the bowel preparations occur, depending on the site performing the bowel evaluation and in some cases the history of the patient. Patients should be given written and verbal instructions for the preparation of having their bowel cleaned properly for the ensuing examination. Asking the patient to repeat the instructions is one good technique to ensure patient understanding. Do not assume that a simple *yes* really means that the patient understands the instructions. A phone number should be included so if they have any questions regarding the preparation and the examination they can have them answered after they leave the facility.

Most preparations consist of the following:

Dietary restrictions: Usually in the form of a minimal- or **low-residue diet**. This diet is designed to reduce the frequency and volume of stools while prolonging intestinal transit time. A low-residue diet is similar to a low-fiber diet, but typically includes restrictions on foods that increase bowel activity, such as milk and milk products, and also restricts the consumption of fruits and vegetables.

Purgation: Using a variety of laxatives, including castor oil, bisacodyl, Milk of Magnesia, or magnesium citrate to evacuate fecal material from the bowel.

Hydration: A clear liquid diet is often prescribed for the 24-hour period before a barium examination. This diet includes carbonated beverages, clear gelatin, clear broth, and coffee and tea with sugar. Whole-grain cereals, bread, vegetables, fried foods, and milk would be excluded. Clear liquids are easily absorbed by the body and reduce stimulation of the digestive system while leaving no residue in the intestinal tract. A diet of clear liquids maintains vital body fluids, salts, and minerals. Consumption of clear liquids also provides some energy for patients when normal food consumption must be interrupted.

Cleansing enemas: This technique is a liquid treatment most commonly used to relieve severe constipation. This process helps to eliminate waste when an individual cannot do so on their own Fig. 19.8. A variety of liquid enemas could be selected, from tap water, saline solutions, hypertonic solutions, and soap suds solutions. Enemas are available for purchase at pharmacies for home use, but discussion with a doctor or a nurse for specific instructions related to need and proper technique should be requested.

Patients with diabetes require special preparation. Diabetic low-calorie drinks may be added to the standard regimen, and patients with insulin-dependent diabetes often forgo their normal morning insulin dose until after the examination has been completed.

Older patients (particularly frail older adults) may require increased education and counseling for preparation for barium enemas because their familiarity with and ability to perform certain portions of the preparation may be compromised. If assessment indicates that the patient will not or may not be able to perform certain aspects of the preparation, then contacting the radiologist or the patient's referring physician may be necessary.

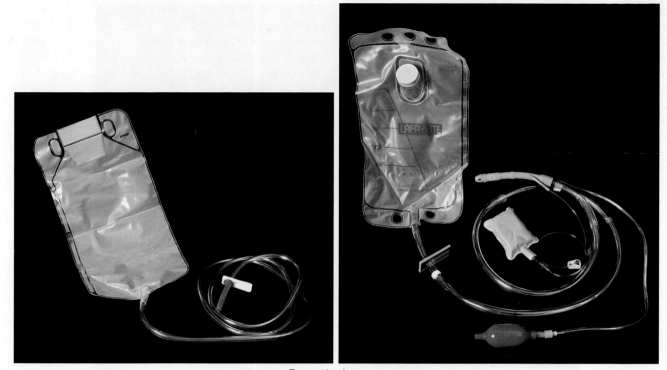

Fig. 19.8 Empty barium enema sets.

Also important to note is that *bowel* preparations and *people* preparations exist. That is, viewing the patient as a bowel rather than a person may lead to a substandard examination because of the lack of patient understanding and cooperation. If, in patient instruction, the radiologic technologist focuses on reciting facts rather than ensuring that the patient understands the preparation, the examination may be less than adequate as a result of poor preparation.

Clinical indications for a fluoroscopic contrast enema examination include, but are not limited to, the following:

- Diverticular disease
- Inflammatory bowel disease (ulcerative colitis or Crohn disease)
- Colon cancer screening
- Incomplete colonoscopy
- Distal intestinal obstruction syndrome or meconium ileus equivalent in cystic fibrosis patients
- Evaluation of questionable findings on other imaging examinations such as CT scanning
- Polyps

Contrast Agents Used in the Radiographic Examination of the Bowel

Barium sulfate is used to help doctors examine the esophagus, stomach, and intestine using x-rays or CT when bowel perforation is not suspected. Barium sulfate is in a class of medications called *radiopaque contrast media*. It works by coating the esophagus, stomach, or intestine with a material that is not absorbed into the body so that diseased or damaged areas can be clearly seen by x-ray examination or CT scan.

When perforation of the bowel is suspected, water-soluble iodine compounds are the only acceptable contrast media

(rather than barium). These compounds, such as diatrizoic acid (Gastrografin), are also used when a more viscous agent such as barium sulfate, which is not water-soluble, is not feasible or is potentially dangerous. Gastrografin does not coat the bowel as well as barium, so it is not commonly used. The situations to use this contrast would include: delineation of an anastomosis in the immediate preoperative period, or outlining of the distal colon and rectum in cases of megacolon and Hirschsprung disease. Hirschsprung disease occurs when nerve cells in the colon don't form completely. Nerves in the colon control the muscle contractions that move food through the bowels, so there is a decrease in the motility of the bowel and its contents. Megacolon and Hirschsprung disease can increase the chance for bowel impaction when barium sulfate is used. Water-soluble contrast agents are hypertonic, which means they draw fluid into the bowel. A hypertonic agent can cause diarrhea and a sudden reduction in blood volume and is particularly dangerous in neonates and in patients with Hirschsprung disease, so the use of this contrast must be done with care.

Barium Enema

For many years, barium enema was the only way to obtain a complete structural examination of the colon. Development of the double-contrast barium enema improved the ability of the method to identify subtle lesions. This is the only kind of barium enema that is appropriate for detecting polyps and potentially curable cancers. Today, colonoscopy, virtual colonoscopy, and magnetic resonance imaging are performed most often due to their overall effectiveness, especially in the identification of polyps, cancers, and detecting colitis.

The sensitivity for colonoscopy in the detection of cancerous and precancerous lesions has been estimated to be greater

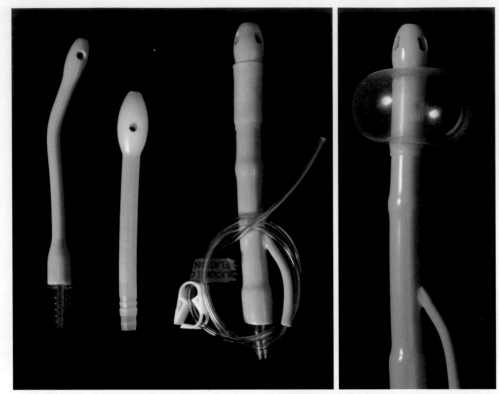

Fig. 19.9 *Left,* Plain barium enema tip. *Right,* Barium enema tip with an inflatable cuff.

than 95%. A major advantage of colonoscopy is that polyps can be excised during the procedure. Specimens that are removed are taken to the clinical laboratory to diagnose cell type.

A barium enema is administered in an examination to investigate and aid in the diagnosis of pathologic conditions that may affect the colon or lower gastrointestinal tract. Single-contrast or double-contrast barium enemas may be ordered.

To administer the barium sulfate solution into the rectum and through the colon, a catheter is needed to allow the viscose solution to travel throughout the large intestine. The catheter end may have a plain tip or an inflatable cuff (balloon) attached (Fig. 19.9). After the tip has been inserted, the cuff may be inflated to hold the catheter in place and to prevent involuntary expulsion of barium and the catheter itself.

Clinical indications for these procedures could include: identification of blood in the stool, abdominal pain, a change in bowel habits, or patients who cannot tolerate the sedation that is used for a colonoscopy.

Rectal tube insertion procedure:

1. Describe the insertion and enema procedure to the patient prior to continuing. Allow the patient time to ask any questions before starting.

2. Barium sulfate solutions are usually available in a prepared, prepackaged powder which must be mixed with water or a suspension (Fig. 19.10). The quantity of barium prepared is large. Most bags hold 3000 mL, although the quantity that is administered varies based on radiologist's techniques and preferences. The barium sulfate solutions should be well mixed. Suspend the bag and let some of the barium flow through the tubing to the tip to remove any air.

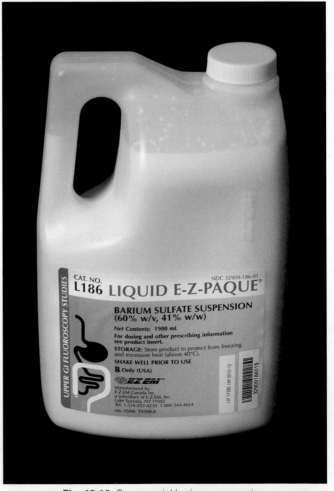

Fig. 19.10 Commercial barium suspension.

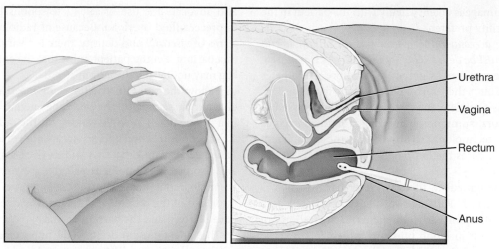

Fig. 19.11 Insertion of an enema tip. Lift the patient's right buttock with the heel of the hand to expose the anus. Insert the enema tip into the rectum toward the umbilicus (anteriorly and superiorly) no more than 3 or 4 inches.

3. Ask the patient to lie on their left side and flex the right knee and hip and place the knee on the table in front of them (Fig. 19.11). This is called the Sims' position.

4. Wear gloves and coat the enema tip well with a water-soluble lubricant.

5. Tell the patient that you are going to insert the tip and it may feel a bit cool. It is important to instruct the patient in the importance of keeping the tip firmly in the rectum. Advise the patient to relax and take in slow deep breaths. Lift the right buttock with the heel of your hand to expose the anus. When the patient exhales, insert the rectal tube gently into the anal orifice and direct the tube anteriorly 1 to 1½ inches (2.5 to 3.8 cm). The depth of the insertion should not exceed 1½ inches. DO NOT force the rectal (enema) tip. The tip of the rectal catheter needs to pass the anal sphincter to have it successfully inserted. If you encounter difficulty in inserting the tip, a qualified professional, such as a supervisor or the department nurse, should be asked to attempt the insertion.

6. After the tube is inserted you may want to tape the tube in place to prevent slipping. (Caution: some patients may be allergic to certain tape). If a retention balloon is being utilized on this tip, do not inflate the balloon unless directed by the radiologist.

7. Make sure that the stopcock is closed on the tubing so that no barium flows into the patient.

8. The patient may lie on their back while waiting for the radiologist.

9. Ensure that the enema bag is not more than 24 inches (60 cm) above the table.

10. Notify the radiologist that everything is ready for the examination.

11. The radiologist will inflate the rectal balloon if necessary, while observing with fluoroscopy to ensure placement proximal to the internal sphincter.

After the colon has been properly prepared, the barium enema or lower GI series begins by introducing barium (a naturally occurring metal that is used in barium sulfate as a contrast material) into the colon through the rectum. As the bowel is visualized with this contrast medium, multiple x-ray images are taken of the entire large bowel. Although it is safe to say that more double-contrast barium enemas examinations are ordered, there are basic reasons that a single-barium enema examination may be preferred in the following situations:

- suspected colon and rectal abnormalities can be identified (i.e., diverticulosis, diverticulitis)
- abnormal colon movements
- narrowing or dilation of the colon
- gross pathologic conditions need to be demonstrated
- when fistulas are thought to be present
- in children, when an intussusception needs to be reduced
- when a volvulus or acute obstruction is to be evaluated

Single-Contrast Barium Enemas

In a typical single-contrast barium enema, the bag containing barium is suspended from an IV pole higher than the level of the patient on the table. The suspension is run in slowly with compression applied to the abdomen. Because greater pressure is required to secure an adequate flow rate, the bag is usually suspended at a greater distance (up to 30 inches) above the table. Due to gravity, the higher the bag is positioned, the faster the suspension liquid enters the rectum and colon. Care must be taken with this due to cramping and the patient's ability to "hold" the enema long enough to completely fill the colon for proper assessment. Approximately 1500 mL of barium is required for the average adult barium enema. Spot views of the cecum, flexures, and sigmoid colon are taken. A variety of views of the abdomen (typically anteroposterior and posteroanterior), a 30-degree caudal angulation of the sigmoid colon, and a lateral rectal view are taken. At the completion of the examination, the excess barium is drained back into the bag that has been placed on the floor. The tip is removed, and the patient is sent to the toilet to evacuate as much of the barium as possible.

A post-evacuation image is taken, usually with the patient in the prone position (facility preference).

When removing a rectal catheter that has an inflatable cuff attached, the cuff must be deflated before the catheter is removed. The barium may be removed by gravity flow before the catheter tip is removed, and air is then permitted to escape from the cuff. After this activity is complete, the catheter is gently removed. If any resistance occurs, summoning another individual such as another radiologic technologist, a supervisor, the department nurse, or in extreme cases the radiologist, may be necessary to remove the catheter.

Always assist the patient to the toilet after barium enemas have been administered. Patients are often dehydrated as a result of the preparation for a barium enema. Dehydration can lead to a postural drop in blood pressure, which might cause the patient to become dizzy and fall. Allowing the patient to evacuate some of the barium into a bedpan before moving may be necessary. To administer the barium sulfate solution into the rectum and through the colon, a much larger catheter is required than is used for cleansing enemas to allow the barium, which is of greater viscosity, to be instilled into the lower bowel. The catheter may have a plain tip or an inflatable cuff (balloon) attached (see Fig. 19.9). After the tip has been inserted, the cuff may be inflated to hold the catheter in place and to prevent involuntary expulsion of barium.

The use of inflatable cuffs (balloon catheters) varies widely among facilities and physicians. Inflating the cuff is done routinely by some physicians, whereas others always use the cuff but inflate only when necessary. Still others believe inflatable cuffs should be used only when absolutely necessary. The most common complication of a barium enema is damage to the rectal wall from improper use of balloon catheters. Balloons should never be overinflated (the amount recommended varies from 30 to 90 mL of air) and are contraindicated in cases of rectal narrowing. Other complications include breaks in the gastrointestinal mucosa caused by trauma or disease, which permit barium to enter the peritoneal cavity or bloodstream. Disease conditions such as ulcers, cancer, and diverticulitis can create minute asymptomatic perforations that can erupt under pressure. Then peritonitis or venous emboli may cause serious complications, including death, fibrosis, and barium granuloma. In addition, allergic reactions to latex tips and cuffs have been reported, which has led to the use of alternative materials.

Barium sulfate solution is usually available in a prepared, prepackaged powder, which must be mixed with water or a suspension (Fig. 19.9). Barium sulfate solutions are also available premixed. Barium suspensions and solutions should have the following characteristics:

- Allow rapid flow
- Allow good adhesion to the mucosa for even coating
- Provide adequate radiographic density in a thin layer
- Lack foam or artifacts

The quantity of barium solution prepared is large. Most bags hold 3000 mL; the actual amount prepared varies. The barium solution may be prepared using warm or cold water. Advocates of the use of cold water maintain that this method reduces irritation to the colon and helps the patient *hold* the enema. Some people also advocate the use of salt (2 teaspoons/1000 mL of water) to prevent fluid overload. Because of radiologist preferences in terms of viscosity and density, there are various correct ways to mix barium. Let the patient know that the entire 3000 mL in the bag may not need to be administered.

Follow the same instructions for inserting the tip as were given in the section on the cleansing enema. The patient may lie in a supine position while waiting for the radiologist.

Patient instruction and reassurance are of utmost importance. Patients must know that they will receive a variety of instructions and also that the radiologist will give a variety of instructions to the radiographer that the patient may ignore. Patients need to be informed of the differences between the cleansing enemas they have received and the barium enema.

The patient must understand the importance of keeping the tip firmly in the rectum. The patient needs to be instructed to try to relax the abdominal muscles to reduce intraabdominal pressure and use deep oral breathing to aid in the prevention of spasms and cramps. As with the cleansing enema, the patient must be informed that the procedure will be suspended if cramping occurs. Student radiographers should carefully observe the interactions among radiographers, radiologists, and patients to develop their own style of patient instruction during the procedure. Although the basic information is consistent from patient to patient, the way it is communicated may vary according to the needs of each patient.

Double-Contrast Barium Enemas

In almost all facilities, the double-contrast barium enema (the addition of air or carbon dioxide to provide for two contrasts—barium and the air) has become more of a routine as compared to a single-contrast enema. This type is highly recommended for patients experiencing diarrhea and in high-risk patients—for example, the patient who has polyps, a family history of colorectal cancer, or a personal history of cancer or rectal bleeding. The patient often receives an injection of a smooth-muscle relaxant such as glucagon immediately before the examination to relieve bowel spasm. A typical routine for a double-contrast barium enema begins with the patient in a prone position and the table tilted slightly head-down. Barium (approximately 300 mL) is instilled into the splenic flexure, and air is then insufflated (added). This action pushes the barium to fill the transverse colon. The bag is lowered, and the head of the table is raised to drain the rectum, which also traps barium in the transverse colon. The patient may be turned to the right side and more air added to bring barium around the hepatic flexure. The patient then is turned prone to bring the barium to the cecum. Once the colon is filled with barium and distended with air, various radiographic views are taken.

Other means of performing double-contrast examinations described in the literature include Miller's seven-pump method; Pochazevsky and Sherman's single-stage, closed system; and Welin's double-stage or Malmo technique, in which the barium is added, the patient evacuates the barium, and air is added. Routines may vary among radiologists.

Postprocedural Instructions

Postprocedural instructions to the patient are extremely important after a barium enema because barium retention can cause fecal impaction or intestinal obstruction. Barium has hydroscopic qualities, which means that it will absorb fluid from the bowel. Extreme dehydration as a result of preparation for the examination is another possible postprocedural complication. Fluid imbalance may lead to altered mental status, especially in older adult patients.

Stools are typically white or light-colored until all of the barium is expelled. Some physicians regularly prescribe a laxative medication or an enema after barium studies. The patient's personal physician should be contacted if there is a lack of a bowel movement within 24 hours after the barium study. The importance of eliminating the barium cannot be stressed enough to the patient.

The patient should increase fluid intake and dietary fiber for several days unless medically contraindicated and should be instructed to rest after the examination. The personal physician should be contacted immediately if any of the following occurs:

- Weakness or fainting
- Abdominal pain, constipation, or rectal bleeding
- Not passing flatus
- Polyuria, nocturia, or abdominal distention

COLOSTOMIES

Because of trauma or a pathologic condition such as cancer, diverticulitis, and ulcerative colitis, formation of a stoma (mouth) from the bowel to the outside of the body may be necessary. A permanent colostomy is performed when a portion of bowel is removed. A temporary colostomy is performed to heal or rest a diseased portion of bowel.

Several types of colostomies have been developed. A *descending* or *sigmoid* colostomy is a permanent colostomy in which the diseased portion of the colon or rectum is removed. In a *transverse* colostomy, a portion of the transverse colon is removed. In a *double-barrel* colostomy, two stomas are formed: the proximal delivers stool, and the distal produces mucus. The longer a colostomy has been in place, the greater will be the consistency of stool.

The radiologic and imaging sciences professional must recognize that an ostomy produces a major change in a patient's body image and that many persons with new colostomies go through the grieving process. The loss of a bowel can be viewed in the same light as any other loss, including death—that is, patients typically pass through various stages, including denial, anger, bargaining, depression, and finally acceptance.

Caring for a patient with a new ostomy requires sensitivity and a matter-of-fact attitude, two seemingly separate entities, both of which must be reconciled for effective care of the ostomy patient. Barbara Mullen, author of *The Ostomy Book* and an ostomate, has said that she appreciated plain speaking over half-hearted platitudes after her own ostomy. The patient can negatively interpret even a hint of revulsion or hesitancy. The radiologic technology student who has never seen an ostomy should observe routines until technical competency, a matter-of-fact attitude (plain speaking), and sensitivity can be combined.

A patient with a colostomy needs special instructions for adequate preparation. In most patients, the stoma is irrigated the night before and the morning of the examination. Irrigation is a type of *enema* for the colostomy that should prevent the expulsion of feces for 24 hours. Dietary and laxative preparations also vary, depending on the ostomy. The ostomate must be instructed, for example, not to take bismuth subgallate tablets—as he or she may normally do to control odor—because these are radiopaque. If available, an enterostomal therapist instructs the patient in preparation. Patients with an ostomy should be instructed to bring an extra pouch with them if they are coming from outside the hospital.

Administering a Barium Enema to a Patient With a Colostomy

The majority of colostomies are performed because of cancerous conditions. Approximately 10% of patients have their bowels removed owing to the recurrence of their cancer, which necessitates follow-up studies.

The radiographic evaluation of the small and large bowel that has been connected to the skin surface as a substitute for the urinary bladder with an ostomy is typically called a loopogram. Obstruction, inflammatory bowel disease, and lesions of the bowel wall such as diverticula, polyps, or certain types of cancers may be the focus of the study; in cases of temporary ostomy placement, examining the bowel before reconnection may also be completed, with subsequent ostomy removal. Wound infection is the most common complication of these procedures.

The patient with a colostomy will have a dressing or drainage pouch securely positioned over the area of the stoma. The dressing must be removed by a radiologic technologist wearing clean gloves and then placed in a plastic bag and discarded in a receptacle intended for contaminated waste. The gloves are then removed, and the hands are washed. A drainage pouch should be removed and set aside in a safe place to be reused after the examination. Gloves are put on again. The patient may want to perform this action or provide direction for the procedure. The pouch must be kept clean and dry.

The procedure for administering a barium enema to a patient with a colostomy differs somewhat from that for the regular examination because of the lack of a sphincter. The main problem with barium administration through a colostomy is trying to prevent leakage without damaging the colostomy. A cone-shaped tip with a long drainage bag that attaches to it is frequently preferred. Nipple colostomy tips and double-barrel (dual tubing that allows for simultaneous study of the proximal and distal colonic loops) colostomy tips are also available. A small catheter with an inflatable cuff is used in some cases. If the patient has had the ostomy for some time, self-insertion of the tip may be preferred.

The radiologic technologist typically lubricates the tip of the cone and hands it to the patient for insertion. If the patient is unable to perform the insertion, the radiologist, who also tapes the device in place, performs the task. Clean disposable gloves should be worn. A much smaller amount of barium solution is often needed, especially when the study is performed for the distal portion of the remaining colon.

The diagnostic procedure is similar to that for other patients once the cone or catheter has been inserted. An intravenous smooth-muscle relaxant is typically necessary to prevent peristalsis, which continually empties the colon. Approximately 250 mL of barium is usually used. Care must be taken not to over distend the colon if air insufflation is used. Prone views are not performed so as not to traumatize the stoma site.

On completion of the procedure, the drainage bag can be attached to the cone and the barium drained. When the drainage is complete, the ambulatory patient can be escorted to the toilet with the drainage bag still in place to be cleaned; the ostomy pouch is then replaced.

Ostomates are often independent if they have had the ostomy for a long time. The patient must be allowed a certain degree of self-control in addition to the direction given to the patient by the radiologic technologist and the physician.

SUMMARY

- NG tubes, male urinals, bedpans, enemas, and colostomies are a part of the daily practice of a radiologic and imaging sciences professional. The detailed routines are described here as they are commonly performed in hospitals and other health care facilities; the actual routine at any given institution may vary slightly.
- The radiologic technologist is most likely to encounter Levin tubes and Salem Sump NG tubes. Patients with NG tubes in place usually experience discomfort and require a great deal of assurance. The radiographer may assist in inserting NG tubes and is sometimes responsible for their removal. Before transporting a patient with an NG tube, the radiographer must ascertain the length of time for which suction may be discontinued.
- Urinals are used by male patients who are unable to walk or stand for urination. These urinals must be rinsed between uses by the same patient and sterilized after each patient. Female urinals are available for those who can stand, but these are not typical. Bedpans are used by female patients for urination and defecation and by male patients for defecation only. The two basic types are the standard bedpan and the fracture bedpan. It is extremely important to maintain a patient's sense of dignity and privacy when he or she is using a bedpan.
- Typical bowel preparations include: dietary restrictions, purgation, hydration, and cleansing enemas. The radiologic and imaging sciences professional focuses on patient understanding of the procedure rather than simply reciting facts to the patient.
- The barium enema is given in an examination to diagnose potential pathologic conditions of the colon.
- The barium sulfate mixture that is used is more viscous than water and is administered differently from the water enema/cleansing enema. It is important to give the patient necessary instructions before, during, and after the procedure to ensure a diagnostic outcome without postprocedural complications. The two main types of barium enemas are the single-contrast examination, in which only barium is used, and the double-contrast examination, in which both barium and air are used to define the colon.

- Colostomies are formed by bringing a portion of the colon to the outside in the form of a stoma, or mouth. The radiologic technologist gains an understanding of the special care that is often required by patients with ostomies through observation and experience. It is important to allow the patient as much control as possible while maintaining control over the examination. It is also important that the radiologic technologist combine technical competency, a matter-of-fact attitude (plain speaking), and sensitivity toward a patient with an ostomy. Owing to the lack of a sphincter and sensitivity of the stoma site, the administration of a barium enema in a patient with a colostomy is different from that in a regular patient.

BIBLIOGRAPHY

American College of Radiology: ACR practice guidelines for the performance of fluoroscopic contrast enema examinations in adult, Reston Va, 2013, The College.

American College of Radiology: ACR appropriateness criteria, Reston Va, 2013, The College.

Best C: Nasogastric tube insertion in adults who require enteral feeding, *Nurs Stand* 21:39, 2007.

Bourgualt A, Haulm M: Assessing placement of feeding tubes, *Am J Crit Care* 18:73, 2009.

Craig M: *Introduction to ultrasonography and patient care*, ed 3, Philadelphia, 2013, Saunders.

Ehrlich RA, Daly J: *Patient care in radiography*, ed 8, St. Louis, 2012, Mosby.

Frank ED, Long BW, Smith BJ: *Merrill's atlas of radiographic positioning and procedures* (vol 1), ed 12, St. Louis, 2011, Mosby.

Grigoleit HG, Grigoleit P: Gastrointestinal clinical pharmacology of peppermint oil, *Phytomedicine* 12:607, 2005.

Hirofuji Y, Aoyama T, Koyama S, Kawaura C, Fujii K: Evaluation of patient dose for barium enemas and CT colonography in Japan, *Br J Radiol* 82:219–227, 2009.

Kim HJ, Kim AY, Lee CW, et al.: Hirschsprung disease and hypoganglionosis in adults: radiologic findings and differentiation, *Radiology* 247(2):428–434, 2008.

Mullen BD, McGinn KA: *The ostomy book: living comfortably with colostomies, iliostomies and urostomies*, ed 3, Palo Alto, Calif, 2008, Bull.

Mulhall BP, Veerappan GR, Jackson JL: Metaanalysis: computed tomographic colonography, *Ann Intern Med* 142:635–650, 2005.

Neri E, Faggioni L, Cerri F, et al.: CT colonography versus double-contrast barium enema for screening of colorectal cancer: comparison of radiation burden, *Abdom Imaging* 35:596, 2010.

Phillips NM: Nasogastric tubes: an historical context, *Medsurg Nurs* 15:84, 2006.

Rockey DC, Paulson E, Niedzwiecki D, et al.: Analysis of air contrast barium enema, computed tomographic colonography, and colonoscopy: prospective comparison, *Lancet* 365:305, 2005.

Sadovsky R: Nebulized lidocaine and nasogastric tube insertion, *Am Fam Physician* 71:1807, 2005.

Stevenson G: Colon imaging in radiology departments in 2008: goodbye to the routine double contrast barium enema, *Canadian Assoc of Rad* 59:174–182, 2008.

Takwoingi YM, Demspter JH: A simple technique for nasogastric feeding tube insertion, *Eur Arch Otorhinolaryngol* 262:423, 2005.

Torres LS, Dutton AE, Watson TA: *Patient care in imaging technology*, ed 8, Philadelphia, 2013, Lippincott.

Winawer SJ, Stewart ET, Zauber AG, et al.: A comparison of colonoscopy and double-contrast barium enema for surveillance after polypectomy, *N Engl J Med* 342:1766, 2000.

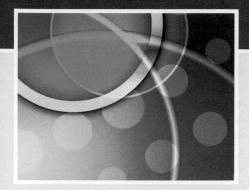

Medical Emergencies

Joanne S. Greathouse, EdS, RT(R), FASRT, FAEIRS

Important to proper evaluation of the critically ill patient is a spirit of cooperation and ongoing communication.

Lawrence Goodman and Charles Putman
Intensive Care Radiology, 1978

OBJECTIVES

On completion of this chapter, the student will be able to:
- Define terms related to medical emergencies.
- List the objectives of first aid.
- List general priorities for working with patients in acute situations.
- Explain the purpose of an emergency cart and its contents.
- Differentiate between the two primary types of external cardiac defibrillators.
- Explain the four levels of consciousness.
- Describe the signs and symptoms of various medical emergencies.

- Discuss methods of avoiding factors that contribute to shock.
- Discuss factors that contribute to the development of hypoglycemia.
- Describe the appropriate procedure for handling patients with various medical emergencies.
- Describe the correct procedure for administration of cardiopulmonary resuscitation.
- Describe the general procedure for the use of an automatic external cardiac defibrillator.
- Demonstrate appropriate principles of cardiopulmonary resuscitation.

OUTLINE

KEY TERMS

Aura Subjective sensation or motor phenomenon that precedes and marks the onset of a paroxysmal attack, such as an epileptic attack

Automatic External Defibrillators (AEDs) Device used for application of external electrical shock to restore normal cardiac rhythm and rate

Cardiac Arrest Sudden stoppage of cardiac output and effective circulation

Cardiopulmonary Resuscitation (CPR) Artificial substitution of heart and lung action as indicated for cardiac arrest or apparent sudden death resulting from electric shock, drowning, respiratory arrest, and other causes

Cerebrovascular Accident (Stroke or Brain Attack) Condition with sudden onset caused by acute vascular lesions of the brain; often followed by permanent neurologic damage

Emergency Unexpected or sudden occasion; an urgent or pressing need

Epistaxis Nosebleed; hemorrhage from the nose

Hemorrhage Escape of blood from the vessels; bleeding

Hyperglycemia Abnormally increased concentration of glucose in the blood

Hypoglycemia Abnormally diminished concentration of glucose in the blood

Lethargy Abnormal drowsiness or stupor; a condition of indifference

Nausea Unpleasant sensation, vaguely referred to the epigastrium and abdomen and often culminating in vomiting

Pallor Paleness; absence of skin coloration

Shock Condition of profound hemodynamic and metabolic disturbance characterized by failure of the circulatory system to maintain adequate perfusion of vital organs

Syncope Temporary suspension of consciousness as a result of generalized cerebral ischemia; faint or swoon

Urticaria Vascular reaction, usually transient, involving the upper dermis, representing localized edema caused by dilatation and increased permeability of the capillaries and marked by the development of wheals; also called hives

Ventricular Fibrillation Disorganized cardiac rhythm

Vertigo Illusion of movement; sensation as if the external world were revolving around the patient or as if the patient were revolving in space

Vomiting Forcible expulsion of the contents of the stomach through the mouth

Wounds Bodily injuries caused by physical means with disruption of the normal continuity of structures

Wound Dehiscence Separation of the layers of a surgical wound; may be partial, superficial only, or complete, with disruption of all layers

MEDICAL EMERGENCY

Definition and Objectives of First Aid

An **emergency** is a situation in which the condition of a patient or a sudden change in medical status requires immediate action. Emergency actions on the part of the radiologic technologist generally have the objectives of preserving life, avoiding further harm to the patient, and obtaining appropriate medical assistance as quickly as possible. Although instances in which a radiologic technologist is required to initiate emergency measures are infrequent, the technologist must be able to recognize emergency situations, maintain a calm and confident presence, and take appropriate action. The recognition of need for assistance is a critical first step; the technologist must be able to recognize when such assistance might be warranted.

General Priorities

Although most patients are sent to the radiology department only after their condition has been stabilized, some patients are not in a stable condition and the status of others may change while they are in the department. Radiologic technologists should never underestimate their ability to contribute to a patient's survival and well-being through quick thinking and appropriate action. The technologist should keep in mind the following priorities when working with patients in emergency situations:

1. Ensure an open airway
2. Control bleeding
3. Take measures to prevent or treat shock
4. Attend to wounds or fractures
5. Provide emotional support
6. Continually reevaluate and follow up appropriately

Emergency Cart

Familiarity with the location of emergency equipment in the radiology department is an important part of being able to respond appropriately. Most radiology departments have at least one emergency cart (often referred to as a *crash cart*). This cart is a wheeled container of equipment and drugs typically required in emergency situations (Fig. 20.1).

The cart itself and its contents—drugs and equipment needed to handle typical life-threatening emergencies—are similar but not identical from one institution to another (Box 20.1). The ready availability of emergency equipment and drugs reduces the time required to respond to a medical crisis. A radiologic technologist's orientation to a department should include learning the location of emergency carts and becoming familiar with the contents and organization of the carts at that particular institution.

Automatic External Defibrillator

Increasingly, radiology departments and other public places have automatic external defibrillators (AEDs) available. This movement has been identified as public access defibrillation and has resulted in significant reduction in mortality from cardiac arrhythmia. AEDs come in the following two primary types:

1. Fully automatic defibrillators, which analyze the patient's cardiac rhythm, determine whether defibrillation is necessary, and, if necessary, deliver a shock
2. Semiautomatic defibrillators, which analyze the patient's cardiac rhythm, determine whether defibrillation is necessary, and, if necessary, advise the operator to deliver a shock by pushing a button

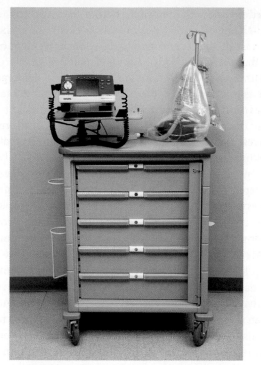

Fig. 20.1 A typical emergency crash cart.

BOX 20.1	**Equipment and Drugs Typically Found on an Emergency Cart**

Standard Equipment

Backboard
Stethoscope
Blood pressure cuff
Ambu bag
Laryngoscope
Flashlight
Batteries
Extension cord
Oxygen flow meter
Tourniquet
Airways
Endotracheal tubes
Nasopharyngeal tubes
Suction catheters
Levine tubing
Jelco cannulas
Tracheal tubes
Cutdown tray
Suction bottle
Hemostat
Scissors
Sterile gloves, various sizes
Syringes, various sizes
Needles, various sizes
Stopcocks and connectors
Tongue blades
Sterile gauze
Adhesive and paper tape
Alcohol swabs
Surgical lubricant
Blood collection tubes

Emergency Drugs Commonly Found on a Crash Cart

Medication	Indication
Adenosine (Adenocard)	Arrhythmias
Amiodarone (Cordarone)	Arrhythmias
Atropine	Bradycardia
Dexamethasone (Decadron)	Allergic reaction
Diphenhydramine (Benadryl)	Allergic reaction
Dobutamine (Dobutrex)	Shock
Dopamine	Shock
Epinephrine	Cardiac arrest, anaphylaxis
Furosemide (Lasix)	Edema
Norepinephrine	Shock
Phenytoin (Dilantin)	Seizures
Procainamide (Pronestyl)	Arrhythmias
Sodium bicarbonate	Metabolic acidosis
Verapamil	Arrhythmias

If such devices are available in the hospital, the technologist should become familiar with the type and specific model, given that each operates somewhat differently.

HEAD INJURIES

Victims of head trauma are often seen in the radiology department. Although diagnosing head injuries is not the responsibility of the radiologic technologist, having knowledge of categorization is useful so that a basic assessment can be made and changes in a patient's status noted. Of the several ways to categorize head injuries, the simplest form of classification is by level of consciousness.

Levels of Consciousness

The patient with the least severe injury is classified as alert and conscious. In most instances, this patient can respond fully to questions and other stimuli. A more seriously injured patient is drowsy but can be roused to response with loud speaking or gentle physical contact. Even more serious injury produces a patient who is unconscious and reacts only to painful stimuli. These patients typically do not respond to verbal stimuli but react to stimuli such as pinches and pinpricks. The most serious condition is that of a patient who is comatose and unresponsive to virtually all stimuli.

Indications of Deteriorating Situations

The technologist should quickly assess a patient when the procedure is begun so that it is readily noticeable if the patient deteriorates from one level of consciousness to another. Findings in an alert or drowsy patient that can signify a deteriorating head injury include irritability, lethargy, slowing pulse rate, and slowing respiratory rate.

When working with an intoxicated patient with a head injury, the technologist is cautioned against assuming that the patient has passed out merely from inebriation. If any doubt exists about the cause of the patient's loss of consciousness, assuming the head injury is more serious and obtaining medical assistance are far better than for a patient to needlessly undergo further deterioration.

Response to Deteriorating Situations

If the radiologic technologist recognizes a deteriorating head injury, the first priority is maintaining an open airway while moving the patient as little as possible. The radiologic procedure should be stopped and medical assistance obtained quickly. The technologist should obtain the patient's vital signs while waiting for help to arrive.

SHOCK

Definition and Types

Another situation typically encountered with emergency patients is shock. **Shock** is a general term that indicates a failure of the circulatory system to support vital body functions. The following types of shock can occur:

Hypovolemic shock, caused by loss of blood or tissue fluid

Cardiogenic shock, caused by a variety of cardiac disorders, including myocardial infarction

Neurogenic shock, caused by spinal anesthesia or damage to the upper spinal cord

Vasogenic shock, caused by sepsis, deep anesthesia, or anaphylaxis

The technologist is most likely to encounter hypovolemic shock or anaphylactic shock, a special type of vasogenic shock, as a result of reaction to contrast media administered in the course of a radiologic procedure.

Prevention

Several factors can contribute to the likelihood that a patient will experience shock or to the degree of shock experienced. Any sudden change in body temperature is one such factor. This change illustrates the importance of keeping patients covered to maintain normal body temperature; to avoid overheating the patient is equally important.

Pain, stress, and anxiety also contribute to the development of shock. Not only is handling patients gently during a procedure an important aspect of good psychologic care, but it also can be a factor in the patient's physical condition. The technologist should also work calmly and confidently, even in a situation of maximum stress; this demeanor helps reassure emergency patients and can contribute to their overall physiologic well-being.

Signs and Symptoms

Signs and symptoms that a patient might be going into shock include restlessness, apprehension or general anxiety, tachycardia, decreasing blood pressure, cold and clammy skin, and **pallor**. If the radiologic technologist believes that such a situation is developing, he or she should stop the procedure, ensure maintenance of the patient's body temperature, call for medical assistance, and measure the patient's vital signs while awaiting assistance.

Contrast Media Reactions (Anaphylactic Shock)

Anaphylactic shock is a type of vasogenic shock and is most commonly encountered in the radiology department in connection with the administration of iodinated contrast media. Although a great deal of debate exists about the nature of contrast media reactions, at least some agreement has been found that these reactions have an element of an allergic reaction. Although such reactions are not common, neither are they so rare as to warrant complacency on the part of the technologist. Reaction to contrast media can range from mild to severe. Because the most severe reaction can result in death from cardiac arrest, contrast media should not be administered without first taking an adequate history.

In general, the longer it takes for a reaction to develop, the less severe it is. Accordingly, the most severe reactions typically arise very quickly. A possibility exists, however, for a severe delayed reaction to occur. Thus, it is important to constantly monitor patients who have had contrast media injections.

Mild reactions are similar to other allergic reactions. Patients develop localized itching and **urticaria** (hives) and may experience nausea and vomiting. Generalized itching and hives are indicative of a systemic reaction, which is generally more serious than most mild reactions. Although none of these reactions is serious in and of itself, they may signal the onset of a more serious reaction. The physician should be notified immediately in the event of any reaction. In most instances, a mild antihistamine is administered to counter the allergic reaction.

The most serious reactions might include laryngeal edema, shock, and cardiac arrest. All of these conditions are life-threatening and should be handled accordingly. The physician must be notified at once and vital signs taken. Patients with cardiac arrest should be treated with cardiopulmonary resuscitation (CPR) which is discussed later in this chapter.

DIABETIC CRISES

Many patients who undergo radiologic procedures are required to have had gastrointestinal (GI) preparation, which might include a special diet or fasting. Most patients can tolerate this preparation fairly easily (if not necessarily comfortably), but such alterations in dietary patterns can be particularly troublesome for patients with diabetes.

In the healthy patient, the body adjusts its insulin production and excretion to meet the demands made on it by the body's intake of carbohydrate. In some patients with diabetes (type 1, typically juvenile onset), however, the insulin is given exogenously, and the patient must adjust dietary intake to balance the insulin taken. The GI preparation can create havoc with this balance.

Hypoglycemia

Hypoglycemia is a condition in which excessive insulin is present. This excess insulin can be the result of a patient taking the usual dose of insulin before a GI study and then not having a normal breakfast. The brain requires glucose for normal metabolism. If no food is eaten, then the administered insulin depletes the body's energy store, leading fairly quickly to insulin shock (sometimes called an *insulin reaction*). Patients who are experiencing this condition are intensely hungry, weak, and shaky and may sweat excessively. They also may become confused and irritable, sometimes to the point of aggression and mild hostility. Most patients, especially those who have lived with the condition for a time, recognize the condition before it becomes serious. The patient needs a quick form of carbohydrate. Some patients carry glucose tablets with them.

If these tablets are not available, then any form of carbohydrate should be administered as long as the patient is conscious. Orange juice sweetened with sugar, a sugared soft drink, a candy bar, or any form of carbohydrate can be consumed. Because physical activity continues to deplete the patient's energy stores, the patient should be encouraged to sit quietly until the food has had a chance to take effect, usually 10 to 15 minutes. No food or fluid should be given to an unconscious patient. If a patient with hypoglycemia becomes unconscious, immediate medical attention is required.

Hyperglycemia

Hyperglycemia is a condition of excessive sugar in the blood and is the characteristic typically associated with diabetes. This condition develops gradually, generally over a period of hours or days, so it is not likely to be noticed by a technologist. These patients exhibit excessive thirst and urination, dry mucosa, rapid and deep breathing, and drowsiness and confusion. The condition leads to diabetic coma if left untreated. The patient needs insulin; if this condition is believed to be present, the technologist should get medical help.

RESPIRATORY DISTRESS AND RESPIRATORY ARREST

Asthma

Respiratory distress is another medical crisis that occasionally occurs in the radiology department. Asthma attacks are often triggered in asthmatic patients when they are exposed to stressful situations, such as might be experienced in a radiology department. A patient in respiratory distress generally exhibits wheezing, a result of dilatation of bronchi on inspiration and collapse on exhalation. Because asthma is a chronic condition, many patients carry an aerosol inhaler or other form of bronchodilator. The radiologic technologist should stop the procedure, assist the patient to a sitting position to support easier respiration, and attempt to reassure the patient. If the patient has medications available, then the technologist should allow the patient to use them. If not, then medical assistance should be obtained.

A calm, confident manner is important when faced with a patient having an asthma attack. When the patient begins to exhibit respiratory distress, the anxiety is likely to increase, which further interferes with respiratory function. The technologist's calm handling of the situation not only comforts the patient but may also be a factor in limiting the severity of the problem.

Choking

Radiologic technologists should also be familiar with the Heimlich maneuver. This maneuver is used in situations in which a person appears to be choking. The technologist should first

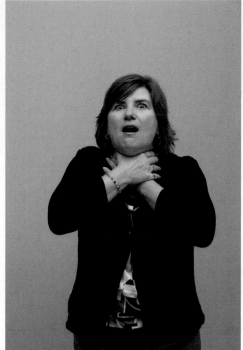

Fig. 20.2 The universal distress signal for choking.

ascertain that the patient is choking by asking the question, "Can you speak?" Patients with partial obstruction can verbalize their problem, but complete obstruction prevents the patient from speaking. A person who is choking and cannot verbalize a response generally clutches the throat with both hands and becomes red in the face. This signal is the universal distress signal for choking (Fig. 20.2). In cases of either partial or complete obstruction, the patient should be encouraged to cough. If coughing is unsuccessful in dislodging the obstruction, the Heimlich maneuver should be used.

Heimlich Maneuver

The purpose of the Heimlich maneuver (abdominal thrusts) is to increase intrathoracic pressure sufficiently to propel the lodged object out of the throat. To apply, the rescuer stands behind the victim and wraps both arms around him or her, clutching one fist with the other hand. The thumb side of the fist is placed in the midline of the victim's abdomen, above the navel and well below the sternum. With the rescuer's elbows held out from the victim, pressure is exerted inward and upward (Fig. 20.3). Although each thrust should be administered separately, the procedure may be repeated quickly 6 to 10 times or until the obstructing object is expelled.

An unconscious patient should be placed in the supine position. If the foreign object is visible in the open mouth, the rescuer should perform a finger sweep (Fig. 20.4). If the object is not visible, or if the finger sweep is unsuccessful, the rescuer should begin CPR (described in the next section). Research has shown that CPR is more effective than abdominal thrusts in increasing intrathoracic pressure. The mouth should be checked for presence of the foreign body before each set of ventilations during CPR. These maneuvers should not be used with women in advanced

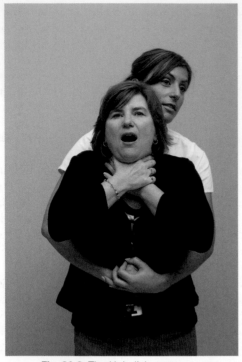

Fig. 20.3 The Heimlich maneuver.

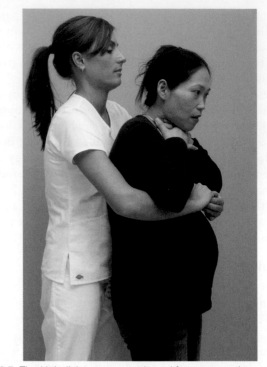

Fig. 20.5 The Heimlich maneuver adapted for a woman in an advanced stage of pregnancy.

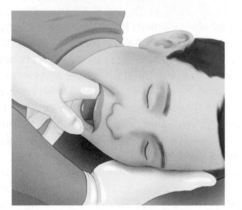

Fig. 20.4 Finger sweep of an unconscious choking patient.

stages of pregnancy or with infants or small children. Variations of the Heimlich maneuver have been developed for such patients.

Modification for Pregnant Patients. Because abdominal thrusts can be dangerous for women in late stages of pregnancy, chest thrusts are used instead. The rescuer again stands behind the patient but places his or her arms under the victim's armpits and around the victim's chest. The thumb side of the fist is placed in the center of the sternum; the second hand is placed over the fist, and backward thrusts are given (Fig. 20.5).

Modification for Infants. In infants younger than 1 year old, a combination of back blows and chest thrusts is recommended. The infant is held by the rescuer along his or her arm with the head lower than the trunk and supported by holding the victim's jaw. With the arm holding the infant resting on the rescuer's thigh, the rescuer uses the heel of the hand to deliver four back blows between the infant's scapulae. While the rescuer continues

to support the head and neck, the infant is turned over, and four chest thrusts are given with two or three fingers (Fig. 20.6). To determine the location of the hand for chest thrusts, the index finger is placed on the sternum just below the intermammary line. Two or three fingers are used to perform the chest thrusts.

CARDIAC ARREST

Signs and Symptoms

Cardiac arrest is the sudden stoppage of cardiac output and leads to permanent organ damage or death if not treated. Death from cardiac arrest has been reduced significantly since the advent of **cardiopulmonary resuscitation (CPR)** and the more recent availability of **automatic external defibrillators (AEDs)**. Patients who are experiencing cardiac arrest generally report crushing chest pain, often described as feeling as though an elephant is standing on the victim's chest. Pain may also radiate down the left arm. However, symptoms may differ significantly.

Cardiopulmonary Resuscitation

The radiologic technologist should be familiar with an institution's protocol for cardiac emergencies. On realization that a patient has experienced cardiac arrest, the rescuer should initiate the appropriate alert before beginning CPR.

Because cerebral function is generally impaired if the brain is deprived of oxygen for more than 4 to 6 minutes, CPR must be initiated immediately on verifying that cardiopulmonary distress exists, but these procedures absolutely must be performed only after determining that true cardiopulmonary distress exists. In October 2010, new guidelines for CPR were released by the American Heart Association. The most significant change is the order in which CPR is started. CPR provides external support

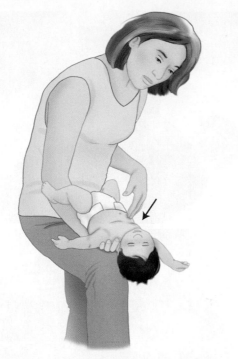

Fig. 20.6 The Heimlich maneuver on an infant. Position the infant face up over the forearm. Use two or three fingers to perform the *abdominal thrust.*

for circulation and respiration and consists of three primary aspects—historically known as the ABCs: *a*irway, *b*reathing, and *c*hest compressions. New guidelines have replaced the ABC order with CAB emphasizing the need, particularly for the non-health care provider, to start chest compressions first. The initial process should begin with 30 compressions at a rate of 100 to 120 compressions/minute followed by the establishment of an airway and rescue breathing. The following abbreviated protocol is based on the standards and guidelines of the American Heart Association and can be found at http://www.heart.org.

One-Person Rescue.

1. *Establish unresponsiveness* by gently shaking and shouting at the victim (Fig. 20.7A). If these actions fail to rouse the person, call for help and proceed with CPR.
2. *Position the patient* on his or her back on a hard surface to facilitate CPR. A radiographic table is suitable. If the patient is lying on a stretcher, then the backboard from the emergency cart should be used.
3. *Perform chest compressions* by positioning yourself to one side of the patient and placing the hands properly. This action is done by using the hand to find the lower edge of the rib cage and running the middle and index fingers along the lower edge to the point where the ribs meet the sternum. Place the middle finger at this notch, and then place the heel of the other hand on the sternum next to the index finger (see Fig. 20.7B). The heel of the hand should rest along the length of the sternum. The other hand is placed on top of the first, and the fingers of both are interlaced and extended to prevent their tips from applying inadvertent pressure on the ribs (see Fig. 20.7C). The elbows are

locked with the arms extended directly over the patient's sternum, and compression is applied straight down from the shoulders (see Fig. 20.7D). The force applied should be smooth and sufficient to depress the sternum a minimum of 2 inches in an adult. Pressure should be released after each compression to allow the sternum to return to its original position, but the hands should not be lifted from the sternum. Thirty compressions should be alternated with two ventilations; the compressions are given at a rate of approximately 100/min.

4. *Open the airway* by tilting the head back, which helps prevent the tongue from falling back and obstructing the airway. Place one hand on the victim's forehead and apply firm backward pressure while placing the fingers of the other hand beneath the bony part of the chin and lifting upward (see Fig. 20.7E). The lips should be close together, but the mouth should not be completely closed.
5. *Establish breathlessness* by placing an ear over the patient's nose and mouth and looking toward the patient's chest (see Fig. 20.7F). In this position, listen for breath sounds, look for any rise and fall in the chest, and feel for flow of air from the victim's nose. If no breath is apparent, then proceed with rescue breathing.
6. *Perform rescue breathing* by putting the palm of the hand on the victim's forehead and using the thumb and fingers to pinch the victim's nostrils shut. Place a facemask tightly over the nose and mouth and take a deep breath (see Fig. 20.7G). Initially, blow two deep breaths, each of 1-second duration, into the mask, while watching to determine whether the chest is rising and falling. Then take another breath between the ventilations. The breaths should not be rapid or forceful. If the mouth is damaged or clogged, sealing the victim's mouth closed and sealing the mask around the nose of the victim is possible (see Fig. 20.7H).
7. *Establish circulatory inadequacy* by palpating the carotid artery (see Fig. 20.7I). If after 5 to 10 seconds the pulse is absent, then proceed with continued closed chest compressions.
8. Continue to perform chest compressions as detailed in step 3.
9. *Reassess* after five complete cycles of compressions and ventilations (30:2 ratio), by taking no more than 7 seconds to reevaluate the patient. If breathing and pulse are still absent, then continue CPR, checking every few minutes for the return of pulse and breathing.

Two-Person Rescue. The protocol for CPR with two rescuers is similar, but each rescuer independently performs compressions or ventilations with periodic switches of position. One rescuer is at the victim's side and performs chest compressions. The second rescuer is at the victim's head and maintains the open airway and provides breathing, usually mouth to mask (Fig. 20.8).

Compressions are delivered at the rate of approximately 100/min, with cycles of 30 compressions and two breaths. The breaths are given during pauses in compression and should be of approximately 1-second duration. When rescuers become fatigued, an organized switch of positions should take place.

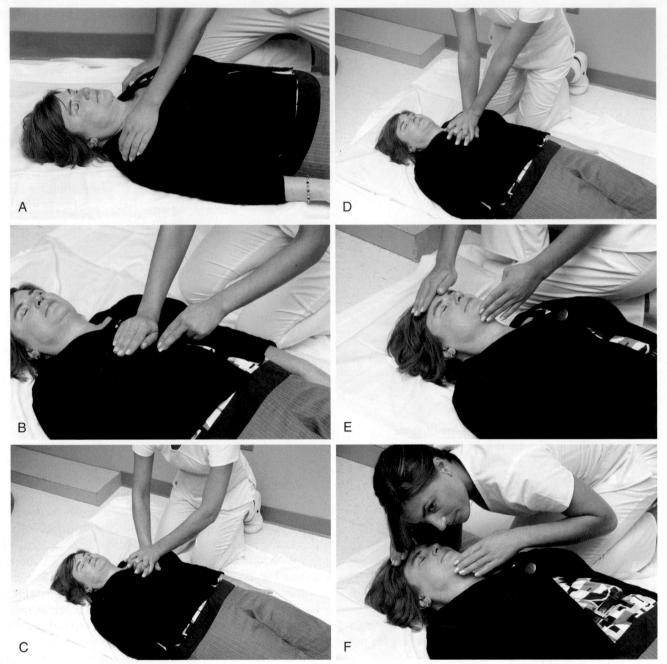

Fig. 20.7 Cardiopulmonary resuscitation: one-person rescue. (A) Establishing unresponsiveness of victim. (B) Correct placement of hand along sternum. (C) Correct placement of hands for external chest compressions. (D) Locked elbows with the arms extended directly over the patient's sternum to apply compression straight down from the shoulders. (E) Head tilt-chin lift maneuver. (F) Proper position for establishing breathlessness.

Infant Rescue. The CPR procedure for infants and children is basically the same as that for adults, with adjustments made in the volume of air delivered during artificial breathing, the placement of the hands, and the depth of depression of the sternum during external chest compressions. When a rescuer is breathing for a pediatric victim, the volume of air should be just enough to cause the rise and fall of the chest.

In performance of chest compressions on infants, the index finger should be placed on the sternum just under the point where it intersects with the intermammary line. Using the third

and fourth fingers, compress the sternum to a depth of ½ to 1 inch at a rate of 100/min. In infants and children, two ventilations are given after 30 compressions. For a child up to 8 years of age, the hand placement is the same as for an adult. The chest, however, is typically compressed with only one hand to a depth of only 1 to 1½ inches, although two hands may be required if the child's size indicates it.

Considerations. CPR is not indicated in all situations of cardiac arrest. If any doubt exists as to its appropriateness, then

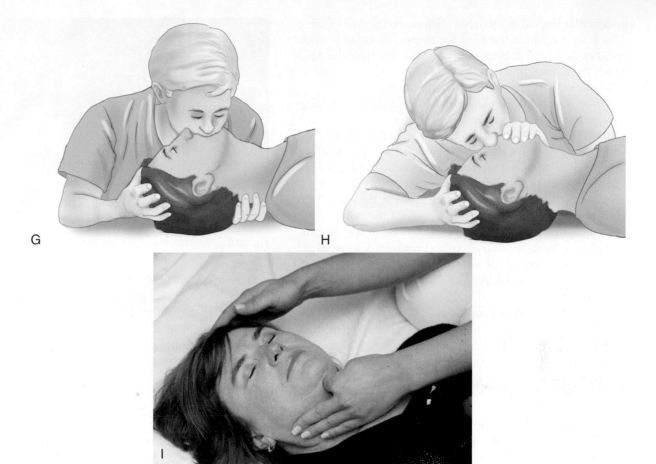

Fig. 20.7, cont'd. (G) Mouth-to-mouth rescue breathing. (H) Mouth-to-nose rescue breathing. (I) Establishing circulatory inadequacy by palpating the carotid artery.

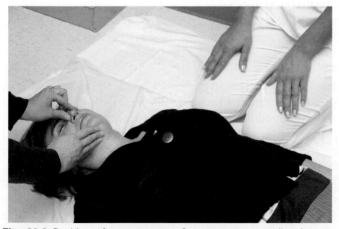

Fig. 20.8 Position of two rescuers for two-person cardiopulmonary resuscitation.

it should be initiated. CPR is clearly *not* indicated in instances in which the patient, the patient's family, or the patient's physician has specifically requested that resuscitation not be done. In these cases, a *do not resuscitate (DNR)* order should be clearly indicated on the patient's chart.

Once begun, basic life support should (and for legal reasons, must) be continued until the victim resumes spontaneous respiration and circulation, a physician or other responsible health care professional calls a halt, or the rescuer is too exhausted to continue.

Improperly performed CPR not only can be ineffective but also can be hazardous. Possible complications from CPR include rib fractures, fractured sternum, pneumothorax, lacerated liver and spleen, and fat emboli. The incidence of complications can be reduced (but not eliminated) by adherence to guidelines.

Changes in recommendations for CPR differentiate between those intended for health care professionals and those intended for laypersons. The abbreviated protocols listed earlier are those for health care professionals. The American Medical Association recommends that health professionals be taught all CPR skills, including single-rescuer, two-rescuer, and infant rescue. The professional technologist is encouraged to become familiar with all required skills and to achieve certification in all CPR procedures.

Automatic External Defibrillation

Ventricular fibrillation is a fluttering or ineffective cardiac rhythm that results in the heart's inability to pump blood. Effective ventricular rhythm must be restored within a few minutes to preserve life. The use of AEDs is one of the few times CPR can be interrupted. One of the most important elements of defibrillation is time; performing it in less than 5 minutes is considered critical to survival.

There are two general types of AEDs—semiautomatic and fully automatic—and there are several different models within each type. The reader is encouraged to become familiar with any defibrillator used in his or her institution. The goal of using AEDs is to determine the need for electric shock and, when necessary, to deliver it. With the fully automatic type, the AED delivers the shock without additional action by the operator.

1. *Determine* that the patient is in cardiac arrest.
2. *Turn on* the defibrillator and prepare the equipment, reading the instructions as necessary.
3. *Attach* the defibrillator cables to the pads if not already connected and place the pads on the patient. One pad should be placed on the upper right area of the chest, and the second pad should be on the lower left ribs.
4. *Initiate rhythm analysis,* usually by pressing the ANALYZE button.
5. If indicated, *deliver the shock.* The need to do so may be indicated by a written message, an audio alarm, a synthesized voice announcement, or a combination of these. After the first shock, press the ANALYZE button again to begin another analysis.
6. If no shock is indicated, continue CPR.
7. After three shocks or three "no shock indicated" messages, CPR should continue uninterrupted.

CEREBROVASCULAR ACCIDENT

A **cerebrovascular accident (stroke or brain attack)** may occur in patients in the radiology department. Strokes are more likely to occur in older patients (over 75 years of age) but can occur in any adult. The onset of a stroke may be sudden, or it may develop gradually over a period of several hours. Warning signs include paralysis on one or both sides, slurred speech or complete loss of speech, extreme dizziness, loss of vision (particularly if only in one eye), and complete loss of consciousness. The symptoms are sometimes only temporary.

If the radiologic technologist observes any of these signs or symptoms, even if they are only temporary, they should be reported to a nurse or physician. Because the potential for paralysis or loss of consciousness is present, the patient should not stand or be moved before further medical assessment can be made. If the patient loses consciousness, CPR may be required and should proceed as described.

MINOR MEDICAL EMERGENCIES

Nausea and Vomiting

Other minor incidents may happen in the radiology department that, although not threatening serious injury, should nevertheless be handled expeditiously. **Nausea** and **vomiting** are frequent occurrences. Nausea tends to be both a psychologic and a physiologic reaction. Patients who feel nauseous often report the feeling to the health care worker. Patients who follow instructions to breathe slowly and deeply through their mouths often become calmer, and nausea and vomiting are avoided.

If the technique does not work and vomiting does occur, the patient should be in a position in which aspiration of vomitus

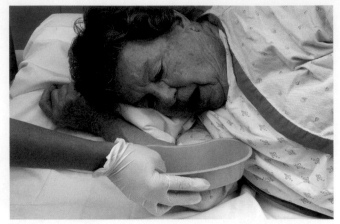

Fig. 20.9 Lateral decubitus position to prevent aspiration of vomitus.

into the lungs is not likely. Recumbent patients should be helped into a lateral decubitus position if possible (Fig. 20.9). If such movement of the patient is contraindicated (e.g., in a patient with a fracture of an arm or leg), the patient should be assisted in turning his or her head to the side. All patients should be provided with an emesis basin and moist cloths.

Epistaxis

Epistaxis, or nosebleed, is another common occurrence. Again, this event is seldom life-threatening. Patients should lean forward and pinch the affected nostril against the midline nasal cartilage with digital pressure (with the fingers). Patients should not be put in a recumbent position or instructed to tilt the head backward because this action allows the blood to flow down the throat, resulting in the patient's swallowing it. If gentle pressure fails to stop the blood flow, a moist compress may also be applied, which will stop most nosebleeds. If these actions are not effective within 15 minutes, medical assistance should be obtained.

Vertigo and Syncope

Many otherwise healthy patients who have been bedridden or who have had limited mobility for a period can often experience **vertigo** (dizziness) or **syncope** (fainting). Vertigo is often a precursor to syncope. A patient who experiences vertigo should be assisted to a seated or recumbent position, which prevents injury from falling as a result of problems with equilibrium. Patients who arise from a radiographic table often experience vertigo as a result of orthostatic hypotension; care should be exercised to not rush these patients, letting them sit on the side of the table for a few minutes before they are escorted from the radiography room.

Syncope is a self-correcting, temporary state of shock and the result of lack of blood flow to the brain. Treatment is aimed at increasing blood flow to the head. The patient should be assisted to a recumbent position with the feet elevated. Any tight clothing should be loosened. These actions assist in increasing overall blood flow. A moist cloth may be applied to the forehead. Patients should remain recumbent until they feel strong enough to undergo the remainder of the procedure or return to their rooms.

Seizures

A seizure in a patient is one of the most frightening events a radiologic technologist might experience. Seizures are caused by a variety of factors, few of which are clearly understood, and may range from mild to severe. A patient who undergoes a mild seizure may experience a brief loss of consciousness or may stare into space for a brief time. This patient may be only slightly confused and weak after such an episode, but the procedure should nevertheless be postponed until another time.

Severe seizures are characterized by involuntary contraction of muscles on either one or both sides of the body. They may last for only a minute or up to several minutes. The patient may drool because of loss of control. The goal is, to the extent possible, to prevent the patient from being injured. No attempt should be made to restrain the patient because the involuntary movements make this not only ineffective but also dangerous. Similarly, no health care worker should ever place his or her hand in a patient's mouth to prevent a backward tongue drop.

Patients who are about to have a seizure will often experience an aura, a physical or mental warning of an impending seizure. The aura is unique for each individual but can be an important help to both the patient and the health care professional. If sufficient warning is given, the patient should be moved to the floor away from objects against which he or she might hit his or her head. A pillow should be placed under the head so it is not banged against the floor. The same precautions should be taken with all patients who experience a seizure, although the absence of a warning aura requires the technologist to be more creative in minimizing the potential for patient harm.

After the patient's seizure, the technologist should be sure that the patient has an open airway, clearing mucus from the mouth as necessary. The patient typically is weak and perhaps disoriented and generally has no memory of the seizure.

Although these experiences are often startling, noting a few things about the seizure itself is helpful to the patient's caregiver. First, make note of where the seizure began, whether it was one-sided or two-sided, and its length. These pieces of information are often important clues in determining the nature of the seizure and may prove helpful in later management and treatment.

Falls

Despite appropriate assistance and care, a patient occasionally falls while in the radiology department. In such a situation the technologist should attempt to minimize the physical impact of the fall to the extent possible by supporting the patient to the floor and then proceed with appropriate emergency action as indicated by the patient's condition.

WOUNDS

Hemorrhage

Some patients come to the radiology department with wounds sustained previously or during surgery. Such wounds may result in hemorrhage (i.e., bleeding outside a vessel). The technologist should always make note of the condition of dressings. If they are clean at the outset of a procedure but become saturated, attention is needed. The saturated dressing should not be removed. Pressure should be applied directly over the saturated dressing, preferably with an additional sterile bandage pressed against it. Because clotting can take up to 10 minutes, the pressure may need to be maintained for some time. Once the bleeding appears to be under control, the bandage should be tied or taped into place.

When a bleeding wound is on an extremity, the affected extremity may be placed above the level of the heart unless other problems that would contraindicate such a procedure exist. This action slows the blood flow to the extremity and may result in less blood loss.

Burns

The radiologic technologist may be required to perform radiologic procedures on patients with burns. Because a burn injury disrupts the normal protective function of the skin, maintaining sterile precautions is imperative. Burns are typically extremely painful injuries; extra gentle care in handling is also indicated.

Dehiscence

Although uncommon, wound dehiscence may happen. *Dehiscence* refers to a situation in which a patient's sutures separate, allowing abdominal contents to spill out of the peritoneal cavity. No attempt should be made to replace tissues inside the wound, but a sterile dressing should be used to cover the area. The patient should be placed in a seated position, somewhat bent forward to relieve any additional pressure on the wound. Medical attention should be obtained quickly.

SUMMARY

- The thought of some of these medical emergencies may be somewhat frightening, but most of them are uncommon. They do occur with enough regularity, however, that the technologist must be aware of typical signs and symptoms associated with the various conditions. The radiologic technologist should be prepared to deal with major medical emergencies, including head injuries, shock, diabetic crises, respiratory distress or arrest, and cardiac arrest. Minor emergencies that may be encountered include nausea and vomiting, epistaxis, syncope and vertigo, seizures, falls, and problems with wounds. An alert technologist who obtains medical assistance quickly may significantly reduce a patient's morbidity and may also play a role in saving a life.
- In addition to the technical knowledge necessary, a calm, confident manner in responding to all of these situations is also important for the radiologic technologist. Thinking and acting appropriately in such periods of stress are difficult, but being able to do so is important to the overall outcome. Moving too quickly and risking a mistake is not worth the potential harm that might result.

BIBLIOGRAPHY

Guidelines for CPR & Emergency Cardiovascular Care, American Heart Association web site, updated. Accessed December 27, 2017, at eccguidelines.heart.org/index.php/circulation/cpr-ecc-guidelines-2.

LeBaudour C, Bergeron JD, Bizjak G: Emergency medical responder: first on scene, ed 10, New York, 2016, Pearson.

Limmer D, O'Keefe MF: Emergency care, ed 13, New York, 2016, Pearson.

Shade BR, Collins TE, Wertz E, et al: Mosby's EMT-intermediate textbook for the 1999 National Standard Curriculum, ed 3 (rev), St. Louis, 2011, Mosby/JEMS/Elsevier.

Pharmacology

Kenya Haugen, DM, MS, RT(R)

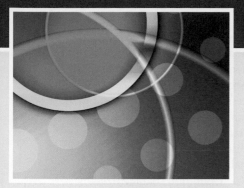

> *It depends only upon the dose whether a poison is poison or not … a lot kills, a little cures.*
>
> **Paracelsus**
> *Grandfather of Pharmacology, 1493–1541*

OBJECTIVES

On completion of this chapter, the student will be able to:

- Recognize common definitions and nomenclature associated with pharmacology.
- Recognize the various classifications of drugs.
- Describe the actions, indications, and precautions related to various drugs.

OUTLINE

KEY TERMS

Analgesics Drugs that relieve pain without causing a loss of consciousness

Anaphylaxis Condition of shock caused by hypersensitivity to a drug or other substance that results in life-threatening respiratory distress and vascular collapse

Anemia Subnormal concentration of erythrocytes or hemoglobin in the blood

Anesthetics Agents that reversibly depress neuronal function, producing loss of ability to perceive pain and/or other sensations

Angina Pectoris Severe constricting pain in the chest, often radiating to the shoulder and down the arm, caused by ischemia (obstruction of blood supply) of the heart muscle, usually a result of coronary disease

Antagonist Substance that tends to nullify the action of another drug

Anticholinergics Drugs that block the passage of impulses through the parasympathetic nerves

Arrhythmias Variations from the normal rhythm of the heartbeat

Atherosclerosis Condition in which thickening of the wall of a blood vessel occurs because of the deposition of plaque (atheroma)

Bronchodilators Drugs that cause expansion of the lumina of the air passages of the lungs

Coagulation Process of clot formation

Contraindications Conditions that render the administration of some drug or some particular line of treatment improper or undesirable

Diabetes Mellitus (DM) Primarily a disorder of carbohydrate, protein,

and fat metabolism secondary to insufficient secretion of insulin or insulin resistance

Diabetic Gastroparesis Form of nerve damage that affects the stomach; food does not move through the stomach in a normal way, resulting in vomiting, nausea, or bloating

Diabetic Peripheral Neuropathy Disorder of the peripheral nervous system, a complication of diabetes

Diuretics Drugs that promote the excretion of urine

Drug Any substance that, when taken into a living organism, may modify one or more of its functions

Edema Presence of abnormally large amounts of fluid in the tissues of the body

Gastroesophageal Reflux Disease (GERD) Inflammation of the lower esophagus from regurgitation of acid gastric contents; symptoms include heartburn

Generic Name Drug name that is usually descriptive of its chemical structure but is not protected as is a brand or trade name

Hematoma Localized collection of blood in the tissue resulting from a break in the wall of the blood vessel

Hyperlipidemia Elevations of plasma lipid concentration

Hypertension Persistently high arterial blood pressure, usually exceeding 140 mm Hg systolic and 90 mm Hg diastolic

Idiosyncratic Reaction Response to a drug that is not normative per its intended action or side effects

Inhalant Breathable chemical vapor that may cause systemic and local effects

Infiltration Diffusion of fluid into a tissue; often used interchangeably with extravasation

Laxatives Agents that promote evacuation of the bowel

Microorganisms Microscopic organisms such as bacteria or viruses

Opioids Drugs, natural or synthetic, that have pain relief activity, example being morphine

Osteoporosis Disease of bone that leads to an increased risk for fracture; bone mineral density is reduced, and bone microarchitecture is disrupted

Parenteral Not through the gastrointestinal tract but by injection

Parkinson Disease (PD) Degenerative neurologic disease of the brain that often impairs motor skills, speech, and other functions

Peristalsis Waves of contraction that propel contents through the gastrointestinal tract

Pharmacist Person who is licensed to prepare and dispense drugs

Pharmacokinetics Study of the metabolism and action of drugs with particular emphasis on the time required for absorption, duration of action, distribution in the body, and method of excretion

Pharmacology Study of drugs and their origin, nature, properties, and effects on living organisms

Physical Dependence State of adaptation exhibited by a withdrawal syndrome specific to a class of drugs and that may be produced by abrupt cessation, rapid dose reduction, or administration of an antagonist

Schizophrenia Chronic mental disorder characterized by periods of hallucinations and paranoia

Shock Condition characterized by profound hypotension and reduced tissue perfusion

Side Effect Consequence other than the one for which a drug is used

Therapeutic Pertaining to the art of healing

Thromboembolic Disorders Conditions involving the partial or complete obstruction of a blood vessel

Tolerance State of adaptation in response to drug exposure that results in a decrease of one or more of the drug's effects over time

Vasoconstrictors Drugs that cause constriction of the blood vessels

Vasodilators Drugs that cause dilatation of the blood vessels

---

The scope of the radiologic technologist includes the practice of identifying, preparing, and/or administering medications as prescribed by a licensed practitioner. The technologist must have an overall knowledge of **drugs**, potential actions, and side effects, as well as the skills necessary to assist with drug administration in many different clinical situations. Pharmacologic knowledge is essential to safe, optimal patient care and competent professional practice. Radiologic technologists may be responsible for administering drugs for contrast media, responding to adverse reactions to contrast, administering pain management medications, sedation, and must be prepared to assist in any life-threatening medical emergency. As the role and responsibilities of the radiologic technologist continue to expand in the area of drug administration, the information presented in this chapter will provide a fundamental framework within which the level of knowledge may increase.

A drug is any chemical substance that produces a biologic response in a living system. More specifically, a drug is a substance used as medicine to aid in the diagnosis, treatment, or prevention of disease. The science concerned with the origin, nature, effects, and uses of drugs is called **pharmacology**.

DRUG NOMENCLATURE

A nomenclature is a classified system of names. In pharmacology, drugs are classified in many different ways. For example, a drug may be classified by its name, its action, or its method of legal purchase. When drugs are classified by name, knowing which kind of name is being used is important because the same drug has at least three different names: (1) a chemical name, (2) a generic name, and (3) a trade name.

Classification by Name

The first name that is likely to be applied to a drug is the chemical name, which identifies the actual chemical structure of the drug. The chemical name is often complex and is seldom of practical importance to the technologist.

The **generic name** is the name given to the drug when it becomes commercially available. The generic name is a simpler name derived from the more complex chemical name. It is usually easier to pronounce than the chemical name and is never capitalized; it is also called the nonproprietary name. Some drugs are best known by the generic name.

A brand name is the name given to a drug manufactured by a specific company. It is usually short and easy to remember. It may or may not reflect any characteristic of the chemical structure of the drug. Because the same drug is manufactured by more than one company, each company selects its own brand name or trademark for the drug. Trademark, brand name, trade name, and proprietary name are all terms used interchangeably to indicate a specific generic drug manufactured by several different companies. An example of the names currently used for a single drug follows:

Chemical name: 2-diphenylmethoxy-*N,N*-dimethylethylamine
Generic name: diphenhydramine
Brand name: Benadryl

Confusion occurs when some physicians use generic names and others use trade names when requesting drugs. Therefore, the radiologic technologist should be aware of drug information resources that are available. One such source is the Physicians' Desk Reference, or PDR as it is frequently called. The PDR is available online for quick and convenient drug searches at www.pdr.net. The PDR provides a drug summary listing the class, drug enforcement agency class, drug description, common brand names, how the drug is supplied, dosage and indications, maximum dosage, dosing considerations, administration storage, **contraindications**/precautions, adverse reactions, drug interactions, pregnancy and lactation, and mechanism of action. If internet access to the PDR is not readily available in the radiology department, then the next best source of drug information is the hospital pharmacist.

Classification by Action

Drugs are also classified according to action or function. Drugs that have similar chemical actions are grouped into categories called *drug families.* For example, drugs that relieve pain are classified as **analgesics,** drugs used to treat high blood pressure are classified as *antihypertensives,* and drugs used to fight inflammation are classified as *antiinflammatories.* Although this system is a convenient way to classify drugs for study purposes, it is not totally reliable or exclusive because one drug may have several different physiologic effects on the body, which means it would be listed under more than one category.

Legal Classification

According to federal laws, drugs are classified legally as either prescription (legend drugs) or non-prescription. Prescription drugs require an order by a legally authorized health practitioner who may be a physician assistant, nurse practitioner, or physician. The prescription is the documentation that specifies precisely the name of the patient, the name of the drug, and the dosage regimen to be followed. Prescription drugs are usually dispensed by a licensed **pharmacist**, although some physicians supply prescription drugs to their patients. Prescription drugs will have the label "Caution: Federal law prohibits dispensing without prescription." Non-prescription drugs, better known as over-the-counter drugs, can be obtained legally without a prescription. Another group of substances that can be obtained without a prescription are called dietary supplements. Vitamins, supplements, and herbal remedies are classified as dietary supplements and by law are not classified as drugs and are therefore not controlled by the US Food and Drug Administration (FDA). This classification means that herbal remedies can be sold without proof of safety or efficacy. The radiologic technologist should be aware that many over-the-counter products and herbal remedies are capable of producing toxic effects if they are misused or used in combination with other drugs. For example, St. John's wort interacts with several prescription medications. Patients with low health literacy may find it difficult to explain prescribed or over-the-counter drugs that are taken. The technologist must take the responsibility of clarifying the types of medications, vitamins, supplements, and herbal remedies the patient is taking by asking a pharmacist or referencing the PDR.

DOSAGE FORMS

The dosage forms of a drug refer to the type of preparation or the way the chemical agent is transported into the human body. A single drug may be available in many different forms to facilitate the administration and action of the drug under a variety of conditions. The dose form may determine the speed, or onset, of the drug's therapeutic effect. Some of the common dosage forms include tablets, capsules, inhalants, suppositories, solutions, suspensions, and transdermal patches.

Tablet

Tablets are the most common oral dose form and one of the easiest to administer. A tablet is a powder or granulated drug that has been compressed into a solid hard disk. Tables vary in size, shape, weight, hardness, thickness, disintegration, and dissolution characteristics. Tablets are single-dose units that may be scored or grooved to facilitate division into halves or quarters. A tablet that is not scored should not be broken into smaller parts. Some tablets are coated with a substance that delays the dissolution of the tablet until it is in the small intestines rather than in the stomach, where it is normally dissolved. These so-called enteric-coated tablets are used for drugs that might irritate the stomach (such as aspirin) or for drugs destroyed by the acid in the stomach. Some tablets are coated with polymers that are designed to produce slow, uniform absorption of the drug for several hours (8 hours or longer). Such products are called sustained-release, extended-release, or controlled-release tablets. Other types of tablet are buccal and sublingual. The sublingual dosage form disintegrates rapidly when placed on the tongue, the buccal tablets dissolve in the buccal pouch, thus eliminating the need to chew, swallow, or take the tablet with liquids. It should be beneficial to pediatric and geriatric patients, to people with conditions related to impaired swallowing, and for treatment of patients when compliance may be difficult.

Capsule

A capsule is a dose form in which a powdered or liquid drug is contained in a gelatin shell. The gelatin shell dissolves in the stomach and releases its contents. Gelatin-coated tablets also facilitate swallowing.

Inhalant

The inhalation route of administration may be used for both local and systemic effects (general anesthetics). Inhalants are used for their local effects in the treatment of asthma or chronic obstructive pulmonary disease. An inhalant allows high concentrations to be deposited in the respiratory mucosa and exert action by producing bronchodilation or reducing inflammation. Local therapeutic effects are optimized, and systemic side effects are minimized.

Suppository

A suppository is a dose form shaped for insertion into a body orifice such as the rectum, vagina, or urethra. Once inserted, the suppository dissolves and releases the drug. It may have a local or systemic effect.

Solution

A solution is a dose form in which one or more drugs are dissolved in a liquid carrier. Solutions are usually rapidly absorbed and may be administered orally or parenterally. Parenteral administration includes any injection of the drug with a needle and syringe beneath the surface of the skin.

Suspension

A suspension is a dose form in which one or more drugs in small particles are suspended in a liquid carrier. Most suspensions are administered orally and should be shaken thoroughly just before administration. Suspensions should never be administered intravenously.

Transdermal Patch

A transdermal patch is a dose form that permits a drug to be applied on the skin surface, where it is absorbed into the bloodstream. The patch-like device containing the drug is applied to the skin with a water-resistant covering. The patch releases the drug gradually over time. Some of these patches contain aluminum or other metals in the backing of the patches. The metals in the patches can overheat during a magnetic resonance imaging scan and cause skin burns.

CLASSIFICATION OF DRUGS

For easy reference, Table 21.1 provides a list of controlled substance schedules. Table 21.2 provides a classification of commonly used drugs listed by drug action. A list of commonly used drugs alphabetically by the trade name and also cross-referenced by generic name is provided in Appendix E. Dietary supplements and herbal remedies commonly used are listed alphabetically in Table 21.3, along with the proposed actions that may occur with prescription and nonprescription drugs.

Controlled Substance Schedules. Drugs and other substances that are considered controlled substances under the Controlled

TABLE 21.1   Federal Drug Scheduling System

Schedule 1 drugs	1. The drug or other substance has a high potential for abuse.
	2. The drug or other substance has no currently accepted medical use in treatment in the United States.
	3. There is a lack of accepted safety for use of the drug or other substance under medical supervision.

Examples: Heroin, lysergic acid diethylamide, marijuana (cannabis), 3,4-methylenedioxymethamphetamine (ecstasy), methaqualone, and peyote

Schedule 2 drugs	1. The drug or other substance has a high potential for abuse.
	2. The drug or other substance has a currently accepted medical use in treatment in the United States or a currently accepted medical use with severe restrictions.
	3. Abuse of the drug or other substances may lead to severe psychological or physical dependence.

Examples: Combination products with <15 mg of hydrocodone per dosage unit (Vicodin), cocaine, methamphetamine, methadone, hydromorphone (Dilaudid), meperidine (Demerol), oxycodone (OxyContin), fentanyl, Dexedrine, Adderall, and Ritalin

Schedule 3 drugs	1. The drug or other substance has a potential for abuse less than the drugs or other substances in schedules I and II.
	2. The drug or other substance has a currently accepted medical use in treatment in the United States.
	3. Abuse of the drug or other substance may lead to moderate or low physical dependence or high psychological dependence.

Example: Products containing <90 mg of codeine per dosage unit (Tylenol with codeine), ketamine, anabolic steroids, testosterone

Schedule 4 drugs	1. The drug or other substance has a low potential for abuse relative to the drugs or other substances in schedule III.
	2. The drug or other substance has a currently accepted medical use in treatment in the United States.
	3. Abuse of the drug or other substance may lead to limited physical dependence or psychological dependence relative to the drugs or other substances in schedule III.

Example: Xanax, Soma, Darvon, Darvocet, Valium, Ativan, Talwin, Ambien, Tramadol

Schedule 5 drugs	1. The drug or other substance has a low potential for abuse relative to the drugs or other substances in schedule III.
	2. The drug or other substance has a currently accepted medical use in treatment in the United States.
	3. Abuse of the drug or other substance may lead to limited physical dependence or psychological dependence relative to the drugs or other substances in schedule III.

Example: Cough preparations with <200 mg of codeine or per 100 mL (Robitussin AC), Lomotil, Motofen, Lyrica, Parepectolin

Substances Act and are divided into five schedules. It is important for the technologist to be familiar with the medications that have a high potential of abuse but may also be a prescribed medication.

Actions, Indications, and Precautions

Health care providers and patients can be at risk for adverse outcomes from mishandling medications. Learning and understanding the use and application of the drugs and safety measures to prevent medication errors should be addressed to protect the patient, technologist, and patient care team. The Institute for Safe Medication Practices biannually issues "Targeted Medication Safety Best Practices for Hospitals." Technologists work in

TABLE 21.2 Commonly Used Drugs by Classification

Classification and Brand Name	Generic Name	Route(s)
Analgesics		
Ecotrin, or various brand names	Aspirin	Oral
Duragesic	Fentanyl	Parenteral, transdermal
MS Contin, or various brand names	Morphine	Oral, parenteral
OxyContin, Roxicodone	Oxycodone	Oral
Percocet	Oxycodone-APAP	Oral
Tylenol	Acetaminophen (APAP)	Oral
Ultram	Tramadol	Oral
Vicodin, Norco	Hydrocodone-APAP	Oral
Anesthetics		
Amidate	Etomidate	Parenteral
Carbocaine	Mepivacaine	Parenteral
Diprivan	Propofol	Parenteral
Ultane	Sevoflurane	Inhalation
Antianemic		
Feraheme	Ferumoxytol	Parenteral
Slo Fe, other various brands	Ferrous Sulfate	Oral
Antianxiety		
Ativan	Lorazepam	Oral, parenteral
Valium	Diazepam	Oral, parenteral
Versed	Midazolam	Oral, Parenteral
Xanax	Alprazolam	Oral
Antiarrhythmics		
Adenocard	Adenosine	Parenteral
Cardizem	Diltiazem	Oral, parenteral
Cordarone	Amiodarone	Oral, parenteral
Lanoxin	Digoxin	Oral, parenteral
Xylocaine	Lidocaine	Parenteral
Antibiotics		
Amoxil	Amoxicillin	Oral
Augmentin	Amoxicillin-clavulanate	Oral
Biaxin	Clarithromycin	Oral
Keflex	Cephalexin	Oral
Cipro	Ciprofloxacin	Oral, parenteral
Levaquin	Levofloxacin	Oral, parenteral
Penicillin VK	Penicillin VK	Oral
Rocephin	Ceftriaxone	Parenteral
Zithromax	Azithromycin	Oral, parenteral
Anticholinergics		
Atropine	Atropine	Oral, parenteral, ophthalmic
Detrol LA	Tolterodine	Oral
Ditropan XL	Oxybutynin	Oral, transdermal
Anticoagulants		
Coumadin	Warfarin	Oral, parenteral
Eliquis	Apixaban	Oral
Heparin	Heparin	Parenteral
Lovenox	Enoxaparin	Parenteral
Pradaxa	Dabigatran	Oral
Xarelto	Rivaroxaban	Oral

Classification and Brand Name	Generic Name	Route(s)
Antidepressants		
Celexa	Citalopram	Oral
Cymbalta	Duloxetine	Oral
Effexor	Venlafaxine	Oral
Lexapro	Escitalopram	Oral
Paxil	Paroxetine	Oral
Prozac	Fluoxetine	Oral
Wellbutrin	Bupropion	Oral
Zoloft	Sertraline	Oral
Antidiabetics		
Actos	Pioglitazone	Oral
Amaryl	Glimepiride	Oral
Glucophage	Metformin	Oral
Glucotrol	Glipizide	Oral
Lantus, Humulin/Novolin	Glargine Insulin, Regular/NPH Insulin	Parenteral
Invokana	Canagliflozin	Oral
Januvia	Sitagliptin	Oral
Micronase	Glyburide	Oral
Onglyza	Saxagliptin	Oral
Victoza	Liraglutide	Parenteral
Antiemetics		
Compazine	Prochlorperazine	Oral, parenteral
Phenergan	Promethazine	Oral, parenteral
Reglan	Metoclopramide	Oral, parenteral
Zofran	Ondansetron	Oral, parenteral
Antiepileptics		
Depakote	Valproate	Oral, parenteral
Dilantin	Phenytoin	Oral, parenteral
Klonopin	Clonazepam	Oral
Lamictal	Lamotrigine	Oral
Lyrica	Pregabalin	Oral
Neurontin	Gabapentin	Oral
Topamax	Topiramate	Oral
Antifungals		
Diflucan	Fluconazole	Oral, parenteral
Fungizone	Amphotericin B	Parenteral
Antihistamines		
Allegra	Fexofenadine	Oral
Benadryl	Diphenhydramine	Oral, parenteral
Claritin	Loratadine	Oral
Vistaril	Hydroxyzine	Oral, parenteral
Antihyperlipidemics		
Crestor	Rosuvastatin	Oral
Lipitor	Atorvastatin	Oral
Zocor	Simvastatin	Oral
Antihypertensives		
Coreg	Carvedilol	Oral
Cozaar	Losartan	Oral
Diovan	Valsartan	Oral
Lopressor	Metoprolol tartrate	Oral, parenteral
Lotensin	Benazepril	Oral

Continued

TABLE 21.2   Commonly Used Drugs by Classification—cont'd

Classification and Brand Name	Generic Name	Route(s)
Norvasc	Amlodipine	Oral
Tenormin	Atenolol	Oral, parenteral
Toprol-XL	Metoprolol succinate	Oral
Vasotec	Enalapril	Oral, parenteral
Zestril	Lisinopril	Oral
Antiparkinson Agents		
Mirapex	Pramipexole	Oral
Requip	Ropinirole	Oral
Sinemet	Levodopa-carbidopa	Oral
Antiplatelets		
Ecotrin, or various brand names	Aspirin	Oral
Plavix	Clopidogrel	Oral
ReoPro	Abciximab	Parenteral
Antipsychotics		
Abilify	Aripiprazole	Oral, parenteral
Haldol	Haloperidol	Oral, parenteral
Risperdal	Risperidone	Oral, parenteral
Seroquel	Quetiapine	Oral
Thorazine	Clorpromazine	Oral, parenteral
Zyprexa	Olanzapine	Oral, parenteral
Antiulcer		
Pepcid	Famotidine	Oral, parenteral
Prevacid	Lansoprazole	Oral, parenteral
Prilosec	Omeprazole	Oral
Zantac	Ranitidine	Oral, parenteral
Antivirals		
Atripla	Efavirenz-emtricitabine-tenofovir	Oral
Zovirax	Acyclovir	Oral, parenteral, topical
Benzodiazepine Antagonist		
Romazicon	Flumazenil	Parenteral
Bronchodilators		
Adrenalin	Epinephrine	Inhalation, parenteral
Advair	Salmeterol-fluticasone	Inhalation
Atrovent	Ipratropium	Inhalation
ProAir HFA	Albuterol	Inhalation
Serevent	Salmeterol	Inhalation
Spiriva	Tiotropium	Inhalation
Antialzheimers		
Aricept	Donepezil	Oral
Namenda	Memantine	Oral
Coagulant		
Mephyton	Phytonadione	Oral, parenteral
Phytonadione	Vitamin K	Oral, parenteral
Corticosteroids		
Decadron	Dexamethasone	Oral, parenteral

Classification and Brand Name	Generic Name	Route(s)
Deltasone	Prednisone	Oral
Depo-Medrol	Methylprednisolone	Parenteral
Flovent	Fluticasone	Inhalation
Solu-Cortef	Hydrocortisone	Parenteral
Diuretics		
Hydrodiuril	Hydrochlorothiazide	Oral, parenteral
Lasix	Furosemide	Oral, parenteral
Hormones		
Premarin	Conjugated estrogens	Oral, vaginal
Synthroid	Levothyroxine	Oral
Laxative		
Dulcolax	Bisacodyl	Oral
Miralax	Polyethylene glycol	Oral
Hypnotics		
Ambien	Zolpidem	Oral
Lunesta	Eszopiclone	Oral
Restoril	Temazepam	Oral
Mood Stabilizer		
Eskalith/Lithobid	Lithium	Oral
Nonsteroidal Antiinflammatories		
Celebrex	Celecoxib	Oral
Motrin	Ibuprofen	Oral
Naprosyn	Naproxen	Oral
Opioid Antagonist		
Narcan	Naloxone	Parenteral, intranasal
Osteoporosis Agents		
Actonel	Risedronate	Oral
Evista	Raloxifene	Oral
Fosamax	Alendronate	Oral
Stimulants		
Adderall	Amphetamine salts	Oral
Dobutrex	Dobutamine	Parenteral
Intropin	Dopamine	Parenteral
Ritalin	Methylphenidate	Oral
Thrombolytics		
Activase	Alteplase (tPA)	Parenteral
Retavase	Reteplase	Parenteral
Vasoconstrictor		
Levophed	Norepinephrine	Parenteral
Vasodilators		
Nitrostat, various other brands	Nitroglycerin	Oral, parenteral, transdermal
Nitropress	Nitroprusside	Parenteral

APAP, N-Acetyl-*para*-amino-phenol (acetaminophen); *AZT*, azidothymidine.

TABLE 21.3 Herbals

Common Name	Proposed Actions and Properties	Adverse Effects	Potential Interaction
Echinacea	Stimulates immune system	Hypersensitivity	Acetaminophen (liver toxicity)
Feverfew	Antiinflammatory, migraine headache	Bleeding, flushing	Aspirin, clopidogrel, warfarin
Garlic	Cholesterol reduction, lowers blood pressure	Bleeding, heartburn	Aspirin, clopidogrel, warfarin
Ginger	Antiemetic	Bleeding	Aspirin, clopidogrel, warfarin
Ginseng	Maintains normal function in time of stress	Insomnia	Digoxin
Ginkgo biloba	Stimulates circulation, increases mental alertness	Bleeding	Aspirin, clopidogrel, warfarin
Kava	Antianxiety, promotes sleep	Liver toxicity	Alprazolam, epinephrine
Saw palmetto	Promotes prostate health	Headache, diarrhea	Oral contraceptives
St. John's wort	Depression	Photosensitivity	Digoxin, antidepressants
Valerian	Promotes sleep	Headache, drowsiness	Benzodiazepines (e.g., lorazepam)

many different areas and it is important to be aware of best practices that may apply to diagnostic, therapeutic, and emergency situations in which the technologist may be involved.

Analgesics. Analgesics are drugs that relieve pain without causing loss of consciousness. Analgesics can be divided into two groups: the nonopioids (non-narcotic) and the opioids (narcotic). Health professionals are encouraged to use the word opioid or opioids rather than narcotic or narcotics. The term opioid is less likely than narcotic to carry a stigma of drug abuse. Opioids, such as morphine and oxycodone ER (OxyContin), are used in the treatment of moderate to severe pain. The FDA has changed the indications for extended-release (ER) and long-acting (LA) opioid analgesics. The updated indication states the ER/LA opioids should be used in the management of pain severe enough to require daily, around-the-clock, long-term treatment and for which alternative treatment options are inadequate.

Whereas physical dependence and tolerance are common with long-term opioid use, addiction is not. Addiction is a chronic neurobiologic disease characterized by one or more of the following behaviors: impaired control over drug use, compulsive use, continued use despite harm, inappropriate use, and craving. Adverse side effects such as nausea, vomiting, and constipation are frequently associated with the administration of opioid analgesics. In cases of opioid overdose, naloxone (Narcan) is administered parenterally or intranasally to terminate respiratory depression. Narcan is an opioid antagonist. Nonopioid analgesics such as acetaminophen (N-acetyl-para-amino-phenol; Tylenol) are relatively safe drugs used in the treatment of mild to moderate pain. They do not cause physiologic dependency.

Anesthetics. Anesthetics are agents that reversibly depress neuronal function, producing loss of ability to perceive pain and/or other sensations. Two types of anesthetic agents are general anesthetics and local anesthetics. General anesthetics can be divided into inhalation agents such as sevoflurane (Ultane) or intravenous agents such as propofol (Diprivan). They act as central nervous system (CNS) depressants by producing muscle relaxation and loss of consciousness. General anesthesia is commonly used on patients undergoing major surgical procedures. Local anesthetics such as mepivacaine (Carbocaine) and lidocaine (Xylocaine) block nerve conduction from an area of the body to the CNS. The extent of their action depends on the area to which they are applied. The FDA issued an advisory about potentially serious hazards associated with overuse of topical anesthetics. Improper use can lead to excessive absorption of drug and may cause life-threatening side effects such as irregular heartbeat, seizures, breathing difficulties, and even death.

Antianemic Agents. Antianemic drugs are used for the treatment of anemia. Anemia is a subnormal concentration of erythrocytes or hemoglobin in the blood. It may be due to iron, folic acid, or vitamin B12 deficiency.

Ferumoxytol (Feraheme) is a parenteral iron product used for the treatment of iron deficiency anemia in adult patients with chronic kidney disease. As a superparamagnetic iron oxide, it may transiently affect magnetic resonance diagnostic imaging studies for up to 3 months after the last dose. It will not affect x-ray, computed tomography, positron emission tomography, single photon emission computed tomography, ultrasound, or nuclear imaging.

Antianxiety Agents. Antianxiety agents, or anxiolytics, are drugs used in the treatment of anxiety. They act on the CNS to calm or relax the anxious patient. Diazepam (Valium) and lorazepam (Ativan) are benzodiazepines prescribed for the treatment of anxiety, muscle spasms, and seizures. They are also used in alcohol detoxification or to prevent seizures and other acute withdrawal reactions. Benzodiazepines are often used as a preoperative drug for various procedures performed in the radiology department. Another benzodiazepine, Midazolam (Versed), is also used as a preoperative drug. Benzodiazepines can be abused, and physical dependence has been documented. Flumazenil (Romazicon) is a benzodiazepine antagonist that reverses the effects of benzodiazepines and therefore may be used in the treatment of a benzodiazepine drug overdose.

Antiarrhythmics. Antiarrhythmics are drugs used to treat arrhythmias, which are variations from the normal rhythm of the heartbeat. The abnormal rhythm may occur in the atria (the upper chambers of the heart) or in the ventricles (the lower chambers of the heart). The antiarrhythmic agent used depends on the type of arrhythmia to be treated. Amiodarone (Cordarone) is mainly used for ventricular arrhythmias. Amiodarone may cause adverse effects such as hypothyroidism and pulmonary fibrosis.

Antibiotics. Antibiotics or antimicrobials are drugs used to kill or inhibit the growth of microorganisms. An antibiotic that is effective against a large number of microorganisms is termed a broad-spectrum antibiotic; if it is effective against only a small number of microorganisms, it is termed a narrow-spectrum antibiotic. Ciprofloxacin (Cipro), a fluoroquinolone, is a broad-spectrum antibiotic, and penicillin VK, a penicillin, is a narrow-spectrum antibiotic used primarily for treating streptococcal pharyngitis ("strep throat"). Allergic reactions to antibiotics are common and range from mild to severe or even fatal.

Anticholinergics. Anticholinergics are drugs that reduce smooth muscle tone, motility of the gastrointestinal (GI) tract, and secretions from respiratory tract and secretory glands. Oxybutynin (Ditropan XL) and tolterodine (Detrol LA) are two commonly used anticholinergics in the treatment of overactive bladder. Atropine is used preoperatively to inhibit the secretions that can be stimulated by general anesthetics and to prevent bradycardia (slowing of the heart) that may result from general anesthesia. The most common side effect of an anticholinergic agent is a dry mouth, but high doses of these drugs can produce serious side effects such as delirium (especially in the older patient), rapid heartbeat, and coma. Many other drugs can have anticholinergic side effects, such as diphenhydramine (Benadryl).

Anticoagulants. Anticoagulants are drugs that inhibit clotting of the blood or increase the coagulation time. They are used primarily to prevent or treat thromboembolic disorders. Anticoagulants are administered orally or parenterally. Heparin and enoxaparin (Lovenox) are commonly used parenteral anticoagulants. Heparin and enoxaparin are not effective when administered orally because they are not absorbed from the GI tract and should not be administered intramuscularly because they may cause a hematoma. There are several oral anticoagulants; warfarin (Coumadin) is an example of an oral anticoagulant. Patients undergoing interventional procedures in the radiology department are often receiving these drugs and should be monitored closely to prevent massive hemorrhage, which can occur with overdose and precipitated with falls.

Anticonvulsants. Anticonvulsants or antiepileptic drugs are drugs used to prevent or control the occurrence of seizures. These drugs do not treat the cause of seizures; they reduce or eliminate seizure activity.

Although divalproex (valproate; Depakote) is an effective oral antiepileptic, it is also used to treat bipolar disease and for the prophylaxis of migraine headaches. It is also available in a parenteral form. Depakote has been associated with liver toxicity, thrombocytopenia (a decrease in the number of platelets), and pancreatitis. Phenytoin (Dilantin) is another

effective antiepileptic that is available in oral or parenteral form. Several antiepileptic drugs are also used for other conditions, such as pregabalin (Lyrica) for fibromyalgia, neuropathic pain associated with diabetic peripheral neuropathy, and postherpetic neuralgia; lamotrigine (Lamictal) for bipolar disorder; and gabapentin (Neurontin) for postherpetic neuralgia.

Antidepressants. *Antidepressants* are drugs used in the treatment of depression. These drugs often require 6 to 12 weeks of administration to achieve their maximal therapeutic effect. When the first depressive episode is treated, antidepressants must be given for an additional 4 to 9 months to prevent a relapse. Withdrawal effects (called *discontinuation syndrome*) after abrupt discontinuation have been reported. Many types of antidepressants are used to treat depression. The selective serotonin reuptake inhibitors fluoxetine (Prozac), sertraline (Zoloft), paroxetine (Paxil), citalopram (Celexa), and escitalopram (Lexapro), the selective serotonin norepinephrine inhibitors (SNRIs) venlafaxine (Effexor) and duloxetine (Cymbalta), and others such as bupropion (Wellbutrin) and mirtazapine (Remeron) are considered drugs of choice in treating clinical depression. The selective serotonin reuptake inhibitors are also used in the treatment of anxiety disorders, and Cymbalta is also used to treat diabetic peripheral neuropathy pain, generalized anxiety, fibromyalgia, chronic musculoskeletal pain resulting from chronic osteoarthritis pain, and chronic low back pain. Nausea, drowsiness, sexual dysfunction, and diarrhea are common side effects. Drug interactions can occur in patients receiving other drugs in combination with antidepressants.

Antidiabetic Agents. Diabetes mellitus (DM) affects approximately 25.8 million Americans (8.3% of the US population). Diabetes mellitus is currently classified as *type 1,* in which insulin is absent, and *type 2,* in which insulin deficiency and insulin resistance exist. Insulin is the only treatment used to treat type 1 diabetes but is also used in the treatment for type 2 diabetes. Glyburide (Micronase), glipizide (Glucotrol), glimepiride (Amaryl), metformin (Glucophage), pioglitazone (Actos), sitagliptin (Januvia), liraglutide (Victoza), and canagliflozin (Invokana) are commonly used for type 2 diabetes. Hypoglycemic (low glucose) reactions are the most common complication of antidiabetic agents. Metformin is associated with lactic acidosis, a rare adverse effect; although rare, it has a mortality rate of approximately 50%. It is recommended that metformin be temporarily discontinued before the use of radiographic contrast agents because of its potential negative effects on renal function.

Antiemetics. *Antiemetics* are drugs used to prevent and treat nausea and vomiting. In general, these agents are more effective in preventing nausea and vomiting than they are in treating the symptoms once they have developed. Thus, they are most effective when given before the onset of symptoms. Prochlorperazine (Compazine) and ondansetron (Zofran) are two commonly used antiemetic agents and are available in both oral and parenteral forms.

Antifungal Agents. *Antifungal agents* are substances that destroy or suppress the growth or multiplication of fungi. Fungal infections are more likely to occur in patients who are immunocompromised. Fungal infections can be divided into two major groups: those that affect the skin or mucosa and those that affect the whole body *(systemic)*. Fungizone (amphotericin B) is usually the drug of choice for treating most serious systemic infections. It must be administered intravenously because it is poorly absorbed from the GI tract. Fungizone can cause a variety of adverse effects, such as chills, fever, and kidney damage. Fluconazole (Diflucan), which is available in oral and parenteral forms, is effective in serious systemic infections and vaginal fungal infections. It is generally well tolerated.

Antihistamines. *Antihistamines* are drugs used primarily to treat allergic disorders, both acute and chronic. They are used to treat the symptoms (e.g., runny nose) of upper respiratory tract infections. Antihistamines fall into two major groups: those that are *sedating* (first generation) and those that are *nonsedating* (second generation). Diphenhydramine (Benadryl) is a sedating antihistamine and is available in oral and parenteral forms. It is administered intramuscularly for moderately severe allergic reactions. Loratadine (Claritin) and fexofenadine (Allegra) are examples of nonsedating antihistamines that are administered orally.

Antihyperlipidemic Agents. Hyperlipidemia is associated with the development of atherosclerosis, which leads to coronary heart disease (CHD). CHD remains the single largest killer of American men and women. Large, randomized, controlled clinical trials have demonstrated that cholesterol lowering significantly reduces CHD mortality and reduces the risk for having a stroke. Drugs called *statins* are usually the drugs of choice in the management of hyperlipidemia. Two common statins, atorvastatin (Lipitor) and simvastatin (Zocor), are used to treat hyperlipidemia. Liver abnormalities and muscle pain can occur. Persistent muscle pain can be a serious side effect. Niacin (Niaspan ER) and ezetimibe (Zetia) are other antihyperlipidemic agents.

Antihypertensives. *Antihypertensives* are drugs used to treat hypertension (high blood pressure). Hypertension is a common disorder that affects approximately 77.9 million (1 in every 3) American adults. If left untreated or improperly treated, hypertension can lead to heart disease, kidney disease, strokes, and blindness. The Seventh Report of the Joint National Committee on Prevention, Detection, Evaluation, and Treatment of High Blood Pressure (the JNC 8 report) recommends a blood pressure less than 140/90 mm Hg in the general population and less than 150/90 mm Hg in patients older than 60 years. Many different drugs are used to treat hypertension because high blood pressure can be caused by many factors. Up to four different antihypertensive agents may be required to control hypertension. Besides lowering blood pressure, many antihypertensive agents are used in the management of other cardiovascular diseases. Angiotensin-converting enzyme inhibitors such as lisinopril

(Zestril) and beta blockers such as metoprolol (Lopressor, Toprol XL) are used in the management of heart failure. A common adverse effect of angiotensin-converting enzyme inhibitors is a cough. Calcium channel blockers such as amlodipine (Norvasc) are used in the management of **angina pectoris**.

Antiparkinson Agents. Parkinson disease (PD) is characterized by a resting tremor, rigidity (inability to initiate movements), and bradykinesia (slowness of movement). Levodopa-carbidopa (Sinemet) is used in the management of PD and is administered orally. Common adverse effects associated with Sinemet are nausea and vomiting. Other medications used in the management of PD include pramipexole (Mirapex) and ropinirole (Requip); they are both administered orally.

Antiplatelets. *Antiplatelet drugs* inhibit platelet aggregation. Antiplatelet drugs are indicated in the prevention of myocardial infarction (MI), stroke, and transient ischemic attacks. Aspirin, clopidogrel (Plavix), and abciximab (ReoPro) are frequently used agents. Aspirin and clopidogrel are administered orally, and abciximab is administered parenterally. The major complication for these drugs is bleeding.

Antipsychotics. *Antipsychotic drugs* (neuroleptics) are used to treat psychiatric disorders such as **schizophrenia**, delusional disorders, acute mania, and agitated states. The antipsychotic agents are divided into two major groups: traditional antipsychotics and atypical (novel) antipsychotics. A well-known traditional antipsychotic is haloperidol (Haldol). It is available in both oral and parenteral forms. Olanzapine (Zyprexa) is a commonly used atypical antipsychotic. It is also available in oral and parenteral forms. A wide variety of adverse side effects, including sedation, orthostatic hypotension, and tremor disorder may be associated with both types of antipsychotic agents.

Antiulcer Agents. *Antiulcer agents* are used to treat peptic ulcers, both gastric and duodenal, and **gastroesophageal reflux disease (GERD)**. GERD is caused by the reflux of acid from the stomach into the esophagus. The most common symptom is heartburn. GERD can cause chest pain, which can be mistaken as a heart attack and trigger an emergency room visit. Ranitidine (Zantac), famotidine (Pepcid), lansoprazole (Prevacid), and omeprazole (Prilosec) reduce the production of acid within the stomach. They are effective in the management of peptic ulcers and GERD. Metoclopramide (Reglan), available in oral and parenteral forms, increases **peristalsis** and accelerates gastric emptying without increasing gastric secretions. Reglan is indicated for the relief of symptoms associated with **diabetic gastroparesis** and may aid in GI barium studies. It is also used as an antiemetic. Reglan can cause Parkinson-like symptoms (e.g., tremors, rigidity).

Antiviral Agents. Unlike most antibiotics, antiviral agents do not destroy their target pathogen; instead, they inhibit its development. Antiviral agents are used to treat herpes simplex, chickenpox, shingles, influenza (flu), hepatitis, and infection with the human immunodeficiency virus (HIV). Acyclovir (Zovirax) is used in the treatment of genital herpes, chickenpox, and shingles and is available in oral, topical, and parenteral forms. A three-drug combination is now the preferred initial treatment for HIV. Efavirenz, tenofovir, and emtricitabine (Atripla) is one of the initial treatments for HIV infections.

Bronchodilators. Bronchodilators are drugs used in the treatment of asthma and chronic obstructive pulmonary disease. These drugs relax bronchial smooth muscles and dilate the respiratory passages. They can be classified as short-acting and LA bronchodilators. Albuterol (ProAir HFA, Ventolin HFA) is the most commonly used fast-acting bronchodilator. It is generally administered by inhalation but can be administered orally. The most common side effects are tremors, nervousness, and increased heart rate (tachycardia). Tiotropium (Spiriva) is an LA bronchodilator, administered by inhalation. The most common side effect is dry mouth.

Cholinesterase Inhibitors. *Cholinesterase inhibitors* increase the levels of acetylcholine, a major neurotransmitter in the CNS. In Alzheimer disease (AD), concentrations of acetylcholine are reduced by 90%. Cholinesterase inhibitors such as donepezil (Aricept) are used in the management of AD. Approximately 4.5 million Americans have AD. The most common side effects are nausea, vomiting, and diarrhea. Cholinesterase inhibitors may exaggerate muscle relaxation under general anesthesia. Although not a cholinesterase inhibitor, memantine (Namenda) is a glutamate antagonist that is also used in the management of AD.

Coagulants. *Coagulants* are drugs used to control hemorrhage or to speed up coagulation. Most coagulants are commercial preparations of vitamin K, a fat-soluble vitamin needed for normal blood coagulation. Phytonadione (Mephyton) is a coagulant available in both oral and parenteral forms.

Corticosteroids. *Corticosteroids* are drugs used to reduce the symptoms associated with chronic inflammatory disorders or for the short-term treatment of acute inflammatory conditions. Dexamethasone (Decadron) and hydrocortisone (Solu-Cortef) are steroidal drugs used systemically, whereas methylprednisolone (Depo-Medrol) is generally injected locally at the inflammatory site, such as a joint or bursa. Fluticasone (Flovent) is administered by inhalation to decrease inflammation in the lungs. Prolonged use of corticosteroids can cause a variety of adverse side effects, such as osteoporosis and cataracts.

Diuretics. Diuretics are drugs that increase the amount of urine excreted by the kidneys, thus removing sodium and water from the body. Furosemide (Lasix) is a loop diuretic often used to treat the edema associated with congestive heart failure. Hydrochlorothiazide is a thiazide diuretic often used as monotherapy or in conjunction with other antihypertensive drugs for the treatment of high blood pressure. Patients receiving diuretics should be monitored for excessive fluid loss and electrolyte imbalance.

Hormones. *Hormones* are drugs that affect the endocrine system. The most important clinical application of these drugs is their use in replacement therapy, such as hypothyroidism. Levothyroxine (Synthroid) is used in the management of hypothyroidism. Conjugated estrogen (Premarin) is a female hormone used in treating moderate to severe vasomotor symptoms (e.g., night sweats, hot flashes) associated with menopause and to prevent osteoporosis. Other agents that affect sex hormones may inhibit the actions of naturally occurring sex hormones. Tamoxifen (Nolvadex) is an antiestrogen used to prevent and treat *breast cancer.*

Laxatives. Laxatives are drugs that act to promote the passage and elimination of feces from the large intestines. Laxatives are frequently used in radiology to prepare patients for both GI procedures and urinary tract procedures. Laxatives such as bisacodyl (Dulcolax), magnesium citrate, and polyethylene glycol electrolyte solution (GoLYTELY) are used to eliminate all fecal matter (stool) from the colon so the physician will have a clear view of the intestinal wall. Miralax (polyethylene glycol) is a powder that can be mixed in a cold or hot beverage to increase the amount of water in the intestinal tract to stimulate bowel movements.

Mood-Stabilizing Drugs. *Mood-stabilizing drugs* prevent mood swings in patients with manic-depressive (bipolar) disorder. Lithium is one agent used in treating bipolar disorder. It is orally administered. Polyuria (large volume of urine), tremor, and hypothyroidism (deficiency of thyroid function) are potential adverse effects.

Nonsteroidal Antiinflammatory Drugs. *Nonsteroidal antiinflammatory drugs* (NSAIDs) have analgesic, antipyretic (fever reducing), and antiinflammatory actions. Most of the NSAIDs available are nonselective. Ibuprofen (Motrin) is an example of a nonselective NSAID commonly used to treat inflammatory conditions, moderate to severe, and fever. Celecoxib (Celebrex) is an example of a COX-2 selective NSAID; it is used to treat inflammatory conditions and moderate to severe pain. All NSAIDs can cause GI irritation, peptic ulcers, GI bleeding, and acute renal failure, although Celebrex causes less GI bleeding and fewer peptic ulcers. All NSAIDs have a black box warning that they may increase the risk for serious and potentially fatal cardiovascular events, MI, and stroke, and this risk may increase with duration of use.

Osteoporosis Drugs. Osteoporosis is characterized by a gradual reduction of bone mass and bone quality that weakens the bone and increases the risk for fractures. The bisphosphonates are considered the drug of choice for the treatment of osteoporosis. The bisphosphonates alendronate (Fosamax) and risedronate (Actonel) are commonly used and are administered orally. Some of their adverse effects include diarrhea, abdominal pain, and esophageal ulcers. Other agents used include raloxifene (Evista), a selective estrogen receptor modulator administered orally.

Sedatives or Hypnotics. The *sedatives,* or *hypnotics,* can produce varying degrees of CNS depression ranging from mild sedation to sleep. Zolpidem (Ambien) and eszopiclone (Lunesta) are commonly used hypnotics. Extended use of these drugs can lead to physical dependence.

Stimulants. CNS stimulants increase the activity of the brain and spinal cord. Amphetamine salts (Adderall) and methylphenidate (Ritalin) are examples of CNS stimulants used to treat attention deficit/hyperactivity disorder. Dobutamine (Dobutrex) and dopamine (Intropin) stimulate the myocardium of the heart and are administered parenterally to treat conditions such as hypotension and **shock**.

Thrombolytics. The *thrombolytics* drugs dissolve thrombi (clots) that have already formed. Alteplase (tPA, Activase), and reteplase (Retavase) are common thrombolytics. They are administered parenterally in cases of acute MI and stroke. The major adverse effect is bleeding complications.

Vasoconstrictors. The **vasoconstrictors** drugs cause blood vessels to constrict, thus increasing heart action and raising blood pressure. Norepinephrine (Levophed) is a potent vasoconstrictor administered parenterally in the treatment of shock. This drug should be injected intravenously because **infiltration** can cause tissue necrosis.

Vasodilators. The **vasodilators** drugs cause blood vessels to dilate. They are useful in treating vascular disease, particularly angina. Nitroglycerin is an effective coronary vasodilator administered sublingually, orally, topically, or parenterally. Nitroprusside (Nitropress) is a peripheral vasodilator that is effective when used in a hypertensive crisis or in treating heart failure.

Pharmacokinetics

The study of how a drug is absorbed into the body, circulates within the body, is changed by the body, and leaves the body is called **pharmacokinetics**. The following four basic factors influence the movement of a drug:

- Absorption: Drug movement from its site of administration into the blood.
- Distribution: Drug movement from the blood to various tissues and organs of the body.
- Metabolism: Chemical alteration of various substances (drugs). The liver is the main organ involved in drug metabolism, taking a drug that is fat soluble and turning it into a water-soluble substance so it can be eliminated from the body.
- Excretion: Drug movement out of the body. The kidney is the most important organ for drug excretion.

Many factors can affect the pharmacokinetics of drugs and therefore affect the intended drug response. A drug's absorption rate is determined by how the drug is administered, the physicochemical properties, and formulation. Older adult patients (65 years of age or older) may respond differently to drugs than younger patients because of decreased absorption, metabolism, and excretion. They generally require a reduction in dose. In addition, children, especially in their first year of life, because of reduced capacity for the metabolism and excretion of drugs, will generally need a reduction in dose. The presence of diseases may decrease the function of vital organs. Liver or kidney disease can influence the metabolism and excretion of drugs, potentially leading to a greater incidence of adverse effects. Modification of a drug's effect by previous or concomitant administration of another drug or food is referred to as a *drug interaction*. If a patient is taking antacids which elevate gastric pH, they will also increase the absorbance of basic drugs and decrease the absorbance of acidic drugs. Other factors that can affect the intended drug effect are sex, genetics, weight, route, and time of administration.

Drugs have a variety of effects in the human body—the clinically desirable actions and the undesirable effects. These adverse drug effects include side effects, toxic effects, allergic reactions, and idiosyncratic reactions. An **idiosyncratic reaction** is a drug reaction that does not occur in most patients who have been treated with the drug and does not include the therapeutic effect of the drug. Essentially, it is impossible to determine who will have an idiosyncratic reaction to a drug. Idiosyncratic reactions are the most dangerous because they are unpredictable and life threatening. A patient's susceptibility is caused by individual genetic differences. A **side effect** results from the drug acting on tissues other than those intended, which causes a response unrelated to the intended action. For example, an antihistamine is intended to counteract an allergic condition, but one of the side effects commonly produced by the drug is drowsiness, which is caused by the drug's unintended effect on the CNS. Toxic effects are adverse drug effects related to the dose of drug administered. Most drugs are capable of producing toxic effects if the therapeutic dose is greatly exceeded. Allergic reactions occur when the body's immunologic system is hypersensitive to the presence of the drug. Allergic reactions can occur only after repeated exposure to the specific drug or a chemically related compound; however, the radiologic technologist must remember that prior sensitization to the drug may have taken place without the knowledge of the patient. An allergic reaction may take one of two forms: immediate or delayed. Immediate reactions may range from a mild response such as hives to a severe life-threatening response such as **anaphylaxis**, which may include respiratory or circulatory collapse. Delayed reactions are usually less severe than immediate reactions and may not become evident for hours or even days after the drug has been administered. The technologist must know the location of the nearest crash cart but also have knowledge of the drugs on the crash cart. Medical errors occur due to the lack of knowledge of drugs and drug administration. The patient has five drug rights regarding medication. It should be that the right patient receives the right drug, the right amount, the right time, and the right route. In addition, the technologist is responsible for accurate documentation and assisting with patient monitoring after a drug is administered, especially in an emergency situation. The

TABLE 21.4 Emergency Drugs Commonly Found on a Crash Cart

Medication	Indication
Adenosine	Cardiac arrhythmias
Amiodarone	Cardiac arrest
Aspirin	Inhibit platelet aggregation, analgesic
Atropine Sulfate	Beta blocker
Benadryl	Allergic reaction
Cardizem	Cardiac dysrhythmias
Dextrose	Restore sugar levels
Epinephrine	Cardiac arrest, anaphylaxis
Lopressor	Beta blocker
Narcan	Opioid overdose
Nitroglycerin Spray	Angina
Pronestyl (Procainamide)	Antiarrhythmic
Solumedrol	Allergic reactions

drugs commonly found on a crash cart for emergency situations are listed alphabetically by trade name in Table 21.4.

In radiology, drugs are often administered to patients, particularly pediatric patients, to sedate them for a lengthy or difficult procedure. The American Society of Anesthesiologists has developed a continuum to describe the various levels of sedation. The sedation levels are as follows:

- Minimal sedation (anxiolysis)
- Moderate sedation/analgesia (conscious sedation)
- Deep sedation/analgesia
- General anesthesia

Minimal sedation is a drug-induced state during which patients will respond normally to verbal commands. Cognitive function and coordination may be affected, but ventilation and cardiovascular function are unaffected. With moderate sedation, a drug-induced depression of consciousness occurs, but patients respond purposefully to verbal commands. This term has replaced the term conscious sedation. Ventilation is adequate and cardiovascular function is usually maintained. With deep sedation, a drug-induced depression of consciousness occurs during which patients cannot be easily aroused. They can respond purposefully after repeated or painful stimuli. Ventilation may be inadequate, but cardiovascular function is usually maintained. General anesthesia is a drug-induced loss of consciousness during which patients are not arousable even to painful stimuli. Ventilation is frequently inadequate, and cardiovascular function may be impaired. Because levels of sedation are along a continuum, predicting how a patient will respond is not always possible. Children, in particular, are prone to slip from one state to another with little warning.

SUMMARY

- Pharmacology is the scientific study of drugs, including the origin, nature, effects, and uses of drugs. The radiologic technologist is expected to have a basic knowledge of pharmacology to prepare and administer drugs under the supervision of a licensed practitioner.

- Drugs are classified in a variety of ways. A drug may be classified by name, action, or how the drug is obtained—either by prescription or over the counter. When drugs are classified by name, a single drug has a chemical name that represents its actual chemical structure; a generic name, which is a simplified version that reflects the chemical structure but is easier to pronounce; and the brand name, which is unique to the company that manufactures the drug. The *PDR*, easily found online, is a reference that lists drugs by both generic and trade names. Drugs are also classified according to proposed action, with drugs that have similar chemical actions grouped together.

- The dosage form indicates the type of preparation for drug administration. Some common dosage forms include tablets, capsules, suppositories, solutions, suspensions, and transdermal patches.

- The radiologic technologist should be familiar with the actions and precautions associated with commonly used drugs. A listing of commonly used drugs arranged alphabetically by trade name and a list of drugs most often found on an emergency cart are provided in this chapter for easy reference. An additional list arranged alphabetically by generic name is also provided.

BIBLIOGRAPHY

Allen L, Ansel HC: *Ansel's pharmaceutical dosage forms and delivery systems*, Baltimore, 2014, Lippincott Williams & Wilkins.

Basch E, Ulbricht C: *Natural standard herb and supplement handbook: the clinical bottom line*, St. Louis, 2005, Elsevier.

Brenner GM, Stevens CW: *Pharmacology*, ed 4, Philadelphia, 2013, Elsevier.

Brunton LL, Lazo JS, Parker KL: *Goodman & Gilman's the pharmacological basis of therapeutics*, ed 12, Chicago, 2010, McGraw-Hill.

Drug Enforcement Agency. www.dea.gov/druginfo/ds.shtml.

Golan DE, Tashjian JRAH, Armstrong EJ, et al.: *Principles of pharmacology: the pathophysiologic basis of drug therapy*, ed 3, Philadelphia, 2012, Lippincott Williams & Wilkins.

Koda-Kimble MA, Young LY, Aldredge BK, et al.: *Applied therapeutics: the clinical use of drugs*, ed 10, Philadelphia, 2013, Lippincott Williams & Wilkins.

Mangoni AA, Jackson SHD: Age-related changes in pharmacokinetics and pharmacodynamics: basic principles and practical applications, *Br J Clin Pharmacol* 57:6, 2003.

Physicians' desk reference, Montvale, NJ, 2014, Thompson.

Reynolds A: Patient-centerd care, *Radiol Technol* 81:2, 2009.

Rodbard HW, Jellinger PS, Davidson JA, et al.: Statement by an American Association of Clinical Endocrinologists/American College of Endocrinology consensus panel on type 2 diabetes mellitus: an algorithm for glycemic control, *Endocr Pract* 15:540, 2009.

Shimbo D, Tanner R, Muntner P: Prevalence and characteristics of systolic blood pressure thresholds in individuals 60 years or older, *JAMA* 178:8, 2014.

Shargel L, Wu-Pong S, Yu ABC: *Applied biopharmaceutics and pharmacokinetics*, ed 5, New York, 2005, McGraw-Hill.

Stedman's medical dictionary for the health profession and nursing, Baltimore, 2005, Lippincott Williams & Wilkins.

Stone NJ, Blum CB: *Management of lipids in clinical practice*, ed 7, West Islip, NY, 2008, Professional Communications.

Thengampallil A, Thengampallil S: Pharmacology in radiology, *Rad Tech* 80:6, 2009.

Uetrecht J, Naisbitt D: Idiosyncratic adverse drug reactions: current concepts, *Pharmacol Rev* 65:2, 2013, https://doi.org/10.1124/pr.113.007450.

You JJ, Singer DE, Howard PA, et al.: Antithrombotic therapy for atrial fibrillation antithrombotic therapy and prevention of thrombosis, 9th ed, american college of chest physicians evidence-based clinical practice guidelines, *Chest* 141(Suppl):e531S, 2012.

22

Principles of Drug Administration

Kenya Haugen, DM, MS, RT(R)

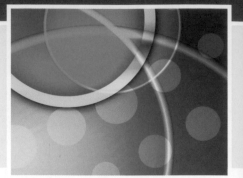

The greatest wealth is health.

Virgil (70 BC–19 BC)

OBJECTIVES

On completion of this chapter, the student will be able to:
- List the five rights of drug administration.
- Identify the common metric systems of measurement.
- List the methods of drug administration.
- Identify the appropriate areas for drug administration.
- Prepare intravenous drugs for injection.

- Perform venipuncture using appropriate universal precautions.
- Describe documentation procedures related to drug administration.
- Identify common standard abbreviations.

OUTLINE

KEY TERMS

Ampule Small sealed glass container that holds a single dose of parenteral solution in a sterile condition

Angiocath Catheter inserted directly into the vein for drug administration

Bolus Concentrated mass of pharmaceutical preparation

Buccal Pertaining to the inside of the mouth

Drip Infusion Infusion of liquid directly into the vein

Enteral Within the gastrointestinal tract

Extravasation Discharge or escape of fluid from a vessel into the surrounding tissue that can cause localized vasoconstriction, resulting in sloughing of tissue and tissue necrosis if not reversed with an antidote

Intradermal Within or between the layers of skin

Intramuscular Within the muscle tissue

Intravenous Within a vein

Intravenous Injection Medication that is delivered by intravenous push (rapid delivery) or intravenous infusion (slow drip of medication over a period of time) directly into the vein

Parenteral or Parenterally Drug administration by a route other than the gastrointestinal (GI) tract, typically by injection through the skin

Rectal Inserted into the rectum

Subcutaneous Beneath the skin

Sublingual Beneath the tongue

Topical Applied to a certain area of the skin and affecting only the area to which it is applied

Transdermal Entering through the skin

Venipuncture Puncture of a vein

Vial Small glass bottle containing multiple doses of a drug

PRINCIPLES OF ADMINISTRATION

As a member of the health care team it is critical to understand how to prepare and administer drugs. Many responsibilities accompany the duties of administering drugs to patients. The radiologic technologist is expected to understand the appropriate dosage, side effects, contraindications, safe injection practices, and potential adverse patient reactions once a drug is administered. The radiography student must be supervised by a licensed professional and adhere to ethical, legal guidelines, and institutional policies when performing drug administration.

Five Rights

In preparing to administer drugs, the radiologic technologist should always follow the golden rules of drug administration, or what are commonly referred to as the *five rights* of drug administration (Box 22.1). When used properly, the five rights reduce medication errors and patient harm. The radiologic technologist's duty is not to only achieve the five rights but also to follow procedural guidelines designed by the organization to produce these outcomes.

> ⚡ **STOP**
>
> Ensure that you have made the check of the five rights before you administer any drug to your patient!

The five rights are as follows:
1. Right drug
2. Right amount
3. Right patient
4. Right time
5. Right route

When determining the *right drug* to administer, there are several precautions to follow. Read the entire label on the drug. *Check the name carefully.* Ensure that you have read the label when drawing up or pouring a medication. To ensure that the right drug is administered, always check the label on the container three times: once when the container is removed from the shelf, again when the drug is removed from the container, and a third time when the container is replaced. Remember that the names of different drugs sometimes sound similar. If you are asked to prepare a drug for another health professional to administer, always show the container to the person who will administer the drug.

> ⚡ **STOP**
>
> Never use a drug that is unlabeled, and always check labels for the expiration date. If the date is expired, do not use, and report it. If you are unsure if the container has been used, do not use and report it.

The *right amount,* or dose, of the drug must be used. To ensure that the right amount of the drug is used, it must be measured carefully and accurately. If drug remains, do not put back into original container; dispose of according to institutional policy. Check the department protocol to ensure that the correct amount is used for the respective examination.

> ## BOX 22.1 Five Rights of Drug Administration
>
> Right drug
> Right amount
> Right patient
> Right time
> Right route

The *right patient* must receive the drug. Use the institution's protocol for patient identifiers before administering the drug. Ask the patient to repeat his or her name; read and ask the patient's identification number, medical record number, and/or check the patient's birth date as it is printed on the patient's armband. If the patient is too young to speak or is unable to speak, ask a parent or someone else present to identify the patient. If the patient's name or any other identifiers do not match, STOP, and get the appropriate corrections made before continuing with the procedure. Once the patient is correctly identified, explain the use of the drug with the patient and how it will be administered for the examination.

The drug must be administered at the *right time.* The physician or practitioner responsible for ordering the drug usually determines the right time for the administration of the drug. As a general rule, the radiologic technologist does not determine the time, but should administer the drug at the time specified. Once the drug is administered, do not leave the patient unattended. A patient may have an allergic reaction, and the radiographer must be familiar with the signs of a mild, moderate, and severe allergic reactions.

The *right route* must be used. Make certain that the drug is administered by the correct route. The physician usually specifies the route by which the drug should be administered. The radiologic technologist must be familiar with the terminology associated with the most common routes.

Finally, document the drug you used, the amount, route of administration, date, and time; if the patient refused to take the medication; and all other pertinent information that would be useful when the examination is reviewed. Document any patient drug allergies before drug administration. Allergies specifically to the cleaning agents that would be applied to the skin prior to injection should also be noted in the patient's record. Ask the patient about latex allergies. Any time a drug is administered to a patient, relevant information must be recorded on the patient's medical record to document the event. If the drug is administered **parenterally,** the site of injection should be included.

Legal Considerations

Increasingly, radiologic technologists are expected to chart a drug that they administered or helped to administer. The technologist must follow the proper precautions and make certain that all information is documented on the patient's chart. If an error occurs in the administration of a drug, or if the patient experiences any adverse effects from the drug, make certain to document the details of the incident thoroughly. Both students and radiologic technologists

TABLE 22.1   Common Abbreviations

Abbreviation	Meaning
ac	Before meals
bid	Twice a day
$\bar{c}$	With
et	And
g	Gram
gtt	Drop(s)
h	Hour
hs	At bedtime
Hypo	Hypodermic(ally)
IM	Intramuscular(ly)
IV	Intravenous(ly)
mg	Milligram
mL	Milliliter
mm	Millimeter
od	In the right eye
os	In the left eye
pc	After meals
PO	By mouth
prn	As needed
qh	Every hour
q2h	Every 2 h
q3h	Every 3 h
qid	Four times a day
$\bar{s}$	Without
SC	Subcutaneous
stat	Immediately
tid	Three times a day

TABLE 22.2   Metric Measurements

Weight	Volume	Equivalents
Microgram (mcg)	Milliliter (mL)	One milliliter (1 mL) is the same as 1 cubic centimeter (1 cc)
Milligram (mg)	Cubic centimeter (cc)	1000 milliliters = 1 liter = 1000 cubic centimeters
		1000 micrograms = 1 milligram
		1000 milligrams = 1 gram
		1000 grams = 1 kilogram
		100 milligrams = 0.1 gram
Gram (g or gm)		10 milligrams = 0.01 gram
Kilogram (kg)	Liter (L)	1 kilogram = 2.2 pounds

must follow these simple rules. Errors associated with drug administration are among the most common legal problems in which radiologic technologists are involved. If an error is made or an adverse drug event occurs, immediately report the incident to a supervisor or physician. Follow facility protocols for drug charting and reporting drug administration errors and adverse drug events.

Common Abbreviations

Health care professionals who order, dispense, or administer drugs often use abbreviations. Becoming thoroughly familiar with the common abbreviations that are used is important to ensure the safe and accurate administration of drugs. The list of abbreviations found in Table 22.1 includes those that are frequently encountered when administering drugs. The Joint Commission has published a *DO NOT USE* list of abbreviations. A current list can be found on their website at http://www.jointcommission.org. For example, the abbreviation *U or u* meaning *unit* has been mistaken for *0* (zero), the number *4* (four), and *cc;* and *IU,* which stands for international unit, has been mistaken for *IV,* which means intravenous, and the number *10* (ten). In addition to the Joint Commission office "Do Not Use" List, the Institute for Safe Medication Practices (ISMP) has also published a list of error-prone abbreviations, symbols, and dose designations, which can be found on their website at http://www.ismp.org. Organizations are expected to standardize the abbreviations, acronyms, and symbols that will be used and

have a list of abbreviations, acronyms, and symbols that should not be used. It is best to spell out the word rather than use abbreviations to avoid potential drug administration errors.

Units of Measurement

The radiologic technologist should understand the units used in administering a drug. Too much of a drug can be deadly, and a small amount of the same drug can be therapeutic. Clinical facilities have established units of measurement for the various types of medications that the technologist may administer. Multiple measurement systems are used in the medical field. A technologist needs to know the different measurements and be able to convert from one unit or system to another. The metric system is commonly used in the United States. The metric system is based on units of 10. The most common units that the technologist encounters are the liter, meter, and gram. The most common unit of measurement for liquid medications is the milliliter, the equivalent of $\frac{1}{1000}$ of a liter (Table 22.2).

DRUG ADMINISTRATION ROUTES

Drugs are administered in a variety of ways, including enterally, topically, and parenterally.

Enteral Routes

Enteral routes include oral, sublingual, buccal, and rectal.

Oral. The oral route is the most common method of drug administration. This method of administration is medically termed PO (by mouth). The drug is taken by mouth and swallowed; it is absorbed from the gastrointestinal (GI) tract. When receiving drugs by the oral route, the patient must be conscious and the head should be elevated to aid in swallowing. Absorption time is longer, which is the reason for oral administration, because the absorption takes place along the entire length of the GI tract.

Oral administration is a safe and convenient method of drug administration if a few simple rules are followed (Box 22.2). When the patient takes a tablet or capsule, ensure that water is available to the patient for ease of swallowing the medication. Remember to always wash your hands thoroughly before

---

BOX 22.2 Rules for Oral Drug Administration

Wash hands thoroughly.
1. Place drug directly into a medicine cup or on a clean paper towel. Do not touch the drug with your hands.
2. Read the label three times.
3. Check two patient identifiers.
4. Explain the procedure to the patient. Ask the patient about any allergies.
5. Elevate the patient's head.
6. Provide water or liquid to aid in swallowing.
7. Allow the patient to take the drug.
8. Chart all relevant information.

BOX 22.3 Rules for Topical Drug Administration

1. Wash hands thoroughly.
2. Put on disposable gloves.
3. Read the label three times.
4. Check two patient identifiers.
5. Explain the procedure to the patient. Ask the patient about any allergies.
6. Apply the amount of drug prescribed.
7. Chart all relevant information.

---

preparing or administering an oral medication. Avoid touching tablets or capsules with your hands. Transfer tablets, capsules, or liquid from the container directly into a medication cup or clean paper towel. When pouring liquids, pour away from the label, and wipe the neck of the bottle with a clean, damp cloth before replacing the cap.

Never leave a patient unattended while the patient is taking an oral medication. Ensure that the medication is completely consumed before leaving the patient.

Sublingual. Administration by the sublingual route means that the drug is placed under the tongue and allowed to dissolve. Drugs intended to be administered sublingually should not be swallowed. One drug commonly given by the sublingual route is nitroglycerin. This allows for rapid absorption for immediate onset of action.

Buccal. Administration by the buccal route means that the drug is placed against the mucous membranes of the cheek of the upper or lower jaw. The buccal drug will dissolve. A lozenge is commonly given by the buccal route. This allows for a local effect.

Rectal. Administration by the rectal route is an option when the patient is not capable of taking a drug orally. The radiologic technologist will have little to no reason to administer a drug rectally. Effectiveness of rectal dosages may be difficult to measure because of varied absorption rates.

Topical Route

The topical route of drug administration involves the application of a drug directly onto the skin. The drug is diffused through the skin and absorbed into the bloodstream. Topical drugs can be applied as lotions or ointments. Drugs for topical application have become available in a unit-dose device called a transdermal patch. The patch is applied to the skin and provides a precise dose of drug released over a specified time. Drugs applied topically include tinctures, ointments, lotions, and sprays. To administer a topical drug to the skin properly, follow the steps outlined in Box 22.3. Drugs administered by this route should not be applied with the bare hand. After topical administration, the skin area must be monitored for any signs of local irritation.

Parenteral Route

The term *parenteral* means that the drug is administered by a route other than the GI tract, typically by injection using a syringe and needle. Parenteral administration is used when drug administration by other means would be ineffective or impractical. The parenteral method is a valuable method for administering drugs in an emergency. Parenteral drugs can be administered in four different routes: intradermal (ID), intramuscular (IM), with rapid onset of action; subcutaneous (subcut), with slow and constant absorption, and intravenous (IV), with immediate onset of action. Strict aseptic technique and Standard Precautions should always be used when drugs are administered with a needle. Infection control is of paramount importance in parenteral therapy because of breaking the skin's protective covering, which increases the risk for infection. The Occupational Safety and Health Administration (OSHA) issued standards on bloodborne pathogens, mandating the use of *universal precautions* and the *Needlestick Safety Prevention* program. If a drug is injected incorrectly, it may cause nerve damage or introduce microorganisms into the patient's system.

Drugs that are injected have a rapid onset of action because they are absorbed directly into the bloodstream. All forms of parenteral administration require the use of a needle, syringe, and container. Because this method of administration involves penetrating the protective layer of the skin, strict aseptic technique and standard precautions should be followed when preparing and administering the drug. In addition, it is important to become oriented with the type of safety needles used within a facility. Selecting the proper equipment and supplies for parenteral administration depends on the specific injection route, as well as the kind and amount of drug to be administered. The patient must be properly identified and the procedure explained to the patient before the injection. Each parenteral route of injection is discussed separately.

SUPPLIES FOR PARENTERAL DRUG ADMINISTRATION

Several types of needles are used to administer parenteral drugs. The different types of syringes include (1) standard hypodermic syringe (Fig. 22.1); (2) insulin syringe (Fig. 22.2); (3) tuberculin syringe (Fig. 22.3); and (4) prefilled syringe (Fig. 22.4). The hypodermic needle may be used for a variety of medications. The insulin syringe is used for the administration of insulin. The tuberculin syringe is best used for TB intradermal injection or Heparin subcutaneous injection. The tuberculin and insulin syringes are designed for situations that require the precise measurement of a small volume of drug. Drugs are injected into the body with a plastic syringe. Syringes may be packaged separately from the needle or packaged together with the needle. Syringes can be prefilled or empty. Plastic syringes are disposed of after being used only once.

A syringe has three parts: (1) the *tip,* where the needle attaches; (2) the *barrel,* where the calibration scales are printed and what holds the medication; and (3) the *plunger,* the inside part that fits into the barrel and changes the pressure within the barrel as it is pulled or pushed in or out of the barrel. The parts of a syringe are shown in Fig. 22.5. Several kinds of syringes have been produced, and they vary in size and shape. The general-purpose syringe comes in a variety of sizes, including 2, 2.5, 3, 5, 10, 20, and 50 mL. Some syringes, such as Luer-Lock syringes (Fig. 22.6), have a locking device on the tip that holds the needle firmly in place. An eccentric tip syringe is one that has the tip located to the side rather than in the center.

Most hospitals are now using needleless systems for intravenous administration of drugs to reduce the number of needle sticks. Many companies are making these systems, and many varieties are available. These systems have a few features in common. All needleless heparin locks have a white ring on the port, shown in Fig. 22.7. This feature identifies the lock as a needleless system, and needles should not be used.

Needles used for injection are made of stainless steel and may or may not be disposable. The needle has three parts: (1) the *hub,* which is the part that attaches to the syringe; (2) the *cannula* or *shaft,* which is the length of the metal part; and (3) the *bevel,* which is the slanted part at the tip of the needle. The parts of a needle are shown in Fig. 22.8. The tip of the needle is what penetrates the skin, and the bevel portion separates the tissues apart for the needle to easily pass through the tissues. Ensure the bevel is always up before insertion into the patient. Needles come in a plastic sheath for safety purposes. Needles are sized according to length and gauge. The *gauge* (G) refers to the thickness or diameter of the needle. The *length* refers to the measurement in inches of the shaft portion. The length will vary from 0.25 to 5 inches, the gauge from 14 to 28. The most common gauge needles are 19, 20, 21, 23, 25 gauge. As a rule, shorter needles are used for subcutaneous injections, and longer needles are used for intramuscular injections. Needles 1 to $1\frac{1}{2}$ inches in length are most commonly used for intravenous injections. The smaller the diameter of the shaft or the finer the needle is, the larger the gauge number will be. For example, a 25-gauge needle has a very small diameter, and an 18-gauge needle has a large diameter. Subcutaneous injections often use a 25-gauge needle, and an intravenous injection generally uses a 20- or 21-gauge needle. A large-diameter needle such as an 18-gauge needle is often used to draw a drug or solution into the syringe but is seldom used to inject the drug into the patient. The package label indicates both the length and the gauge of the needle. Two examples of prepackaged needles are shown in Fig. 22.9. Thus, a package labeled *20 g/1½* indicates that the needle is 20 gauge and 1½ inches long. The bevel of the needle may also vary from long to short. Fig. 22.10 illustrates the difference between a long-bevel needle and a short-bevel

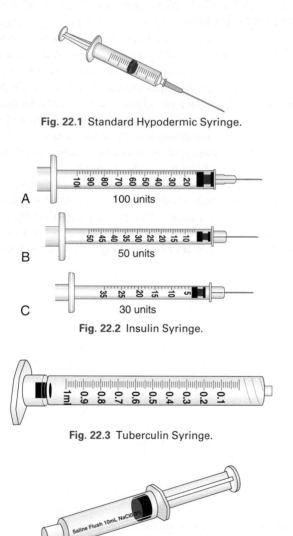

Fig. 22.1 Standard Hypodermic Syringe.

A   100 units

B   50 units

C   30 units

Fig. 22.2 Insulin Syringe.

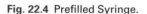

1ml

Fig. 22.3 Tuberculin Syringe.

Saline Flush 10mL NaCl 0.9%

Fig. 22.4 Prefilled Syringe.

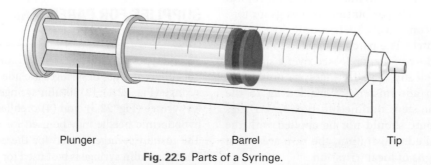

Plunger   Barrel   Tip

Fig. 22.5 Parts of a Syringe.

needle. Long-bevel needles are generally used for subcutaneous and intramuscular injections, and short-bevel needles are used for intravenous injections. The type of patient may also determine the length of the needle used for drug administration. The pediatric patient may require a shorter needle for subcutaneous injections compared with that for a patient with increased fatty deposits.

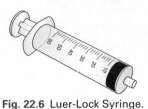

Fig. 22.6 Luer-Lock Syringe.

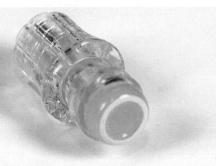

Fig. 22.7 A Needleless Injection System.

An **angiocath** is a safer device compared with other systems to use when performing venipuncture (Fig. 22.11). An angiocath, also called an intravenous catheter, is used the same as any other needle to puncture the vein. It differs from other systems in that after venipuncture, the user pulls on a sheath, which extracts the needle up through a catheter and into the protective sheath, where it cannot accidentally puncture anyone (Fig. 22.12). When using an angiocath, do not insert the catheter into a bifurcated vein or near a vein valve.

Drugs intended for use by parenteral administration are packaged in two different kinds of containers: ampules and vials. An **ampule** is a sealed glass container designed to hold a single dose of a drug and is intended for use only once. It is made of clear glass and has a shape with a scored constricted neck that is weakened so that it breaks more easily than other parts of the glass structure. The scoring line of the neck of the ampule is marked with a colored band indicating the breaking point. Wash hands and work on a clean surface; it may require the technologist to wear gloves. To prepare the ampule, it should be held upright and the top of the neck lightly flicked with a finger until all the drug is in the bottom part of the ampule (Fig. 22.13A). Then a dry gauze pad is wrapped around the neck of the ampule and the top snapped off (see Fig. 22.13B and C). Caution

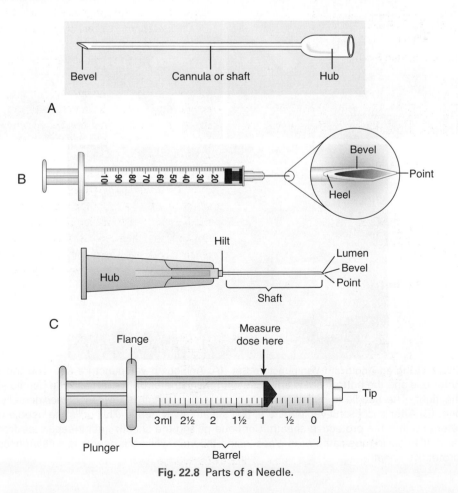

Fig. 22.8 Parts of a Needle.

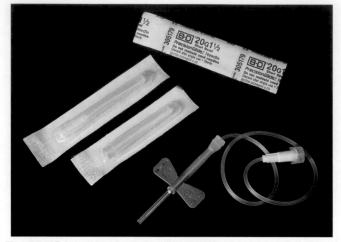

Fig. 22.9 Prepacked needles and winged or butterfly infusion sets showing the gauge and length of the needle.

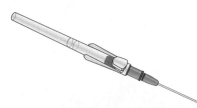

Long bevel for intramuscular or subcutaneous injection

Short bevel for intravenous injection

Fig. 22.10 **Needle Bevels.** Long or regular bevels are usually used for intramuscular or subcutaneous injections. Short bevels are commonly used for intravenous injections.

Fig. 22.11 Intravenous Catheters.

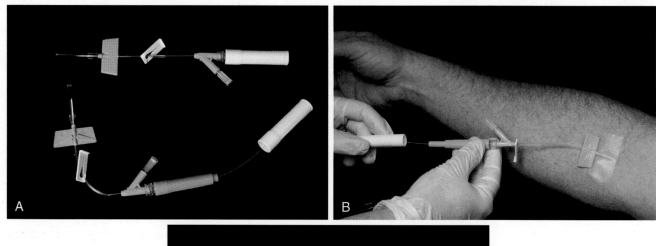

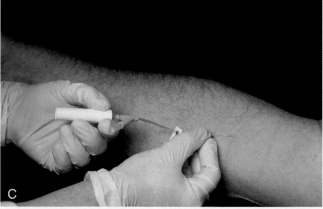

Fig. 22.12 **Using an Angiocath Venipuncture Set.** (A) Angiocath venipuncture set. The top set is ready for use and the bottom set is after use with the catheter on the left and the needle sheath on the right. The needle is pulled inside the protective sheath so it cannot accidentally stick anyone. (B) After successful venipuncture, pull sheath away gently. This pulls the needle up the catheter and into the protective sheath. Continue pulling the sheath until it separates from the catheter. (C) Leaving the catheter in place inside the vein while the needle is safely encased in the protective sheath.

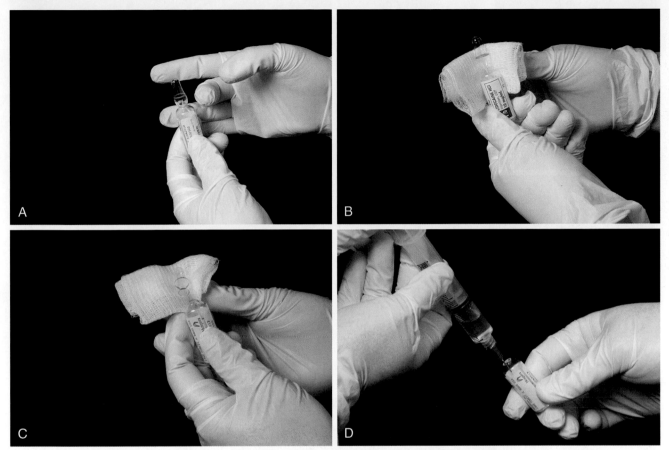

Fig. 22.13 Withdrawing a Drug From a Glass Ampule. (A) Flick the top of the neck until all liquid is in the bottom of the container. (B and C) With a gauze pad, snap off the top. (D) Withdraw the contents, being careful not to let the shaft of the needle touch the broken edge of the ampule. One person opens and holds the ampule while a second person withdraws the drug.

should be taken to avoid contaminating the needle by touching the outer broken edge of the ampule with the shaft of the needle when inserting it to draw out the contents. This task is best accomplished by letting the tip of the needle rest on the inside of the ampule (see Fig. 22.13D). The procedure is most easily performed when one person opens and holds the ampule while a second person withdraws the drug. When drawing medication from a glass ampule, you must use a filter needle and then change the needle before injecting.

A **vial** is a small glass or plastic bottle with a sealed rubber cap. Vials are manufactured in different sizes and may contain multiple doses of a drug. Wash hands and work on a clean surface; it may require the technologist to wear gloves. To prepare the vial, the metal cap is removed without breaking the outside metal seal, and the exposed rubber stopper is wiped with an alcohol wipe. This allows for decontamination before the entry of the needle. After a syringe package has been opened, the syringe plunger is pulled back to pull air into the syringe equal to the amount of drug that will be withdrawn from the vial. After the needle package is open, the needle is inserted on the end of the syringe without letting the end of the syringe and the end of the needle touch anything but each other. Carefully remove the needle cap and do not touch the needle. The vial is held securely in the nondominant hand and the vial inverted; with the dominant hand the needle can be inserted without letting the tip of the needle touch anything but the rubber stopper of the vial as shown in Fig. 22.14. With the tip of the needle in the fluid, air is injected equal to the volume of drug to be removed.

If the needle is above the fluid level in the vial, air instead of solution will be drawn into the syringe. The plunger is pulled back until the correct amount of drug has been drawn into the syringe. The needle can be withdrawn and the syringe held with the needle pointing up while the technologist is tapping it with his or her finger to move any air bubbles toward the hub, where it can be expelled by gently pushing on the plunger of the syringe. After use, the entire syringe and needle *must* be discarded into an acceptable sharps biohazard container (Fig. 22.15).

PARENTERAL ADMINISTRATION METHODS

Intradermal Injection

Intradermal injections are usually administered by injecting the contents of the syringe between the layers of the skin. Intradermal injection sites are on the inside of the lower arm, as for testing for exposure to tuberculin. Another site of administration includes the upper back below the shoulder blades and the chest, which is usually a site for allergy testing. Fig. 22.16 demonstrates proper needle placement for intradermal injections.

Intramuscular Injection

For an **intramuscular** injection, the drug is placed into muscle tissue that lies under the subcutaneous tissue layer. It is

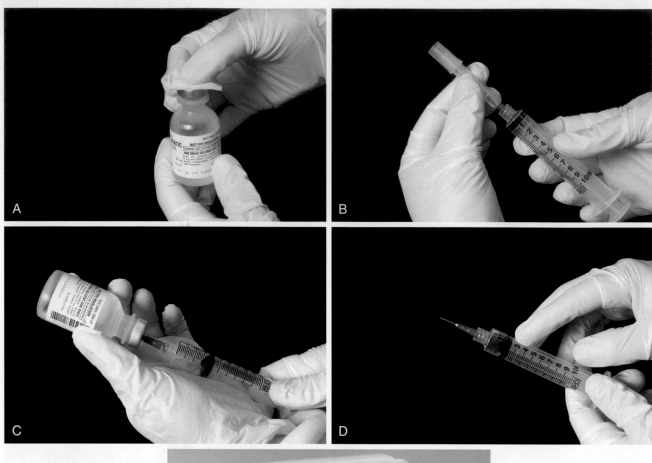

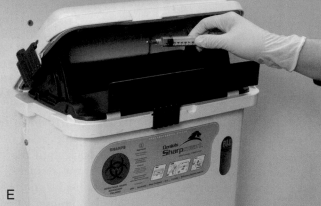

Fig. 22.14 Withdrawing a Drug From a Vial. (A) Break the seal, expose the rubber stopper, and wipe the stopper with an alcohol swab. (B) Open a syringe package and pull back the syringe plunger to pull air into the syringe equal to the amount of drug that will be withdrawn from the vial. Open a needle package and insert the needle on the end of the syringe without letting the end of the syringe and the end of the needle touch anything but each other. (C) Invert the vial, and with the dominant hand, insert the needle without letting the tip of the needle touch anything but the rubber stopper of the vial. With the tip of the needle in the fluid, inject air equal to the volume of drug to be removed. Pull back on the plunger until the correct amount of drug has been drawn into the syringe. (D) Remove the needle and hold the syringe with the needle pointing up while tapping it with your finger to move any air bubble toward the hub, where it can be expelled by gently pushing on the plunger of the syringe. (E) After use, dispose of the entire syringe and needle into an acceptable *sharps* biohazard container.

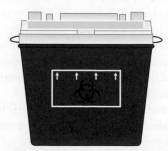

Fig. 22.15 Sharps Container.

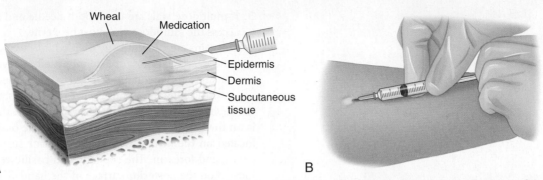

Fig. 22.16 Intradermal Injections. A, cross section view of the intradermal injection into the dermis of the skin. B, visual of the wheal formation when intradermal injection into the dermis of the skin.

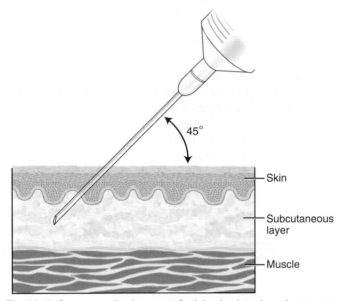

Fig. 22.17 Proper needle placement for injection into the subcutaneous tissue. The needle is inserted at a 45-degree angle.

BOX 22.4 Steps Involved in Intramuscular Drug Injection

1. Wash hands thoroughly.
2. Put on disposable gloves.
3. Check two patient identifiers.
4. Explain the procedure to the patient. Ask the patient about any allergies.
5. Prepare the site by cleansing the skin with an alcohol swab using a circular motion and moving from the center to the outside.
6. Inspect the needle for any frayed or sheared areas. If this is noted, properly dispose of the defective needle.
7. With your free hand, retract the skin approximately 1 inch to either side of the site and hold it firmly.
8. Insert the needle at a 90-degree angle.
9. Continue to hold the skin while you gently pull back on the plunger to make certain the needle is not in a blood vessel.
10. If blood does not appear in the syringe, slowly inject the drug. If blood appears in the syringe, remove the needle and prepare another site for injection.
11. Withdraw the needle while releasing the tension on the skin.
12. Apply gentle pressure to the site with a gauze.
13. Unless contraindicated, massage the injection site.
14. Dispose of the syringe and needle properly.
15. Chart all relevant information.

---

necessary to locate the appropriate injection site for intramuscular injection. It is possible to damage a blood vessel when injecting deeply into the muscle. The most commonly used intramuscular injection sites include the deltoid muscle in the upper arm, the vastus lateralis muscle in the lateral thigh, and the gluteus maximus muscles in the buttocks.

In general, the needle length is 1 to 3 inches with a 19 to 25 gauge, depending on the viscosity of the drug to be injected. Intramuscular injections allow for a larger amount of drug to be administered—up to 3 mL. The muscle can absorb medications faster than other tissues. This route is also effective for patients who are unable to swallow. Fig. 22.17 demonstrates the proper placement of the needle for an intramuscular injection. A 90-degree angle of insertion is used for intramuscular injections. Box 22.4 lists the steps involved in intramuscular injection.

Subcutaneous Injection

When a subcutaneous injection is administered, the drug is placed under the skin into the subcutaneous tissue that lies under the epidermal layers. The thickness of the subcutaneous tissue depends on whether the patient is obese and, if so, to what degree. In some pediatric and older patients, this layer of thickness is difficult to identify. The most commonly used subcutaneous sites include the anterior thigh, upper back below the shoulder blades, outer upper arm, and abdomen. Subcutaneous absorption is slower than the intramuscular route because of the lack of vascularity. The needle length and angle of insertion depend on the thickness of the subcutaneous tissue. Fig. 22.18 illustrates the proper placement of the needle for a subcutaneous injection. For average-size patients, a 25-gauge, 5/8-inch needle at a 45-degree angle of insertion is generally used. For above-average-size patients, a 25-gauge, 1/2-inch needle at a 90-degree angle of insertion is generally used. Box 22.5 lists the steps involved in subcutaneous injection.

Intravenous Injection

When an intravenous injection is administered, the drug is placed directly into a vein and a rapid action occurs in minutes. Intravenous drug administration is effective for the patient when the other parenteral routes would not be as effective. When injecting an intravenous drug or contrast agent, the patient cannot be left alone. Reactions can occur immediately, and any changes in the patient's vital signs or behavior must be reported to a physician immediately and recorded in the patient's chart.

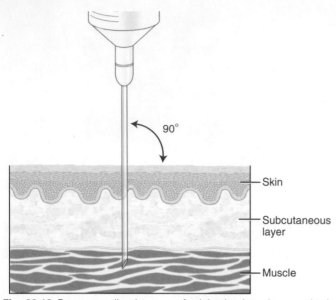

90°

— Skin

— Subcutaneous layer

— Muscle

Fig. 22.18 Proper needle placement for injection into the muscle tissue. The needle is inserted at a 90-degree angle. (The picture for this image is reversed with the picture for Fig. 22.17).

BOX 22.5 Steps Involved in Subcutaneous Drug Injection

1. Wash hands thoroughly.
2. Put on disposable gloves.
3. Check two patient identifiers.
4. Explain the procedure to the patient. Ask the patient about any allergies.
5. Prepare the site by cleansing it with an alcohol swab using a circular motion and moving from the center to the outside.
6. Inspect the needle for any frayed or sheared areas. If this is noted, properly dispose of the defective needle.
7. With your free hand, pinch the skin gently together, and insert the needle quickly at the appropriate angle for the patient's size.
8. Release the skin and pull back on the syringe plunger to make certain the needle is not in a blood vessel.
9. Inject drug slowly, and quickly withdraw the needle at the same angle used for insertion.
10. Dispose of the syringe and needle properly.
11. Chart all relevant information.

⚡ STANDARD PRECAUTIONS

With any injection it is necessary to perform adequate standard precautions because all patients are considered potentially infectious with bloodborne pathogens. Always follow all universal precautions before attempting any parenteral drug administration. Safe injection practices are part of standard precautions and are a set of measures taken to maintain basic levels of patient safety, health care providers, and others.

Injection Safety
1. Adhere to facility protocols for infection control and aseptic technique.
2. Do not administer drugs or medications from a syringe to multiple patients. One needle, one syringe, one patient.
3. Use intravenous or drip infusion sets for one patient only and dispose after use.
4. Use single-dose vials whenever possible.

---

5. If multidose vials are used, both needle and syringe used to access the multidose vial must be sterile.

The veins are anatomically divided into two groups: superficial and deep. The most commonly used intravenous injection sites include the median cubital vein, the superficial vein that lies over the cubital fossa and serves as an anastomosis between the cephalic and basilic veins. The location of the cephalic vein is on the lateral side of the forearm and the basilic vein can be located on the medial side of the anterior surface of the arm, elbow, and forearm. The cephalic and basilic veins can also be located on the posterior surface of the hand. The cephalic vein and basilic veins are the best choices when available. Fig. 22.19 shows the sites commonly used for **venipuncture.** Veins in the arms and hands should be selected for most common procedures. The veins in the lower extremities should be used only in an emergency. If using the vein that lies over the cubital fossa, ensure that the patient's arm is immobilized unless an intravenous catheter is used instead of a needle. The palm side of the wrist should be avoided because of the close proximity of the radial nerve. The needle length and gauge depend on the viscosity of the drug, the site selected, and the specific method of injection. Injection of contrast with a small-gauge needle may cause leakage of the contrast into surrounding tissues. It is best to use a larger gauge needle—18 to 20 gauge—when injecting contrast.

⚡

If you are injured or pricked by a needle or other sharp object or get blood or other potentially infectious materials in the eyes, nose, mouth, or on broken skin, flood the area with water, clean with soap and water, report the incident immediately, and follow facility protocols for a needle stick.

⚡ INAPPROPRIATE SITES FOR VENIPUNCTURE

Scarred areas, arm on side of mastectomy, edematous areas, hematomas, arm getting a blood transfusion, arm with a fistula or vascular graft, bifurcated vein, vein valve, and sites above an intravenous access device.

One of the most commonly used intravenous needles is the winged-tip or butterfly needle, which is manufactured in lengths of ¼ to 1¼ inch and 18 to 25 gauge. An 18- to 20-gauge butterfly needle is commonly used for adults and 22- to 23-gauge devices are more commonly used for pediatric patients. It has tubing 3 to 12 inches long that extends from the needle to the hub. Winged needles are usually 21 g (green) or 23 g (blue) and best used for shallow veins. A butterfly needle is shown in Fig. 22.20. Box 22.6 identifies the steps involved in venipuncture and intravenous injection. During injection of a drug into the vein, observing the site closely for any signs of extravasation or infiltration is important—the tissue will swell around the area of the injection site, and the area will become edematous and painful for the patient. If extravasation occurs, the first step is to remove the needle, apply pressure to the injection site, and apply moist heat pack to relieve the discomfort. If the extravasation involves a corrosive drug, immediate attention is needed to prevent tissue necrosis. When a corrosive drug infiltrates the tissue, a cold pack rather than heat should be applied to the site, and the physician and pharmacy must be notified. It is important for the technologist to understand the effects of the drug if extravasation occurs because appropriate treatment management varies depending on the type of infused drug. Box 22.7 explains how to appropriately apply a tourniquet.

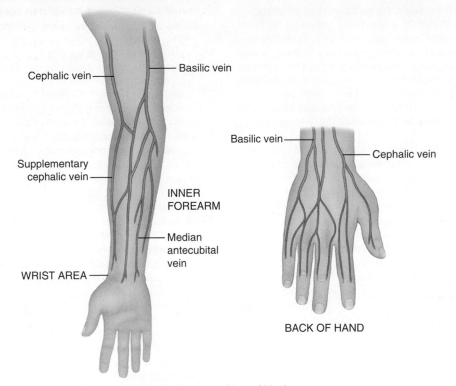

Fig. 22.19 Common Sites of Venipuncture.

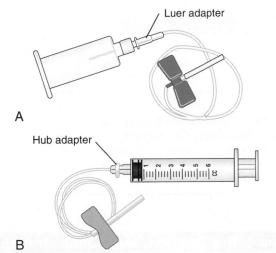

Fig. 22.20 Butterfly Winged Infusion Set. A, winged infusion set (butterfly needle) with plastic holder. B, winged infusion set (butterfly needle) with syringe.

Intravenous Injection Methods. Drugs that are administered by the intravenous route may be injected using one of three methods. One method involves a single administration in which the drug is injected slowly. A second method involves the administration of a drug by intravenous bolus or intravenous push. The term **bolus** refers to the amount of fluid injected, and *intravenous push* refers to a rapid injection. This method is generally used in an emergency when immediate drug action is required. The third method of administration involves the intravenous infusion of a large volume of fluid. This method

is sometimes called a **drip infusion,** and it requires some additional equipment to ensure accurate delivery of the intravenous solution. A drip infusion also includes the delivery of a certain amount of medication over a certain period.

An administration set for infusion of the solution and an intravenous pole are needed. Box 22.8 outlines the steps involved in preparing for drip infusion. The proper procedure for setting up drip infusion solutions is demonstrated in Fig. 22.21.

When a standard administration set is used, adjusting the clamp below the drip chamber controls the flow rate or drip rate. Unless otherwise instructed by a physician, 10 to 20 drops per minute is an acceptable flow rate. Patients receiving intravenous infusion should be monitored closely. If the flow stops, the site of injection should be checked for signs of infiltration. If evidence such as swelling and pain around the injection site exists, the infusion must be stopped immediately, the needle removed, and a warm pack applied to the area.

Patients receiving medication by the intravenous infusion method may come to the radiology department with additional equipment attached to the administration set. An intravenous pump and controller are devices used to regulate the flow rate electronically (Fig. 22.22). A controller regulates the flow rate by counting the drops and compressing the intravenous tubing to adjust the flow. A pump propels the solution through the tubing at the desired rate under pressure. The pump is more accurate than the controller. Both devices have alarms that sound a beep or flash a light when the infusion fails to flow at the prescribed flow rate.

BOX 22.6 Steps Involved in Venipuncture and Intravenous Drug Injection

1. Wash hands thoroughly.
2. Check two patient identifiers.
3. Explain the procedure to the patient. Ask the patient about any allergies.
4. Assemble all needed supplies for venipuncture to include but not limited to a topical anesthetic spray, gauze, tape, and/or adhesive bandage strip, tourniquet, appropriate needle or butterfly, syringe or intravenous catheter. Inspect the bevel for any frayed or sheared areas. If this is noted, properly dispose of the defective needle. Ensure the needle size is appropriate for the patient. Pediatric patients may require a smaller needle gauge in comparison with one for an adult. If using a butterfly needle, include in the preparation flushing the needle with saline before administering the drug.
5. Put on disposable gloves.
6. Once an appropriate site for venipuncture has been selected, clean it with an alcohol swab using a circular motion while moving from the center to the outside. Allow the area to dry before inserting the needle. Thirty seconds is appropriate amount of drying time. Do NOT blow or fan the area in an attempt to dry the area. Inadequate drying may cause the patient to feel a stinging sensation from the alcohol swab. Once the site has been cleaned, you cannot touch the venipuncture site with or without gloves. This is contaminating the area, and you will need to alcohol swab the area again.
7. Apply a tourniquet above the site using sufficient tension to impede the flow of blood in the vein. Ensure that the ends of the tourniquet do not dangle over the proposed venipuncture site. Geriatric patients may have extremely sensitive skin that may tear under the pressure of the tourniquet. Ask the patient to open and close the fist to distend the vein fully. Palpate the vein if necessary. When the vein has been identified, ask the patient to hold the fist in a clenched position.
8. To stabilize the median cephalic vein, place your thumb on the tissue just above or below the site and gently pull the skin and vein toward the patient's hand if below and toward the patient's shoulder if above. Stabilizing the vein prevents the vein from rolling under the pressure of the needle entering the vein. Geriatric patients have veins that tend to roll and may be more fragile.
9. Hold the needle with the bevel facing upward. You should see the opening of the bevel. When using a butterfly needle, pinch the wings together tightly toward you. The reason the wings of the needle are held is to allow the technologist to grasp the needle close to the end to ensure accurate placement in the vein.
10. Insert the needle next to the vein at a 15–30 degree angle and gently advance it into the vein. Blood flows back into the tubing when the needle is correctly positioned. If there is only a flash of blood in the tubing of the butterfly, gently reposition the needle. If the needle is pulled out during the reposition, you will need to start again. DO NOT reinsert the needle if it has exited the vein and skin.
11. If the tubing of the butterfly needle has not previously been filled with solution, allow the blood to flow from the hub before attaching the syringe to ensure that no air bubbles are contained in the system.
12. If using an intravenous catheter to inject the solution, insert the needle next to the vein at a 15–30 degree angle, and gently advance into the vein once the flashback of blood is seen in the chamber of the catheter.
13. On flashback visualization, lower the catheter to be parallel with the skin. Advance the entire catheter unit before threading the flexible plastic portion of the catheter into the vein. Advance the plastic sheath of the catheter into the vein while pulling the needle back away from the sheath while maintaining a taut pressure on the patient's skin. Most catheters have a spring release button to retract the needle. Once the needle is retracted, blood will flow freely. Dispose of the needle properly.
14. Remove the tourniquet and inject the drug. If using the catheter, you will need to apply a syringe to administer the drug. Use facility procedure.
15. Unless otherwise instructed, remove the needle and apply gentle pressure to the site with a gauze.
16. If using the catheter, remove the plastic sheath that is in the patient's vein and apply gentle pressure with gauze once the catheter is removed.
17. Dispose of the syringe and needle or butterfly needle properly.
18. Chart all relevant information.

BOX 22.7 Proper Tourniquet Application

The purpose of the tourniquet is to minimize venous blood flow back to the heart while allowing arterial blood to continue to flow to the extremity.

1. Ask the patient about any allergies to latex. Do not use a latex tourniquet if the patient has a latex allergy. If possible, use disposable, single-use tourniquets.
2. Apply the tourniquet 3–4 inches above the area for venipuncture or IV drug injection. The vein will fill with blood which will make vein location and identification easier.
3. If using the median cephalic vein in the patient's arm, place the tourniquet under the patient's arm with an end in each hand. The tourniquet should be flat under the patient's arm.
4. Holding tension on both ends of the tourniquet, swap the two ends. Pull the ends upward, forming a "X."
5. Pinch the "X" with the left thumb and index finger. Fold one end on the right side over itself. The left side should be slightly tighter than the other.
6. Tuck the right double-folded end halfway under the left next to the pinched "X," leaving both ends point away from the injection site.
7. Do not leave the tourniquet on for more than two minutes. If using the tourniquet for vein selection, a minute or less is appropriate.

BOX 22.8 Steps Involved in Setting Up an Intravenous or Drip Infusion Drug Administration

1. Wash hands thoroughly.
2. Check two patient identifiers.
3. Explain the procedure to the patient.
4. Assemble all needed supplies.
5. Check the expiration date. Remove the administration set from the box and straighten the tubing while checking for any cracks or holes.
6. Slide the clamp up to the drip chamber and close it.
7. If the intravenous solution to be infused is contained in a bottle, place the bottle on a hard surface and remove the metal cap and rubber diaphragm that covers the rubber stopper. Wipe the rubber stopper with an alcohol sponge. Remove the protective cap from the spike on the drip chamber, and firmly insert the spike into the center of the bottle's rubber stopper. Check to make certain the clamp is closed and invert the bottle. Hang the bottle on the intravenous pole and squeeze the drip chamber until it is half full.
8. If the intravenous solution to be infused is contained in a plastic bag rather than a bottle, place the bag on a hard surface, remove the protective cap from the tubing insertion port on the bag, and wipe it with an alcohol sponge. Remove the protective cap from the spike on the drip chamber of the tubing and insert the spike into the port. Check again to make certain the clamp is closed, hang the bag on the intravenous pole 18–24 inches above the site, and squeeze the drip chamber until it is half full.
9. Prime all tubing before using the intravenous setup by removing the protective cap from the end of the tubing and holding it over a sink or wastebasket. Take care to preserve the sterility of the cap and end of the tubing.
10. Release the clamp and allow the solution to run freely until all air bubbles are cleared from the tubing.
11. Reclamp the tubing to stop the flow and replace the protective cap over the end of the tubing.
12. Loop the tubing over the intravenous pole until the injection site has been selected and the venipuncture is complete.
13. Chart all relevant information.

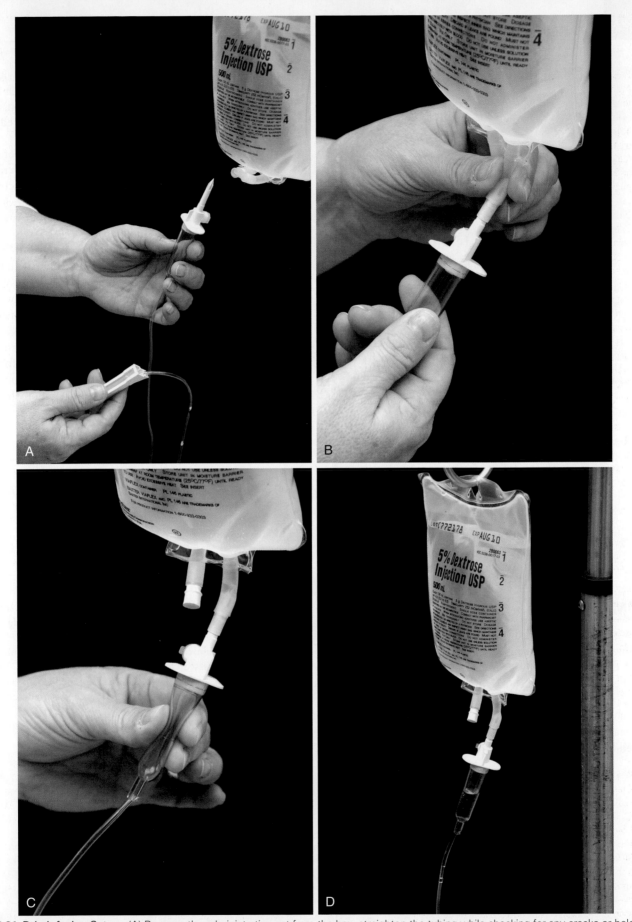

Fig. 22.21 Drip Infusion Setup. (A) Remove the administration set from the box, straighten the tubing while checking for any cracks or holes, and slide the clamp up to the drip chamber and close it. (B) Place the bag on a hard surface, remove the protective cap from the tubing insertion port on the bag, and wipe it with an alcohol sponge. Remove the protective cap from the spike on the drip chamber of the tubing and insert the spike into the port. (C) Check again to make certain the clamp is closed, hang the bag on the intravenous pole, and squeeze the drip chamber until it is half full. (D) Prime the intravenous setup by removing the protective cap from the end of the tubing and holding it over a sink or wastebasket. Taking care to preserve the sterility of the cap and end of the tubing, release the clamp and allow the solution to run freely until all air bubbles are cleared from the tubing. Reclamp the tubing to stop the flow and replace the protective cap over the end of the tubing.

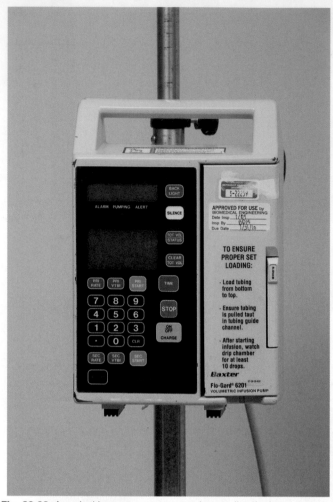

Fig. 22.22 A typical intravenous pump and controller device.

SUMMARY

- The golden rules of drug administration should always be followed when preparing to administer or when assisting with drug administration. Simply stated, the rules remind us to check for the right drug, right amount, right patient, right time, and right route. Drugs can be administered enterally, which includes oral, sublingual, buccal, and rectal routes, topically, or parenterally. Parenteral drugs can be administered by four routes: intradermal (ID); intramuscular (IM),

with rapid onset of action; subcutaneous (subcut), with slow and constant absorption; and intravenous (IV), with immediate onset of action. In all four methods of injection, appropriate injection practices should always be followed when preparing and administering the drug.

- Syringes and needles are manufactured in a variety of shapes and sizes. Selecting the proper needle and syringe is important when preparing drugs. Drugs that are to be injected may come in two kinds of containers. One type is an ampule, which usually holds a single dose, and the other is a vial, a small bottle that holds multiple doses.

- Numerous factors affect the patient's response to a drug, which may be undesirable. Adverse effects include side effects, toxic effects, allergic reactions, and idiosyncratic reactions. After drug administration by any route, the patient should be monitored closely for any signs of adverse effects.

- Guidelines for enteral and parenteral administration are included in this chapter. Instructions are provided for intradermal, subcutaneous, intramuscular, and intravenous injections. After administration, relevant information should be recorded on the patient's medical record.

BIBLIOGRAPHY

Al-Benna S, O'Boyle C, Holley J. Extravasation injuries in adults, *ISRN Dermatol* 2013, 2013: 856541. Doi:10, 1155/2013/856541.

Beyea S: Best practices for abbreviation use, *AORN J* 79:3, 2004.

CDC's Role in Safe Injection Practices. www.cdc.gov/injectionsafety/cdcsrole.html.

Fulcher E, Frazier M: *Introduction to intravenous therapy for healthcare professionals*, St. Louis, 2007, Saunders.

Gauwitz D: *Pharmacology for health careers*, ed 2, New York, 2009, McGraw Hill.

Pierce ET, Kumar V, Zheng H, et al: Micro-drip intravenous infusion: potential variations during "wide open" flow, *Anesth Analg* 116:3, 2013.

The Joint Commission: *Sentinel Even Alert,* Issue 52. , www.jointcommission.org, Accessed October 10, 2017.

Wolf Z, Hicks R, Serembus J: Characteristics of medication errors made by students during the administration phase: a descriptive study, *J Prof Nurs* 22:1, 2006.

Weinstein S, Hagle M: *Plumer's Principles and Practice of Infusion Therapy*, ed 9th, New York, 2014, McGraw Hill.

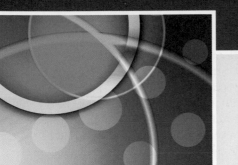

Contrast Media and Introduction to Radiopharmaceuticals

Norman E. Bolus, MSPH, MPH, CNMT, FSNMMI-TS, Elizabeth Cloyd, BS, RT(R)(CT)(MR)

To array a person's will against their sickness is the supreme art of medicine.

Henry Ward Beecher

OBJECTIVES

On completion of this chapter, the student will be able to:

- State the purpose of contrast media.
- Differentiate between low and high subject contrast.
- Compare negative and positive contrast agents.
- Name the general types of contrast media used for specific radiographic procedures.
- List the serious complications of the administration of barium sulfate.
- Match specific procedures to particular patient instructions.
- Explain the importance of osmosis as it relates to various effects of iodinated ionic contrast media.
- Discuss the advantages of nonionic iodinated contrast media.
- Differentiate among the major adverse effects of various contrast agents.
- Recognize clinical symptoms of adverse reactions to iodinated contrast media to the level of treatment required.
- Relate the patient history to the possibility of adverse reactions.
- Introduce general concerns and issues when using contrast agents in children.
- Introduce the concept of radiopharmaceuticals.

OUTLINE

KEY TERMS

Acid Group Contains carbon double bonded to an oxygen, single bonded to another oxygen, and a negative charge at the pH of the body

Amine Group Contains nitrogen bonded to two hydrogen atoms

Anaphylactoid Resembling an immune system response to foreign material (antigen)

Atomic Numbers Numbers of protons in the nuclei of the different elements

Blood Urea Nitrogen (BUN) BUN test can reveal whether the urea nitrogen levels are higher than normal, suggesting that the kidneys or liver may not be working properly

Bond Interactions between electrons of atoms that hold the atoms together in a stable group; line drawn between atoms indicates a bond H-O-H

Bronchospasm Involuntary constriction of the bronchial tubes usually resulting from an immune system reaction to a foreign particle or molecule

Compound Substance composed of two or more elements combined in definite ratios that give the substance specific properties

Contraindications Factors of a patient's history or present status that indicate that a medical procedure should not be performed or that a medication should not be given

Creatinine Nitrogen-containing waste products of metabolism excreted by the kidney's filtration system; high blood plasma levels indicate poor filtration by the kidney

Dimer Compound formed by bonding of two identical simpler molecules

Extravasation Leakage from a vessel into the tissue

Flocculation Formation of flaky masses resulting from precipitation or coming out of a suspension or solution

Histamine Molecular substance containing an amine group; causes bronchial constriction and a decrease in blood pressure

Hydroxyl Common chemical group, part of the water molecule, containing one atom of hydrogen and one atom of oxygen; carries a negative charge (anion) when not a part of a molecule

Ionic Atom or molecule having a negative charge (anion) or positive charge (cation)

Methyl Groups Common biochemical groups containing one carbon atom and three hydrogen atoms

Molecules Stable groups of bonded atoms having specific chemical properties

Monomers Simple molecules of a compound of relatively low molecular weight

Osmolality Measurement of the number of particles (molecules or ions or cations) that can crowd out water molecules in a measured mass (kilogram) of water

Osmosis Movement of water from an area of high concentration to an area of low concentration through

a semipermeable membrane such as blood vessel walls and cell membranes

pH Relative acidity or basicity (alkalinity) of a solution; pH below 7.0 is acidic and has more hydrogen cations than hydroxyl anions, whereas pH above 7.0 is alkaline and has more hydroxyl anions than hydrogen cations

Radiopharmaceutical Pharmaceutical compound that is attached to a radioisotope

Shock Inadequate blood flow within the body with resulting loss of oxygen and therefore energy

Solution Uniform mixture of two or more substances composed of molecule-sized particles that do not react together chemically

Suspension Nonuniform mixture of two or more substances, one of which is composed of larger-than-molecule-size particles that have a tendency to cluster together

INTRODUCTION TO CONTRAST MEDIA

Historical Aspects of Contrast Agents

Air, a negative contrast medium, was initially used in 1918 by Walter Dandy, a neurosurgeon who did injections of air to study the cerebral ventricles of children with hydrocephalus. Dandy's published articles initiated the use of air to localize tumors within the brain and spinal cord. Later, carbon dioxide, nitrous oxide, and oxygen came into use.

Immediately after Roentgen's discovery of x-rays, physiologists realized that the functions of the digestive system could be monitored by giving animals food mixed with compounds of high atomic number and watching the mixture's passage by way of a fluorescent screen. In 1896, lead subacetate was used to study the digestive system of the guinea pig. However, it later proved to be toxic. In the same year, Walter Cannon, then a Harvard medical student, began a series of experiments to study the digestive system using bismuth subnitrate. His subjects included geese, cats, and a 7-year-old girl. Although bismuth subnitrate eventually proved to be toxic, Cannon is credited with awakening the medical profession to the realization that diseases of the gastrointestinal (GI) tract could be studied by watching the movement of radiopaque media through the tract.

Toxicity remained a problem with many of the compounds with high atomic numbers in those early years. In fact, Thorotrast, which incorporated thorium, proved to be radioactive. By 1910, articles about the advantages of the inert and insoluble

compound barium sulfate began to appear in the medical literature. Its use increased rapidly because of its lack of toxicity, low cost, and availability.

Water-soluble iodinated contrast media were introduced by Egas Moniz in 1927 when he injected sodium iodide into the cerebrovascular circulation by way of the carotid arteries. Sodium iodide proved to be a blood vessel irritant.

During the 1930s, chemical methods improved. Atoms with high atomic numbers, such as iodine, could be placed on nontoxic water-soluble carrier molecules. Eventually, more iodine atoms per molecule were added, which increased visualization of the vascular and urinary systems. The 1950s saw the beginning of the use of three iodine atoms per carrier molecule. These triiodinated molecules are the basic chemical structures from which both ionic and nonionic water-soluble iodine contrast media originate.

Purpose of Contrast Media

For anatomic detail to be visualized, the area of interest must differ in radiographic density from its surrounding tissues. The ability to distinguish between radiographic densities enables differences in anatomic tissues to be visualized. Factors that affect the degree of radiographic density differences include absorption characteristics of the tissues that comprise the anatomic part, technical factors used, characteristics of the image receptor, automatic image processing, and the use of contrast media agents.

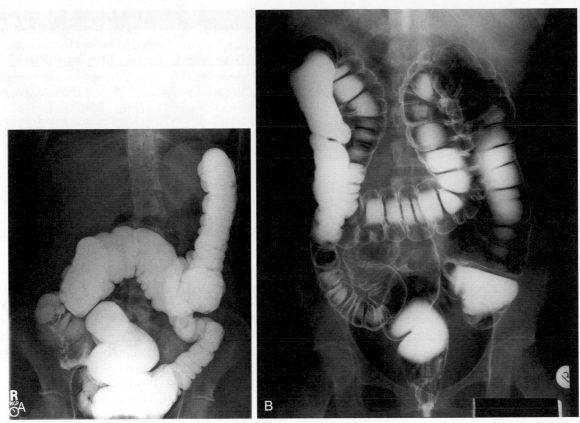

Fig. 23.1 (A) Radiopaque barium sulfate fills the colon in a lower gastrointestinal study. (B) Barium sulfate and air are used together to visualize the lumen of the colon.

The body absorbs x-ray photons according to the various tissue **atomic numbers** and the amount of matter per volume of tissue. Tissues with higher atomic numbers absorb more x-ray photons than those with low atomic numbers. For example, increased absorption of x-ray photons occurs with bone because calcium has a high atomic number, whereas soft tissues transmit or scatter x-ray photons more easily, resulting in decreased x-ray absorption.

Radiographic images of anatomic areas classified as low in subject contrast result in few density differences and are difficult to visualize. Instilling a contrast medium into the area of interest will change the absorption characteristics of the anatomic area and alter its subject contrast and the radiographic density differences. Enhancing the density differences within the area of interest will improve visualization of the anatomic detail.

Contrast media are diagnostic agents that are instilled into body orifices or injected into the vascular system, joints, and ducts to enhance subject contrast in anatomic areas where low subject contrast exists. The ability of the contrast media used in radiographic procedures to enhance subject contrast depends greatly on the atomic number of the element used in a particular medium and the concentration of atoms of the element per volume of the medium.

Contrast media are generally classified as negative or positive contrast agents. Negative contrast agents decrease attenuation of the x-ray beam and produce areas of increased density on the radiograph, whereas positive contrast agents increase the attenuation of the x-ray beam and produce areas of decreased density on the radiograph.

General Types of Contrast Agents

Radiolucent (Negative). X-ray photons are easily transmitted or scattered through radiolucent contrast media. As the name implies, these media are relatively lucent to x-rays. Because the anatomic areas filled by these agents appear dark (increased density) on radiographs, they are also called *negative contrast agents*. These media are composed of elements with low atomic numbers.

Radiopaque (Positive). X-ray photons are absorbed by radiopaque contrast media because these media are opaque to x-rays. Because the anatomic areas filled by these agents appear light (decreased density) on radiographs, they are also called *positive contrast agents*. These media are composed of elements with high atomic numbers.

In some instances, negative and positive agents are used together so that the lumen of organs, such as the colon (Fig. 23.1), can be visualized or so that anatomic structures within a space, such as the menisci of the knee, can be visualized.

Specialty Contrast Agents. Contrast agents of varying types are also being used in other modalities, such as magnetic resonance imaging (MRI) and diagnostic medical sonography. A common intravenous contrast agent used in MRI studies

TABLE 23.1	**Common Double-Contrast Studies**			
Area	Contrast Agent	Method of Administration	Patient Preparations	Patient Instructions and Care During Procedure
Stomach	Barium sulfate Carbon dioxide as tablets, crystals, or soda water	Oral	Nothing to eat or drink after midnight before examination	Patient should not belch after carbon dioxide is given so that the lumen of the stomach can be seen.
Large intestine	Barium sulfate Air	Rectal	Large amount of fluid before examination or fluid diet Nothing to eat or drink after midnight before examination Cleansing enema before examination	Provide supportive communication so that the patient does not lose control.
Arthrography: Shoulder, knee, wrist, hip	Water-soluble iodine media Air	Injection into joint space	None	Provide supportive communication because stress views performed during procedure can be painful.

is gadolinium diethylenetriaminepentaacetic acid (gadolinium-DTPA). This contrast agent is a metallic and magnetic agent that will affect the signal intensity used to image the anatomic area of interest. Ultrasound contrast agents are generally gas-filled microbubbles that affect the sound wave to enhance ultrasound contrast. Although not the focus of this chapter, these agents have a purpose similar to that of radiographic contrast agents—that is, of enhancing the subject contrast of the area of interest.

NEGATIVE CONTRAST MEDIA

Physical Properties

Negative contrast media are composed of low-atomic-number elements and are administered as gas (air) or gas-producing tablets, crystals, or soda water (carbon dioxide). Because cells absorb oxygen quickly, this gas is rarely used alone as a contrast agent.

Specific Procedures

Air alone provides negative contrast for laryngopharyngography because upper respiratory tract structures contain air naturally. Otherwise, radiolucent contrast media are used in combination with radiopaque media to outline the lumens of, or spaces within, body structures. Table 23.1 lists common double-contrast studies, contrast media used, method of administration, patient preparations, instructions, and patient care.

Adverse Reactions

Generally, complications from the administration of negative contrast agents are minimal, although air can cause emboli. These small air masses can enter the circulatory system and become lodged in blood vessels, causing pain and loss of oxygen to the area. Patients who receive barium sulfate with air should be instructed to drink plenty of fluids after the procedure to dilute and eliminate the barium sulfate. Administration of water-soluble iodine contrast media along with air in the joint spaces usually does not result in complications.

POSITIVE CONTRAST MEDIA

Barium Sulfate Contrast Media

Physical Properties. The element barium has an atomic number of 56; thus, it is radiopaque. Barium sulfate is an inert powder composed of crystals that is used for examining the digestive system. The chemical formula is $BaSO_4$, which indicates a ratio of one atom of barium to one atom of sulfur to four atoms of oxygen; thus, it is a compound. Because barium sulfate is not soluble in water, it must be mixed or shaken into a suspension in water. Depending on the environment of the barium sulfate, such as acid within the stomach, the powder has a tendency to clump and come out of suspension. This action is called flocculation. Stabilizing agents such as sodium carbonate or sodium citrate are usually used to prevent flocculation. These ingredients are listed as suspending agents on the container labels. Other ingredients used in orally administered barium sulfate include vegetable gums, flavoring, and sweeteners to increase palatability. Barium sulfate suspensions must be concentrated enough that x-rays are absorbed. These suspensions must flow easily and yet coat the lining of organs.

For studies of the small intestine, oral formulations of barium sulfate and methylcellulose, a nondigestible starch, have been introduced. These preparations are designed to give a *see-through* effect to better diagnose small lesions.

For lower GI studies, general recommendations are that barium sulfate be mixed with *cold* tap water to reduce irritation to the colon and to aid the patient in holding the enema during the examination. The cold tap water reduces spasm and cramping, although mixing the barium sulfate with room temperature water has also been recommended for maximal patient comfort.

A primary function of the colon is to absorb water from waste; however, increased water absorption by the colon can result in excess fluid entering the circulatory system (hypervolemia), a serious, sometimes fatal, complication. The addition of 2 teaspoons of table salt per liter of water used in the enema preparation reduces the risk for hypervolemia. Following the manufacturer's directions is critical when mixing barium sulfate suspensions so that diagnostic

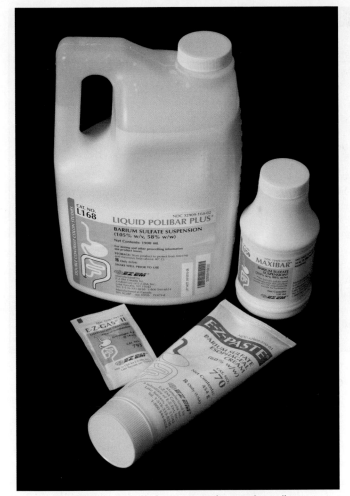

Fig. 23.2 Various barium preparations and supplies.

TABLE 23.2 Patient History Factors in Barium Sulfate Examinations

Factor	Importance
Age	Ability to communicate, hear, and follow directions
	↑ Risk for colon perforation caused by loss of tissue tone
Diverticulitis or ulcerative colitis	↑ Difficulty in holding an enema
	↑ Risk for colon perforation
Long-term steroid therapy	↑ Risk for colon perforation
Colon biopsy within previous 2 weeks	Lower gastrointestinal series contraindicated
Pregnancy	Inform radiologist before proceeding with examination
Mental retardation, confusion, or dizziness	↑ Risk for aspiration during upper gastrointestinal series
Recent onset of constipation or diarrhea	↑ Risk for colon perforation or tumor rupture
Nausea and vomiting	↑ Risk for aspiration during upper gastrointestinal series

↑, Increased.

radiographs will be obtained. Fig. 23.2 shows various barium sulfate preparations and carbon dioxide crystals used for double-contrast studies.

Specific Procedures. The administration of barium sulfate can result in complications, generally as a result of preexisting patient disease or status. If a patient is thought to have a perforation in the digestive tract, barium sulfate is contraindicated because the body does not absorb barium sulfate naturally. If it enters the peritoneal or pelvic cavity, barium sulfate can cause peritonitis and must be surgically removed. In place of barium sulfate, a water-soluble iodine contrast agent is recommended. The body is capable of absorbing this type of agent.

In certain patients, the administration of barium sulfate can result in trauma such as perforation of the colon. The radiologic technologist must obtain a detailed patient history to give appropriate patient care. Table 23.2 outlines patient history factors that should be considered before barium sulfate is administered. Table 23.3 lists the specific procedures that use a barium sulfate suspension.

Adverse Reactions. As previously mentioned, patients should be instructed to drink plenty of fluids after receiving barium sulfate. All barium sulfate suspensions transit the colon. Because one function of the colon is to absorb water from waste, barium sulfate residue within the colon can dry and cause an obstruction. The major symptom of obstruction is constipation.

A complication related to the administration of barium sulfate during a lower GI examination is perforation of the colon with **extravasation** (leakage through a duct or vessel) into the abdominal cavity. Extravasation results in inflammation of the abdominal cavity, termed *barium peritonitis*. Older adult patients or persons receiving long-term steroid medication are at increased risk for colon perforation because their tissues have become *atrophic* (lost elasticity and muscle tone). Also at risk are patients with diverticulitis and ulcerative colitis because these diseases result in inflammation and degradation of the colon tissues. Patients with toxic megacolon should not have lower GI procedures because this serious complication of ulcerative colitis results in a dilated colon that can rupture. Recent biopsy of the colon is a contraindication to a lower GI series until the area heals. The barium retention catheter can be a source of colon perforation. The radiologic technologist should use one or two gentle squeezes (or one full squeeze) to inflate the retention cuff (consult with the physician in charge for best practices).

Vaginal rupture, a rare complication of barium sulfate administration, is caused by incorrect placement of the catheter before lower GI examinations. Knowing the anatomy of the female pelvis in the anteroposterior and lateral configurations is critical. Female patients should be asked whether they can feel the enema tip in the rectum.

Water absorption from the colon is a serious complication of lower GI administration of barium sulfate suspensions. Water from the cleansing enema and the barium enema can be shifted from the colon into the circulatory system with a resulting increase in blood volume. Consequences of this fluid overload are pulmonary edema (fluid in the lungs), seizures, coma, and death. The table salt **solution** previously discussed reduces the possibility of hypervolemia. The radiologic technologist must

TABLE 23.3 **Common Procedures for Which Barium Sulfate Suspensions Are Used**

Area	Concentration (wt/vol%)	Method of Administration	Patient Preparation	Patient Instructions and Care During Procedure
Esophagus: Esophagram	30–50	Oral	None	Provide supportive communication. For esophageal varices, the patient should exhale, swallow barium, and then hold his or her breath on that exhalation for that exposure.
Stomach: Upper gastrointestinal series	30–50	Oral	Nothing to eat or drink after midnight before examination	Provide supportive communication. Provide explanation of reasons for various positions.
Small intestine: Small bowel series	40–60 if included with stomach examination	Oral	If included with a stomach examination, low-residue diet eaten for 2 days before examination	Provide supportive communication. Provide explanation for length of procedure. In most patients, the transit time of the barium sulfate suspension through the small intestine is approximately 1 h.
Large intestine: Colon or barium enema	12–25	Rectal	Large amount of fluid or fluid diet day before examination. Nothing to eat or drink after midnight before examination. Cleansing enema before examination	Provide supportive communication so that the patient does not lose control. Watch patient for changes in mental status that may indicate fluid overload.
Stomach: Computed tomography[a]	12–25	Oral	Nothing to eat or drink after midnight before examination	Provide supportive communication. The patient should believe that the radiographer is constantly watching the procedure.

[a]Generally used to accent contrast in the abdomen.

observe patients for changes in mental status, such as apathy and drowsiness, that would indicate onset of hypervolemia. Symptoms of fluid overload are masked in sedated patients; therefore, sedative premedication is contraindicated for lower GI examinations.

Sedated patients should not undergo upper GI examinations because the swallowing reflex is diminished, which greatly increases the risk for aspiration (inhalation) of the barium sulfate suspension with resultant barium pneumonia. Aspiration is also a risk for mentally handicapped patients and persons with altered mental status because of age or disease.

A few allergic-type reactions have been noted, but these may have been caused by preservatives in the particular barium sulfate preparation or by latex used in barium enema retention catheters. Occasionally, barium sulfate has collected within the appendix. No directly related complications have resulted from this occurrence.

Water-Soluble Iodine Contrast Media

Physical Properties

Ionic Iodine Contrast Media. The element iodine has an atomic number of 53, making it relatively radiopaque. Ionic media dissociate into two molecular particles in water or blood plasma, just as table salt does. These media are **ionic** because one particle, called an *anion,* has a negative charge and the other particle, called a *cation,* has a positive charge. The anion part of the molecule begins with a six-carbon bonded hexagon called *benzene.* A carbon atom is located at each corner of the hexagon but is not usually drawn because the molecular diagram would appear cluttered. Every other carbon **bond** site of the benzene is bonded to an iodine atom; therefore, each anion portion contains three iodine atoms and is therefore triiodinated. Of the three remaining carbon bond sites, one is

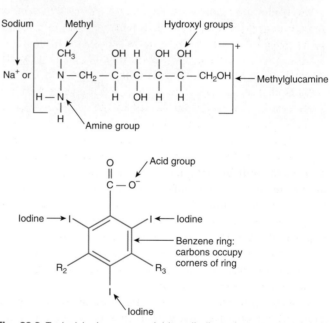

Fig. 23.3 Typical ionic, water-soluble, triiodinated contrast molecule. The anion is the benzene ring with the negatively charged acid group attached. The groups R_2 and R_3 aid in solubility and excretion. The positively charged cations are sodium or methylglucamine. Some media contain both cations.

occupied by an **acid group.** The acid group carries the negative charge at physiologic **pH.**

At the acid group, the anion and cation dissociate on injection. The other two carbon bond sites are occupied by chemical structures that increase the solubility or the excretion rate of the contrast by the body. These two carbon bond sites result in the different classes of ionic media: *diatrizoate, metrizoate,* and *iothalamate* (Fig. 23.3). The cation part of the molecule is either a sodium atom or a more complex

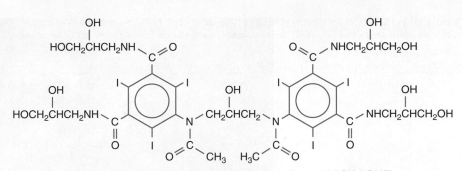

Fig. 23.4 Nonionic, water-soluble dimer iodixanol (VISIPAQUE).

structure, methylglucamine. Its rather long name describes its structure. The six carbons bonded to one another in a straight line and bonded to oxygens and hydrogens (**hydroxyl** groups) come from glucose, a common biologic sugar. The hydroxyl groups increase solubility. The nitrogen on the left is part of an **amine group.** (Amines are found in amino acids, and ammonia contains nitrogen.) Finally, a one-carbon, three-hydrogen group is attached to a nitrogen on the left. These one-carbon, three-hydrogen **methyl groups** are extremely common.

Methylglucamine is sometimes identified as *meglumine* on package inserts. Most ionic iodine contrast media are identified as *higher osmolality contrast media* because of their osmotic effects. **Osmolality** is a measure of the total number of particles in solution per kilogram of water. The osmolality of contrast media is of great biologic significance. Most adverse reactions to contrast media have been related to the osmolality of the media because the osmolality of a solution determines osmotic pressure, which controls the movement of water in the body. High-osmolality contrast media have an increased number of particles in solution, such as blood plasma, which pull water toward them.

Nonionic Iodine Contrast Media. Efforts to decrease the many side effects of ionic iodine contrast media resulted in the development of molecules that do not dissociate into anions and cations (nonionics) or that are ionic but too big to have osmotic effects, such as ioxaglate (Hexabrix). These agents are identified as *lower osmolality contrast media.*

Ioxaglate is an ionic molecule composed of two connected benzene hexagons, one that carries an acid group that dissociates on injection. This contrast agent is a **dimer** because it is composed of two identical simpler molecules. Ioxaglate carries six iodine atoms per molecule. It is ionic because it dissociates into two particles in blood plasma. Most ionic iodine contrast media are **monomers,** or simple molecules of relatively low molecular weight. Because dimers are large molecules, their osmotic effects are low. Because of their high molecular weights, they are viscous.

Recently, a nonionic dimer, iodixanol (VISIPAQUE), was introduced. Iodixanol is made to be isomolar (having the same number of particles) to blood plasma by the addition of electrolytes, small anions, and cations, which are normally present in blood plasma. Fig. 23.4 shows the molecular structure of the nonionic dimer iodixanol.

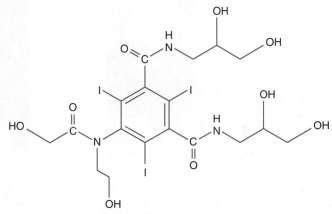

Fig. 23.5 Nonionic, water-soluble, triiodinated contrast molecule ioversol (Optiray).

An additional advantage of the lower osmolality contrast media is that they are more hydrophilic (water soluble) than the higher osmolality contrast media. As a result, they may be less likely to be reactive with the cells that can trigger allergic effects. Fig. 23.5 shows the molecular structure of one of the water-soluble nonionic iodine contrast agents, ioversol (Optiray). It is a triiodinated benzene ring and does *not* carry an acid group. Many oxygen-hydrogen hydroxyl groups surround the benzene ring. These groups increase the solubility of the media in blood plasma. Fig. 23.6 shows radiographs of some procedures performed using water-soluble nonionic iodine contrast agents.

Fig. 23.7 shows a photograph of various nonionic agents. Iodine in its elemental form is chemically reactive and can be toxic in the body. Consequently, both ionic and nonionic agents contain additives such as citrate and calcium disodium edetate. These compounds prevent iodine atoms from being removed from the contrast molecules.

General Effects. Water-soluble iodine contrast media have known physiologic effects. High osmolality and the aspects of chemical structure are the major characteristics of the water-soluble media that are responsible for these effects. Although both ionic and nonionic iodine media have physiologic effects on the body, most ionic agents are higher osmolality contrast media and therefore have shown greater effects and adverse reactions. Viscosity, or *friction,* of a medium is influenced by the concentration and size of the molecule. It affects the injectability, or delivery, of the medium. Heating the medium to body temperature significantly reduces the viscosity and

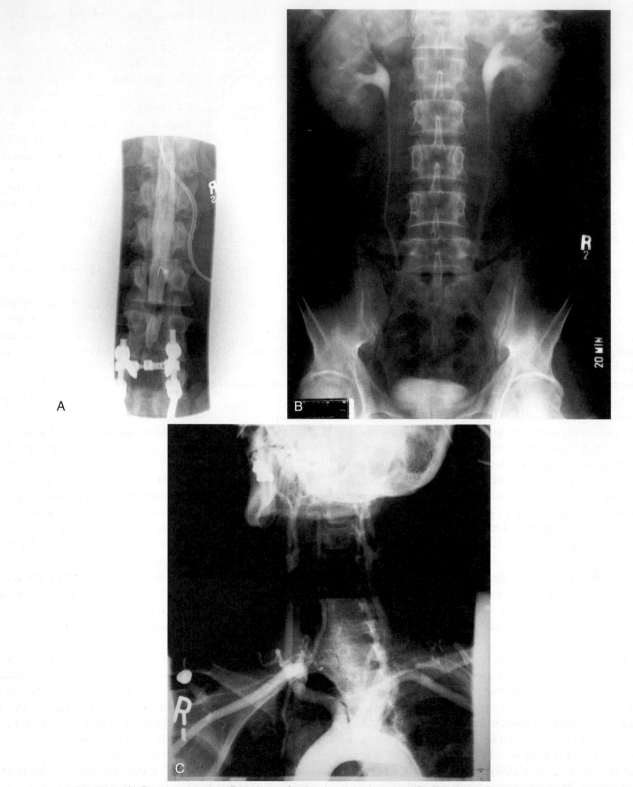

Fig. 23.6 (A) Posteroanterior (PA) view of a lumbar myelogram. (B) PA view of an excretory urogram. (C) Aortic arch angiogram.

facilitates the ability for rapid injection. Heating is commonly accomplished through the use of a *contrast warmer*.

Osmotic Effects. Because ionic media dissociate in water, their injection into the blood plasma results in a great increase in the number of particles present in the plasma, which has the effect of displacing water. Water moves from an area of high concentration to an area of low concentration; the process is called osmosis. When the plasma water is displaced by contrast particles, water from body cells moves into the vascular system. This movement results in hypervolemia and blood vessel

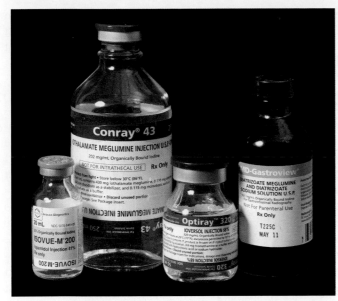

Fig. 23.7 Various iodinated contrast agents.

dilatation, producing pain and discomfort. Blood pressure may decrease because of vessel dilatation, or it may increase as a result of hypervolemia and the effects of hormones in the kidneys.

When higher osmolality contrast media are given for imaging of the intestinal tract, fluid from cells is drawn into these areas. This osmotic effect can aid in reducing obstructions because the increase in fluid increases peristalsis. In dehydrated patients, however, the osmotic effect further reduces body cell volume and can result in shock. Consequently, obtaining a patient history and conveying any contraindications to the radiologist or other physician are important. The number of molecular particles of a particular contrast medium is shown on the package insert in units of milliosmoles per kilogram of water at 37°C. The higher the number is, the greater will be the number of particles that can produce osmotic effects. As an example, the osmolality of iodixanol at 300 mg of iodine per milliliter in milliosmoles per kilogram is 290, equal to that of blood plasma.

Allergic-like Effects (Anaphylactoid). Allergic reactions to water-soluble iodinated contrast media resemble allergic reactions to foreign substances, such as pollen grains. Reactions of typical allergic patients may be minor, such as urticaria (hives). Some patients, however, experience wheezing and edema in the throat and lungs, with accompanying bronchospasm. Other anaphylactoid effects of water-soluble iodinated contrast media are nausea and vomiting. These reactions are thought to be caused by the release of a substance called histamine from certain cells found in the lungs, stomach, and lining of blood vessels. Although some radiologists believe that the allergic-like effects are caused by extreme anxiety, the radiologic technologist should consider these effects as serious. Premedication with steroids and antihistamines (to prevent the release of histamine) can reduce or eliminate allergic effects.

Renal Effects. High-osmolality contrast media can cause the arteries of the kidneys to expand as a result of the osmotic effect. Arterial expansion results in the release of vasoconstrictors.

These substances cause constriction of the renal arteries. Therefore, injection of the contrast media results in dilatation and then constriction of the renal arteries. The end result is diminished blood supply to the kidneys.

Osmotic effects are also presumed to cause an increase in the amount of molecular substances that cannot be reabsorbed by the renal tubules. This increase results in *osmotic diuresis* (increased secretion of urine) and dehydration. Increased blood urea nitrogen (BUN) and creatinine (waste product of metabolism) levels indicate that the patient may have renal disease and are good indicators for possible contrast medium-induced renal effects. Patients with renal disease or diabetes and older patients are at increased risk for these complications. Intravenous fluid given before and during procedures can reduce the severity of renal effects. Theophylline, a substance found in tea, is currently being investigated as a preventive of toxic renal effects by increasing the filtering action of the kidneys.

Other Effects. Carotid artery injection of water-soluble iodine contrast media can alter the blood-brain barrier (separation between brain capillaries and support cells for the neurons) by causing the capillary cells to shrivel because of water loss. Some of these media can stimulate areas in the carotid artery that help control heart rate and blood pressure. Clinical symptoms of these effects include increased blood pressure, bradycardia (slow heartbeat), and tachycardia (fast heartbeat).

In patients with sickle cell anemia and those who carry the trait but who are asymptomatic, injection of high-osmolality contrast media can cause the red blood cells to shrink and to *sickle* (assume an elongated shape). These sickled cells may be trapped in small-diameter blood vessels and capillaries, causing pain and blood clots. A common effect is a sensation of warmth and pain on injection into the arterial vessels. Theories suggest that this effect is caused by dissociation of the contrast media into anions and cations.

In helical computed tomography (CT) procedures, a large amount of contrast material is injected at a rate of at least 2.5 mL/sec. This amount increases the probability of nausea and vomiting and extravasation of the contrast with patient motion as a result.

Drug Interactions and Considerations. One class of drugs used to treat hypertension is the beta-adrenergic blockers. These drugs reduce cardiac output, but they also reduce dilatation of bronchial smooth muscle and block the effect of epinephrine. Patients who take these drugs are at increased risk for anaphylactoid reactions during procedures in which water-soluble iodine contrast media are used.

Calcium-channel blockers reduce hypertension by relaxing electrical conduction of cell membranes in arterioles (small arteries) and in heart muscle. Patients who take these drugs are at risk for heart block and abrupt decrease in blood pressure if ionic contrast media are used during cardiac catheterization.

Metformin (Glucophage) is a type of drug used to treat non-insulin-dependent diabetes. Metformin should be discontinued for 48 hours before and 48 hours after the use of iodine contrast media. Although metformin does not interact with the iodine contrast agents, if renal failure should occur as an effect of iodine contrast administration, drug levels of metformin would accumulate in the patient and lactic acidosis might develop. (Metformin increases the uptake of glucose in body cells. One end product of glucose metabolism is lactic acid. Consequently, increased levels of metformin will increase lactic acid production and decrease the pH in body cells: acidosis.)

Considerations in the Use of Nonionic Contrast Media. Most adverse reactions associated with water-soluble ionic iodine contrast media are significantly decreased with the use of the nonionic media. This decrease is attributed to the decreased osmolality of the nonionic media. In addition, the injection of nonionics during angiography is much less painful compared with injection of ionic media; however, kidney toxicity has not been reduced. Including the patient's BUN and creatinine level in the history is therefore important. Nonionic iodine contrast media cost two to three times more than ionic media. Therefore, decisions about which patients will receive nonionic media are controversial. Some institutions have decided to use low-osmolality contrast media on all patients regardless of cost. Other institutions have established a selective use of these agents.

Sample criteria for the use of low-osmolality (nonionic) contrast media might include the following:

- Patients with a history of adverse reactions to contrast media, excluding mild reactions such as the sensation of heat or flushing
- Patients with a history of asthma or allergies
- Patients with known cardiac problems
- Patients with generalized severe debilitating conditions
- Patients who will undergo helical CT procedures

These criteria include patients with diabetes mellitus, renal disease or elevated creatinine levels, or sickle cell disease.

Specific Procedures. A wide variety of radiologic procedures use water-soluble iodine contrast media. These agents are important in visualizing the urinary and cardiovascular systems in particular. They are also commonly used in CT studies of the brain, chest, and abdomen. Table 23.4 provides a list of the common procedures that use water-soluble iodine contrast agents.

The most important patient care aspect before administration of water-soluble iodine contrast media is the patient history. The possibility of patient reaction is closely related to the patient's disease state or age. Moreover, the chemical nature of these contrast media can provoke severe reactions. The radiologic technologist is responsible for observation of patient well-being. Table 23.5 lists some patient history factors to consider before administering water-soluble iodine contrast media.

Adverse Reactions. As discussed in the section on the general effects of water-soluble iodine contrast media, these media have physiologic effects that may result in adverse reactions. The responsibility of the radiologic technologist in patient surveillance is critical in assessing the severity of these effects. Box 23.1 lists adverse reactions divided into three categories: mild, moderate, and severe. A discussion of treatment is also provided. Box 23.2 details the management of patients with

acute reactions. Although adverse reactions can occur when using low-osmolality (nonionic) contrast media, they are most often associated with the higher osmolality (ionic) contrast media.

CONTRAST MEDIA IN CHILDREN

Some considerations need to be made when working with children and contrast media. Although many principles are the same as for adults, there are some differences to consider. If pediatric cases are rare in your facility, you may want to contact a children's hospital for recommendations and guidance. Contrast media osmolality is of particular importance in neonates and small children. These patients can be especially susceptible to fluid shifts that could in extreme cases lead to cardiac failure and pulmonary edema. In children who have significant pre-existing conditions such as cardiac dysfunction, consideration should be given to use iso-osmolality intravascular contrast agents. Another consideration is contrast media viscosity with pediatric patients. If a rapid injection rate is desired through a small angiocatheter with a high-viscosity agent, two issues could occur. The proper injection rate may not be possible, and the catheter could burst, causing vessel injury in the pediatric patient. Other common issues with pediatric patients and contrast agent use include small volumes used, small-gauge angiocatheters, and unusual vascular access sites. Care should also be used because children may not effectively communicate pain at the injection site if a dose extravasation occurs.

RADIOPHARMACEUTICALS
General Characteristics

A radiopharmaceutical is not a contrast agent. A **radiopharmaceutical** is a radionuclide that is attached (chemically bound) to a pharmaceutical that has a specific biodistribution in the human body. This biodistribution depends on many factors, such as route of administration; gas, liquid, or solid state of the radiopharmaceutical; and sensitivity, as well as specificity, of the pharmaceutical in the body as it is taken up. The radioisotope attached to the pharmaceutical is imaged using a gamma camera, which *sees* or detects where the radiopharmaceutical is in the body and forms an image of more or less concentration of the radiopharmaceutical. Physicians read the images knowing the normal biodistribution patterns and look for pathologic conditions within the body based on where the radiopharmaceuticals concentrate. The functionality of this procedure lies in the ability of many radiopharmaceuticals to be taken up by an organ of interest and then be metabolized and used or eliminated by the body. A prime example would be renal imaging, whereby the radiopharmaceutical is taken up by the kidneys, metabolized into urine, and collected in the bladder. If a patient has a kidney stone that is blocking the path of urine in one of the ureters, this stone would show up while the study is being performed. Physicians can also determine the rate of uptake and elimination of the radiopharmaceutical in the kidneys and determine if they are functioning normally or not. This method is how an effective renal plasma flow is determined. Table 23.6 lists several radionuclides, their

TABLE 23.4 Some Procedures for Which Water-Soluble Iodine Contrast Media Are Used

Area	Contrast Agent	Method of Administration	Patient Preparation	Patient Instructions and Care During Procedure
Brain: Cerebral angiography, computed tomography	Usually nonionic	Injection into vein or artery	Usually liquid diet to minimize nausea Premedication for sedation Intravenous fluids to aid hydration	Provide supportive communication. Tell the patient that he or she may feel warm and sense a metallic taste on injection. Explain what is being done as it is being done. Watch the patient for adverse reactions. Apply pressure to injection site after procedure is completed.
Thorax: Thoracic angiography or four-vessel study	Usually nonionic	Injection into vein or artery	Usually liquid diet to minimize nausea Premedication for sedation Intravenous fluids to aid hydration	Provide supportive communication. Tell the patient that he or she may feel warmth and sense a metallic taste on injection. Explain what is being done as it is being done. Watch the patient for adverse reactions. Apply pressure to injection site after procedure is completed.
Lower limbs: Venography	Usually nonionic	Injection into vein	Sometimes premedication for sedation Intravenous fluids for hydration	Provide supportive communication. Tell the patient that he or she may feel warmth and sense a metallic taste on injection. Explain what is being done as it is being done; some pain may be present. Watch the patient for adverse reactions. Apply pressure to injection site after procedure is completed.
Spinal canal: Myelography	Only nonionic	Injection into subarachnoid space	Usually liquid diet Usually premedication for sedation	Provide supportive communication. Explain the use of shoulder braces and that the table will be tilted but the patient's head must be kept in extension. Explain what is being done as it is being done. Watch the patient for adverse reactions. Advise nursing staff and patient that patient should remain in bed with the head up for 24 h to prevent headache and nausea.
Kidneys, ureters, and bladder: Excretory urography, renal angiography, cystography	Usually nonionic	Injection into vein or artery For cystography, usually through catheter in urinary bladder	Liquid diet day before examination to reduce gas formation Laxatives or a cleansing enema may be given Bladder should be emptied before the examination begins	Provide supportive communication. Tell the patient that he or she may feel warmth and sense a metallic taste during and just after injections; several injections may be performed. Explain the timing of the radiographs and the x-ray tube movement if tomography is done. Watch the patient for adverse reactions. Angiography: Apply pressure to the injection site after procedure is completed.
Heart and coronary arteries: Cardiac catheterization	Usually nonionic	Usually through catheter	Liquid or low-residue diet usually ordered the evening before the procedure Antibiotics usually ordered Premedication for sedation Intravenous fluids for hydration Blood clotting (prothrombin) time must be within a range acceptable to the physician Catheter may be inserted in femoral artery; therefore, strength of dorsal pedal pulses is evaluated	Provide supportive communication. Tell the patient that he or she may feel warmth and sense a metallic taste on injection. Explain what is being done as it is being done. The patient may be apprehensive about the movements of the x-ray tube around the body or the use of two x-ray tubes. Lead glass shielding should be explained. Nursing procedures: Monitoring of peripheral pulses and blood pressure. Watch the patient for adverse reactions. Advise nursing staff that temperature may be elevated after procedure.

TABLE 23.5 Patient History Factors in Water-Soluble Iodine Contrast Examinations

q	Importance
Age	↑ Risk with increased age
Allergies or asthma	↑ Risk for allergic-like reactions
Diabetes	Insulin usually given before procedure; these patients should be scheduled before others
Coronary artery disease	↑ Risk for tachycardia, bradycardia, hypertension, myocardial infarction (heart attack)
Hypertension	Hypertension with tachycardia
Renal disease	Inform radiologist if creatinine level is above 1.4 mg/dL
Multiple myeloma	Abnormal protein binds with contrast and can cause renal failure
	Patients must be hydrated
Confusion or dizziness	Blood-brain barrier effects
Sickle cell anemia or family history of chronic obstructive pulmonary disease	↑ Risk for blood clots
	↑ Risk for dyspnea (difficulty in breathing)
Previous iodine contrast examinations	Did the patient have difficulties with procedure?
Pregnancy	Inform radiologists before proceeding
History of blood clots	↑ Risk for blood clots
Use of beta blockers	↑ Risk for anaphylactoid reactions
Use of calcium-channel blockers	↑ Risk for heart block
Use of metformin (Glucophage)	↑ Risk for lactic acidosis if renal failure occurs

↑, Increased.

BOX 23.1 Categories of Acute Reactions to Contrast Media

Allergic-Like	Physiologic	Treatment

Mild

Signs and symptoms are self-limited without evidence of progression. Mild reactions include:

Allergic-Like	Physiologic	Treatment
Limited urticaria/pruritus	Limited nausea/vomiting	Requires observation to confirm resolution and/or lack of progression but usually no treatment. Patient reassurance is usually helpful.
Limited cutaneous edema	Transient flushing/warmth/chills	
Limited "itchy"/"scratchy" throat	Headache/dizziness/anxiety/altered taste	
Nasal congestion	Mild hypertension	
Sneezing/conjunctivitis/rhinorrhea	Vasovagal reaction that resolves spontaneously	

Moderate

Signs and symptoms are more pronounced and commonly require medical management. Some of these reactions have the potential to become severe if not treated. Moderate reactions include:

Allergic-Like	Physiologic	Treatment
Diffuse urticaria/pruritus	Protracted nausea/vomiting	Clinical findings in moderate reactions frequently require prompt treatment. These situations require close, careful observation for possible progression to a life-threatening event.
Diffuse erythema, stable vital signs	Hypertensive urgency	
Facial edema without dyspnea	Isolated chest pain	
Throat tightness or hoarseness without dyspnea	Vasovagal reaction that requires and is responsive to treatment	
Wheezing/bronchospasm, mild or no hypoxia		

Severe

Signs and symptoms are often life-threatening and can result in permanent morbidity or death if not managed appropriately.

Cardiopulmonary arrest is a nonspecific end-stage result that can be caused by a variety of the following severe reactions, both allergic-like and physiologic. If it is unclear what caused the cardiopulmonary arrest, it may be judicious to assume that the reaction is/was an allergic-like one.

Pulmonary edema is a rare severe reaction that can occur in patients with tenuous cardiac reserve (cardiogenic pulmonary edema) or in patients with normal cardiac function (noncardiogenic pulmonary edema). Noncardiogenic pulmonary edema can be allergic-like or physiologic; if the cause is unclear, it may be judicious to assume that the reaction is/was an allergic-like one.

Severe reactions include:

Allergic-Like	Physiologic	Treatment
Diffuse edema, or facial edema with dyspnea	Vasovagal reaction resistant to treatment	Requires *prompt* recognition and aggressive treatment; manifestations and treatment frequently necessitate hospitalization.
Diffuse erythema with hypotension	Arrhythmia	
Laryngeal edema with stridor and/or hypoxia	Convulsions, seizures	
Wheezing/bronchospasm, significant hypoxia	Hypertensive emergency	
Anaphylactic shock (hypotension + tachycardia)		

BOX 23.2	**Management of Acute Reactions in Adults**	
	Treatment	**Dosing**
Hives		
Mild (scattered and/or transient)	No treatment often needed; however, if symptomatic, can consider:	
	Diphenhydramine (Benadryl)[a]	25–50 mg PO
	or	
	Fexofenadine (Allegra)[b]	180 mg PO
Moderate (more numerous/bothersome)	Monitor vitals	
	Preserve IV access	
	Consider diphenhydramine (Benadryl)[a]	25–50 mg PO
	or	
	Fexofenadine (Allegra)[b]	180 mg PO
	or	
	Consider diphenhydramine (Benadryl)[a]	25–50 mg IM or IV (administer IV dose slowly over 1–2 min)
Severe (widespread and/or progressive)	Monitor vitals	
	Preserve IV access	
Consider	Diphenhydramine (Benadryl)[a]	25–50 mg IM or IV (administer IV dose slowly over 1–2 min)
Can also consider	Epinephrine (IM)	IM 0.3 mg (0.3 mL of 1 : 1000 dilution)
		or
		IM EpiPen or equivalent (0.3 mL of 1: 1000 dilution, fixed)
	or	
	Epinephrine (IV)	IV 1–3 mL of 1 : 10 000 dilution; administer slowly into a running IV infusion of saline
Diffuse Erythema		
All forms	Preserve IV access	
	Monitor vitals	
	Pulse oximeter	
	O_2 by mask	6–10 L/min
Normotensive	No other treatment usually needed	
Hypotensive	IV fluids 0.9% normal saline	1000 mL rapidly
	or	
	Lactated Ringer solution	1000 mL rapidly
If profound or unresponsive to fluids alone can also consider	Epinephrine (IV)[c]	IV 1–3 mL of 1 : 10 000 dilution; administer slowly into a running IV infusion of saline; can repeat every few minutes as needed up to 10 mL (1 mg) total
	or (if no IV access available)	
	Epinephrine (IM)[c]	IM 0.3 mg (0.3 mL of 1 : 1000 dilution); can repeat up to 1 mg total
		or
		IM EpiPen or equivalent (0.3 mL of 1: 1000 dilution, fixed); can repeat every 5-15 minutes up to three times
	Consider calling emergency response team or 911	
Bronchospasm		
All forms	Preserve IV access	
	Monitor vitals	
	Pulse oximeter	
	O_2 by mask	6–10 L/min
Mild	Beta-agonist inhaler (Albuterol)	2 puffs (90 mcg/puff) for a total of 180 mcg; can repeat up to three times
	Consider sending patient to emergency department or calling emergency response team or 911, based on the completeness of the response	
Moderate	Consider adding epinephrine (IM)[c]	IM 0.3 mg (0.3 mL of 1: 1000 dilution; administer slowly into a running IV infusion of saline; can repeat every 5-15 minutes up to 1 mL (1mg) total
		or
	Consider sending patient to emergency department or calling emergency response team or 911, based on the completeness of the response	IM EpiPen or equivalent 0.3 mL of 1: 1000 dilution, fixed (0.3mg); can repeat every 5-15 minutes up to three times
		or Epinephrine (IV)
		IV 1 mL of 1:10,000 dilution (0.1 mg); administer slowly into a running IV infusion of fluids or use saline flush; can repeat every few minutes as needed up to 10 mL (1 mg) total

Continued

BOX 23.2 Management Of Acute Reactions In Adults—cont'd

	Treatment	Dosing
Severe	Epinephrine IV[c]	IV 1 mL of 1:10,000 dilution (0.1 mg); administer slowly into a running IV infusion of fluids or slow IV push followed by a slow saline flush; can repeat every few minutes as needed up to 10 mL (1 mg) total
	or	
	Epinephrine IM[c]	IM 0.3 mg (0.3 mL of 1 : 1000 dilution); can repeat every 5-15 minutes up to 1 mL (1mg) total
		or
	and	IM EpiPen or equivalent (0.3 mL of 1 : 1000 dilution, fixed); can repeat every 5-15 minutes up to three times
	Beta agonist inhaler (Albuterol) (may work synergistically)	
	2 puffs (90 mcg/puff) for a total of 180 mcg; can repeat up to 3 times	
	Call emergency response team or 911	
Laryngeal Edema		
All forms	Preserve IV access	
	Monitor vitals	
	Pulse oximeter	
	O$_2$ by mask	6–10 L /min
	Epinephrine (IV)[c]	IV 1–3 mL of 1 : 10 000 dilution; administer slowly into a running IV infusion of saline; can repeat every few minutes as needed up to 1 mg total
	or	
	Epinephrine (IM)[c]	IM 0.3 mg (0.3 mL of 1 : 1000 dilution); can repeat every 5-15 minutes up to 1 mg total
		or
		IM EpiPen or equivalent (0.3 mL of 1 : 1000 dilution, fixed); can repeat every 5-15 minutes up to three times
	Consider calling emergency response team or 911 based on the severity of the reaction and the completeness of the response	
Hypotension (Systolic Blood Pressure <90 mm Hg)		
	Preserve IV access	6–10 L/min
	Monitor vital signs	
	Pulse oximeter	
	O$_2$ by mask	
	Elevate legs at least 60 degrees	
	Consider IV fluids: 0.9% normal saline	1000 mL rapidly
	or	
	Lactated Ringer solution	1000 mL rapidly
Hypotension With Bradycardia (Pulse <60 bpm) (Vasovagal Reaction)		
Mild	No other treatment usually necessary	
Severe (patient remains symptomatic despite above measures)	In addition to above measures, IV atropine	0.6–1 mg; administer slowly, followed by saline flush; can repeat up to 3 mg total
	Consider calling emergency response team or 911	
Hypotension With Tachycardia (Pulse >100 bpm) (Anaphylactoid Reaction)		
If hypotension persists	Epinephrine IV[c]	IV 1–3 mL of 1 : 10 000 dilution; administer slowly in a running IV infusion of saline; can repeat every few minutes up to 1 mg total
	or	
	Epinephrine IM[c]	IM 0.3 (0.3 of 1 : 1000 dilution); can repeat every 5-15 minutes up to 1 mg total
		or
		IM EpiPen or equivalent (0.3 mL of 1 : 1000 dilution, fixed); can repeat every 5-15 minutes up to three times
	Consider calling emergency response team or 911 based on the severity of the reaction and the completeness of the response	

BOX 23.2 Management of Acute Reactions in Adults—cont'd

	Treatment	Dosing
Hypertensive Crisis (Diastolic BP >120 mm Hg; Systolic BP >200 mm Hg; Symptoms of End-Organ Compromise)		
All forms	Preserve IV access	
	Monitor vital signs	
	Pulse oximeter	
	O$_2$ by mask	6–10 L/min
	Labetalol (IV)	IV 20 mg; administer slowly over 2 min; can double the dose every 10 min (e.g., 40 mg 10 min later; 80 mg 10 min after that)
	or if labetalol not available	
	Nitroglycerin tablet (SL)	0.4-mg tablet; can repeat every 5–10 min
	and	
	Furosemide (Lasix) (IV)	IV 20–40 mg; administer slowly over 2 min
	Call emergency response team or 911	
Unresponsive and Pulseless		
	Check for responsiveness	
	Activate emergency response team (call 911)	
	30 compressions at the rate of 100-120/min, then 2 respirations	
	Get defibrillator or automated electronic defibrillator (AED); apply as soon as available; shock as indicated	
	Epinephrine (between 2-min cycles)	IV 10 mL of 1 : 10 000 dilution (administer entire ampule quickly)
Pulmonary Edema		
	Preserve IV access	
	Monitor vital signs	
	Pulse oximeter	
	O$_2$ by mask	6–10 L/min
	Elevate head of bed if possible	
	Furosemide (Lasix)	IV 20–40 mg; administer slowly over 2 min
	Morphine (IV)	IV 1–3 mg; repeat every 5–10 min, as needed
	Call emergency response team or 911	
Seizures		
	Observe and protect the patient	
	Turn patient on side to avoid aspiration	
	Suction airway as needed	
	Preserve IV access	
	Monitor vitals	
	Pulse oximeter	
	O$_2$ by mask	6–10 mL/min
If unremitting	Call emergency	
	Lorazepam (IV)	IV 2–4 mg; administer slowly, to maximum dose of 4 mg
	Call emergency response team or 911	
Hypoglycemia		
	Preserve IV access	
	O$_2$ by mask	6–10 L/min
If patient is able to swallow safely	Oral glucose	Two sugar packets or 15 g of glucose tablet/gel or ½ cup (4 oz) of fruit juice or any sugary soda
If patient is unable to swallow safely and IV access available	Dextrose 50% (IV)	IV D$_{50}$W 1 ampule (25 g); administer over 2 min
	D$_5$W or D$_5$NS (IV) as adjunct therapy	Administer at a rate of 100 mL/h
If no IV access is available	Glucagon (IM)	IM 1 mg

Continued

BOX 23.2 Management of Acute Reactions in Adults—cont'd

	Treatment	Dosing
Anxiety (Panic Attack)	Diagnosis of exclusion Assess patient for developing signs and symptoms that might indicate another type of reaction Preserve IV access Monitor vital signs Pulse oximeter If no identifiable manifestations and normal oxygenation, consider this diagnosis Reassure patient	
Reaction Rebound Prevention *Note:* Although IV corticosteroids may help prevent a short-term recurrence of an allergic-like reaction, they are not useful in the acute treatment of any reaction. However, these may be considered for patients having severe allergic-like manifestations before transportation to an emergency department or inpatient unit.	Hydrocortisone (Solu-Cortef) (IV)	IV 5 mg /kg; administer over 1-2 minutes
	or Methylprednisolone (Solu-Medrol) (IV)	IV; 1 mg/kg; administer over 1-2 minutes

Reprinted with permission of the American College of Radiology. No other representation of this material is authorized without expressed, written permission from the ACR. Refer to the ACR website for the most current and complete version of the ACR Manual on Contrast Media at the link http://www.acr.org/~/media/ACR/Documents/PDF/QualitySafety/Resources/Contrast%20Manual/2013_Contrast_Media.pdf. *Note:* Please also see BLS and ACLS booklets published by the American Heart Association.

TABLE 23.6   Selected Radiopharmaceuticals

Radionuclide	Pharmaceutical	Main Energy	Half-Life	Main Organ of Interest
^{99m}Tc	Medronate	140 keV	6.02 h	Bone
^{99m}Tc	Mertiatide	140 keV	6.02 h	Kidneys
^{99m}Tc	Sulfur colloid	140 keV	6.02 h	Liver, spleen
^{99m}Tc	Mebrofenin	140 keV	6.02 h	Hepatobiliary
^{99m}Tc	Albumin aggregated	140 keV	6.02 h	Lung perfusion
^{99m}Tc	Tetrofosmin	140 keV	6.02 h	Myocardial perfusion
^{99m}Tc	Fanolesomab	140 keV	6.02 h	Appendix
^{201}Tl	Thallous chloride	68–80 keV	3.04 days	Myocardial perfusion
^{131}I	Sodium iodide	364 keV/gamma beta used for therapy	8.02 days	Thyroid imaging or therapy ablation
^{67}Ga	Citrate	93, 184, 300, 393 keV	3.26 days	Infection, inflammation
^{133}Xe	Xenon gas	81 keV	5.243 days	Lung ventilation

characteristics, and associated pharmaceuticals for some typical nuclear medicine studies.

Positron Emission Tomography Agents

A positron is a positive electron, which is also known as *antimatter*. Antimatter cannot exist for long because when it comes into contact with a negative electron, it annihilates itself into two 511-keV photons of energy that are approximately 180 degrees apart from each other. Positron emission tomography (PET) imaging takes advantage of these two 511-keV photons nearly 180 degrees opposite each other to do coincidence imaging, whereby the gamma camera accepts only two 180-degree opposing events to form an image. Positron emitters are formed in a cyclotron and often have very short half-lives. Table 23.7 lists several different PET agents. When using contrast media for a PET/CT scan for a diagnostic CT, one should do the PET study first and then the CT examination. There is a small possibility that the contrast media could attenuate or interfere with the PET scan if the area of interest is a place in the body that concentrates the contrast media.

Special Considerations When Working With Unsealed Radiation Sources

The primary concern when working with short-lived (small half-lives of hours, minutes, or seconds) unsealed radiation sources is contamination, which can occur on patients,

TABLE 23.7	Selected Positron Emission Tomography Agents			
Radionuclide	Pharmaceutical	Main Energy	Half-Life	Main Organ of Interest
^{18}F	Fluorodeoxyglucose	511 keV	109.71 min	Brain, heart, tumors
^{11}C	Raclopride	511 keV	20.3 min	Neurologic and psychiatric disorders, Parkinson's disease
^{15}O	Saline	511 keV	122 s	Myocardial and cerebral perfusion
^{13}N	Acidic saline	511 keV	9.97 min	Myocardial and cerebral perfusion

personnel, floors, tables, or imaging equipment, that might be misconstrued as part of the image produced for physicians to read. These artifacts may not be easily ascertained and might be misinterpreted by a physician as a pathologic abnormality in a patient when reading a study. Another concern with contamination of unsealed sources is increased radiation exposure to personnel and patients that might occur. This contamination might be in the form of external or internal contamination. External contamination would be dropped, splashed, or spilled unsealed sources deposited on someone or something. Internal contamination might occur if these dropped, splashed, or spilled unsealed sources were internalized via inhalation, absorption, or ingestion. Unsealed sources must be contained as much as possible before, during, and after their use. This contamination is why nuclear medicine personnel recap needles on a syringe or otherwise secure the needle and syringe after use, whereas all other medical personnel do not.

Magnetic Resonance Contrast Media Agents

There are several commercially available MRI contrast media on the market. Examples and their uses include:

Omniscan—used to primarily help diagnose certain disorders of the brain.

Eovist—used to primarily diagnose disorders of the liver.

Gadavist—used mainly for magnetic resonance angiography's (MRA's) to allow blood vessels, organs, and other non-bony tissues to be seen more clearly.

Magnevist—used to see blood vessels, organs, and non-bony tissues more clearly.

Ablavar—this contrast raises the chance of the health problem NSF (nephrogenic systemic fibrosis (NSF)) in some people. This may lead to very bad and sometimes deadly skin, muscle, and organ problems.

Dotarem—raises the chance of health problem NSF, same as the contrast agent mentioned above.

Feridex—this is the only MRI contrast agent that can be used while breast feeding.

GastoMark—This an oral suspension contrast used to visualize the stomach, small bowel, and large intestines.

Multihance—this contrast has the same properties as Ablavar and Dotarem.

Optimark—this is used to diagnose certain disorders of the brain & spine (the entire central nervous system).

Prohance—this contrast has the same properties as Ablavar, Dotarem, and Multihance.

Teslascan—this contrast is used to provide a clear picture in the MRI machine itself. It uses magnets and computers to create images or pictures of certain areas inside the body.

Vasovist—this is primarily used in MRA imaging and to help diagnose certain disorders of the heart.

NSF or nephrogenic fibrosing dermopathy (NFD) is a rare and serious syndrome that involves fibrosis of skin, joints, eyes, and internal organs. The first cases were identified in 1997 and its cause is not fully understood. However, evidence suggests that NSF is associated with exposure to gadolinium-based MRI contrast agents being frequently used as contrast agents for MRI in patients with severe kidney failure. Symptoms can occur 6 months after a procedure. If patients are diagnosed with NSF due to the use of MRI contrast, these patients develop large areas of hardened skin with fibrotic nodules and plaques. NSF may also cause joint pain and limitation in range of motion. In its most severe form, NSF may cause severe systemic fibrosis affecting internal organs including the lungs, heart, and liver. Concerns associated with the possibility of NSF development requires proper patient history taking of any renal disease and sometimes requires a creatinine blood test to assess renal function.

Gadolinium contrast agents have received some negative publicity due to evidence that it accumulates in brain tissue; however, to date there is no evidence of any clinically significant symptoms associated with this issue. It is concerning because it was assumed that it cleared the body with no accumulation. Further research and long-term studies are underway to investigate this phenomenon.

HEALTH PROFESSIONAL RESPONSIBILITIES

Qualifications of Personnel Who Handle Contrast Media

The supervising physician should be a licensed physician with the following qualifications:

1. Certification in radiology or radiation oncology by the American Board of Radiology, the American Osteopathic Board of Radiology, the Royal College of Physicians, or Surgeons of Canada

2. A minimum of 6 months of documented formal dedicated training in the interpretation and formal reporting of general radiographs or, if the residency or fellowship did not include formal training in the interpretation and formal reporting of general radiographs, the ability to demonstrate sufficient knowledge of pharmacology, indications, contraindications, and safe administration and the ability to initiate treatment in the event of adverse reactions

3. Familiarity with the various risk factors, premedication strategies, and preprocedural screening

4. Immediate availability to respond in the event of an adverse reaction

5. Knowledge of appropriative alternate imaging methods
6. Awareness of the signs and symptoms of adverse reactions and how to monitor the patient having a contrast reaction

The technologist is responsible for patient comfort throughout the duration of the procedure, as well as for being able to identify the signs and symptoms of adverse reactions and having adequate knowledge of how to treat any adverse reaction.

Patient Preparation

The general considerations for the patient have two aims: contrast media reaction prevention and preparedness in the event of an adverse reaction. The prevention of contrast media reactions depends on obtaining a thorough patient history that can indicate contrast media contraindications or an increased likelihood of adverse reactions, patient preprocedural preparations and instructions to include adequate hydration and appropriate premedication when indicated, and adequate knowledge regarding treatment and use of emergency equipment in cases of adverse reactions.

Sources of Information

In almost no other medical specialty do practitioners inject, or have the patient ingest, such large amounts of nonbiologic substances over a short time as in radiology. Obviously, the chemical structures of these agents greatly influence the (1) ability of the agents to enhance subject contrast, (2) types of agents used for specific procedures, and (3) reasons for adverse reactions that can occur in patients.

The discussion presented in this chapter about the physical properties of contrast media aids in interpreting the package inserts. The technologist should look at the chemical structure presented and locate the common chemical groups discussed. Then the radiologic technologist can consider other information in the package inserts about specific procedures, doses, and adverse reactions.

Technical representatives from pharmaceutical companies that supply contrast agents can also supply journal articles as important sources of information. Problems arising from specific contrast media examinations should be discussed with the radiologist. Valuable insights for effective patient care are gained in this manner.

Patient Care and Surveillance

The setup for any contrast media procedure, patient positioning, and radiographic technique are important professional responsibilities. The patient must remain the focus of the procedure, however. The patient is usually anxious about the procedure and the reasons that made the procedure necessary. In many instances the patient has an empty stomach; therefore, he or she may be irritable. These feelings, combined with the reasons for the adverse reactions from contrast media, may result in an increased possibility of these reactions.

Due to an increase in outpatient procedures that use water-soluble iodine contrast media, instances of adverse reactions occurring hours later have been reported. These reactions have been poorly communicated to radiologists because of a lack of patient knowledge. The radiographer might develop an instruction sheet about mild adverse reactions and discuss these issues with the patient after the procedure is complete but before the patient leaves. Such instructions might include calling the department (direct telephone number) if any of the following occurs within 24 hours: hives, flushing, chills, nasal stuffiness, swelling of the eyes or face, or wheezing.

A calm, supportive manner on the part of the radiologic technologist is a necessity. Continued communication, with questions regarding patient comfort, allows observation of the patient's physical and emotional status. A professional demeanor can increase the well-being of the patient and thereby reduce the possibility of adverse reactions.

Many procedures require patient preparation at home, such as enemas before lower GI procedures and fasting after midnight before some procedures. The diagnostic quality of procedures that require patient preparation is diminished by patient failure to follow instructions. Before beginning the examination, the radiologic technologist must ask the patient if he or she followed the instructions for it. Some patients comply with some but not all the instructions. Therefore, the radiologic technologist must also find out to what extent the patient complied. This information can usually be obtained by one question, "What did you do at home to prepare for your x-ray today?" If the patient forgets an aspect of the instructions, then the radiologic technologist should use prompts such as, "What about the pills, Mr. Jones?"

Many referring physicians do not tell their patients what to expect during contrast media procedures. In addition, many people have only a rudimentary knowledge of body functions. Explaining to the patients, in simple terms, what will be done is the radiologic technologist's responsibility. The radiologic technologist must also convey to the patient *a sense of being cared for* and *a sense of being safe* during the procedure. These subjective qualities can be communicated by addressing the patient by name (e.g., Mr. Jones, Mrs. Green), by using blankets or sheets for warmth and modesty, by using pillows when possible, and by asking questions such as, "Are you warm enough?" Many patients exhibit reduced anxiety if the radiologic technologist explains the procedure as it is performed. Finally, a universal form of supportive communication is touch.

SUMMARY

- Radiographic contrast media are used to visualize areas within the body that otherwise might not be seen well. These agents are not drugs; however, they can affect the physiologic status of patients.
- Radiolucent contrast media transmit x-rays and are usually used with radiopaque contrast media to visualize the lumina of organs and joint spaces. Radiopaque contrast media absorb x-rays and are used to demonstrate the GI, biliary, urinary, circulatory, lymphatic, and respiratory systems.
- Most adverse reactions encountered by patients are associated with the use of radiopaque contrast agents. Serious complications from the administration of barium sulfate include hypervolemia and colon and vaginal rupture. Water-soluble iodine contrast agents can cause allergic-like effects and can increase the severity of sickle cell anemia, renal disease, and

diabetes. The patient history obtained by the radiologic technologist gives information about preexisting disease that can increase the possibility of some adverse reactions. Appropriate patient preparation and care can then be given to eliminate or decrease these adverse reactions.

- The radiologic technologist should be familiar with the general chemical structure of contrast media and the relationship of the structure to the formal and trade names of the particular medium. The radiologic technologist absolutely must relate the various media to examinations for which they are best suited. Knowledge of specific patient preparations and adverse reactions associated with each agent is imperative.
- The radiologic technologist should be aware that radiopharmaceuticals are not contrast agents, and he or she must be aware of the special considerations for using PET agents and any unsealed radiation sources in a nuclear medicine department.
- The manner in which patient care is given can decrease the possibility of adverse reactions and can increase the diagnostic quality of the examination by increasing patient cooperation.

BIBLIOGRAPHY

Benison S, Walter B: *Cannon: the life and times of a young scientist*, Cambridge, Mass, 1987, Harvard University Press.

Bettmann M: Ionic versus nonionic contrast agents for intravenous use: are all the answers in? *Radiology* 175:616, 1990.

Cornuelle AG, Gronefild DH: *Radiographic anatomy positioning: an integrated approach*, East Norwalk, Conn, 1998, Appleton & Lange.

Curry NS, Schabel SI, Reiheld CT, et al.: Fatal reactions to intravenous nonionic contrast media, *Radiology* 178:361, 1991.

Dawson P, Cosgrove DO: *Textbook of contrast media*, ed 2, New York, 2009, Informa HealthCare.

Garcia-Bournissen F, Shrim A, Koren G: Safety of gadolinium during pregnancy, *Can Fam Physician* 52:309–310, 2006. PMC 1479713. PMID 16572573.

Grobner T: Gadolinium - a specific trigger for the development of nephrogenic fibrosing dermopathy and nephrogenic systemic fibrosis? *Nephrol Dial Transplant* 21(4):1104–1108, 2005, https://doi.org/10.1093/ndt/gfk062.PMID16431890.

International Society For Magnetic Resonance in Medicine: Questions and Answers (PDF). Found at: http://www.ismrm.org/special/EMEA2.pdf.

Jacobson PD: Who decides who gets low-osmolar contrast? *Diagn Image* 13:77, 1991.

Katayama H, Yamaguchi K, Kozuka T, et al.: Adverse reactions to ionic and nonionic contrast media: a report from the Japanese committee on the safety of contrast media, *Radiology* 175:621, 1990.

Kowalsky RJ, Falen SW: *Radiopharmaceuticals in nuclear pharmacy and nuclear medicine*, ed 2, Washington, DC, 2004, American Pharmacists Association.

Lentschig MG, Reimer P, Raush-Lentschig UL, Allkemper T, Oelerich M, Laub G: Breath-hold gadolinium-enhanced MR angiography of the major vessels at 1.0 T: dose-response findings and angiographic correlation, *Radiology* 208(2):353–357, 1998. https://doi.org/10.1148/radiology.208.2.9680558. PMID 9680558.

Long BW, Rollins JH, Smith BJ: *Merrill's atlas of radiographic positions and radiologic procedures*, ed 13, St. Louis, 2016, Elsevier.

Manual on contrast media, version 10.3, Reston, Va, 2017, American College of Radiology.

McClennan B: Ionic and nonionic iodinated contrast media: evolution and strategies for use, *AJR Am J Roentgenol* 155:225, 1990.

Murray RK, Bender DA, Botham KM, et al.: *Harper's illustrated biochemistry*, ed 28, Columbus, Ohio, 2009, McGraw-Hill.

Radioisotope decay tables, Ottawa, Ontario, Canada, 2002, MDS Nordion.

Saha GB: *Fundamentals of nuclear pharmacy*, ed 6, New York, 2010, Springer-Verlag.

Torsten A: Relations between chemical structure, animal toxicity and clinical adverse effects of contrast media. In Enge I, Edgren J, editors: *Patient safety and adverse events in contrast medium examinations*, New York, 1989, Elsevier.

Wang, Yi-Xiang J: Superparamagnetic iron oxide based MRI contrast agents: current status of clinical application. *Quant Imaging Med Surg* 1(1):35–40, 2011. https://doi.org/10.3978/j.issn.2223-4292.2011.08.03. PMC 3496483. PMID 23256052.

PART IV

Ethical and Legal Issues

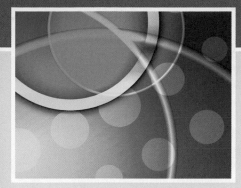

Professional Ethics

James M. Ketchum, MSEd, DHA, RT(R)

Knowing what's right doesn't mean much unless you do what's right.

Anonymous

OBJECTIVES

On completion of this chapter, the student will be able to:

- Explain the ethics of the radiologic technology profession.
- Differentiate the systems of ethics, law, and morals.
- Explain the four-step problem-solving process of ethical analysis.
- Explain two sources of moral judgment that underlie ethical decision making.
- Identify moral dilemmas encountered in patient relationships.
- Identify moral dilemmas encountered in physician relationships.
- Identify moral dilemmas encountered in relationships with other health professionals.
- Recognize values associated with ethical decision making in the practice of radiologic technology.
- Apply critical analysis to ethical decision making.

OUTLINE

KEY TERMS

Autonomy Person's self-reliance, independence, liberty, rights, privacy, individual choice, freedom of the will, and self-contained ability to decide

Beneficence Doing of good; active promotion of goodness, kindness, and charity

Caring Care for; an emotional commitment to and a willingness to act on behalf of a person with whom a caring relationship exists

Codes of Ethics Articulated statements of role morality as seen by the members of a profession

Confidentiality Belief that health-related information about individual patients should not be revealed to others; maintenance of privacy

Consequentialism Belief that the worth of actions is determined by their ends or consequences; actions are right or wrong according to the balance of their good and bad consequences

Duties Obligations placed on individuals, groups, and institutions by reason of the so-called moral bond of our interdependence with others

Ethical Dilemmas Situations requiring moral judgment between two or more equally problem-fraught alternatives; two or more competing moral norms are present, creating a challenge about what to do

Ethical Outrage Gross violation of commonly held standards of decency or human rights

Ethical Theories Bodies of systematically related moral principles used to resolve ethical dilemmas

Ethics Systematic study of rightness and wrongness of human conduct and character as known by natural reason

Ethics of Care Ethical reflections that emphasize an intimate personal relationship value system that includes such virtues as sympathy, compassion, fidelity, discernment, and love

Fidelity Strict observance of promises or duties; loyalty and faithfulness to others

Justice Equitable, fair, or just conduct in dealing with others

Laws Regulations established by government and applicable to people within a certain political subdivision

Legal Rights Rights of individuals or groups that are established and guaranteed by law

Liberal Individualism Basis for rights-based ethical theory; each individual is protected and allowed to pursue personal projects

Moral Principles General, universal guides to action that are derived from so-called basic moral truths that should be respected unless a morally compelling reason exists not to do so; also referred to as ethical principles

Moral Rights Rights of individuals or groups that exist separately from governmental or institutional guarantees; usually asserted based on moral principles or rules

Moral Rules Statements of right conduct governing individual actions

Morals Generally accepted customs, principles, or habits of right living and conduct in a society and the individual's practice in relation to these

Nonconsequentialism Belief that actions themselves, rather than consequences, determine the worth of actions; actions are right or wrong according to the morality of the acts themselves

Nonmaleficence Ethical principle that places high value on avoiding harm to others

Norms Standards set by individuals or groups of individuals

Principle-Based Ethics Use of moral principles as a basis for defending a chosen path of action in resolving an ethical dilemma; also see Principlism

Principlism Belief system based on a set of moral principles that are embedded in a common morality

Professional Ethic Publicly displayed ethical conduct of a profession, usually embedded in a code of ethics; affirms the professional as an independent, autonomous, responsible decision maker

Professional Ethics Internal controls of a profession based on human values or moral principles

Professional Etiquette Manners and attitudes generally accepted by members of a profession

Rights Justified claims that an individual can make on individuals, groups, or society; divided into legal rights and moral rights

Rights-Based Ethics Belief that individual rights provide the vital protection of life, liberty, expression, and property

Rules of Ethics ARRT's mandatory standards of minimally acceptable professional conduct. These are enforceable and can result in sanctions should the ARRT determine the certificate holder has violated any of the rules.

Social Contract Relationship that exists when two mutually dependent groups in a society recognize certain expectations of each other and conduct their affairs accordingly

Standards of Professional Conduct Practice behaviors that are defined by members of a profession

Values Ideals and customs of a society toward which the members of a group have an affective regard; a value may be a quality desirable as an end in itself

Value System Collection or set of values that an individual or group has as each person's personal guide

Veracity Duty to tell the truth and avoid deception

Virtues Traits of character that are socially valued, such as courage

Virtue-Based Ethics Ethical theory that emphasizes the agents who perform actions and make choices; character and virtue form the framework of this ethical theory

IMPORTANCE OF A PROFESSIONAL ETHIC

Health care professionals often encounter situations in their practices that they find deeply disturbing. These situations, which are usually unrelated to clinical procedures or medical intervention, may involve such basic human rights as the right to privacy and dignity or even the simple right to be told the truth. Professionals may encounter conflicting value or belief systems that can compromise patient care. They also must make difficult choices that depend on their understanding of such moral principles as justice and beneficence, such virtues as compassion and caring, and such fundamental responsibilities as honesty and loyalty to both patients and physicians.

All of these situations are generally encompassed under the term professional ethics. Principles of professional ethics may be reduced to a written code, but professionals who attempt to apply such unyielding standards to their daily practice often become dismayed and frustrated because the code does not address their specific problems. When faced with an ethical problem or dilemma, many professionals simply obey the rules of their institution, follow the policies of their supervisor, or choose the least objectionable course of action among a bewildering array of choices, each of which may have profound consequences for patient care.

As emerging health care professionals in their own right, radiologic technologists play a critical supportive role between the physician and the patient. They assist in providing valuable information that enables physicians to make accurate diagnoses and establish sound therapeutic plans. Accordingly, radiologic technologists must comply with established standards of professional conduct as professional persons, standards that support the emotional and physical needs of the patients with whom they come in contact. The professional conduct of radiologic technologists, as that of all health care professionals, should be based on complete, uncompromised devotion to patients as individuals in providing them with the highest possible quality of medical care.

The public expects all professionals to exhibit self-discipline within a system of self-regulation. This sense of self-discipline is particularly important within the health care professions, in which errors in judgment can have serious, even life-threatening, consequences. Furthermore, despite the increasing sophistication among segments of the American public, few individuals are able to judge the quality of the professional services they receive. Patients who submit to radiologic procedures, for example, have no way of determining whether the procedures have been performed properly or even whether they have been injured in the process. As a result, a professional ethic is one of several generally accepted criteria that serve to distinguish a profession from other occupations or trades.

State licensing laws reflect the public's demand that it be served by qualified health care practitioners. The professional

TABLE 24.1	Comparison of Systems of Ethics, Law, and Morals			
System	**Application**	**Control**	**Enabling Source**	**Sanctions**
Ethics	Specific group	Within group	Codes of ethics	Expulsion
Law	Political subdivision	Outside group	Legislation	Fines, prison
Morals	Individuals	Conscience	Religious writing	Shame, guilt

licensing boards that enforce these and other professional practice laws provide one element of self-regulation. Professionals are given certain prerogatives by society, such as a quasi-monopoly to operate in a certain professional arena. In return for granting these prerogatives, society expects professionals to be guided by a standard of conduct beyond mere conformity to law. This standard of conduct, this common concern for collective self-discipline, this control of the profession from within is known as ethics.

In philosophy, *ethics* is often defined as the science of rightness and wrongness of human conduct as known by natural reason. Professional ethics, however, may be defined as rules of conduct or standards by which a particular group regulates its actions and sets standards for its members. The system of ethics is closely related and overlaps two other systems designed to control society: law and morals. Laws are regulations established by a government that are applicable to people within a certain political subdivision; morals are generally accepted customs of right living and conduct and an individual's practice in relation to these customs. Table 24.1 summarizes these distinctions.

At first glance, the system of laws, with its sanctions of fines and imprisonment for noncompliance, would seem to have the greatest payoff to society. Moreover, the system of laws is dynamic, subject to the ever-changing will of the people and their legislators; however, the system of laws does not cover all areas of professional conduct or potential risks a professional may encounter. No matter how broadly laws and regulations are written or how detailed they may seem, areas still exist that must be covered by a system of voluntary self-discipline, the system of ethics.

Society expects a profession, through its collective members, to generate its own statement of acceptable and unacceptable behavior, usually in the form of a code of ethics; practice behaviors that are defined by the members of a profession are standards of professional conduct. The code of ethics adopted by the American Registry of Radiologic Technologists (ARRT) is Part A of the ARRT Standards of Ethics and is reproduced in Appendix D; the code comprises 10 principles, which are intended to be aspirational. Part B of the Standards contains the Rules of Ethics, which are the mandatory rules of acceptable professional conduct for radiologic technologists, and these rules are enforceable through ARRT-prescribed sanctions. Similarly, the American Society of Radiologic Technologists has a 10-point Code of Ethics that is essentially the same as that of the ARRT.

Ideally, all radiologic technologists subscribe to the ethical principles contained in these documents and apply them to problems in their professional practice. These codes serve the profession well by providing the practitioner with a detailed, explicit, operational blueprint of norms of professional conduct. Unfortunately, some of these principles are stated in abstract or idealized terms that provide little in the way of concrete guidance for young practitioners. For example, Principle 9 of the ARRT Code of Ethics states that the radiologic technologist "reveals confidential information only as required by law or to protect the welfare of the individual or the community." Under what circumstances, if any, might a patient's right to privacy be infringed? What standards are used to determine when the welfare of the community supersedes the welfare of the individual? What information can be released, to whom, and under what circumstances? The answers to these questions, of course, are not usually found in codes of ethics. Furthermore, you may encounter situations that are not even remotely related to the statements in the codes, reflecting the static nature of any professional code. Finally, do the principles that make up the code take into consideration the role of human values and virtues in deciding professional practice behavior? This question suggests that a more serviceable method for determining the correct conduct in professional practice involves something beyond mere reflection on a code of ethics.

ETHICAL EVALUATIONS

Before we can develop our own personal set of internal guidelines for determining what constitutes right conduct in our professional practice, we must clarify a few additional concepts. Professional etiquette, the manners and attitudes toward patients generally accepted by practitioners, should not be confused with professional ethics. For example, rudeness to patients or insensitivity to their need to preserve modesty may violate our sense of professional propriety but are not considered breaches in professional ethics. We will consider professional ethics as rules of conduct or standards beyond conformance to either law or etiquette, the internal controls of a profession based on human values or moral principles.

Next, we must develop some skill in both recognizing and analyzing ethical dilemmas. Although we all may agree on what constitutes patently unethical conduct, the so-called ethical outrage, the true ethical dilemma invites a wide range of personal opinion among colleagues in a profession, each of which is based on a highly individualistic, strongly held value system. For example, we might agree that refusing to provide services to dirty, unkempt patients or to those with acquired immunodeficiency syndrome is unethical, but we might hold a variety of opinions on what degree of loyalty we owe to our fellow workers on the health care team. When does our loyalty to physicians or administrators overshadow our loyalty to our patients? On the other hand, if our loyalty to our patients' autonomy interferes with their decisions to accept needed medical treatment, we may wish to set aside this value temporarily so that a higher human value, the resulting benefit to these patients, is served. To a greater or lesser extent, all professional decisions in radiologic technology and other health care practices involve a consideration of human values. By the same token, every ethical decision also involves human values, values that often conflict and compete for recognition and acceptance among our professional colleagues.

Once we have identified an ethical dilemma and the human values that may be associated with the dilemma, how should we proceed to analyze the situation? The process of ethical analysis generally contains the following four components:

- Identifying the problem
- Developing alternative solutions
- Selecting the best solution
- Defending the selection

Many students encounter difficulty in *identifying the problem* simply because they are eager to proceed with the problem-solving process. Thoroughness in problem identification—that is, looking at every possible twist or nuance in a given situation—is absolutely essential for successful resolution of any ethical dilemma. In *developing alternative solutions,* we attempt to exhaust all possible pathways to a resolution of the dilemma, taking care to view the dilemma from the perspective not only of the patient and the patient's family, but also of the health care professionals and administrators to whom they entrust their care. The most challenging step in the problem-solving process is *selecting the best solution,* a highly personal activity that involves choosing an alternative that not only is based on widely held moral standards but also is in full accord with your own individual value system. Finally, by *defending your selection,* you can explain the basis for your ethical decision in terms that you can justify to both colleagues and patients. Although this process may seem difficult or even impossible at first glance, we can approach it with confidence once we have considered the underlying sources of moral judgment that allow us to move beyond feelings, emotions, and intuitions toward more structured foundations for our ethical decision making. These sources of moral judgment are discussed under the general headings of moral rules and ethical theories.

Moral Rules

In making ethical decisions, we might rely on widely held **moral rules.** The Bible contains the *golden rule* and the Ten Commandments, schools teach that cheating is wrong, and our professional associations promulgate codes of ethics that encourage practitioners to *do no harm.* Many individuals successfully use moral rules to guide their behavior, but this approach has its limitations. The most serious limitation to using moral rules as a primary guide to moral behavior is that most people lack access to a complete set of moral rules or that a complete set of moral rules simply does not exist. Another concern when attempting to use one's own moral code is that beliefs and cultures vary and what may be seen as moral or immoral by one person may not necessarily be viewed as such by another. As noted, most codes of ethics are incomplete and

do not speak to all ethical issues that radiologic technologists and other health care professionals encounter.

Ethical Theories

Another approach to establishing a foundation on which to base ethical decision making involves normative ethical systems—that is, sets of principles that tell us what actions are right or wrong, or **ethical theories.** These systems are usually divided into two groups. **Consequentialism** evaluates the rightness or wrongness of ethical decisions by assessing the consequences of these decisions on the patient—that is, producing a good effect for the patient or at least avoiding some potential harm. **Nonconsequentialism** holds that other right-making characteristics of our actions beyond consequences exist and must be examined to determine whether a given behavior is right or wrong. For example, persons who use the consequentialist system for ethical decision making may lie to a patient if he or she thinks the lie might ultimately benefit the patient; persons using the nonconsequentialist system would caution against lying to a patient under any circumstances because the act of lying is generally accepted as morally wrong in our society.

Recently, modifications to these ethical theories have been developed, including such concepts as social contracts, the ethics of care, rights-based ethics, principle-based ethics, and virtue-based ethics. These refinements are being used increasingly in medical practices to analyze and defend actions and their outcomes, especially practices that attempt to fulfill the ethical mandates of high-quality patient care.

Social contract theory attempts to describe the relationship that exists between two mutually dependent persons or groups of persons in a society. Under this theory, these persons or groups—radiologic technologists and patients, in our context—recognize certain expectations of each other and act accordingly. For example, patients expect their radiologic technologist to tell them the truth; by the same token, radiologic technologists expect their patients to tell them the truth. Whereas social contract theory sounds simple and straightforward, social contracts can be perplexing. Unlike legal contracts, with their precise language and implicit sanctions, social contracts are unwritten, leaving the specific duties and actions expected of health care practitioners and their patients to be resolved through a process of reasoning and discernment.

The **ethics of care** cautions that our actions should not be examined as isolated events; instead, our actions should be considered an integral part of the context of specific situations. For example, lying to a patient is not an isolated event; rather, this act is surrounded by a web of circumstances—who the patient is, what his or her particular ills might be, how he or she relates to us, what beliefs we have, and so on. Furthermore, a caring ethic requires us to make moral judgments that reflect the values of the communities within which we live. The ethics of care require the decision maker to focus as clearly as possible on such basic moral skills as kindness, sensitivity, attentiveness, tact, patience, and reliability. Indeed, the ethics of care emphasizes the need for an accurate understanding of moral competence, a clear vision of the meaning of a *virtuous person,* and finely honed skills in human relations.

TABLE 24.2 Selected Ethical Principles

Moral Principle	Your Aspiration
Beneficence (bringing about good)	Perform actions that benefit others. Decide and act always to benefit the patient.
Nonmaleficence (preventing harm)	Above all, do no harm. Never perform or allow acts that may harm the patient.
Autonomy (acting with personal self-reliance)	Perform actions that respect the independence of other persons. The patient must decide what is done to his or her person.
Veracity (telling the truth)	Being truthful is right. To tell the truth is expected.
Fidelity (being faithful)	Performing acts that observe covenants or promises is right. Be faithful.
Justice (acting with fairness or equity)	Performing acts that ensure the fair distribution of goods and harm are right. Be fair.

Rights-based ethics, one of the increasingly popular approaches to ethical reasoning, is based on an understanding of *human rights*. Advocates often express their human rights openly and forcefully, claiming a *right to health care*. Advocates who are medical practitioners often champion the *rights of the health professions*. The importance of human rights is reflected in the tenets of **liberal individualism,** a belief that an individual in a democratic society is shielded from undue forces and allowed to enjoy and pursue personal projects—that is, the individual has certain *rights*.

Rights are justified claims that an individual can make on others (individuals or groups) or on society and may be considered as either **legal rights** or **moral rights.** *Legal rights* are claims that have a foundation in legal principles and rules; *moral rights* are claims that are justified by moral principles and rules. Moreover, a right, whether legal or moral, carries with it a corresponding duty that is placed on someone. **Duties** may be considered as obligations placed on individuals, groups, and institutions by reason of the so-called *moral bond* of our interdependence with others. We expect to receive positive responses to our own needs and to be treated humanely. In addition, we form special relationships with our parents, our children, our spouses, our teachers, and our health care professionals. Realizing our duties as radiologic technologists helps us know to whom and for what we are accountable. For this reason, rights-based ethical reasoning can have great appeal to beginning practitioners; however, radiologic technologists who attempt to apply rights theory to ethical dilemmas must be cautious because they may encounter considerable tension between what they envision as professional duties and what their patients claim as human rights.

Principle-based ethics, or **principlism,** the use of moral principles as a basis for defending a chosen path of action in resolving an ethical dilemma, has been widely accepted by medical communities. **Moral principles** (also referred to as *ethical principles*) are general, universal guides to action that are derived from so-called "basic moral truths" that should be respected unless a morally compelling reason exists not to do so. Moral principles include not only the two principles traditionally associated with the health care professions, **beneficence** and nonmaleficence, but also several newer principles such as **justice, autonomy, veracity,** and **fidelity.** Most professional codes of ethics are based primarily on the principle of *beneficence*—that is, the codes encourage practitioners to engage in actions that ultimately benefit their patients. For example, the Code of Ethics for radiologic technologists states that the ethical radiologic technologist "acts in the best interest of the patient," a clear appeal to beneficence. Although these principles seem forbidding and difficult to grasp, they can be understood with some careful reading and reflection. Table 24.2 provides some definitions and examples of ethical principles to help clarify these difficult concepts.

Living a good life, becoming a good person, and acquiring certain desirable characteristics (called **virtues**) have been the main goals of ethics during most of its long history. **Virtue-based ethics,** the use of virtues in establishing right reason in action, offers the opportunity to include the character of each participant involved in an ethical dilemma and is an especially important consideration when linked to principlism. Virtues include such character traits as caring, faith, trust, hope, compassion, courage, and fidelity. Principle 2 of the ARRT Code of Ethics emphasizes this call to virtue by pledging the intent of the profession "to provide services to humanity with full respect for the dignity of mankind."

PATIENT CARE AND INTERPROFESSIONAL RELATIONSHIPS

As do members of the other allied health professions, radiologic technologists place a high value on high-quality patient care and solid interprofessional relationships. This section will help you explore these relationships in the context of ethical dilemmas that you may face in your professional practice. We have also provided several case studies to help you work through the problem-solving approach outlined earlier. We have analyzed the first case for you by way of illustration; the other cases give you an opportunity to practice using the problem-solving approach.

Patient Relationships

Some of the most frequently encountered ethical issues that affect the relationship between radiologic technologists and their patients involve maintaining patient faithfulness (i.e., keeping faith with our patients), maintaining patient **confidentiality,** and preserving professional boundaries. The following cases illustrate the types of problems associated with these ethical issues.

Case 1: Maintaining Patient Faithfulness. Radiologic technologists are often confronted by situations that test their ability to deal with sensitive patient care information. In many instances, the duty to respect the patient's confidences is compromised by pressures from authority figures or other persons who may not share the radiologic technologist's value system (Box 24.1).

Identifying the Problem. In this case, Mrs. Brown is seeking information that you may or may not be at liberty to provide. On one hand, as a health care professional you sense a duty to

BOX 24.1　**"Do You Think My Doctor Is Doing the Right Thing?"**

Mrs. Brown, a 27-year-old patient of Dr. Smith, looks apprehensive as you begin your radiologic procedure. Mrs. Brown found a lump in her breast and is worried about the possibility of having to undergo a mastectomy. Your mammographic examination reveals that Mrs. Brown probably has a small fibroid cyst. Mrs. Brown confides to you that Dr. Smith has mentioned the possibility of surgery. You are also aware that, given a choice, Dr. Smith nearly always operates. As you conclude your procedure, Mrs. Brown asks you whether surgery is indicated, adding, "Do you think my doctor is doing the right thing?"

BOX 24.2　**"Does Mr. Gray Have Cancer?"**

The images you took of Mr. Gray do not look good. As a matter of fact, you overheard Dr. Jones mutter about the "advanced stage" of Mr. Gray's condition. The transporting aide wheels Mr. Gray back to his room and returns with your next patient. The patient slips behind a screen to change into an examination gown and is out of earshot. "Mr. Gray seemed real depressed," the aide volunteers. "How did his film look? Does Mr. Gray have cancer?" The aide is a good friend of yours and always has seemed committed to good patient care. How do you respond?

BOX 24.3　**"Can We Connect?"**

You have performed multiple imaging procedures on Ms. Gold over the course of her stay in the hospital. During this time, you have developed a friendly rapport with Ms. Gold and often spend a few extra minutes chatting with her when you can spare the time. She then tells you that she is being released from the hospital the next day and asks if she can connect with you on a social media site. How do you respond?

provide Mrs. Brown with all the information available to you at this point about her condition. On the other hand, you feel professional loyalty toward Dr. Smith and all the other health professionals involved with Mrs. Brown's case.

Developing Alternative Solutions. You might respond to Mrs. Brown's question truthfully by revealing your understanding of her medical condition and your concerns about Dr. Smith's tendency to use surgery as a primary treatment. Alternatively, you might try to avoid answering her questions directly. Finally, you might refer Mrs. Brown's questions to Dr. Smith or to some other physician in whom you have more confidence.

Selecting the Best Solution. The first alternative forces you to choose between being truthful to Mrs. Brown (veracity), possibly saving her from some harm (nonmaleficence), or maintaining your loyal relationship with Dr. Smith. The second alternative forces you to be evasive (and possibly untruthful) with your answers, thereby compromising your respect for Mrs. Brown's right to make informed decisions about her care (autonomy). The final alternative seems to be the best solution because it not only allows you to include Dr. Smith (or another physician) in Mrs. Brown's decision-making process, but it also places a high value on actions that may ultimately benefit Mrs. Brown (beneficence).

Defending Your Selection. Principle 5 of the ARRT Code of Ethics states that the radiologic technologist "assesses situations; exercises care, discretion and judgment; assumes responsibility for professional decisions; and acts in the best interest of the patient." In this particular case, being completely truthful to Mrs. Brown may create unnecessary anxiety or cause her to question Dr. Smith's competence. By referring Mrs. Brown's questions to Dr. Smith and tactfully suggesting that she may wish to seek a second opinion if she has lingering concerns, we support Dr. Smith's treatment plan while allowing Mrs. Brown to increase her involvement in making decisions affecting her personal health care.

Case 2: Maintaining Patient Confidentiality. Of the values associated with radiologic practice, patient confidentiality is the most easily identified and the most prevalent. On the surface it seems that the trust that patients place in their health care providers cannot be compromised. Information obtained directly from the patient, observed, or obtained from other sources should be kept strictly confidential. The radiologic technologist should be alert to situations that may compromise patient confidences (Box 24.2).

Identifying the Problem. Is Mr. Gray's condition confidential? Is an aide considered a member of the health care team? Does your friendship with the aide (loyalty) play a role in this case?

Developing Alternative Solutions. Would Mr. Gray's confidence be compromised by telling the aide the truth? Should you refer the aide to Mr. Gray or to Mr. Gray's physician? Is Mr. Gray's condition none of the aide's business?

Selecting the Best Solution. What solution would satisfy your professional ethics, the aide's curiosity, and Mr. Gray's right to privacy? Is any action possible that would benefit Mr. Gray?

Defending Your Selection. What principles in the ARRT Code of Ethics apply to this case? Is it possible to take an action that will strike a balance between providing a benefit to Mr. Gray and protecting his right to privacy?

Case 3: Preserving Professional Boundaries. While it is important to develop a rapport with patients, strict adherence to professional boundaries is essential. Social networking platforms may be used to enhance patient care and education; however, they can also lead to ethical issues such as violations of patient privacy. In addition, many organizations have strict guidelines for employee use of social media. Failure to follow these guidelines could irreparably damage a technologist's professional image (Box 24.3).

Identifying the Problem. Do you consider this a true friendship or are you just being courteous? Would you have any interactions with Ms. Gold outside of the social media platform? What harm can occur should you accept the friend request? What benefits can be gained?

Developing Alternative Solutions. Are there opportunities for other means to continue the friendship? Would your actions be affected if you and Ms. Gold shared mutual friends?

Selecting the Best Solution. Is there a compromise that will allow you to continue the friendship with Ms. Gold and not jeopardize your employment? What action is ultimately the best solution for everyone involved?

Defending Your Selection. What is your employer's policy on initiating social media contact with patients? Does it make a difference that Ms. Gold has requested the interaction? Can you guarantee that your professional and personal communication will be separate?

Physician Relationships

As a radiologic technologist, your relationships with physicians will be one of the most important aspects of your professional practice. Loyalty, faithfulness, and fairness are virtues all health professionals need to share with one another. Observing professional discretion in your relationships with physicians, recognizing your professional limitations in practice, and balancing the safety and needs of the patient with physician demands will serve as a firm foundation for maintaining your ethical standards.

Case 4: Observing Professional Discretion. Radiologic technologists see, hear, and experience a wide variety of personal and sensitive patient care activities. Radiologic technologists must both respect the confidences of their patients and safeguard the knowledge they obtain through their everyday practice activities. Questions concerning the competency or professional judgment of the physicians working with you often raise serious ethical issues and should be handled with professional discretion (Box 24.4).

Identifying the Problem. Do you have an equal degree of loyalty to both Mrs. Green and Dr. Jones? Are conflicting professional duties present in this case?

Developing Alternative Solutions. Is this situation a personal matter between you and Dr. Jones? Should you discuss the issue with Dr. Jones's chief resident? The medical board? Mrs. Green or her family?

Selecting the Best Solution. Does a radiologic technologist have a professional obligation to point out a physician's possible errors? Does Mrs. Green have a right to know about her possible serious condition?

Defending Your Selection. Principle 6 of the ARRT Code of Ethics states that "interpretation and diagnosis are outside the scope of practice" for radiologic technologists. Does this principle apply in this case?

Case 5: Recognizing Professional Limitations. As do other health professionals, radiologic technologists have a specific role to perform on the health care team. *Teamwork* implies cooperation, as well as a sharing of professional functions. Radiologic technologists should be aware of the limitations of their professional practice (Box 24.5).

Identifying the Problem. How do radiologic technologists identify the boundaries of their professional practice? Does your compassion for Mr. Black supersede your duty to respect your boundary of professional practice?

Developing Alternative Solutions. Do you have a duty to respond to Mr. Black's questions? Should you follow your first impulse and simply reassure Mr. Black? Should you alert Dr. Roe to Mr. Black's concerns?

Selecting the Best Solution. Does Mr. Black share your value system? Do all your alternative solutions respect the values of the individuals associated with this case?

Defending Your Selection. Principle 5 of the ARRT Code of Ethics states that radiologic technologists should always act "in the best interest of the patient." Can your decision be justified by this principle?

Case 6: Balancing the Safety and Needs of the Patient With Physician Demands. The goal of the physician, indeed the entire health care team, is to care for the patient in an efficient and timely manner. Sometimes the demands of the physician may be in opposition to what the technologist believes is best for the patient (Box 24.6).

Identifying the Problem. To whom do you owe more of a duty, Dr. Williams or the patient? How can the needs of both the patient and Dr. Williams be adequately addressed?

Developing Alternative Solutions. Are there any other imaging procedures that can be performed using mobile equipment that can provide some information to Dr. Williams until help with transport is available? Are there personnel from other areas that could provide assistance?

Selecting the Best Solution. What is the best way to approach Dr. Williams with your concerns? Should others be involved in the conversation for additional advice and support?

Defending Your Selection. Does Principle 5 of the ARRT Code of Ethics apply in the case as well? Does the institution have policies in place to promote a "culture of safety" as discussed in Chapter 13?

Relationships With Other Health Professionals

Although your primary professional responsibilities are to the physicians with whom you work, the radiologic technologist also interacts with a wide range of other health professionals. These relationships often provide a source of satisfaction and support but can be marred by so-called "turf battles" or role conflicts and unrealistic practice expectations. Although most of us have grown up with a sense of loyalty and a corresponding aversion to reporting bad behavior in others, health care professionals have a special obligation to place the interests of their patients before such personal loyalty.

Case 7: Reporting Unethical Conduct of Others. Radiologic technologists have an ethical obligation to provide *high-quality patient care* and act *in the best interest of the patient.* Taken to its logical extension, this obligation includes the reporting of unethical conduct in other health professionals (Box 24.7).

Identifying the Problem. You have met the initial obligation to identify unprofessional conduct. Do you have an obligation to carry your complaint to Nurse Smith's superiors? What competing loyalties are involved in this case?

Developing Alternative Solutions. Once you have confronted Nurse Smith, can you let the matter rest? Should Miss White become involved as a witness or complainant? Should you tell Nurse Smith's supervisor? Someone in the hospital administration? Should you call the police?

Selecting the Best Solution. What solution would both best serve Nurse Smith and improve patient care on her ward? Can you choose between your ethical obligation to report unprofessional behavior and good patient care? What balance should exist between *doing no harm* to the patient and loyalty to your colleagues?

Defending Your Selection. Principle 9 of the ARRT Code of Ethics states that the radiologic technologist "respects confidences entrusted in the course of professional practice." Does this principle apply in this case? Do other personal values that you hold apply?

Dealing With Mistakes

All humans make mistakes, and health care professionals are no exception. Because of the life-and-death nature of medical practice, mistakes made by health care professionals can create considerable, though unintentional, harm to patients. A full response to the human dimensions of health care requires that all persons involved be prepared to act faithfully and honestly when a patient-care mistake has been made. Radiologic technologists will make mistakes because of the lack of attention to detail, preoccupation with other matters, or even a lack of professional commitment. A mistake can place significant emotional, financial, and psychological burdens on everyone involved in addition to the possible harm caused to the patient.

Case 8: Dealing With Mistakes. Including patients in the resolution of a practice error also presents an opportunity for them to practice the virtue of forgiveness. Nonetheless, developing safeguards in your practice that will prevent mistakes is far more desirable. Dealing with mistakes openly in such a way that the patient and others involved know all aspects, including your remorse and proposed outcome, tests the mettle of the most experienced radiologic technologist and will require virtuous action, as the case in Box 24.8 demonstrates.

Identifying the Problem. A potentially serious error has been made, but by the time it is discovered, it seems clear that no real harm has been done to either patient. The real benefit and harm in this case, however, may not be with the patients involved; rather, others may gain or lose, including the radiologic technologist who made the mistake and even the department head who authorized the management shift. More important, future patients may receive greater benefits if a more rigorous set of controls is instituted.

Developing Alternative Solutions. Agreeing to the suggested silence would be the easiest alternative to follow. Another approach might be to ask the department head to expand the meeting to include the two patients, their physicians, and the radiologists and to discuss the situation fully. Finally, you might request that an *incident report* be completed and filed with the medical center administration.

Selecting the Best Solution. Following the advice of the department head seems to ignore certain rights of the patients while at the same time shielding both the radiologic technologist and the department head from possible censure. Informing the medical center administration through an incident report may prompt beneficial management changes. The inclusion of the patients' physicians in the full discussion of the regrettable incident allows for the participation of both the concerned physicians and the radiologic technologists in the resolution of the incident.

Defending Your Solution. As mentioned in an earlier case, Principle 5 of the ARRT Code of Ethics pledges the radiologic technologist to act "in the best interests of the patient." Cases dealing with mistakes often require the balancing of patient interests with the interests of others involved. Patients' interests in this case include not only physical well-being, but also certain rights that need to be addressed.

SUMMARY

- The profession of radiologic technology shares the ethical concerns of other health professions toward promoting good patient care. Radiologic technologists have emerged as health care professionals in their own right, as witnessed by their educational programs, licensure requirements, professional associations, journals, and a unique code of ethics that reflects their professional function in the health care arena.
- Beyond subscribing to the principles contained in a professional code of ethics, however, radiologic technologists need to reflect on a broader base of moral principles in their ethical decision making.
- Moreover, ethical radiologic technologists must possess a keen sense of the role that human values can play in resolving

ethical dilemmas that arise in their professional practice, both in their dealings with patients and in their interactions with physicians and other health professionals. By practicing the ethical problem-solving technique of identifying the problem, developing alternative solutions, selecting the best solution, and defending that solution, radiologic technologists not only can improve their professional stature but also can enhance the health outcomes of the patients in their care.

BIBLIOGRAPHY

American Registry of Radiologic Technologists: *Standards of ethics*, St. Paul, Minn, 2017, The Registry, p 1.

American Society of Radiologic Technologists: *Code of ethics*, Albuquerque, NM, 2017, The Society.

Ashcroft RE, Goddard PR: Ethical issues in teleradiology, *Br J Radiol* 73:578, 2000.

Dowd SB, Durick D: Elder abuse: the RT's role in diagnosis and prevention, *Radiol Technol* 68:23, 1997.

Doherty F, Purtilo R: *Ethical dimensions in the health professions*, ed 6, Philadelphia, 2015, Saunders.

Golden DG: Medical ethics courses for student technologists, *Radiol Technol* 62:452, 1991.

Haddad AM: Teaching ethical analysis in occupational therapy, *Am J Occup Ther* 42:300, 1988.

Lynn SD: Ethics and law for the radiologic technologist, *Radiol Technol* 70:257, 1999.

Maestri WF: *Basic ethics for the health care professional*, Lanham, Md, 1982, University Press of America.

Reed J: A review of ethics for the radiologic technologist, *Radiol Technol* 82:519, 2011.

Veatch RM, Flack HE: *Case studies in allied health ethics*, Upper Saddle River, NJ, 1997, Prentice-Hall.

Veatch RM: *Hippocratic, religious, and secular medical ethics: the points of conflict*, Washington, DC, 2012, Georgetown University Press.

Ventola CL: Social media and health care professionals: benefits, risks, and best practices, *J Clin Pharm Ther* 39, 2014.

Warner SL: Code of ethics: legal implications, *Radiol Technol* 52:485, 1981.

25

Health Records and Health Information Management

Linda C. Galocy, MS, RHIA, FAHIMA

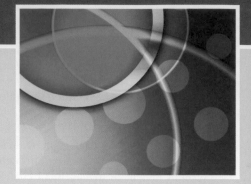

Health information is indeed a strategic resource crucial to the health of individual patients and the population, as well as to the success of the institution or enterprise.

Mervat Abdelhak Health Information: Management of a Strategic Resource, 2016

OBJECTIVES

On completion of this chapter, the student will be able to:

- Identify major health information management department functions.
- List the key components of a patient health record in acute care.
- List the key components of a patient health record in alternative health care settings, including ambulatory care and long-term care.
- Describe how health record documentation affects health care facilities and physician reimbursement.
- Describe the prospective payment system, including diagnosis-related groups, ambulatory payment classifications, and coding and classification systems.

- Identify coding as it relates to radiologic procedures and the reimbursement impact for health care facilities.
- Identify components of performance improvement and the relationship of performance improvement to all hospital departments.
- Differentiate between confidential and nonconfidential information.
- Explain the Health Insurance Portability and Accountability Act privacy and security requirements in a radiologic setting.
- Discuss the procedure for correcting or amending documentation errors in a patient health record.

OUTLINE

KEY TERMS

Ambulatory Patient Classifications (APCs) Classification system of patients based on the International Classification of Diseases, clinical modification codes for diagnoses, current procedural terminology evaluation and management codes, and procedure codes, age, sex, and visit disposition used for reimbursement

for health care provided in the hospital outpatient setting

Current Procedural Terminology, 4th Edition (CPT-4) Comprehensive listing of medical terms and codes for the uniform designation of diagnostic and therapeutic procedures; used in the United States for coding for physician reimbursement and

hospital outpatient and ambulatory surgical procedures

Diagnosis-Related Groups (DRGs) System that categorizes into payment groups patients who are medically related with respect to diagnosis and treatment and statistically similar with regard to length of stay

Electronic Health Record (EHR)/ Electronic Medical Record (EMR) Electronic health record system generally considered as the portal through which clinicians access a patient's health record, order treatments or therapy, and document care delivered to patients; allows providers to gather multiple types of data about a patient (clinical, financial, administrative, and research)

Healthcare Facilities Accreditation Program (HFAP) An accreditation program "authorized by the Centers for Medicare and Medicaid Services (CMS) to survey" all hospitals and many other types of health care settings (Healthcare Facilities Accreditation Program, 2017)

Health Information Management Practitioners Term used to encompass both registered health information administrators and registered health information technicians as individuals with either of these credentials who hold a variety of positions within the health information management profession

Health Insurance Portability and Accountability Act of 1996 (HIPAA) Federal legislation passed to improve the efficiency and effectiveness of the health care system; components that affect health information include privacy, security, and the establishment of standards and requirements for the electronic transmission of certain health information

Health Records Permanent or long-lasting documentation of all patient care information that applies to individual patients

International Classification of Diseases, 9th edition, Clinical Modification (ICD-9-CM) The classification system used in the United States to report morbidity and mortality information until September 30, 2015

International Classification of Diseases, 10th revision, Clinical Modification (ICD-10-CM) The classification system that replaced ICD-9-CM, Volumes 1 and 2 on October 1, 2015. This classification system is used for diagnosis coding in all health care settings in the United States

International Classification of Diseases, Procedure Coding System (ICD-10-PCS) A classification system used in the United States for reporting of inpatient hospital procedures. This classification system replaces the ICD-9-CM Volume 3 procedure codes on October 1, 2015

The Joint Commission Organization that accredits and certifies health care organizations and other programs in the United States (The Joint Commission, 2017)

Performance Improvement Process by which the quality of the care and services provided to patients within a health care facility is monitored and evaluated

Prospective Payment System (PPS) System for Medicare patients by which a predetermined level of reimbursement is established before services are provided

Registered Health Information Administrators (RHIAs) Professionals who possess the expertise to develop, implement, and/or manage individual, aggregate, and public health care data in support of patient safety and privacy, as well as the confidentiality and security of health information

Registered Health Information Technicians (RHITs) Professionals who are technical experts in health data collection, analysis, monitoring, maintenance, and reporting activities in accordance with established data-quality principles, legal and regulatory standards, and professional best practice guidelines

HEALTH INFORMATION MANAGEMENT AND TECHNOLOGY

Hospitals, ambulatory care facilities, physician practices, emergency and trauma centers, rehabilitation centers, long-term care facilities, home care programs, and all other health care settings maintain health records on all persons receiving health care services. Although these settings vary with regard to the type and range of medical and health-related services they provide, they all have a common need to concentrate, within a single record, all patient care information that applies to an individual patient. Such a concentration promotes effective communication among all health care professionals involved in the care of the patient, as well as provide for continuity of patient care.

Every health care institution needs a health information management department that has been organized and staffed to provide adequate health information management systems and practices. These systems facilitate the collection of health information, ensure complete documentation, maintain health data, and protect the content of the record against unauthorized disclosure.

The functions of the health information management department are service oriented and support the optimal standards set forth for quality of care and services in the health care institution. Although the functions of the health information management department and specific demands for its services vary according to the type of institution, the common function of these departments is the maintenance of health information systems in one or more forms to provide for the availability, accuracy, and protection of the clinical information that is needed to deliver health care services and to make appropriate health care–related decisions. Health records are more commonly electronic, but they can be scanned and stored as computerized images. Some records may still be found as hard copy or in miniaturized form (microfilm). The health information department's functions support the current and continuing care of patients; the institution's administrative processes; patient billing and accounting processes; medical education programs; health services research; utilization management, risk management, and quality management or performance improvement programs; privacy and security issues related to the *Health Insurance Portability and Accountability Act of 1996 (HIPAA)*; legal requirements; and extraneous patient services.

Because clinical decision making and financial reimbursement depend on the information contained in the health record, maintaining a complete and accurate record is essential. An error in recording the medications administered to a patient, for example, might lead to a life-threatening situation. An error in data reporting might mean a sizable financial loss for the health care institution.

Since the implementation by the federal government of the Prospective Payment System (PPS) and diagnosis-related groups (DRGs) in 1983, the importance of several health information management functions has grown significantly. The coding of inpatient and outpatient diagnoses and procedures is of highest priority. Coding involves converting diagnoses and procedures into a numeric classification system. The codes are reported to Medicare and other third-party payers, such as insurance companies. Coding must be complete and accurate so that claims can be processed within prescribed time frames. The record has to be designed so that the physician can easily provide complete patient information throughout the encounter or inpatient stay and provide a comprehensive recording of patient diagnoses and procedures at discharge.

The health record must also be complete and readily accessible to anyone who has a right to the information and the need to use it. The record is used for patient care, hospital statistics and research, and activities such as quality and performance improvement, and risk and utilization management. Health information management practitioners (i.e., registered health information technicians and registered health information administrators) must communicate needed data to departments such as radiology. Radiology department staff may also make requests from health information management departments for data used for administrative, research, and applied health informatics activities. Hospitals and other types of health care facilities need high-quality health care data for operations. Whether an electronic (or e-health) environment, or a more traditional paper system is used, robust and relevant clinical information supports decision makers and all persons involved in patient care. It should be noted that health records and radiology records are retained by a facility for a specific amount of time according to the Code of Federal Regulations, state law, and accreditation requirements. The length of time that a record must be retained in original or miniaturized form varies from state to state. Each state hospital association can provide information on the state's legal requirements for record retention. A very useful resource is the AHIMA Practice Brief "Retention and Destruction of Health Information" (Galocy, 2017). When determining a retention schedule it is important to involve the organization's legal counsel, as well as health information management personnel.

According to the *Mammography Quality Standards Act*, a facility must keep a mammogram in the permanent medical record of the patient for no less than 5 years or no less than 10 years if a patient has had no other mammograms at that facility, or longer if mandated by state law. A facility must also, on request, transfer the mammogram to another medical institution, to a physician, or to the patient directly.

PATIENT RECORD IN ACUTE CARE

Standards for the maintenance and the documentation within health records have been established by accrediting agencies such as The Joint Commission (TJC) and the Healthcare Facilities Accreditation Program (HFAP). One of the responsibilities of the health information management practitioner is to keep abreast of the standards for Information Management and Record of Care, Treatment, and Services from TJC and medical record documentation guidelines from HFAP, all published in the latest editions of the accreditation manuals for the appropriate organizations. These organizations are authorized by the Centers for Medicare and Medicaid Services (CMS) to survey health care facilities under Medicare. These accrediting agencies are also recognized by state governments, insurance carriers, and managed care organizations.

Health Record Content

Regardless of the method used to record health information, the content of each health record depends on which health care facility department is treating the patient and recording the information. All departments that take part in the care of a patient must document that care in the health record. Documenting in the patient's record, or *charting*, should be done by radiologists and radiographers when a patient receives either diagnostic or therapeutic radiologic services. Charting information about the procedure is appropriate, particularly about contrast media administration, along with the patient's condition during an examination. This charting is routinely done as a part of most special procedures, especially invasive procedures such as angiography and myelography. Any time a patient has an unusual reaction during a procedure, this information should be documented as well.

- Neither various accrediting agencies nor the American Hospital Association recommends any specific format or forms for use in health records. Health care organizations use forms and established electronic health record (EHR)/electronic medical record systems to best fit their needs; however, TJC, for example, has established standards for health record content. The health record, per TJC, must contain sufficient information to identify the patient, support the diagnoses, justify the treatment, document the course and results, and facilitate continuity of care. Briefly, standards for inpatient records require that the records include the following information:
- Patient identification data
- Medical history of the patient, provided by the patient, including chief complaint, history of present illness or injury, relevant family and social histories, and inventory by body system
- Report of relevant physical examination findings
- Diagnostic and therapeutic orders

- Clinical observations, including results of therapy
- Reports of diagnostic and therapeutic procedures and tests, as well as their results
- Evidence of appropriate informed consent (when consent is not obtainable, the reason should be entered in the record)
- Conclusions at termination of hospitalization or evaluation of treatment, including any pertinent instructions for follow-up care

Radiographers should be familiar with the health record format at their place of employment. Reviewing the chart or accessing the health information system is often necessary for radiographers to gather information, such as laboratory results, about their patients. A radiology department, in addition to using the hospital mainframe or electronic health information system for the master patient index or billing information, may have a departmental film-tracking system. A computerized system tracks film and folders with a bar code system. Film control is a key issue because lost or missing film can have a negative effect on patient care.

TJC standards require that the health record contain evidence of informed consent for procedures and treatment for which hospital policy requires informed consent. The policy on informed consent is typically developed by the medical staff and the hospital governing board, consistent with legal requirements for appropriate informed consent. The term *informed consent* implies that the patient has been informed of the procedure or operation to be performed, the risks involved, and the possible consequences. By signing the consent form, the patient or the patient's representative indicates that he or she has been informed of and consents to the procedure or treatment.

An authorization for treatment, signed at the time of admission or registration, is not to be confused with informed consent. If, for some reason, the informed consent is not filed with the record, the record must then indicate that informed consent was obtained for a given procedure or treatment and must indicate where the informed consent form is located.

Incident reports contain information relative to patient incidences or event occurrences. Incident reports must be completed after an event; however, the reports themselves should not be a part of the patient record. Rather, they are administrative documents and are typically maintained by hospital legal counsel or the risk management team. The event should be completely documented in the patient health record. This documentation should include information about the incident, patient reaction, notification of health personnel, patient progress, and so on. The incident report, on the other hand, would include information relative to perhaps actual equipment failure rather than what happened to the patient because of the equipment failure.

Health Record in Radiology

Before a radiologic procedure is performed, a radiology order for service is completed. This order includes the patient demographic information (name, health record number, other identifying information) along with the name of the specific procedure being requested. The physician ordering the procedure is also identified. Typically, these orders are sent to the radiology department by means of the computerized information system within the hospital. For documentation of medical necessity, a diagnosis or sign or symptom for which the test is being performed *must* be included on the order. Failure of the attending physician to report such a diagnosis, or sign or symptom, will result in a delay in performing the procedure. Hospital and billing requirements under medical necessity require that the medical necessity be justified before a procedure is performed. This requirement applies to inpatient and outpatient procedures. If Medicare does not cover the procedure, then the patient must be notified and is required to sign an advance beneficiary notice. The patient then assumes responsibility for payment when Medicare denies the claim.

The results of the procedure are documented on a radiology report (diagnostic and therapeutic). These reports must be included in the patient record to describe the radiologic services the patient received. A physician, usually a radiologist, writes or dictates and authenticates a description of what is seen on the radiograph and the implications for the patient (Fig. 25.1). A written report must be completed for every service for which a medical claim will be filed. The name of the study must be on the report. With therapeutic radiology, required documentation includes the amount of the dose of the x-ray or radioactive material administered, as well as the date and time. Again, authentication is required on the report before it becomes a part of the patient's permanent record.

Any special reports documenting evaluation or treatment of a patient must be made a part of the patient's permanent record. The radiology department usually maintains a copy of the information submitted to the patient record with the hard copy images; however, the original document should be placed in the patient's permanent health record. Radiology reports are almost always transcribed, and the radiologist electronically signs or otherwise authenticates the report before permanent placement in the record. Increasingly, radiology departments are implementing speech recognition technology. This is a process whereby a radiologist dictates the report and as he or she is speaking the speech is converted automatically to text. Either the radiologist can make corrections to the text immediately or a transcriptionist will listen to the dictation and edit the text for later review and authentication by the radiologist. In either case, the original document is placed into the patient's permanent health record.

Requirements of Health Record Entries

Federal requirements and accrediting bodies, such as TJC, require that the medical staff of an institution have bylaws, rules, and regulations that include a provision for accurate and complete medical records, with the original copies of documents in the patient record. Medical records must incorporate all significant clinical information regarding a patient. The record is the means of communication between the attending physician and all others rendering patient care.

Various regulations and standards exist throughout federal, state, and accrediting bodies that address signatures in the patient record. TJC, for example, requires that all health record entries be dated and authenticated and their authors identified.

University Radiological Group, Inc.
1234 Main Street
Los Angeles, CA 90012-0000

NAME: Jane Doe DOB: 03/17/50 RM/BD: 513301 EDP# 75033 ORD# 00034
REFERRING PHYSICIAN: John Smith, M.D. PERFORMED BY CMK
DATE: 04/16/XXXX TIME: 1735
MJ DATE: 04/17/XXXX TIME: 1012
RADIOLOGIST: James Jones, M.D.
DATE AND TIME OF FINAL REPORT: 04/18/XX 1036
X-RAY# 000097959

EXAMINATION: CHEST PA & LATERAL

The heart size and contour are normal. There is streaky infiltration in the left infraclavicular region extending back down toward the left hilar area. There is somewhat similar interstitial infiltration in the projection of the 2nd right anterior interspace. There are several smooth, rounded areas of radiolucency within the infiltrate.

There are also interstitial infiltrations in the right, mid, and left paracardiac regions.

The costophrenic angles are clear.

Impression: BILATERAL UPPER LOBE INFILTRATIONS WITH PROBABLE CAVITY FORMATION WITH BRONCHOGENIC SPREAD TO THE RIGHT, MID, AND LEFT LOWER LUNG FIELDS.

THE FINDINGS ARE MOST LIKELY ON THE BASIS OF TUBERCULOSIS, BUT THE EXACT ETIOLOGY AND ACTIVITY MUST BE ESTABLISHED CLINICALLY.

_____
James Jones, M.D.

JJ/alb
D: 4/18/XX
T: 4/18/XX

Fig. 25.1 Sample radiology report for a chest procedure.

The use of an electronic signature is of significance to radiology departments because most radiologists choose this method of authenticating radiology reports. All entries made in a patient health record should be in ink when information is written. Pencil documentation is not legal in any state. In the electronic patient record, this is not an issue, but it is important should the EHR not be available for any reason. Regulations also address other health record documentation issues such as abbreviations used in the record, a list of do-not-use abbreviations, timeliness of documentation, record legibility, and correction of errors or omissions. Basically, an abbreviation in the record can be used only if it has been approved by the medical staff and if an abbreviation list is on file that explains the abbreviations. In 2004 TJC created a do-not-use abbreviation list. This list includes commonly misinterpreted or confusing abbreviations. TJC reviews and updates this list annually, and it applies to all orders and medication-related documentation in handwritten format. Providers are encouraged to work to eliminate the do-not-use abbreviations from all EHR systems, but, as of 2017, the requirement is only enforced for handwritten records. Federal requirements mandate that current and discharged patient records be completed promptly. Record reports such as x-ray examination findings should be documented and completed as soon as possible after the procedure takes place.

In a paper record, the person who makes an error in documentation is responsible for correcting the error. The individual should draw a single line through the erroneous documentation, write an explanatory note such as "ERROR" near it, and then document the correct information. The note should be dated and signed. Facilities with an EHR will have specific procedures for the correction or amendment of erroneous documentation. Communication with the health information management department will be necessary to understand the process that a health care facility must follow.

A long-standing basic principle of health record documentation is the adage *not documented, not done*. This tenet applies to all health care practitioners who make entries in the patient health record. If the record is submitted in court in any type of legal case, the statement holds true. In the absence of the requisite documentation in the health record of what was done to the patient, the assumption is that the event did not take place.

HEALTH RECORD AND RADIOLOGY IMPLICATIONS IN ANCILLARY HEALTH SYSTEMS

Radiology reports generated by a patient's encounter with health services need to be maintained in the patient's record, whether that is a hospital-based ambulatory care record, or a record used in a freestanding facility. Examples of other health care areas in which radiology reports are often generated include emergency department encounters, ambulatory surgery centers, ambulatory care facilities, physician offices, and urgent care centers. Ambulatory care records have requirements similar to those for inpatient care records. Federal and state regulations need to be followed, as well as those of any other accrediting body such as HFAP or TJC. TJC, for example, specifies that ambulatory records include items such as patient identification; relevant history of the illness or injury; physical findings; diagnostic and therapeutic orders; clinical observations; reports of tests, procedures, and results; diagnostic impression; patient disposition and pertinent follow-up instructions; immunization records; allergy history; growth charts for pediatric patients; and information regarding referral to and from any other health care facilities.

A long-term care health record is similar to an inpatient record. The long-term care facility can be subject to state, federal, and accreditation agency regulations. In a long-term care facility, radiology services may be provided through a contract with an outside provider. The record must contain a physician order for the service and the reason for the service. The actual radiology report should be dated, authenticated, and placed in the patient record. The attending physician is notified of the findings of the diagnostic service.

HEALTH RECORDS IN REIMBURSEMENT

Prospective Payment System

Health record data serve as the basis for hospital reimbursement in the PPS using the DRG system in the inpatient setting and ambulatory patient classifications (APCs) in the outpatient setting. The concept of the DRG is that patients fall into statistically similar, diagnostically related groups. Therefore the hospital receives payments based on the group into which the patient fits. The health information professional uses the diagnosis terminology provided by the physician and codes this information into the classification system of the *International Classification of Diseases*, 10th revision, Clinical Modification (ICD-10-CM). The use of the International Classification of Diseases, Procedure Classification System (ICD-10-PCS) is used for procedural classification of inpatient procedures. Using a computer program called a *grouper*, the health information practitioner computes the patient's DRG. For Medicare and for some other payers, the hospital hopes to receive this DRG amount as payment for its services. The alpha numeric ICD-10-CM and ICD-10-PCS codes are the basis for the DRG to which the inpatient is classified. Before October 1, 2015, the United States has been using the International Classification of Diseases, 9th edition, Clinical Modification (ICD-9-CM) volumes 1 and 2 for the diagnosis classification of diseases and volume 3 for the procedural classification.

Current Procedural Terminology, 4th Edition (CPT-4) codes are used to code procedures for outpatient encounters and coding for ancillary services such as radiology and laboratory. Using a computer program called a grouper, the health information practitioner computes the patient's APC. This payment system can result in one, or a number of APC's for which the facility hopes to receive reimbursement.

The coding and classification functions of the health information services department have become complex, and significantly more important since the implementation of PPS-based DRGs and APCs. The DRG classification is based on an inpatient classification scheme that categorizes patients who are medically related with respect to diagnosis and treatment and who are statistically similar in their lengths of stay. The health information management professional must be knowledgeable in the various case-mix classification systems used to measure the categories of patients and the types of patients treated by a health care institution.

A criticism of DRGs has been that the system does not take into account the severity of a patient's disease. Existing and available severity of illness methodologies go beyond DRGs to classify the extent of a patient's illness. Clinical differences in patients with the same diagnosis can account for varying levels of care rendered and varying amounts of resources used. As of October 1, 2007, CMS implemented the Medicare Severity DRG system, which takes into account the level of severity of a patient's condition and the amount of resources used to care for him or her.

The management personnel in a radiology department must understand communication through the diagnostic codes of ICD-10-CM and procedural codes of CPT-4. The correct billing process in a major revenue-producing department of a hospital, such as radiology, is critical to a hospital's financial solvency. Payers carefully review radiology services for medical necessity. The diagnosis code provided by the ordering physician is critical to the payment and is the reason to either justify or deny reimbursement. Technologists generally obtain a patient history before an examination. This information cannot be used for coding purposes, but can be very helpful in determining the severity of illness and communicating with the ordering physician when necessary to obtain appropriate reimbursement. Hospitals may use a computer program called a *chargemaster* to report radiologic procedures. When a radiologic procedure is ordered and performed, the computer automatically assigns the CPT-4 code and applies the charge. Chargemaster codes must be correct to reflect the code and payment for all radiology procedures accurately. Radiology must work with both health information management and billing departments for chargemaster updating and maintenance.

APCs constitute an ambulatory case-mix system used for prospective payment in ambulatory care. The system is a patient-classification scheme that explains the amounts and types of resources used in an ambulatory visit. Patients in each APC have similar clinical characteristics, resource use, and costs. ICD-10-CM diagnosis codes and CPT procedure codes drive the procedural and ancillary APCs. Radiologic procedures are all coded via CPT and affect the APC assigned for each patient. Again, accuracy in the documentation of the procedure performed leads to accuracy in the CPT procedure coded, and appropriate reimbursement for the outpatient facility.

Coding Function

The ICD-10-CM and PCS classification systems are used for inpatient reporting effective October 1, 2015. Prior to this date the ICD-9-CM classification system was in use. For outpatients, hospitals must report the diagnosis using the ICD-10-CM codes and CPT-4 codes for the procedures. The physician's office uses the ICD codes for the diagnosis and the CPT coding system for the procedures.

Radiology codes in CPT include diagnostic and therapeutic radiology, nuclear medicine, diagnostic ultrasonography, and radiation oncology. The code numbers range from 70010 to 79999. For example, a chest radiograph, single view, frontal, would be coded as 71010. A magnetic resonance image of the cervical spine with contrast material is coded to 72142.

The health information management department would use an ICD-10-CM code to report a diagnosis for billing and information management purposes. In this system, the code assigned would be C40.20. This code indicates a malignant neoplasm of the long bones of the lower limb.

Radiology departments may use the Index of Radiologic Diagnoses (IRD) of the American College of Radiology to "classify teaching cases according to the underlying anatomy and pathology." This information can be used for statistics, for follow-up, or for evaluation of patient care. TJC requires that information about important aspects of diagnostic radiology or therapy services be collected.

The IRD is a database that contains four data tables: Anatomical, Sub-anatomical, Pathological, and Sub-pathological. Pathologic findings as well as imaging techniques can be indexed in the Pathological and Sub-pathological tables. There is a 4-digit coding scheme for the anatomy table and a 5-digit scheme for pathology and imaging techniques.

PERFORMANCE IMPROVEMENT

Performance improvement is a process by which the quality of the care and services provided to patients within a health care facility are monitored and evaluated. The terms *quality assurance*, *quality assessment*, and *performance improvement* are all used to encompass activities related to performance improvement, including utilization and risk management, infection control, surgical case review, medication usage evaluation, health record review, blood usage review, pharmacy and therapeutic review, and case management. Performance improvement activities include work performed by various committees and the medical staff, as well as other professional staff from various ancillary departments. A separate performance improvement or quality management department exists in many hospitals. In other types of facilities, a unit or section within the health information management department is responsible for performance improvement.

TJC standards discussed here are specific to acute care, but similar standards exist in other accrediting bodies, as well as for other types of health care organizations. TJC's standards require that hospitals have a planned, systematic, and hospital-wide approach for monitoring, evaluating, and improving the quality of care, and of key governance, managerial, and support activities. TJC's current standards, for example, require a written performance improvement plan as a separate document, or it can be incorporated into other planning documents within an organization. Many items commonly included within a performance improvement plan are the following:

- Statement of mission or vision
- Objectives
- Values
- Leadership
- Organizational structure
- Methodologies
- Performance measures
- Communication
- Annual plan review

Data are collected in areas such as operative; other invasive and noninvasive procedures that put the patient at risk; significant discrepancies in operative documentation; processes related to medication and use of blood; adverse events; resuscitation efforts; behavioral management; the needs, expectations, and satisfaction of patients; and the staff's views regarding performance and improvement opportunities.

TJC's standards also encourage the use of multiple data sources to identify problems, and discourage the use of performance management studies for the sole purpose of documenting high-quality care. Examples of performance improvement activities in radiology departments can include adverse events, medication errors, adverse drug reactions, patient perception of the safety and quality of care, treatment, or services, patient thermal injuries that occur during MRI exams, and any other priority identified by the leadership (The Joint Commission, 2017).

TJC's 10-step process was created to help organizations make the transition from quality assurance to continuous quality improvement. Facilities that use the 10-step process are required to do the following:

1. Assign responsibility for the department's or service's monitoring and evaluation activities
2. Delineate the scope of care or service that the department provides
3. Identify the most important aspects of that care or service
4. Identify indicators of quality and appropriate nature for the recognized important aspects of care
5. Establish thresholds (levels, patterns, trends) for evaluation (maximum allowable error rates)
6. Collect and organize relevant data, compare the data with preestablished criteria, and analyze the findings
7. Evaluate care (compare actual rate to thresholds)
8. Take action to improve care and services
9. Assess the effectiveness of the actions and maintain the gain
10. Communicate results to affected individuals and groups

Dimensions of Performance

TJC requires the medical and professional staff to participate in review functions. Many approaches should be used to analyze and evaluate performance. TJC has defined various dimensions of performance that need to be addressed in performance improvement activities in health care organizations. These dimensions include the following:

Efficacy: Have our activities achieved desired outcomes?

Appropriateness: Is the activity relevant to our clinical needs?

Availability: Is intervention available and accessible?

Timeliness: Is activity done at the most beneficial time?

Effectiveness: Do care and resources achieve the desired outcome?

Continuity: How are activities or interventions coordinated among providers and over time?

Safety: What is the degree to which associated risks are minimized?

Efficiency: How do we maximize the relationship between outcomes and resources?

Respect and caring: What are the degree of patient involvement in care decisions and the degree of sensitivity shown for individual needs?

Operation of a Performance Improvement Program

Each department or service is responsible for documenting the effectiveness of its performance improvement activities and for reporting such activities to the organization-wide program. In turn, the staff members who perform the performance improvement coordinating function should be responsible for demonstrating that the overall hospital program is functional and effective. The data must be consolidated and reported to the medical staff and the organization's governing body. Such a report might include a description of a process identified for improvement, the method used to identify that process, the department or service involved, the person assigned to perform the study, the data sources used, the cause of any identified

variation, any corrective action taken, the person who implemented the action, the timetable for implementation, whether the process was improved, plans for a monitoring procedure, and plans for restudy. The persons involved must remember that quality management activities are confidential matters, and special procedures should be followed to avoid or minimize possible incrimination of the parties involved. TJC uses the evaluation, or clinical outcomes, as part of the accreditation process. The hospital must work to systematically improve its performance and must take action if it has identified a person with performance problems who is unable or unwilling to improve. This action may mean a modification in a staff member's clinical privileges.

LEGAL ASPECTS OF HEALTH RECORDS

The patient record is an important legal document that the health care institution uses to define what was or was not done to the patient. The record may be submitted as evidence in court cases and used in any litigation in which the institution is involved. Principles of both common law and statutory law have an impact on the legal aspects of medical records. Federal regulations affect an institution's participation in Medicare and Medicaid programs. Radiographers may be required to give depositions or testimony regarding information in the health record or, in the case of a radiograph, testimony regarding the procedures involved.

Correcting or Amending the Health Record

The proper method for correcting an error that an author makes, as mentioned earlier, is for the author to draw a single line through the error, write "ERROR," and then record the correct information. The individual then should date and authenticate the entry. Patients have the right to review and request an amendment to their health record. Original entries cannot be altered; therefore the patient must request an amendment in writing to the facility. This request should include a reason for the amendment. The physician has the right to review the request and respond back to the patient in writing. All documentation is made part of the patient's legal health record. Facilities will have procedures in place for when patients request amendment of their health records.

Correcting or amending an entry in the EHR is a bit more complicated. There are several factors to consider, such as the functionality of the electronic system in use, whether the entry has been signed and is considered complete, and the policies of the facility. It is important for the person responsible for entering information into the EHR to understand the steps required when needing to correct or amend an entry, and the procedure will most likely vary from facility to facility.

Confidentiality of Health Records

Radiographers and students bear the same responsibility as all other hospital personnel to safeguard the confidentiality of health record information. Computerized information systems are a significant part of these records. Employers require that all employees or students who have access to the medical record sign a confidentiality statement. Technologists may be asked to release information to patients concerning results of procedures. Informing patients of examination results is the physician's responsibility, and the technologist should refer the patient to his or her physician.

The Health Insurance Portability and Accountability Act

The HIPAA regulations ensure the health care industry is focused on the need to protect health information from inappropriate access or use. The federal regulations generated by HIPAA support the need for timely access to health information, and the EHR remains secure and patient information remains private. The health care facility makes health care information available in an automated form that benefits the facility without sacrificing the privacy of the patient. HIPAA regulations require that health care facilities design and maintain systems to protect the security and privacy of electronically transmitted data. The systems must prevent unauthorized individuals from accessing, creating, or modifying information while at the same time allowing authorized users to have access.

Privileged Communication

States can enact statutes specifically recognizing physician–patient privilege. If this legislation exists, a physician cannot testify in court or in any legal proceeding without the consent of the patient. A patient can waive this privilege through specific actions, such as bringing the subject of the medical condition into evidence.

Consent to Release Information

It is very important that a radiology department or facility abide by HIPAA privacy rules. When a patient desires to have his or her health information released to him or her or another entity, it is important to follow facility policy very carefully. The patient, or legal representative, must sign a release of information form for consenting to release information. The consent must contain items such as to whom the information is to be released; the patient's name, address, and birth date; the extent of the information to be released; the reason for the release; the date; and the signature of the patient or legal representative. It is important that a department or facility work with a health information professional or risk manager to ensure that a release of information consent form and policy are consistent with HIPAA requirements.

Facsimile Transmission of Health Information

The use of a facsimile (fax) machine is commonplace in health care communications. The instant transmission of data enhances patient care, but also presents confidentiality issues. Every health care organization must have a policy in place, to which all employees must adhere, when faxing health information with patient-identifiable information included.

If the policy is not available to the radiology department, one should query the health information management department for the policy.

Information Security

The confidential nature of electronic or paper health records is paramount in this information-driven age. Hospitals and other institutions must protect patient information in the health information system. All health care organizations have security policies in place to ensure staff is able to access the minimum necessary patient information to perform their job duties. Mechanisms, such as access to physical locations by way of keypads or door locks, must be in place to ensure the safety and confidentiality of patient records. There are policies in place for password management and the prohibited use of sharing those passwords. Audit mechanisms are in place to ensure all policies are being followed and are still effective.

There are many facets to information security, and it is important for employees and students to be fully aware of all organizational policies related to security, and ramifications for violation of any policy.

Patient Access to the Health Record

HIPAA regulations mandate the confidentiality of health information. A patient or patient representative should have access to, the right to request a copy of, and the right to request an amendment or correction of information to the health care record; however, requests for the information within the health record should be restricted only to the specific information required to carry out the legitimate purpose of the request. HIPAA contains penalties for wrongful disclosure of individually identifiable health information.

Because of federal laws, patients have a right to access their medical records. Health care facilities have the right to charge a copy fee to the patient for this record. The facility also has the right to require a properly completed and signed patient authorization. A facility does have the right to prohibit patient access when the provider reasonably believes that having access is not in the best interest of the patient's health, or if the knowledge of the health care information might cause danger to the life or safety of any person. Patients sometimes ask radiographers whether they can examine their records while in transit, waiting for a procedure, or undergoing an examination. The record information should not be shared with the patient in this fashion because misinterpretation of information can occur. Again, the technologist should refer the patient to the physician for discussion of record documentation.

Health Record in Court

The health record is a legal document that is admissible as evidence in court. A health information manager may be required to honor a subpoena for the record and take the record to court. The original record is never left in court; rather, a photocopy is used. The original record is then retained in the hospital health information management department. A more common approach is that a copy of the record is sent by certified mail.

SUMMARY

- The health information management department is a key hospital department that affects many other departments. Health information management departments do not render patient care but are identified as a support service department. Because of the coding function, health information management departments directly affect hospital revenue and therefore facility operations. The health record is the document that communicates information pertaining to patient care. The record is a valuable tool in preparing health service statistics; substantiating patient care services and treatment provided; supporting medical education, health services, and clinical research; maintaining quality assessment and risk management; and making financial planning decisions. Health information management professionals manage health data and information resources. The health information management professionals ensure the availability of health information for health care delivery, and information for critical decisions across various organizations, settings, and disciplines. The profession serves the health care system, including patient care organizations, payers, research and policy agencies, and other health care–related industries.
- The health record is the legal document that attests to the care that was rendered to the patient. The record is a recapitulation of all patient care events. The radiology department contributes to this complete record by thorough documentation of all care provided.

BIBLIOGRAPHY

Abdelhak M, Hankin MA: *Health information: management of a strategic resource*, ed 5, Philadelphia, 2016, Saunders.

A web-based ACR index for radiological diagnoses: *Am J Roentgenol*, 2017. http://www.ajronline.org/doi/full/10.2214/ajr.183.5.1831517#abstract. Accessed November 7.

LaTour K, Eichenwald-Maki S: *Health information management: concepts, principles, and practice*, ed 4, Chicago, 2013, American Health Information Management Association.

Shaw P, Elliot C, Isaacson P, et al.: *Quality and performance improvement in healthcare*, ed 5, Chicago, 2012, American Health Information Management Association.

Skurka M: *Health information management: principles and organization for health information services*, Chicago, 2017, Jossey-Bass.

Galocy L: The Health Record: electronic and paper. In Skurka MA, editor: *Health information management principles and organization for health information services (p. 71)*, San Francisco, 2017, Jossey-Bass.

Healthcare Facilities Accreditation Program: *Frequently asked questions*, 2017. Retrieved from HFAP https://www.hfap.org/about/faq.aspx.

The Joint Commission: *About The Joint Commission*, 2017. Retrieved from The Joint Commission https://www.jointcommission.org/about_us/about_the_joint_commission_main.aspx.

The Joint Commission: *Accreditation requirements, performance Improvement*, Oak Brook, IL, 2017, US.

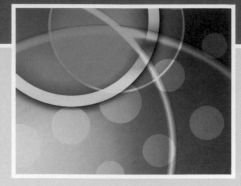

26

Medical Law

Ann M. Obergfell, JD, RT(R)

The liability of the technologist is not the same as the radiologist involved, but the liability is potentially real.

Albert Bundy, MD, JD, 1988

OBJECTIVES

On completion of this chapter, the student will be able to:
- Differentiate among the various types of law.
- Outline how the standard of care is established for radiologic technologists.
- Discuss the concept of tortious conduct and causes of action that may arise from the behavior of a health care practitioner.
- Argue the importance of privacy of records and the relationship between privacy of records and patient confidentiality issues.

- Explain negligence and the four elements necessary to meet the burden of proof in a medical negligence claim.
- Explain the legal theory of res ipsa loquitur and how an attorney may use it in a claim of medical negligence.
- Illustrate how a hospital may be liable under the doctrine of respondeat superior.
- Justify the need for informed consent.
- Outline the information a patient must have before an informed consent may be given.

OUTLINE

KEY TERMS

Assault Any willful attempt or threat to inflict injury on the person of another, when coupled with the apparent present ability to do so, and any intentional display of force such as would give the victim reason to fear or expect immediate bodily harm

Battery Any unlawful touching of another that is without justification or excuse

Contract An agreement between two or more persons or parties which creates an obligation to do or not to do a particular thing.

Defamation Holding up a person to ridicule, scorn, or contempt in a respectable and considerable part of the community

False Imprisonment Conscious restraint of the freedom of a person without proper authorization, privilege, or consent

Fraud Intentional perversion of truth for the purpose of inducing a person to rely on the false information to his or her detriment

Implied Consent Person's agreement to allow something to happen which

is not expressly given but rather inferred from a person's actions or inactions

Informed Consent Person's agreement to allow something to happen (such as surgery) that is based on a full disclosure of the facts needed to make the decision intelligently—that is, knowledge of risks involved, alternatives, benefits, and other information needed by a reasonable person to make a decision

Negligence Failure to do something that a reasonable person guided by the ordinary considerations that ordinarily regulate human affairs would do or the doing of something a reasonable and prudent person would not do

Res Ipsa Loquitur Meaning the thing speaks for itself; legal theory requiring three elements(1) that the type of injury did not occur except for negligence, (2) that the activity

was under the complete control of the defendant, and (3) that the plaintiff did not contribute to his or her own injury in any way

Respondeat Superior Meaning let the superior respond or the master speaks for the servant; the physician, supervisor, or employer may be liable in certain cases for the wrongful acts of employees or subordinates

Standard of Care Degree of skill (proficiency), knowledge, and care ordinarily possessed and employed by members in good standing within the profession

Tort Private or civil wrong or injury, other than breach of contract, for which the court provides a remedy in the form of an action for damages

LAW

Today's litigious society requires that all health care professionals, including radiologic technologists, be aware of the areas of the law that may affect the delivery of health care services. A basic principle of the law was defined in *Schloendorf v. Society of New York Hospital* in 1914 and lays a foundation for the relationship between patients and health care practitioners:

Every human being of adult years and sound mind has a right to determine what shall be done with his or her own body, and a surgeon who performs an operation without his or her patient's consent commits an assault, for which he or she is liable in damages.

This doctrine serves six functions. It (1) protects individual autonomy, (2) protects the patient's status as a human being, (3) avoids fraud and duress, (4) encourages health care practitioners to consider their decisions carefully, (5) fosters rational decision making by the patient, and (6) involves the public in medicine. Despite this carefully formed doctrine and its well-articulated functions, many members of the health care team take a paternalistic role in their practice and forget the patient's right to be informed of and to make decisions about his or her own health care diagnosis and treatment. The violation of this fundamental right, as articulated in the American Hospital Association's Patient Care Partnership (Appendix F), is improper not only from a moral and ethical standpoint but also may be construed as improper from a legal perspective. Although health care practitioners clearly need to inspire confidence in their patients, they must remember the fundamental principle of patient autonomy underlying the delivery of health care in the United States.

Medicine and the law are sometimes in conflict because each looks at a situation from a different perspective. One entity is looking to see that the patient's physical needs are being met through diagnosis and treatment, whereas the other attempts to control the abuse of patients, make sure that the patient's care is being met according to recognized standards of practice, and ensure patients are compensated for injuries received at the hands of negligent health care practitioners. Both processes are necessary to ensure that the patient receives the best possible care. To gain a better understanding of the relationship between law and the delivery of health care, looking at the law and how it may be applied to everyday situations in radiology is helpful.

TYPES OF LAW

The law is multifaceted and draws its principles from several foundations. The first and probably most important foundation is the *Constitution of the United States*. This document, considered as the supreme law of the land, was written to separate powers of the three branches of government: the Executive (the Presidency), the Legislative (Congress), and the Judiciary (a system of Courts). The separation of powers offers a system of checks and balances that prohibits any one branch from becoming more powerful than another. The Constitution also protects the individual rights of citizens of the United States. Much like the federal government, each state has a constitution that defines its government and articulates the rights of its citizens.

The second form of law is that enacted by legislative bodies or administrative agencies. This system of statutes and regulations is written at local, state, and federal levels and runs the gamut from who will drive cars to how citizens will be taxed. Many areas of health care are defined and regulated by these statutes and regulations. For instance, state legislators adopt a statute that defines radiation machine operators and may, through the statute, delegate power to an administrative agency, such as a board of health or environmental and radiation safety office, to establish regulations and guidelines that define the practice. Examples of such definitions may include restrictions on who may operate medical imaging equipment, how radionuclides are to be transported and handled, and how ionizing radiation equipment is registered and inspected. These statutes and regulations may change from time to time at the discretion of the legislature or agency as needs, scope of practice, and knowledge regarding the profession changes. Legislators and administrators may also be persuaded to make changes if the profession or others find that the statutes or regulations need to be modified to meet the changing needs of professional practice or the constituencies being served.

A third area of the law is case law, which is derived from the Common Law of England. This type of law is decided on a case-by-case basis by either a judge or a jury. The decisions in these cases determine an outcome for the parties and may be precedent setting for future cases with similar fact patterns.

Whereas the Constitution defines individual rights and statutes and regulations define the practice, case law will determine if there is liability for the health care practitioner who has been sued for medical negligence, malpractice or other cause of action.

An additional area of law which will not be covered in depth but plays an important role on all health care relationships is contract law. A contract is a legally enforceable agreement between parties creating mutual obligations. An example might be when a health care facility contracts with a radiologist's practice group to interpret images or with a manufacturer to purchase a piece of equipment. In contract law, the parties must mutually agree to the terms based on a valid offer and acceptance of the offer. There must be adequate consideration and the parties must be legally able to enter into a contract.

CAUSES OF ACTION

Newspaper headlines proclaim huge monetary awards given to an individual as a result of medical negligence. These headlines are followed by stories of horrendous injuries patients received at the hands of negligent physicians, nurses, or other health care professionals. These cases are quite disturbing, but they are generally found to be the exception instead of the rule. Even if these cases are the exception, the general public will clearly not tolerate actions by health care practitioners that are less than the generally accepted standard of care. An estimated 10% of all medical negligence claims are somehow related to diagnostic imaging, either by improper diagnosis or by injuries to patients sustained during diagnostic procedures. Therefore any radiographer may be called to testify at some time, either as a defendant or as a witness to the practice of another.

TORTS

A patient's claim that he or she has been wronged or has sustained some injury, other than a breach of contract, and for which cause may exist for an action to receive compensation for damages is known as a tort. This type of claim arises from a violation of a duty imposed by general law on all persons involved in a transaction or situation. For a patient to have a claim, some breach of duty must have occurred on the part of the health care practitioner. When the patient or their representative makes the decision to bring a cause of action they become a plaintiff in the litigation. Those entities, either persons or organizations, who the plaintiff believes has caused the injury become defendants.

In a case against a radiologic technologist, the patient contacts an attorney with the belief that an injury has occurred during a procedure or while the patient was present in the radiology department. The patient may also look for legal guidance if the care received has been less than optimal or threatening in any way. Although these legal inquiries may not lead to lawsuits, many of the complaints are based on legitimate concerns about negligent care or claims of assault, battery, false imprisonment, defamation, or fraud.

Assault

An assault claim may arise when a patient believes he or she has been threatened in such a way that reason to fear or to expect immediate bodily harm exists. This fear may arise from comments made by a technologist to the patient before or during the examination. For example, threatening to repeat a painful examination if the patient does not hold still may be construed as an assault. This type of threat may appear to be harmless on the part of the technologist; however, if the patient truly believes that he or she is threatened, the claim may be valid. Another example may be raising a fist in an angry or menacing way.

Battery

In a similar context, if a technologist performs an examination or touches a patient without that patient's permission, battery may occur even if no injury arises from such contact. Any unlawful touching may constitute battery if the patient thinks that the technologist has touched him or her in an offensive way. Such a touch may occur if a procedure is performed on the wrong patient or if a patient is moved roughly about the radiographic table while being positioned for an examination.

False Imprisonment

The common claim of false imprisonment arises when a person is restrained or believes he or she is being restrained against his or her will. The individual must be aware of the confinement and have no reasonable means of escape. This phenomenon is most prevalent with people who are unable to cooperate, such as inebriated, senile, or pediatric patients. Each of these types of patients poses an interesting and often confusing set of problems that must be handled without compromising the quality of medical care.

Inebriated patients pose a problem in that they are unable to consent to treatment and may oppose restraint. The general practice in such cases is to speak with the physician who has ordered the examination to determine whether the requested procedure is of the utmost importance and must be completed immediately or whether the examination may be delayed until the patient is coherent enough to make informed decisions. If the examination must be done immediately or if the patient is in such a condition that he or she may bring harm to self, the technologist, or others, appropriate immobilization devices or restraints may be applied.

In the case of senile, pediatric, or other incompetent patients, obtaining consent to restrain or immobilize from someone authorized to give consent is important. This person may be a parent or guardian who has the legal right to make decisions about the treatment and care of the patient. This person must be informed as to the reasons for the restraint and the possible risks that may occur if restraints are not used before any such devices may be applied. In either of these cases, the radiographer or other provider should document the use of restraint or immobilization device as well as the rationale for use and evidence of consent, if available.

Defamation

Health care professionals have an obligation to maintain patient confidentiality and are required to keep all protected health information concerning the patient, including diagnosis and prognosis, in strictest confidence. This information should be shared only with persons who need to know and who have an authorized health care relationship with the patient, or whom the patient has authorized to receive information. If information concerning a patient was released to unauthorized individuals, and if the information was disseminated in such a way that the patient became subject to ridicule, scorn, or contempt or was injured in some other way such as loss of business, job, or home, then an action for defamation might be brought against the individual responsible for the breach of patient confidence.

Two types of defamation are generally recognized: (1) slander, which involves the spoken word, and (2) libel, which involves written or published comments or pictures. In the case of slander, it may involve releasing information about a patient in a way that causes harm to the individual or gossiping about a co-worker or other professional colleague in a way that causes some injury to the person in his or her professional or personal life. Libel may include writing inappropriate comments about a patient in the health record or indicating that a professional colleague has done something wrong, such as failing to treat a patient properly or failing to order the proper procedure. In either case, the allegedly injured party must prove that he or she has been defamed and that the defamation has caused an injury.

The increased usage of social media has allowed for easy and irresponsible dissemination of information related to patients and health care facilities. Health care providers must know that posting information and/or images on social media sites that identify patients or health care organizations may lead to claims of defamation.

An employer may also be able to take action against an employee for social media posts which release patient information or cause harm to the reputation of the employer. Such action may include suspension or termination of employment

Fraud

Fraud in health care is on the rise and occurs in the areas of health care financing, as well as during attempts to cover up wrongdoing or errors on the part of the patient or provider. Fraud is generally defined as a willful and intentional misrepresentation of facts that may cause harm to an individual or result in loss of an individual right or property. Cases of fraud may arise when a pathologic condition is missed on a radiograph or when a study is not completed with optimal images and a health care provider attempts to cover up the error by destroying or altering images or records. Other areas of fraud may include altering personnel records, changing patient's medical records, billing for procedures that were not performed, or altering other documentation in an attempt to mislead or cover up some wrongdoing. For a plaintiff to prevail in a claim of fraud, the alleged injured party must show that (1) an untrue statement, known to be untrue by the party making it, was made so as to mislead, (2) the injured party relied on the statement, and (3) damages were incurred as a result of the reliance. An example of such conduct may be modifying the patient's health information to receive compensation for a procedure that was not medically indicated.

PRIVACY OF RECORDS

Privacy of records and confidentiality are two principles clearly articulated in the American Hospital Association's Patient Care Partnership. Although the patient's health records belong to the hospital or health care facility, the information contained in the records belongs to the patient and therefore may not be distributed without the patient's consent. The records, which include radiographic images, should be kept in a secured area with access given only to persons who need to know what is contained in them. The patient generally has a right to see what is contained in his or her records, but each provider may determine a reasonable method for releasing this information to the patient. In some limited cases, the physician may determine that the patient should not have access to the files. Such a case may arise when a physician believes that a patient may not be emotionally stable enough to understand or handle the information contained in the health record.

The issue of acquired immunodeficiency syndrome or other communicable diseases has brought attention to the importance and sensitivity of patient health information. Information disclosed from records of a patient who is human immunodeficiency virus positive or has another communicable disease may cause the individual to lose a job or to experience discrimination, or in the alternative, fear of improper release of information may lead the patient to not seek necessary care. A claim of defamation, invasion of privacy, or a *Health Insurance Portability and Accountability Act* of 1996 (HIPAA) violation may be made if a person's records are released or used in a way contrary to the standard established by the health care community.

HIPAA calls for the standardization of electronic data interchange, the protection of confidentiality, and the security of individually identifiable health information. The confidentiality standards establish guidelines for the storage, access, and transmission of individuals' health information. Under these guidelines, patients must authorize the release of health information, and a knowing misuse of health information by a health professional may result in fines and/or imprisonment. Every health provider must understand the rules for release of patient health information and follow the policies established by the employer for access and release. Any questions that arise about the appropriateness of the release of information should be directed to the facility's compliance officer.

NEGLIGENCE

The existence of a medical injury shall not create any inference or presumption of negligence against the health-care provider, and the claimant must provide the burden of proving that the injury was proximately caused by the breach in the prevailing professional standard of care.
McDonald v. Medical Imaging Center of Boca Raton, 662So2d733 (Fla App 1995)

Medical malpractice litigation is predominantly founded in the negligence theory of liability. Negligence is a failure to use such care as a reasonably prudent person would use under like or similar circumstances. Medical negligence uses this theory, but instead of the prudent person, the reasonably prudent health care professional or, in the case of radiologic technology, the reasonably prudent radiographer is used as a model.

For a patient (plaintiff) to recover damages for injuries sustained because of alleged negligence, four elements must be proved: (1) a duty to the patient by the health care practitioner (in medical-related cases this is defined as the standard of care), (2) breach of this duty by an act or by failing to perform some act (deviation from the standard of care), (3) a compensable injury, and (4) a causal relationship between the injury and the breach of duty.

For example, a patient arrives in the radiology department on a stretcher. After the radiographer has completed the examination, the patient is transferred back to the stretcher but the side rails are not raised. In moving about, the patient falls and fractures a hip. The radiographer has a duty to protect the patient from falls by following the standard practice of raising the side rails, and this duty was breached by the radiographer's failure to lock the side rails in the raised position. The injury element is demonstrated by the fact that the patient has fractured a hip as a result of the fall. The causation factor is generally the most difficult to prove; however, the fractured hip was apparently a direct result of the fall from the cart, which, most likely, but for the failure of the radiographer to place the side rails in the raised position, would not have occurred.

Another example of negligence in medical imaging may arise when a radiographer fails to properly assess an individual before administration of a contrast medium, and after administration a situation arises that requires medical intervention and results in a long-term complication for the patient. Does the standard of care require a radiographer to assess a patient in an attempt to determine the appropriateness of administering contrast media? Is there a case in which the injury may not have been the result of the radiographer's failure to assess? What if the radiographer had assessed properly and there was still a complication?

Each of the four elements must be proved before the radiographer can be found negligent. The evidence requirements may vary from one jurisdiction to another, and other legal factors may affect the outcome. However, generally speaking, the four elements—duty (standard of care), breach of duty, injury, and causation—must be proved no matter where the case is filed.

STANDARD OF CARE

The term "standard of care" in common law is generally understood to mean a measure or rule against which a defendant's conduct is to be measured. … The established standard of care for all professionals is stated as use of the same degree of knowledge, skill, and ability as an ordinarily careful professional would exercise under similar circumstances.

**Advincula v United Blood Services,
678 NE2d 1009 (Ill 1996)**

Each profession or area in the health care delivery system has a standard of care. The standard for radiologic technology is not written in stone and is constantly changing because of the dynamic nature of the technology. Regardless of the changing nature of the discipline, guidelines are established to help define the standard of care for medical imaging.

The general definition of the standard of care is the degree of skill (proficiency), knowledge, and care ordinarily possessed and employed by members in good standing within the profession. The test of whether the standard of care has been met by an individual under certain circumstances is to determine what a reasonable, prudent practitioner would have done under the same or similar circumstances. The court looks to the profession for guidance as it tries to establish the standard of care for a particular practice. Information that may be used to determine the standard include federal and state regulations, position descriptions, curriculum guides, institutional policies and procedures, professional customs, standards of practice, and rules of ethics.

Practice Standards for Medical Imaging and Radiation Therapy were developed by members of the American Society of Radiologic Technology (ASRT) in order to help define the expectations of the profession for those who practice in the professions. These standards outline the practice for medical imaging and radiation therapy professionals in clinical, quality, and professional performance and include the scope of practice for each area such as radiography, radiation therapy, radiologist assistants, computed technology, nuclear medicine, and mammography. Each section of the standards offer a framework for performance that helps direct the practitioner while allowing for variations in different localities and areas of practice. The standards outline minimum expectation of performance as determined by the profession. For example, an individual providing patient assessment will be measured against the general and specific criteria of Standard One, including patient identification, verification of appropriate procedure, gathering relevant patient information, and determining indication or contraindication for the procedure. A review of actual practice as compared to the guidance in the standards will be used to determine whether an individual is compliant with acceptable professional practice. Expert witnesses, who are generally educators or long-term practitioners in the field, may be asked to testify as to the standard of care based on these standards established by the profession. Appendix A contains the Practice Standards for Radiography. The standard of care will be modified as the profession grows; therefore all radiologic technologists must keep abreast of current trends in the profession because the standards adopted by the profession are likely to be the principles against which practice will be measured.

A governing body known as the Practice Standards Council has been established with the purpose of continually reviewing and updating the practice standards. Upon review and modification by the Council, the proposed revisions of the standards are brought before the House of Delegates of the ASRT for final approval. This Council is also charged with researching practice questions and rendering opinions as to the current standard based on an analysis of professional literature, research, statute, regulation, and professional best practice.

OTHER LEGAL THEORIES

Whereas negligence is the primary theory of liability in medical malpractice claims, attorneys may use other legal theories to switch the burden of proof from the plaintiff to the defendant or to bring additional parties into the litigation. Such theories include res ipsa loquitur, respondeat superior, and corporate liability.

Res Ipsa Loquitur

The legal doctrine of res ipsa loquitur sometimes arises in cases of medical negligence and is used to switch the burden of proof from the plaintiff to the defendant. Res ipsa loquitur translates to *the thing speaks for itself* and describes how a patient is injured through no fault of his or her own while in the complete control of another. In these cases the plaintiff must show that the action causing the injury was in the exclusive control of the defendant and that the injury is a type that would not have occurred but for the negligent activity of the defendant. This type of case occurs most often in the surgical setting in which a patient is anesthetized and sustains an injury that would not have happened in the ordinary course of the operation. Radiology may be involved in such a case—for example, when a patient sustains a burn from a portable machine when the field light remains on while in contact with the patient's skin or from excessive radiation exposure in the case of fluoroscopy.

In a case in which the theory of res ipsa loquitur is raised, the burden of proof shifts from the patient's obligation to prove negligence to the defendant health care practitioner who must prove that negligence did not occur.

Respondeat Superior. If the radiographer in the previous scenario was sued for negligence, then more often than not the hospital and surgeon would also be named as defendants. This legal theory is known as respondeat superior or *the master speaks for the servant*. In cases of medical negligence, the well-established theory asserts that the physician or the health care facility is responsible for the negligent acts of its employees. Many critics of this theory claim that this action is a *deep pocket* approach to legal recovery based primarily on the fact that a physician or health care facility has more money than an individual technologist. Although this circumstance may be true in many cases, other reasons and strategies are used when determining whom to name as defendants in a medical negligence complaint. One such theory is that a lone technologist on the stand is a more sympathetic character than a wealthy physician or hospital corporation.

An example in which individual liability and supervisory liability for the organization that employs the radiographer may arise is in the negligent performance of a procedure, such as a radiographer who administers excessive amounts of radiation to a pediatric patient during a procedure because the child continues to move and repeat images are performed. What is the radiographer's obligation to minimize radiation exposure of a patient? What is the organization's responsibility in establishing policies and procedures to prevent this type of activity or in selecting qualified clinical competent personnel? Might both the individual and the organization be liable for an injury sustained by the patient?

Corporate Liability. The theory of corporate liability requires the hospital or health care entity to be responsible for the quality of care delivered to patients in their facilities. This liability extends not only to the actions of actual employees of the corporation, but also to independent contractors, such as physicians who practice within the facility.

Courts have in recent years expanded the concept of corporate liability to include the following:
1. Duty of reasonable care in the selection and retention of employees and medical staff
2. Duty of reasonable care in the maintenance and use of equipment
3. Availability of equipment and services

Liability may arise if an organization uses equipment that exposes a patient to excessive amounts of radiation through some type of automatic exposure control or preprogrammed delivery. Should the organization be responsible for equipment programming errors? What is their obligation to perform technical surveys on the equipment to ascertain optimal performance factors? Is the responsibility solely that of the manufacturer?

Under these guidelines, the health care corporation has the responsibility to assess and evaluate the quality of care delivered and must be prepared to make changes as needed to protect the consumer of health care services. The corporation may be required to intervene if suboptimal care is being provided by one of its employees, independent contractors, or equipment manufacturers.

CONSENT

When patients enter a health care facility for examination or treatment, they place their trust in health care professionals. This trust includes an assumption that the correct procedures are being performed and that the professional is meeting the appropriate standard of care. This trust does not mean, however, that patients relinquish their right to make decisions about their own health care. They rely on the fact that health care professionals will give them all of the information necessary to make an informed decision regarding the consent to care.

Implied Consent

Implied consent results when an individual appears at the imaging department and allows the radiographer to perform a simple procedure such as a chest or extremity radiograph. This is the most common form of consent in medical imaging. It does not require a signed statement of consent but still allows the patient to ask questions or refuse the procedure. On the other hand, invasive or complex procedures that include a certain level of risk require a more extensive consent process.

Informed Consent

Only when patients have all the information they need to make decisions about their health care will they be able to give an informed consent for examination and treatment. Informed consent is required when a patient is subjected to any type of invasive procedure. In medical imaging departments, this consent requirement runs the gamut from excretory urography to interventional vascular examinations.

When patients are informed that a particular procedure would assist the physician in making a diagnosis, they should also be informed of the techniques that will be used to complete the examination, the possible risks associated with them, the benefits, and any alternative procedures that might be performed. A good example may be the patient who is scheduled for a myelogram. The patient should receive a careful explanation of how the procedure is to be performed, along with an enumeration of the benefits and risks that may be associated with it. The patient should also be informed of alternatives such as computed tomography or magnetic resonance imaging and should be informed of the risks and benefits of each alternative. All this information must be relayed to patients in language they can understand. A patient cannot understand the explanation of a procedure if the health care practitioner uses medical terminology that is foreign to the patient. This situation is similar to explaining something to a Spanish-speaking individual in English and expecting him or her to understand. Current guidelines recommend that consent be given in layperson's terms in the primary language of the patient. Hospitals are required to have interpreters who will be able to relay procedural and other health care information to patients.

After the physician has given the patient all the information necessary to make an informed decision, a consent form should be signed that documents the information that has been given. These forms are usually prepared by the health care facility. As a general rule, a consent form should contain (1) an authorization clause to permit the physician or other health care professional to perform the examination; (2) a disclosure clause to explain the procedure, its risks and benefits, and possible alternatives to the procedure; (3) an anesthesia clause, if required; (4) a no-guarantee clause for therapeutic procedures; (5) a tissue-disposal clause if the removal of tissue may be necessary; (6) a patient understanding clause, which usually states that all the information contained in the consent form has been carefully explained to the patient; and (7) a signature clause, which calls for the signature of the patient, as well as that of a witness. The witness should be a disinterested third party who will not be involved in the actual performance of the procedure.

The amount of information given to the patient must be evaluated on a case-by-case basis. Because every individual is different, the need for information differs from patient to patient. The health care professional who is obtaining the consent must assess the patient as the information is received and base the disclosure of information on the responses and history of the patient. The circumstances surrounding the signing of consent forms are also important, and the department should establish a policy as to how consent forms are to be signed. The evaluation process in determining the policy should include when the consent should be signed, who will be available to answer questions from the patient, who will obtain the signature, and how it will be determined whether the patient is mentally and physically able to make an informed consent.

The patient's autonomy should always be considered when performing diagnostic or therapeutic procedures. If the patient consents to a procedure and then revokes the consent, the health care practitioner must then recognize the patient's right to revoke and must stop the procedure at a point at which the patient will not be injured in any way. Such a case may arise during a barium enema procedure when a patient with discomfort determines that he or she does not want to proceed with the examination. The radiologist and radiographer must comply with the patient's wishes by stopping the flow of barium and allowing any barium already administered to flow back into the enema bag. Simply stopping the procedure without allowing the barium to flow back may cause a subsequent injury to the patient because barium that is not evacuated in a timely fashion may cause a perforated colon or other injury.

SUMMARY

- Radiologic technologists are legally liable for their actions in the daily performance of diagnostic procedures and patient management. They must know, understand, and follow the appropriate standard of care and should be well versed in current practice, recommended procedural considerations, and patient rights. They should understand the liability of such actions as assault, battery, false imprisonment, and negligence. Any information the radiographer acquires during the course of an examination must be kept in strictest confidence. The basic right of the patient to determine the course of diagnosis and treatment must always be recognized. Therefore the patient must be given information that allows for high-quality decision making and the ability to give informed consent.

- Health care practitioners who do not remain current in the field or who do not follow the accepted standards may be liable, under several legal theories including but not limited to medical negligence, for their actions if a patient is injured. Similarly, the health care facility and the supervising physician may be liable under the theory of respondeat superior or corporate liability for the actions of their employees.

BIBLIOGRAPHY

Advincula v United Blood Services: 678 NE2d 1009 (Ill 1996).

Berlin L: *Malpractice issues in radiology*, ed 2, Leesburg, Va, 2003, American Roentgen Ray Society.

Berlin L: Radiologic errors and malpractice: a blurry distinction, *AJR Am J Roentgenol* 189:517, 2007.

Fremgan B: *Medical law and ethics*, ed 5, Upper Saddle River, NJ, 2015, Pearson Prentice Hall.

Furrow BR, Greaney TL, Johnson SH, et al.: *Health law: cases, materials, and problems*, ed 7, St. Paul, Minn, 2013, West Wadsworth Publishing.

Furrow BR, Greaney TL, Johnson SH, et al.: *Liability and quality issues in health care*, ed 6, St. Paul, Minn, 2008, West Information Publishing Group.

Health Insurance Portability and Accountability Act of 1996 as amended 2013, Available at: https://www.hhs.gov/hipaa/index.html

Pozgar GD: *Legal and ethical issues for health professionals*, ed 4, Sudbury, Mass, 2014, Jones & Bartlett.

Pozgar GD: *Legal aspects of health care administration*, ed 11, Sudbury, Mass, 2011, Jones & Bartlett Learning.

Practice standards for medical imaging and radiation therapy: adopted as amended by American Society of Radiologic Technology, 2017. Available at: http://www.asrt.org/main/standards-regulations/practice-standards.

Sanbar SS, editor: *Legal medicine: American College of Legal Medicine*, ed 5, St. Louis, 2001, Mosby.

Schloendorf v: In *Society of New York Hospital*, 211 NY, 125, 1914, p 105. (NE 92.)

The Practice Standards for Medical Imaging and Radiation Therapy
Radiography Practice Standards

PREFACE TO PRACTICE STANDARDS

A profession's practice standards serve as a guide for appropriate practice. The practice standards define the practice and establish general criteria to determine compliance. Practice standards are authoritative statements established by the profession for evaluating the quality of practice, service, and education provided by individuals who practice in medical imaging and radiation therapy.

Practice standards can be used by individual facilities to develop job descriptions and practice parameters. Those outside the imaging, therapeutic, and radiation science community can use the standards as an overview of the role and responsibilities of the individual as defined by the profession.

The individual must be educationally prepared and clinically competent as a prerequisite to professional practice. Federal and state laws, accreditation standards necessary to participate in government programs, and lawful institutional policies and procedures supersede these standards.

FORMAT

The Practice Standards are divided into six sections: introduction, scope of practice, clinical performance, quality performance, professional performance, and advisory opinion statements.

Introduction. The introduction provides definitions for the practice and the minimum qualifications for the education and certification of individuals in addition to an overview of the specific practice.

Scope of Practice. The scope of practice delineates the parameters of the specific practice.

Clinical Performance Standards. The clinical performance standards define the activities of the individual responsible for the care of patients and delivery of diagnostic or therapeutic procedures. The section incorporates patient assessment and management with procedural analysis, performance, and evaluation.

Quality Performance Standards. The quality performance standards define the activities of the individual in the technical areas of performance, such as equipment and material assessment safety standards and total quality management.

Professional Performance Standards. The professional performance standards define the activities of the individual in the areas of education, interpersonal relationships, self-assessment, and ethical behavior.

Advisory Opinion Statements. The advisory opinions are interpretations of the standards intended for clarification and guidance of specific practice issues.

Each performance standards section is subdivided into individual standards. The standards are numbered and followed by a term or set of terms that identify the standards, such as "assessment" or "analysis/determination." The next statement is the expected performance of the individual when performing the procedure or treatment. A rationale statement follows and explains why an individual should adhere to the particular standard of performance.

Criteria. Criteria are used to evaluate an individual's performance. Each set is divided into two parts: the general criteria and the specific criteria. Both should be used when evaluating performance.

General Criteria. General criteria are written in a style that applies to imaging and radiation science individuals. These criteria are the same in all of the practice standards, with the exception of limited x-ray machine operators and medical dosimetry, and should be used for the appropriate area of practice.

Specific Criteria. Specific criteria meet the needs of the individuals in the various areas of professional performance. While many areas of performance within imaging and radiation sciences are similar, others are not. The specific criteria were drafted with these differences in mind.

INTRODUCTION TO RADIOGRAPHY PRACTICE STANDARDS

Definition

The practice of radiography is performed by health care professionals responsible for the administration of ionizing radiation for diagnostic, therapeutic, or research purposes. A radiographer performs radiographic procedures at the request of and for interpretation by a licensed practitioner.

The complex nature of disease processes involves multiple imaging modalities. Although an interdisciplinary team of clinicians, radiographers, and support staff plays a critical role in the delivery of health services, it is the radiographer who performs the radiographic procedure that creates the images needed for diagnosis.

Radiography integrates scientific knowledge, technical competence, and patient interaction skills to provide safe and accurate procedures with the highest regard to all aspects of patient care. A radiographer recognizes patient conditions essential for the successful completion of the procedure.

Radiographers must demonstrate an understanding of human anatomy, physiology, pathology, and medical terminology.

Radiographers must maintain a high degree of accuracy in radiographic positioning and exposure technique. They must possess, apply, and maintain knowledge of radiation protection and safety. Radiographers independently perform or assist the licensed practitioner in the completion of radiographic procedures. Radiographers prepare, administer, and document activities related to medications in accordance with state and federal regulations or lawful institutional policy.

Radiographers are the primary liaison between patients, licensed practitioners, and other members of the support team. Radiographers must remain sensitive to the needs of the patient through good communication, patient assessment, patient monitoring, and patient care skills. As members of the health care team, radiographers participate in quality improvement processes and continually assess their professional performance.

Radiographers think critically and use independent, professional, and ethical judgment in all aspects of their work. They engage in continuing education to include their area of practice to enhance patient care, public education, knowledge, and technical competence.

Education and Certification

Only medical imaging and radiation therapy professionals who have completed the appropriate education and obtained certification(s) as outlined in these standards should perform radiographic procedures.

Radiographers prepare for their roles on the interdisciplinary team by successfully completing a program in radiologic technology that is programmatically accredited or part of an institution that is regionally accredited, and by attaining appropriate primary certification from the American Registry of Radiologic Technologists (ARRT).

Those passing the ARRT examination use the credential R.T.(R).

Medical imaging and radiation therapy professionals performing multiple modality hybrid imaging should be registered by certification agencies recognized by the ASRT and be educationally prepared and clinically competent in the specific modality(ies) they are responsible to perform. Medical imaging and radiation therapy professionals performing diagnostic procedures in more than one imaging modality will adhere to the individual practice standard for each.

To maintain ARRT certification, radiographers must complete appropriate continuing education and meet other requirements to sustain a level of expertise and awareness of changes and advances in practice.

Overview

Radiographers are part of the interdisciplinary team that plays a critical role in the delivery of health services as new modalities emerge and the need for imaging procedures increases. A comprehensive procedure list for the radiographer is impractical because clinical activities vary by the practice needs and expertise of the radiographer. As radiographers gain more experience, knowledge, and clinical competence, the clinical activities for the radiographer may evolve.

State statute, regulation, or lawful community custom may dictate practice parameters. Wherever there is a conflict between these standards and state or local statutes or regulations, the state or local statutes or regulations supersede these standards. A radiographer should, within the boundaries of all applicable legal requirements and restrictions, exercise individual thought, judgment, and discretion in the performance of the procedure.

RADIOGRAPHER SCOPE OF PRACTICE

The scope of practice of the medical imaging and radiation therapy professional includes:

- Providing optimal patient care.
- Receiving, relaying, and documenting verbal, written, and electronic orders in the patient's medical record.
- Corroborating a patient's clinical history with procedure and ensuring information is documented and available for use by a licensed practitioner.
- Verifying informed consent for applicable procedures.
- Assuming responsibility for patient needs during procedures.
- Preparing patients for procedures.
- Applying principles of ALARA to minimize exposure to patient, self, and others.
- Performing venipuncture as prescribed by a licensed practitioner.
- Starting, maintaining, and/or removing intravenous access as prescribed by a licensed practitioner.
- Identifying, preparing, and/or administering medications as prescribed by a licensed practitioner.
- Evaluating images for technical quality, ensuring proper identification is recorded.
- Identifying and responding to emergency situations.
- Providing education.
- Educating and monitoring students and other health care providers.
- Performing ongoing quality assurance activities.
- Applying the principles of patient safety during all aspects of patient care. The scope of practice of the radiographer also includes:
  1. Performing diagnostic radiographic and noninterpretive fluoroscopic procedures as prescribed by a licensed practitioner.

2. Optimizing technical exposure factors in accordance with the principles of ALARA.
3. Assisting the licensed practitioner with fluoroscopic and specialized radiologic procedures.

RADIOGRAPHY CLINICAL PERFORMANCE STANDARDS

Standard One—Assessment

The radiographer collects pertinent data about the patient and the procedure

Rationale. Information about the patient's health status is essential in providing appropriate imaging and therapeutic services.

General Stipulation. The individual must be educationally prepared and clinically competent as a prerequisite to professional practice. Federal and state laws, accreditation standards necessary to participate in government programs, and lawful institutional policies and procedures supersede these standards.

General Criteria. The radiographer:
1. Obtains relevant information from all available resources and the release of information as needed.
2. Verifies patient identification and the procedure requested or prescribed.
3. Verifies that the patient has consented to the procedure.
4. Reviews all available patient medical record information to verify the appropriateness of the procedure requested or prescribed.
5. Verifies the patient's pregnancy status.
6. Assesses factors that may negatively affect the procedure, such as medications, patient history, insufficient patient preparation, or artifact-producing objects.
7. Recognizes signs and symptoms of an emergency.

Specific Criteria. The radiographer:
1. Assesses patient risk for allergic reaction(s) to medication prior to administration.
2. Locates and reviews previous examinations for comparison.
3. Identifies and removes artifact-producing objects.

RADIOGRAPHY CLINICAL PERFORMANCE STANDARDS

Standard Two—Analysis/Determination

The radiographer analyzes the information obtained during the assessment phase and develops an action plan for completing the procedure.

Rationale. Determining the most appropriate action plan enhances patient safety and comfort, optimizes diagnostic and therapeutic quality, and improves efficiency.

General Stipulation. The individual must be educationally prepared and clinically competent as a prerequisite to professional practice. Federal and state laws, accreditation standards necessary to participate in government programs, and lawful institutional policies and procedures supersede these standards.

General Criteria. The radiographer:
1. Selects the most appropriate and efficient action plan after reviewing all pertinent data and assessing the patient's abilities and condition.
2. Employs professional judgment to adapt imaging and therapeutic procedures to improve diagnostic quality and therapeutic outcomes.
3. Consults appropriate medical personnel to determine a modified action plan.
4. Determines the need for and selects supplies, accessory equipment, shielding, positioning, and immobilization devices.
5. Determines the course of action for an emergent situation.
6. Determines that all procedural requirements are in place to achieve a quality diagnostic or therapeutic procedure.

Specific Criteria. The radiographer:
1. Reviews lab values prior to administering medication and initiating specialized radiologic procedures.
2. Determines type and dose of contrast agent to be administered, based on the patient's age, weight, and medical/physical status.
3. Verifies that exposure indicator data for digital radiographic systems has not been altered or modified and is included in the Digital Imaging Communications in Medicine header and on images exported to media.
4. Analyzes images to determine the use of appropriate imaging parameters.

RADIOGRAPHY CLINICAL PERFORMANCE STANDARDS

Standard Three—Education

The radiographer provides information about the procedure and related health issues according to protocol.

Rationale. Communication and education are necessary to establish a positive relationship.

General Stipulation. The individual must be educationally prepared and clinically competent as a prerequisite to professional practice. Federal and state laws, accreditation standards necessary to participate in government programs, and lawful institutional policies and procedures supersede these standards.

General Criteria. The radiographer:
1. Provides an accurate explanation and instructions at an appropriate time and at a level the patient and their care providers can understand. Addresses questions and concerns regarding the procedure.
2. Refers questions about diagnosis, treatment, or prognosis to a licensed practitioner.
3. Provides patient education.
4. Explains effects and potential side effects of medications.

Specific Criteria. The radiographer:
1. Provides pre-, peri-, and post-procedure education.
2. Educates the patient about the risks and benefits of radiation.

RADIOGRAPHY CLINICAL PERFORMANCE STANDARDS

Standard Four—Performance

The radiographer performs the action plan.

Rationale. Quality patient services are provided through the safe and accurate performance of a deliberate plan of action.

General Stipulation. The individual must be educationally prepared and clinically competent as a prerequisite to professional practice. Federal and state laws, accreditation standards necessary to participate in government programs, and lawful institutional policies and procedures supersede these standards.

General Criteria. The radiographer:
1. Performs procedural timeout.
2. Implements an action plan.
3. Explains to the patient each step of the action plan as it occurs and elicits the cooperation of the patient.
4. Uses an integrated team approach.
5. Modifies the action plan according to changes in the clinical situation.
6. Administers first aid or provides life support.
7. Uses accessory equipment.
8. Assesses and monitors the patient's physical, emotional, and mental status.
9. Applies principles of sterile technique.
10. Positions patient for anatomic area of interest, respecting patient ability and comfort.
11. Immobilizes patient for procedure.
12. Monitors the patient for reactions to medications.

Specific Criteria. The radiographer:
1. Employs proper radiation safety practices.
2. Optimizes technical factors according to equipment specifications to meet the ALARA principle.
3. Uses pre-exposure collimation and proper field-of-view selection.
4. Uses appropriate uniquely identifiable pre-exposure radiopaque markers for anatomical and procedural purposes.
5. Selects the best position for the demonstration of anatomy.
6. Injects medication into peripherally inserted central catheter lines or ports.
7. Coordinates and manages the collection and labeling of tissue and fluid specimens.
8. Performs appropriate postprocessing on digital images in preparation for interpretation.

RADIOGRAPHY CLINICAL PERFORMANCE STANDARDS

Standard Five—Evaluation

The radiographer determines whether the goals of the action plan have been achieved.

Rationale. Careful examination of the procedure is important to determine that expected outcomes have been met.

General Stipulation. The individual must be educationally prepared and clinically competent as a prerequisite to professional practice. Federal and state laws, accreditation standards necessary to participate in government programs, and lawful institutional policies and procedures supersede these standards.

General Criteria. The radiographer:
1. Evaluates the patient and the procedure to identify variances that might affect the expected outcome.
2. Completes the evaluation process in a timely, accurate, and comprehensive manner.
3. Measures the procedure against established policies, protocols, and benchmarks.
4. Identifies exceptions to the expected outcome.
5. Develops a revised action plan to achieve the intended outcome.
6. Communicates the revised action plan to appropriate team members.

Specific Criteria. The radiographer:
1. Evaluates images for positioning to demonstrate the anatomy of interest.
2. Evaluates images for optimal technical exposure factors.
3. Reviews images to determine if additional images will enhance the diagnostic value of the procedure.

RADIOGRAPHY CLINICAL PERFORMANCE STANDARDS

Standard Six—Implementation

The radiographer implements the revised action plan.

Rationale. It may be necessary to make changes to the action plan to achieve the expected outcome.

General Stipulation. The individual must be educationally prepared and clinically competent as a prerequisite to professional practice. Federal and state laws, accreditation standards necessary to participate in government programs, and lawful institutional policies and procedures supersede these standards.

General Criteria. The radiographer:
1. Bases the revised plan on the patient's condition and the most appropriate means of achieving the expected outcome.
2. Takes action based on patient and procedural variances.
3. Measures and evaluates the results of the revised action plan.
4. Notifies the appropriate health care provider when immediate clinical response is necessary, based on procedural findings and patient condition.

Specific Criteria. The radiographer:
1. Performs additional images that will produce the expected outcomes based upon patient condition and procedural variances.

RADIOGRAPHY CLINICAL PERFORMANCE STANDARDS

Standard Seven—Outcomes Measurement

The radiographer reviews and evaluates the outcome of the procedure.

Rationale. To evaluate the quality of care, the radiographer compares the actual outcome with the expected outcome.

General Stipulation. The individual must be educationally prepared and clinically competent as a prerequisite to professional practice. Federal and state laws, accreditation standards necessary to participate in government programs, and lawful institutional policies and procedures supersede these standards.

General Criteria. The radiographer:
1. Reviews all diagnostic or therapeutic data for completeness and accuracy.
2. Uses evidence-based practice to determine whether the actual outcome is within established criteria.
3. Evaluates the process and recognizes opportunities for future changes.
4. Assesses the patient's physical, emotional, and mental status prior to discharge.

Specific Criteria. None added.

RADIOGRAPHY CLINICAL PERFORMANCE STANDARDS

Standard Eight—Documentation

The radiographer documents information about patient care, the procedure, and the final outcome.

Rationale. Clear and precise documentation is essential for continuity of care, accuracy of care, and quality assurance.

General Stipulation. The individual must be educationally prepared and clinically competent as a prerequisite to professional practice. Federal and state laws, accreditation standards necessary to participate in government programs, and lawful institutional policies and procedures supersede these standards.

General Criteria. The radiographer:
1. Documents diagnostic, treatment, and patient data in the medical record in a timely, accurate, and comprehensive manner.
2. Documents unintended outcomes or exceptions from the established criteria.
3. Provides pertinent information to authorized individual(s) involved in the patient's care.
4. Records information used for billing and coding procedures.
5. Archives images or data.
6. Verifies patient consent is documented.
7. Documents procedural timeout.

Specific Criteria. The radiographer:
1. Documents fluoroscopic time.
2. Documents radiation exposure.
3. Documents the use of shielding devices and proper radiation safety practices.

RADIOGRAPHY QUALITY PERFORMANCE STANDARDS

Standard One—Assessment

The radiographer collects pertinent information regarding equipment, procedures, and the work environment.

Rationale. The planning and provision of safe and effective medical services relies on the collection of pertinent information about equipment, procedures, and the work environment.

General Stipulation. The individual must be educationally prepared and clinically competent as a prerequisite to professional practice. Federal and state laws, accreditation standards necessary to participate in government programs, and lawful institutional policies and procedures supersede these standards.

General Criteria. The radiographer:
1. Determines that services are performed in a safe environment, minimizing potential hazards.
2. Confirms that equipment performance, maintenance, and operation comply with the manufacturer's specifications.
3. Verifies that protocol and procedure manuals include recommended criteria and are reviewed and revised.

Specific Criteria. The radiographer:
1. Controls access to restricted areas during radiation exposure.
2. Follows federal and state guidelines to minimize occupational and patient radiation exposure levels.
3. Maintains and performs quality control on radiation safety equipment.
4. Develops and maintains standardized exposure technique guidelines for all equipment.
5. Participates in radiation protection, patient safety, risk management, and quality management activities.
6. Reviews digital images for the purpose of monitoring radiation exposure.

RADIOGRAPHY QUALITY PERFORMANCE STANDARDS

Standard Two—Analysis/Determination

The radiographer analyzes information collected during the assessment phase to determine the need for changes to equipment, procedures, or the work environment.

Rationale. Determination of acceptable performance is necessary to provide safe and effective services.

General Stipulation. The individual must be educationally prepared and clinically competent as a prerequisite to professional practice. Federal and state laws, accreditation standards necessary to participate in government programs, and lawful institutional policies and procedures supersede these standards.

General Criteria. The radiographer:
1. Evaluates services, procedures, and the environment to determine if they meet or exceed established guidelines and revises the action plan.
2. Monitors equipment to meet or exceed established standards and revises the action plan.
3. Assesses and maintains the integrity of medical supplies.

Specific Criteria. None added.

RADIOGRAPHY QUALITY PERFORMANCE STANDARDS

Standard Three—Education
The radiographer informs the patient, public, and other health care providers about procedures, equipment, and facilities.

Rationale. Open communication promotes safe practices.

General Stipulation. The individual must be educationally prepared and clinically competent as a prerequisite to professional practice. Federal and state laws, accreditation standards necessary to participate in government programs, and lawful institutional policies and procedures supersede these standards.

General Criteria. The radiographer:
1. Elicits confidence and cooperation from the patient, the public, and other health care providers by providing timely communication and effective instruction.
2. Presents explanations and instructions at the learner's level of understanding.
3. Educates the patient, public, and other health care providers about procedures and the associated biological effects.
4. Provides information to patients, health care providers, students, and the public concerning the role and responsibilities of individuals in the profession.

Specific Criteria. None added.

RADIOGRAPHY QUALITY PERFORMANCE STANDARDS

Standard Four—Performance
The radiographer performs quality assurance activities.

Rationale. Quality assurance activities provide valid and reliable information regarding the performance of equipment, materials, and processes.

General Stipulation. The individual must be educationally prepared and clinically competent as a prerequisite to professional

practice. Federal and state laws, accreditation standards necessary to participate in government programs, and lawful institutional policies and procedures supersede these standards.

General Criteria. The radiographer:
1. Maintains current information on equipment, materials, and processes.
2. Performs ongoing quality assurance activities.
3. Performs quality control testing of equipment.
4. Participates in safety and risk management activities.
5. When appropriate, wears one or more personal radiation monitoring devices at the location indicated on the personal radiation monitoring device or as indicated by the radiation safety officer or designee.

Specific Criteria. The radiographer:
1. Consults with the medical physicist when performing the quality assurance tests.
2. Monitors image production to determine technical acceptability.
3. Verifies archival storage of image data as appropriate.
4. Routinely reviews patient exposure records and reject analyses as part of the quality assurance program.

RADIOGRAPHY QUALITY PERFORMANCE STANDARDS

Standard Five—Evaluation
The radiographer evaluates quality assurance results and establishes an appropriate action plan.

Rationale. Equipment, materials, and processes depend on ongoing quality assurance activities that evaluate performance based on established guidelines.

General Stipulation. The individual must be educationally prepared and clinically competent as a prerequisite to professional practice. Federal and state laws, accreditation standards necessary to participate in government programs, and lawful institutional policies and procedures supersede these standards.

General Criteria. The radiographer:
1. Validates quality assurance testing conditions and results.
2. Evaluates quality assurance results.
3. Formulates an action plan.

Specific Criteria. None added.

RADIOGRAPHY QUALITY PERFORMANCE STANDARDS

Standard Six—Implementation
The radiographer implements the quality assurance action plan for equipment, materials, and processes.

Rationale. Implementation of a quality assurance action plan promotes safe and effective services.

General Stipulation. The individual must be educationally prepared and clinically competent as a prerequisite to professional practice. Federal and state laws, accreditation standards necessary to participate in government programs, and lawful institutional policies and procedures supersede these standards.

General Criteria. The radiographer:
1. Obtains assistance to support the quality assurance action plan.
2. Implements the quality assurance action plan.

Specific Criteria. None added.

RADIOGRAPHY QUALITY PERFORMANCE STANDARDS

Standard Seven—Outcomes Measurement

The radiographer assesses the outcome of the quality management action plan for equipment, materials, and processes.

Rationale. Outcomes assessment is an integral part of the ongoing quality management action plan to enhance diagnostic and therapeutic services.

General Stipulation. The individual must be educationally prepared and clinically competent as a prerequisite to professional practice. Federal and state laws, accreditation standards necessary to participate in government programs, and lawful institutional policies and procedures supersede these standards.

General Criteria. The radiographer:
1. Reviews the implementation process for accuracy and validity.
2. Determines that actual outcomes are within established criteria.
3. Develops and implements a revised action plan.

Specific Criteria. The radiographer:
1. Reviews and evaluates quality assurance processes and tools for effectiveness.

RADIOGRAPHY QUALITY PERFORMANCE STANDARDS

Standard Eight—Documentation

The radiographer documents quality assurance activities and results.

Rationale. Documentation provides evidence of quality assurance activities designed to enhance safety.

General Stipulation. The individual must be educationally prepared and clinically competent as a prerequisite to professional practice. Federal and state laws, accreditation standards necessary to participate in government programs, and lawful institutional policies and procedures supersede these standards.

General Criteria. The radiographer:
1. Maintains documentation of quality assurance activities, procedures, and results.
2. Documents in a timely, accurate, and comprehensive manner.

Specific Criteria. The radiographer:
1. Reports any out-of-tolerance deviations from quality assurance activities to appropriate personnel.

RADIOGRAPHY PROFESSIONAL PERFORMANCE STANDARDS

Standard One—Quality

The radiographer strives to provide optimal patient care.

Rationale. Patients expect and deserve optimal care during diagnosis and treatment.

General Stipulation. The individual must be educationally prepared and clinically competent as a prerequisite to professional practice. Federal and state laws, accreditation standards necessary to participate in government programs, and lawful institutional policies and procedures supersede these standards.

General Criteria. The radiographer:
1. Collaborates with others to elevate the quality of care.
2. Participates in ongoing quality assurance programs.
3. Adheres to standards, policies, and established guidelines.
4. Applies professional judgment and discretion while performing the diagnostic study or treatment.
5. Anticipates, considers, and responds to the needs of a diverse patient population.

Specific Criteria. None added.

RADIOGRAPHY PROFESSIONAL PERFORMANCE STANDARDS

Standard Two—Self-Assessment

The radiographer evaluates personal performance.

Rationale. Self-assessment is necessary for personal growth and professional development.

General Stipulation. The individual must be educationally prepared and clinically competent as a prerequisite to professional practice. Federal and state laws, accreditation standards necessary to participate in government programs, and lawful institutional policies and procedures supersede these standards.

General Criteria. The radiographer:
1. Assesses personal work ethics, behaviors, and attitudes.
2. Evaluates performance and recognizes opportunities for educational growth and improvement.
3. Recognizes and applies personal and professional strengths.
4. Participates in professional societies and organizations.

Specific Criteria. None added.

RADIOGRAPHY PROFESSIONAL PERFORMANCE STANDARDS

Standard Three—Education

The radiographer acquires and maintains current knowledge in practice.

Rationale. Advancements in the profession and optimal patient care require additional knowledge and skills through education.

General Stipulation. The individual must be educationally prepared and clinically competent as a prerequisite to professional practice. Federal and state laws, accreditation standards necessary to participate in government programs, and lawful institutional policies and procedures supersede these standards.

General Criteria. The radiographer:
1. Maintains credentials and certification related to practice.
2. Advocates for and participates in continuing education related to area of practice to maintain and enhance clinical competency.
3. Advocates for and participates in vendor-specific applications training to maintain clinical competency.

Specific Criteria. The radiographer:
1. Maintains knowledge of the most current practices and technology used to minimize patient dose while producing diagnostic quality images.

RADIOGRAPHY PROFESSIONAL PERFORMANCE STANDARDS

Standard Four—Collaboration and Collegiality

The radiographer promotes a positive and collaborative practice atmosphere with other members of the health care team.

Rationale. To provide quality patient care, all members of the health care team must communicate effectively and work together efficiently.

General Stipulation. The individual must be educationally prepared and clinically competent as a prerequisite to professional practice. Federal and state laws, accreditation standards necessary to participate in government programs, and lawful institutional policies and procedures supersede these standards.

General Criteria. The radiographer:
1. Shares knowledge and expertise with others.
2. Develops and maintains collaborative partnerships to enhance quality and efficiency.
3. Promotes understanding of the profession.

Specific Criteria. None added.

RADIOGRAPHY PROFESSIONAL PERFORMANCE STANDARDS

Standard Five—Ethics

The radiographer adheres to the profession's accepted ethical standards.

Rationale. Decisions made and actions taken on behalf of the patient are based on a sound ethical foundation.

General Stipulation. The individual must be educationally prepared and clinically competent as a prerequisite to professional practice. Federal and state laws, accreditation standards necessary to participate in government programs, and lawful institutional policies and procedures supersede these standards.

General Criteria. The radiographer:
1. Provides health care services with consideration for a diverse patient.
2. Acts as a patient advocate.
3. Accepts accountability for decisions made and actions taken.
4. Delivers patient care and service free from bias or discrimination.
5. Respects the patient's right to privacy and confidentiality.
6. Adheres to the established practice standards of the profession.
7. Adheres to the established ethical standards of recognized certifying agencies.

Specific Criteria. The radiographer:
1. Reports unsafe practices to the radiation safety officer (RSO), regulatory agency, or other appropriate authority.

RADIOGRAPHY PROFESSIONAL PERFORMANCE STANDARDS

Standard Six—Research and Innovation

The radiographer participates in the acquisition and dissemination of knowledge and the advancement of the profession.

Rationale. Scholarly activities such as research, scientific investigation, presentation, and publication advance the profession.

General Stipulation. The individual must be educationally prepared and clinically competent as a prerequisite to professional practice. Federal and state laws, accreditation standards necessary to participate in government programs, and lawful institutional policies and procedures supersede these standards.

General Criteria. The radiographer:
1. Reads and evaluates research relevant to the profession.
2. Participates in data collection.
3. Investigates innovative methods for application in practice.
4. Shares information through publication, presentation, and collaboration.
5. Adopts new best practices.
6. Pursues lifelong learning.

Specific Criteria. None added.

RADIOGRAPHY ADVISORY OPINION STATEMENTS

Administering Medication in Peripherally Inserted Central Catheter Lines or Ports with a Power Injector.

Medication Administration by Medical Imaging and Radiation Therapy Professionals. Medication Administration through Existing Vascular Access.

Placement of Personal Radiation Monitoring Devices.

Use of Post-Exposure Shuttering, Cropping, and Electronic Masking in Radiography.

Professional Organizations

ACCREDITING AGENCIES

Joint Review Committee on Education in Diagnostic Medical Sonography
6021 University Boulevard, Suite 500
Ellicott City, MD 21043
443-973-3251
http://www.jrcdms.org

Joint Review Committee on Education in Radiologic Technology
20 North Wacker Drive, Suite 2850
Chicago, IL 60606-3182
312-704-5300
http://www.jrcert.org

Joint Review Committee on Education Programs in Nuclear Medicine Technology
2000 West Danforth Road, #B1
Edmond, OK 73003
405-285-0546
http://www.jrcnmt.org

REGISTRIES AND OTHER CERTIFICATION AGENCIES

American Registry of Diagnostic Medical Sonographers
1401 Rockville Pike, Suite 600
Rockville, MD 20852-1402
800-541-9754 or 301-738-8401
http://www.ardms.org

American Registry of Radiologic Technologists
1255 Northland Drive
St. Paul, MN 55120-1155
612-687-0048
http://www.arrt.org

Nuclear Medicine Technology Certification Board
3558 Habersham at Northlake
Building I
Tucker, GA 30084-4009
404-315-1739
http://www.nmtcb.org

STATE LICENSING AGENCIES

See Appendix C.

PROFESSIONAL SOCIETIES

American Association of Medical Dosimetrists
2201 Cooperative Way, Suite 600
Herndon, VA 20171
Phone: 703-677-8071
http://www.medicaldosimetry.org/

American Society of Radiologic Technologists
15000 Central Avenue, Southeast
Albuquerque, NM 87123-3909
505-298-4500 or 800-444-2778
http://www.asrt.org

Association of Educators in Imaging and Radiologic Sciences
526 Kingwood Drive #412
Kingwood, TX 77339-4473
936-647-1443
http://www.aeirs.org

The Association for Medical Imaging Management
Formerly American Healthcare Radiology Administrators
490B Boston Post Road, Suite 200
Sudbury, MA 01776
800-334-2472
http://www.ahra.org

Association of Vascular and Interventional Radiographers
8485 Lantana Ct.
Toano, VA 23168
571-252-7174
http://www.avir.org

International Society for Clinical Densitometry
955 South Main Street Building C
Middletown, CT 06457
Telephone: 860-259-1000
http://www.iscd.org

International Society for Magnetic Resonance in Medicine, Society for MR Radiographers and Technologists
2300 Clayton Road Suite 620
Concord, CA 94520
924-825-7678
http://www.ismrm.org/smrt

International Society of Radiographers and Radiological Technologists
Visit the ISRRT website for contact information and member national organization contacts
http://www.isrrt.org

Medical Dosimetrist Certification Board
1120 Route 73, Suite 200
Mt. Laurel, NJ 08054
856-439-1631
http://www.mdcb.org/

Society of Breast Imaging
1891 Preston White Drive
Reston, VA 20191
703-715-4390
http://www.sbi-online.org

Society of Diagnostic Medical Sonographers
2745 Dallas Parkway, Suite 350
Plano, TX 75093-8730
800-229-9506 or 214-473-8057
www.sdms.org

Society for Imaging Informatics in Medicine
19440 Golf Vista Plaza, Suite 330
Leesburg, VA 20176-8264
703-723-0432
http://www.siim.org

Society of Nuclear Medicine and Molecular Imaging—Technologist Section
1850 Samuel Morse Drive
Reston, VA 20190-5316
703-708-9000
http://www.snmmi.org

STATE AND LOCAL RADIOLOGIC TECHNOLOGY SOCIETIES

Because many state societies do not maintain an executive office, we suggest contacting the American Society of Radiologic Technologists for current addresses and telephone numbers. Local societies can usually be contacted through local radiologic technology educators or administrators or through the state society.

Radiologist, Physician, and Physicist Organizations

American Association of Physicists in Medicine
1631 Prince Street
Alexandria, VA 22314
571-298-1300
http://www.aapm.org

American Board of Radiology
5441 East Williams Boulevard, Suite 200
Tucson, AZ 87511-7412
520-790-2900
http://www.theabr.org

American College of Radiology
1891 Preston White Drive
Reston, VA 20191
703-648-8900
http://www.acr.org

American Institute of Ultrasound in Medicine
14750 Sweitzer Lane, Suite 100
Laurel, MD 20707
301-498-4100
http://www.aium.org

American Medical Association
330 North Wabash Avenue Suite 39300
Chicago, IL 60611
312-464-5000 or 800-621-8335
http://www.ama-assn.org

American Roentgen Ray Society
44211 Slatestone Court
Leesburg, VA 20176-5109
866-940-2777
http://www.arrs.org

American Society for Radiation Oncology
251 18th Street South, 8th Floor
Arlington, VA 22202
703-502-1550
http://www.astro.org

Radiological Society of North America
820 Jorie Boulevard
Oak Brook, IL 60523-2670
630-571-2670
http://www.rsna.org

C APPENDIX

State Licensing Agencies

Most states (including the territory of Puerto Rico and the District of Columbia) have licensing laws in effect for radiographers. Although the laws and regulations vary widely from state to state, in general, states that require licenses accept the Examination in Radiography of the American Registry of Radiologic Technologists (ARRT) to obtain a license to practice.

Students or radiographers desiring information should contact the appropriate agency for the particular state. A current listing of contacts for state licensing agencies is maintained by the American Society of Radiologic Technologists on their website at http://www.asrt.org and at the ARRT website at https://www.arrt.org/State-Licensing/State-Contacts. The ARRT always maintains a current listing of the agencies in each state that control the credentialing of radiologic science professionals.

Radiologic and imaging sciences professionals should be aware that some states have credentialing requirements that are not universal—for example, Michigan requires only mammography and computed tomography technologists to have credentials. It is the professional's responsibility to ascertain the credentialing requirements and to meet them in order to practice.

The American Registry of Radiologic Technologists Code of Ethics

The Code of Ethics forms the first part of the *Standards of Ethics*. The Code of Ethics shall serve as a guide by which Certificate Holders and Candidates may evaluate their professional conduct as it relates to patients, healthcare consumers, employers, colleagues, and other members of the healthcare team. The Code of Ethics is intended to assist Certificate Holders and Candidates in maintaining a high level of ethical conduct and in providing for the protection, safety, and comfort of patients. The Code of Ethics is aspirational.

1. The radiologic technologist acts in a professional manner, responds to patient needs, and supports colleagues and associates in providing quality patient care.
2. The radiologic technologist acts to advance the principal objective of the profession to provide services to humanity with full respect for the dignity of mankind.
3. The radiologic technologist delivers patient care and service unrestricted by the concerns of personal attributes or the nature of the disease or illness, and without discrimination on the basis of sex, race, creed, religion, or socio-economic status.
4. The radiologic technologist practices technology founded upon theoretical knowledge and concepts, uses equipment and accessories consistent with the purposes for which they were designed, and employs procedures and techniques appropriately.
5. The radiologic technologist assesses situations; exercises care, discretion, and judgment; assumes responsibility for professional decisions; and acts in the best interest of the patient.
6. The radiologic technologist acts as an agent through observation and communication to obtain pertinent information for the physician to aid in the diagnosis and treatment of the patient and recognizes that interpretation and diagnosis are outside the scope of practice for the profession.
7. The radiologic technologist uses equipment and accessories, employs techniques and procedures, performs services in accordance with an accepted standard of practice, and demonstrates expertise in minimizing radiation exposure to the patient, self, and other members of the healthcare team.
8. The radiologic technologist practices ethical conduct appropriate to the profession and protects the patient's right to quality radiologic technology care.
9. The radiologic technologist respects confidences entrusted in the course of professional practice, respects the patient's right to privacy, and reveals confidential information only as required by law or to protect the welfare of the individual or the community.
10. The radiologic technologist continually strives to improve knowledge and skills by participating in continuing education and professional activities, sharing knowledge with colleagues, and investigating new aspects of professional practice.

E APPENDIX

Commonly Used Drugs by Brand and Generic Names

Commonly Used Drugs by Brand Name

Brand Name	Generic Name	Route(s)	Classification
Abilify	Aripiprazole	Oral, parenteral	Antipsychotic
Activase	Alteplase	Parenteral	Thrombolytic
Actonel	Risedronate	Oral	Osteoporosis
Actos	Pioglitazone	Oral	Antidiabetic
Adderall	Amphetamine salts	Oral	Stimulant
Adenocard	Adenosine	Parenteral	Antiarrhythmic
Adrenalin	Epinephrine	Parenteral	Stimulant
Advair	Salmeterol-fluticasone	Inhalation	Bronchodilator, corticosteroid
Allegra	Fexofenadine	Oral	Antihistamine
Amaryl	Glimepiride	Oral	Antidiabetic
Ambien	Zolpidem	Oral	Hypnotic
Amidate	Etomidate	Parenteral	Anesthetic
Amoxil	Amoxicillin	Oral	Antibiotic
Augmentin	Amoxicillin-clavulanate	Oral	Antibiotic
Aricept	Donepezil	Oral	Antialzheimer
Ativan	Lorazepam	Oral, parenteral	Anxiolytic atropine
Atripla	Efavirenz-emtricitabine-tenofovir	Oral	Antibiotic
Atropine	Atropine	Oral, parenteral, opthalmic	Anticholinergic
Atrovent	Ipratropium	Inhalation	Bronchodilator
Benadryl	Diphenhydramine	Oral, parenteral	Antihistamine
Biaxin	Clarithromycin	Oral	Antibiotic
Carbocaine	Mepivacaine	Parenteral	Local anesthetic
Cardizem	Diltiazem	Oral, parenteral	Antiarrhythmic
Celebrex	Celecoxib	Oral	Antiinflammatory
Celexa	Citalopram	Oral	Antidepressant
Claritin	Loratadine	Oral	Antihistamine
Cipro	Ciprofloxacin	Oral, parenteral	Antibiotic
Compazine	Prochlorperazine	Oral, parenteral	Antiemetic
Cordarone	Amiodarone	Oral, parenteral	Antiarrhythmic
Coreg	Carvedilol	Oral	Antihypertensive
Coumadin	Warfarin	Oral, parenteral	Anticoagulant
Cozaar	Losartan	Oral	Antihypertensive
Crestor	Rosuvastatin	Oral	Antihyperlipidemic
Cymbalta	Duloxetine	Oral	Antidepressant
Decadron	Dexamethasone	Oral, parenteral	Corticosteroid
Deltasone	Prednisone	Oral	Corticosteroid
Depakote	Valproate	Oral, parenteral	Antiepileptic
Depo-Medrol	Methylprednisolone	Parenteral	Corticosteroid
Detrol LA	Tolterodine	Oral	Anticholinergic
Diflucan	Fluconazole	Oral, parenteral	Antifungal
Dilantin	Phenytoin	Oral, parenteral	Antiepileptic
Diovan	Valsartan	Oral	Antihypertensive
Diprivan	Propofol	Parenteral	Anesthetic
Ditropan XL	Oxybutynin	Oral, transdermal	Anticholinergic
Dobutrex	Dobutamine	Parenteral	Stimulant
Dulcolax	Bisacodyl	Oral	Laxative

Commonly Used Drugs by Brand Name—cont'd

Brand Name	Generic Name	Route(s)	Classification
Duragesic	Fentanyl	Parenteral, transdermal	Analgesic
Ecotrin, or various brand names	Aspirin	Oral	Analgesic, antiplatelets
Effexor	Venlafaxine	Oral	Antidepressant
Eliquis	Apixaban	Oral	Anticoagulant
Eskolith/LithoBid	Lithium	Oral	Mood Stabilizer
Evista	Raloxifene	Oral	Osteoporosis
Feraheme	Ferumoxytal	Parenteral	Antianemia
Flovent	Fluticasone	Inhalation	Corticosteroid
Fosamax	Alendronate	Oral	Osteoporosis
Fungizone	Amphotericin B	Parenteral	Antifungal
GoLytely	Polyethylene glycol electrolyte solution	Oral	Laxative
Glucophage	Metformin	Oral	Antidiabetic
Glucotrol	Glipizide	Oral	Antidiabetic
Haldol	Haloperidol	Oral, parenteral	Antipsychotic
Heparin	Heparin	Parenteral	Anticoagulant
Hydroduril	Hydrochlorothiazide	Oral	Diuretic
Intropin	Dopamine	Parenteral	Stimulant
Invokana	Canagliflozin	Oral	Antidiabetic
Januvia	Sitagliptin	Oral	Antidiabetic
Keflex	Cephalexin	Oral	Antibiotic
Klonopin	Clonazepam	Oral	Antiepileptic, antianxiety
Lamictal	Lamotrigine	Oral	Antiepileptic
Lanoxin	Digoxin	Oral, parenteral	Antiarrhythmic
Lasix	Furosemide	Oral, parenteral	Diuretic
Lantus, Humulin/ Novolin	Glargine Insulin, Regular/NPH Insulin	Parenteral	Antidiabetics
Levophed	Norepinephrine	Parenteral	Vasoconstrictor
Levaquin	Levofloxacin	Oral, parenteral	Antibiotic
Lexapro	Escitalopram	Oral	Antidepressant
Lipitor	Atorvastatin	Oral	Antihyperlipidemic
Lopressor	Metoprolol	Oral, parenteral	Antihypertensive
Lotensin	Benazepril	Oral	Antihypertensive
Lovenox	Enoxaparin	Parenteral	Anticoagulant
Lyrica	Pregabalin	Oral	Antiepileptic
Lunesta	Eszopiclone	Oral	Hypnotic
Magnesium Citrate	Magnesium Citrate	Oral	Laxative
Mephyton	Phytonadione	Oral, parenteral	Coagulant
Micronase	Glyburide	Oral	Antidiabetic
Miralax	Polyethylene glycol	Oral	Laxative
Mirapex	Pramipexole	Oral	Antiparkinson
Motrin	Ibuprofen	Oral	Antiinflammatory
MS Contin, or various brand names	Morphine	Oral, parenteral	Analgesic
Namenda	Memantine	Oral	Antialzheimer
Naprosyn	Naproxen	Oral	Antiinflammatory
Narcan	Naloxone	Parenteral, intranasal	Opioid antagonist
Neurontin	Gabapentin	Oral	Antiepileptic
Nitropress	Nitroprusside	Parenteral	Vasodilator
Nitrostat, various other brands	Nitroglycerin	Oral, parenteral, transdermal	Vasodilators
Norvasc	Amlodipine	Oral	Antihypertensive
Onglyza	Saxagliptin	Oral	Antidiabetic
OxyContin, Roxi-codone	Oxycodone	Oral	Analgesic
Paxil	Paroxetine	Oral	Antidepressant

Continued

Commonly Used Drugs by Brand Name—cont'd

Brand Name	Generic Name	Route(s)	Classification
Penicillin VK	Penicillin VK	Oral	Antibiotic
Pepcid	Famotidine	Oral, parenteral	Antiulcer
Percocet	Oxycodone-APAP	Oral	Analgesic
Phenergan	Promethazine	Oral, parenteral	Antiemetics
Phytonadione	Vitamin K	Oral, parenteral	Coagulant
Plavix	Clopidogrel	Oral	Antiplatelet
Pradaxa	Dabigatran	Oral	Anticoagulant
Premarin	Conjugated estrogen	Oral	Oral, vaginal
Prevacid	Lansoprazole	Oral, parenteral	Antiulcer
Prilosec	Omeprazole	Oral	Antiulcer
Proair HFA	Albuterol	Inhalation	Bronchodilator
Prozac	Fluoxetine	Oral	Antidepressant
Reglan	Metoclopramide	Oral, parenteral	Antiemetic
ReoPro	Abciximab	Parenteral	Antiplatelet
Requip	Ropinirole	Oral	Antiparkinson
Restoril	Temazepam	Oral	Hypnotic
Retavase	Reteplase	Parenteral	Thrombolytic
Risperdal	Risperidone	Oral, parenteral	Antipsychotic
Ritalin	Methylphenidate	Oral	Stimulant
Rocephin	Ceftriaxone	Parenteral	Antibiotic
Romazicon	Flumazenil	Parenteral	Benzodiazepine antagonist
Serevent	Salmeterol	Inhalation	Bronchodilator
Seroquel	Quetiapine	Oral	Antipsychotic
Sinemet	Levodopa-carbidopa	Oral	Antiparkinson
Slo Fe, other various brands	Ferrous Sulfate	Oral	Antianemic
Solu-Cortef	Hydrocortisone	Parenteral	Corticosteroid
Spiriva	Tiotropium	Inhalation	Bronchodilator
Synthroid	Levothyroxine	Oral, parenteral	Thyroid hormone
Tenormin	Atenolol	Oral	Antihypertensive
Thorazine	Chlorpromazine	Oral, parenteral	Antipsychotic
Topamax	Topiramate	Oral	Antiepileptic
Toprol-XL	Metoprolol Succinate	Oral	Antihypertension
Tylenol	Acetaminophen	Oral	Analgesic
Ultane	Sevoflurane	Inhalation	Anesthetic
Ultram	Tramadol	Oral	Analgesic
Valium	Diazepam	Oral, parenteral	Antianxiety
Vasotec	Enalapril	Oral, parenteral	Antihypertensive
Verapamil	Verapamil	Oral, parenteral	Antiarrhythmic
Versed	Midazolam	Oral, parenteral	Antianxiety
Vicodin, Norco	Hydrocodone-APAP	Oral	Analgesic
Victoza	Liraglutide	Parenteral	Antidiabetic
Vistaril	Hydroxyzine	Oral, parenteral	Antihistamines
Wellbutrin	Bupropion	Oral	Antidepressant
Xanax	Alprazolam	Oral	Antianxiety
Xarelto	Rivaroxaban	Oral	Anticoagulant
Xylocaine	Lidocaine	Parenteral	Antiarrhythmic, local anesthetic
Zantac	Ranitidine	Oral, parenteral	Antiulcer
Zestril	Lisinopril	Oral	Antihypertensive
Zithromax	Azithromycin	Oral, parenteral	Antibiotic
Zocor	Simvastatin	Oral	Antihyperlipidemic
Zofran	Ondansetron	Oral, parenteral	Antiemetic
Zoloft	Sertraline	Oral	Antidepressant
Zovirax	Acyclovir	Oral, parenteral	Antiviral
Zyprexa	Olanzapine	Oral, parenteral	Antipsychotic

APAP, N-acetyl-para-amino-phenol (acetaminophen).

Commonly Used Drugs by Generic Name

Generic Name	Brand Name	Route(s)	Classification
Abciximab	ReoPro	Parenteral	Antiplatelet
Acetaminophen	Tylenol	Oral	Analgesic
Acyclovir	Zovirax	Oral, parenteral	Antiviral
Adenosine	Adenocard	Parenteral	Antiarrhythmic
Albuterol	Proair HFA	Inhalation	Bronchodilator
Alendronate	Fosamax	Oral	Osteoporosis
Alprazolam	Xanax	Oral	Antianxiety
Alteplase	Activase	Parenteral	Thrombolytic
Amiodarone	Cordarone	Oral, parenteral	Antiarrhythmic
Amlodipine	Norvasc	Oral	Antihypertensive
Amoxicillin	Amoxil	Oral	Antibiotic
Amoxicillin-clavulanate	Augmentin	Oral	Antibiotic
Amphetamine salts	Adderall	Oral	Stimulant
Amphotericin B	Fungizone	Parenteral	Antifungal
Apixaban	Eliquis	Oral	Anticoagulant
Aripiprazole	Abilify	Oral, parenteral	Antipsychotic
Aspirin	Ecotrin, or various brand names	Oral	Analgesic, antiplatelet
Atenolol	Tenormin	Oral	Antihypertensive
Atorvastatin	Lipitor	Oral	Antihyperlipidemic
Atropine	Atropine	Oral, parenteral, opthalmic	Anticholinergic
Azithromycin	Zithromax	Oral, parenteral	Antibiotic
Benazepril	Lotensin	Oral	Antihypertensive
Bisacodyl	Dulcolax	Oral	Laxative
Bupropion	Wellbutrin	Oral	Antidepressant
Canagliflozin	Invokana	Oral	Antidiabetic
Carvedilol	Coreg	Oral	Antihypertensive
Ceftriaxone	Rocephen	Parenteral	Antibiotic
Celecoxib	Celebrex	Oral	Antiinflammatory
Cephalexin	Keflex	Oral	Antibiotic
Chlorpromazine	Thorazine	Oral, parenteral	Antipsychotic
Ciprofloxacin	Cipro	Oral, parenteral	Antibiotic
Citalopram	Celexa	Oral	Antidepressant
Clarithromycin	Biaxin	Oral	Antibiotic
Clonazepam	Klonopin	Oral	Antiepileptic
Clopidogrel	Plavix	Oral	Antiplatelet
Conjugated estrogens	Premarin	Oral, vaginal	Female hormone
Dabigatran	Pradaxa	Oral	Anticoagulant
Dexamethasone	Decadron	Oral, parenteral	Corticosteroid
Diazepam	Valium	Oral, parenteral	Antianxiety
Digoxin	Lanoxin	Oral, parenteral	Antiarrhythmic
Diltiazem	Cardizem	Oral, parenteral	Antiarrhythmic
Diphenhydramine	Benadryl	Oral, parenteral	Antihistamine
Dobutamine	Dobutrex	Parenteral	Stimulant
Donepezil	Aricept	Oral	Antialzheimer
Dopamine	Intropin	Parenteral	Stimulant
Duloxetine	Cymbalta	Oral	Antidepressant
Efavirenz-emtricitabine-tenofovir	Atripla	Oral	Antiviral
Enalapril	Vasotec	Oral, parenteral	Antihypertensive
Enoxaparin	Lovenox	Parenteral	Anticoagulant
Epinephrine	Adrenalin	Parenteral	Stimulant
Escitalopram	Lexapro	Oral	Antidepressant
Eszopiclone	Lunesta	Oral	Hypnotic
Etomidate	Amidate	Parenteral	Anesthetic
Famotidine	Pepcid	Oral	Antiulcer
Fentanyl	Duragesic	Parenteral, transdermal	Analgesic
Ferrous Sulfate	Slo Fe, other various brands	Oral	Antianemic

Continued

Commonly Used Drugs by Generic Name—cont'd

Generic Name	Brand Name	Route(s)	Classification
Ferumoxytal	Feraheme	Parenteral	Antianemia
Fexofenadine	Allegra	Oral	Antihistamine
Fluconazole	Diflucan	Oral, parenteral	Antifungal
Flumazenil	Romazicon	Parenteral	Benzodiazepine antagonist
Fluoxetine	Prozac	Oral	Antidepressant
Fluticasone	Flovent	Inhalation	Corticosteroid
Furosemide	Lasix	Oral, parenteral	Diuretic
Gabapentin	Neurontin	Oral	Antiepileptic
Glargine Insulin, Regular/ NPH Insulin	Lantus, Humulin/Novolin	Parenteral	Antidiabetics
Glimepiride	Amaryl	Oral	Antidiabetic
Glipizide	Glucotrol	Oral	Antidiabetic
Glyburide	Micronase	Oral	Antidiabetic
Haloperidol	Haldol	Oral, parenteral	Antipsychotic
Heparin	Heparin	Parenteral	Anticoagulant
Hydrochlorothiazide	Hydroduril	Oral, parenteral	Diuretic
Hydrocodone-APAP	Vicodin, Norco	Oral	Analgesic
Hydrocortisone	Solu-Cortef	Parenteral	Corticosteroid
Hydroxyzine	Vistaril	Oral, parenteral	Antihistamine
Ibuprofen	Motrin	Oral	Antiinflammatory
Ipratropium	Atrovent	Inhalation	Bronchodilator
Lamotrigine	Lamictal	Oral	Antiepileptic
Lansoprazole	Prevacid	Oral, parenteral	Antiulcer
Levodopa Carbidopa	Sinemet	Oral	Antiparkinson
Levofloxacin	Levaquin	Oral, parenteral	Antibiotic
Levothyroxine	Synthroid	Oral	Thyroid hormone
Lidocaine	Xylocaine	Parenteral	Antiarrhythmic, local anesthetic
Liraglutide	Victoza	Parenteral	Antidiabetic
Lisinopril	Zestril	Oral	Antihypertensive
Lithium	Eskolith/LithoBid	Oral	Mood stabilizer
Loratadine	Claritin	Oral	Antihistamine
Lorazepam	Ativan	Oral, parenteral	Antianxiety
Losartan	Cozaar	Oral	Antihypertensive
Magnesium Citrate	Magnesium Citrate	Oral	Laxative
Memantine	Namenda	Oral	Antialzheimer
Mepivacaine	Carbocaine	Parenteral	Local anesthetic
Metformin	Glucophage	Oral	Antidiabetic
Methylphenidate	Ritalin	Oral	Stimulant
Methylprednisolone	Depo-Medrol	Parenteral	Corticosteroid
Metoclopramide	Reglan	Oral, parenteral	Antiemetic
Metoprolol Tartrate	Lopressor	Oral, parenteral	Antihypertensive
Metoprolol Succinate	Toprol-XL	Oral	Antihypertensive
Midazolam	Versed	Oral, parenteral	Antianxiety
Morphine	MS Contin, or various brand names	Oral, parenteral	Analgesic
Naloxone	Narcan	Parenteral, intranasal	Opioid antagonist
Naproxen	Naprosyn	Oral	Antiinflammatory
Nitroglycerin	Nitrostat, various other brands	Oral, parenteral, transdermal	Vasodilator
Nitroprusside	Nitropress	Parenteral	Vasodilator
Norepinephrine	Levophed	Parenteral	Vasoconstrictor
Olanzapine	Zyprexa	Oral, parenteral	Antipsychotic
Omeprazole	Prilosec	Oral	Antiulcer
Ondansetron	Zofran	Oral, parenteral	Antiemetic
Oxybutynin	Ditropan XL	Oral, transdermal	Anticholinergic
Oxycodone	OxyContin, Roxicodone	Oral	Analgesic
Oxycodone-APAP	Percocet	Oral	Analgesic
Paroxetine	Paxil	Oral	Antidepressant

Commonly Used Drugs by Generic Name—cont'd

Generic Name	Brand Name	Route(s)	Classification
Penicillin VK	Penicillin VK	Oral	Antibiotic
Phenytoin	Dilantin	Oral, parenteral	Antiepileptic
Phytonadione	Mephyton	Oral, parenteral	Coagulant
Pioglitazone	Actos	Oral	Antidiabetic
Polyethylene glycol	Miralax	Oral	Laxative
Pramipexole	Mirapex	Oral	Antiparkinson
Prednisone	Deltasone	Oral	Corticosteroid
Pregabalin	Lyrica	Oral	Antiepileptic
Prochlorperazine	Compazine	Oral, parenteral	Antiemetic
Promethazine	Phenergan	Oral, parenteral	Antiemetics
Propofol	Diprivan	Parenteral	Anesthetic
Quetiapine	Seroquel	Oral	Antipsychotic
Raloxifene	Evista	Oral	Osteoporosis
Ranitidine	Zantac	Oral, parenteral	Antiulcer
Reteplase	Retavase	Parenteral	Thrombolytic
Risedronate	Actonel	Oral	Osteoporosis
Risperidone	Risperdal	Oral, parenteral	Antipsychotic
Rivaroxaban	Xarelto	Oral	Anticoagulant
Ropinirole	Requip	Oral	Antiparkinson
Rosuvastatin	Crestor	Oral	Antihyperlipidemic
Salmeterol	Serevent	Inhalation	Bronchodilator
Salmeterol-fluticasone	Advair	Inhalation	Bronchodilator, corticosteroid
Saxagliptin	Onglyza	Oral	Antidiabetic
Sertraline	Zoloft	Oral	Antidepressant
Sevoflurane	Ultane	Inhalation	Anesthetic
Simvastatin	Zocor	Oral	Antihyperlipidemic
Sitagliptin	Januvia	Oral	Antidiabetic
Temazepam	Restoril	Oral	Hypnotic
Tiotropium	Spiriva	Inhalation	Bronchodilator
Tolterodine	Detrol LA	Oral	Anticholinergic
Topiramate	Topamax	Oral	Antiepileptic
Tramadol	Ultram	Oral	Analgesic
Valproate	Depakote	Oral, parenteral	Antiepileptic, mood stabilizer
Valsartan	Diovan	Oral	Antihypertensive
Venlafaxine	Effexor	Oral	Antidepressant
Vitamin K	Phytonadione	Oral, parenteral	Antialzheimer
Warfarin	Coumadin	Oral, parenteral	Anticoagulant
Zolpidem	Ambien	Oral	Hypnotic

APAP, N-acetyl-para-amino-phenol (acetaminophen).

The Patient Care Partnership: Understanding Expectations, Rights, and Responsibilities

When you need hospital care, your doctor and the nurses and other professionals at our hospital are committed to working with you and your family to meet your health care needs. Our dedicated doctors and staff serve the community in all its ethnic, religious, and economic diversity. Our goal is for you and your family to have the same care and attention we would want for our families and ourselves.

The sections explain some of the basics about how you can expect to be treated during your hospital stay. They also cover what we will need from you to care for you better. If you have questions at any time, please ask them. Unasked or unanswered questions can add to the stress of being in the hospital. Your comfort and confidence in your care are very important to us.

WHAT TO EXPECT DURING YOUR HOSPITAL STAY

High-Quality Hospital Care

Our first priority is to provide you the care you need, when you need it, with skill, compassion, and respect. Tell your caregivers if you have concerns about your care or if you have pain. You have the right to know the identity of doctors, nurses, and others involved in your care, and you have the right to know when they are students, residents, or other trainees.

Clean and Safe Environment

Our hospital works hard to keep you safe. We use special policies and procedures to avoid making mistakes in your care and keep you free from abuse or neglect. If anything unexpected and significant happens during your hospital stay, you will be told what happened, and any resulting changes in your care will be discussed with you.

Involvement in Your Care

You and your doctor often make decisions about your care before you go to the hospital. At other times, especially in emergencies, those decisions are made during your hospital stay. When decision making takes place, it should include the following:

- **Discussing your medical condition and information about medically appropriate treatment choices.** To make informed decisions with your doctor, you need to understand:
  - The benefits and risks of each treatment.

- Whether your treatment is experimental or part of a research study.
- What you can reasonably expect from your treatment and any long-term effects it might have on your quality of life.
- What you and your family will need to do after you leave the hospital.
- The financial consequences of using uncovered services or out-of-network providers.
- *Please tell your caregivers if you need more information about treatment choices.*
- **Discussing your treatment plan.** When you enter the hospital, you sign a general consent to treatment. In some cases, such as surgery or experimental treatment, you may be asked to confirm in writing that you understand what is planned and agree to it. This process protects your right to consent to or refuse a treatment. Your doctor will explain the medical consequences of refusing recommended treatment. It also protects your right to decide if you want to participate in a research study.
- **Getting information from you.** Your caregivers need complete and correct information about your health and coverage so that they can make good decisions about your care. That includes:
  - Past illnesses, surgeries, or hospital stays.
  - Past allergic reactions.
  - Any medicines or dietary supplements (such as vitamins and herbs) that you are taking.
  - Any network or admission requirements under your health plan.

Understanding your health care goals and values. You may have health care goals and values or spiritual beliefs that are important to your well-being. They will be taken into account as much as possible throughout your hospital stay. Make sure your doctor, your family, and your care team know your wishes.

Understanding who should make decisions when you cannot. If you have signed a health care power of attorney stating who should speak for you if you become unable to make health care decisions for yourself, or a "living will" or "advance directive" that states your wishes about end-of-life care, give copies to your doctor, your family, and your care team. If you or your family need help making difficult decisions, counselors, chaplains, and others are available to help.

Protection of Your Privacy

We respect the confidentiality of your relationship with your doctor and other caregivers, and the sensitive information about your health and health care that are part of that relationship.

State and federal laws and hospital operating policies protect the privacy of your medical information. You will receive a *Notice of Privacy Practices* that describes the ways that we use, disclose, and safeguard patient information and that explains how you can obtain a copy of information from our records about your care.

Preparing You and Your Family for When You Leave the Hospital

Your doctor works with hospital staff and professionals in your community. You and your family also play an important role in your care. The success of your treatment often depends on your efforts to follow medication, diet, and therapy plans. Your family may need to help care for you at home. You can expect us to help you identify sources of follow-up care and to let you know if our hospital has a financial interest in any referrals. As long as you agree that we can share information about your care with them, we will coordinate our activities with your caregivers outside the hospital. You can also expect to receive information and, where possible, training about the self-care you will need when you go home.

Help with Your Bill and Filing Insurance Claims

Our staff will file claims for you with health care insurers or other programs such as Medicare and Medicaid. They will also help your doctor with needed documentation. Hospital bills and insurance coverage are often confusing. If you have questions about your bill, contact our business office. If you need help understanding your insurance coverage or health plan, start with your insurance company or health benefits manager. If you do not have health coverage, we will try to help you and your family find financial help or make other arrangements. We need your help with collecting needed information and other requirements to obtain coverage or assistance.

While you are here, you will receive more detailed notices about some of the rights you have as a hospital patient and how to exercise them. We are always interested in improving.

Student Labs

CHAPTER 13 SAFE PATIENT MOVEMENT AND HANDLING TECHNIQUES

Patient Care Laboratory Activities

STUDENT NAME: _____ DATE: _____

LAB 13.1 Patient Transfer Techniques

Objective
- To demonstrate proper wheelchair and cart transfer techniques

Equipment
- Wheelchair, cart, transfer belt, Hoyer lift, transfer sheet, moving device

Procedures
- On completion of this laboratory activity, the student will be able to perform the following procedures:
  - Before doing any transfer, the person playing the role of the clinician should introduce herself/himself, explain what will happen during the transfer, and ask the person playing the role of the patient how much assistance is required. In a standby assist transfer, "patients" should answer "I think I can do this myself." "Patients" in transfers requiring more assistance should answer, "I think that I need some help."

Standby Assist Wheelchair Transfer	Yes	No
1. Move the wheelchair footrests out of the way.	_____	_____
2. Position the wheelchair at a 45-degree angle to the table, and be sure that the wheel locks are locked.	_____	_____
3. Instruct the patient to sit on the edge of the wheelchair seat.	_____	_____
4. Instruct the patient to push down on the arms of the chair to assist in rising and then to stand up slowly.	_____	_____
5. Direct the patient to reach out and hold onto the table with the hand closest to the table and then to turn slowly until he or she feels the table behind him or her.	_____	_____
6. Instruct the patient to hold onto the table with both hands and then to sit down.	_____	_____

Assisted Standing Pivot Wheelchair Transfer	Yes	No
1. Move the wheelchair footrests out of the way.	_____	_____
2. Position the wheelchair at a 45-degree angle to the table with the patient's strongest side closest to the table. If the patient has loose-fitting clothes, place a transfer belt around the patient's waist.	_____	_____
3. Be sure that the wheel locks are locked.	_____	_____
4. Direct the patient to sit on the edge of the wheelchair seat, providing assistance as needed.	_____	_____
5. Instruct the patient to push down on the arms of the wheelchair to assist in rising.	_____	_____
6. Bend at the knees, keeping the back stationary, and grasp the transfer belt with both hands. Block the patient's feet and knees to provide stability, especially for patients who are paraplegic and hemiplegic.	_____	_____
7. Assist the patient in rising to a standing position.	_____	_____
8. Ask the patient whether he or she is feeling all right. If the patient reports any feelings of dizziness or exhibits any of the other signs of orthostatic hypotension, let him or her stand for a moment, taking slow deep breaths until the feeling subsides.	_____	_____
9. Pivot the patient toward the table until the patient can feel the table against the back of the thighs.	_____	_____
10. Ask the patient to support himself or herself on the table with both hands and sit down, assisting as necessary.	_____	_____

Two-Person Wheelchair Lift	Yes	No
1. Plan for the lift by locating an assistant, who will lift the patient's feet as you lift the patient's torso.	_____	_____
2. Remove the armrests, swing away or remove the leg rests, apply wheel locks, and direct the patient to cross his or her arms over the chest.	_____	_____
3. Stand behind the patient, reach under the patient's axillae, and grasp the patient's crossed forearms. Direct the assistant to squat in front of the patient and cradle the patient's thighs in one hand and the calves in the other hand.	_____	_____
4. On command, lift the patient to clear the wheelchair, and move the patient as a unit to the desired place.	_____	_____

LAB 13.1   Patient Transfer Techniques—cont'd

Cart Transfer with a Moving Device	Yes	No
1. Move the cart alongside the table, preferably on the patient's strong or less affected side. Place it as close to the table as possible, and then secure it by depressing the wheel locks. In addition, place sandbags or other devices on the floor to block the wheels satisfactorily.	_____	_____
2. Place the patient at an oblique angle away from the table while the moving device is placed to the midpoint of the back.	_____	_____
3. Return the patient to a supine position so that he or she is halfway onto the moving device.	_____	_____
4. Grab the draw sheet, and use it to move the patient slowly onto the table.	_____	_____
5. Remove the moving device, turning the patient obliquely if necessary.	_____	_____

Cart Transfer without a Moving Device	Yes	No
1. Move the cart alongside the table, preferably on the patient's strong or less affected side. Place it as close to the table as possible, and then secure it by depressing the wheel locks. In addition, place sandbags or other devices on the floor to block wheels satisfactorily.	_____	_____
2. Begin by rolling up the draw sheet on both sides of the patient. Be sure that the draw sheet is completely under the patient and straightened before the transfer.	_____	_____
3. Support the patient's head and upper body from the far side of the radiographic table. Direct a second assistant to support the patient's pelvic girdle from the cart side and a third assistant to support the patient's legs from the table side.	_____	_____
4. Cross the patient's arms over the chest to avoid injury or interfering with a smooth transfer.	_____	_____
5. Direct the second assistant supporting the pelvic girdle to stand on the opposite side of the cart, and make sure that the cart does not move away from the table during the transfer.	_____	_____
6. On command, grasp the rolled-up draw sheet and slowly pull the patient to the edge of the cart. On a second command, slowly lift and pull the patient onto the table.	_____	_____

Comments: _____

_____

_____

Evaluator's Signature: _____

Student's Signature: _____

CHAPTER 14 IMMOBILIZATION TECHNIQUES

Patient Care Laboratory Activities

STUDENT NAME: _____ DATE: _____

LAB 14.1   Immobilization Devices

Objective

- To demonstrate proper technique for patient immobilization

Equipment

- Oblique sponge
- Finger sponge
- Strap
- Compression bands
- Sandbags
- Head clamp

Procedure

- On completion of this laboratory activity, the student will be able to perform the following procedure:

Immobilization Devices	Yes	No
1. Position a patient with a sponge for an oblique lumbar spine position.	_____	_____
2. Position a patient's hand in a fan lateral position on a sponge.	_____	_____
3. Position a patient for an axial calcaneus position using a strap.	_____	_____
4. Position a patient on a table in a semi-erect position using compression bands.	_____	_____
5. Position a patient in an erect lateral cervical position using sandbags.	_____	_____
6. Position a patient for an anteroposterior (AP) skull radiograph using head clamps.	_____	_____

Comments: _____

_____

_____

Evaluator's Signature: _____

Student's Signature: _____

CHAPTER 14 IMMOBILIZATION TECHNIQUES

Patient Care Laboratory Activities

STUDENT NAME: _____ DATE: _____

LAB 14.2   Pediatric Immobilization Techniques

Objective
- To demonstrate proper techniques for pediatric immobilization

Equipment
- Pediatric patient or doll
- Sheet
- Pigg-O-Stat
- Velcro restraint board
- Octostop

Procedures
- On completion of this laboratory activity, the student will be able to perform the following procedures:

Sheet Restraint/Mummy Wrap	Yes	No
1. Position the child in the center of a triangularly folded sheet so that the shoulders are just above the top fold.	_____	_____
2. Bring the left corner of the sheet over the left arm and under the body so that approximately 2 feet of the sheet extends beyond the right side of the body. Make sure the child is not lying on the left arm.	_____	_____
3. Tuck the 2 feet of sheet over the right arm and under the body. Again, make sure the child is not lying on the arm.	_____	_____
4. Bring the remaining sheet over the body, tucking the sheet securely under the left side of the body. Secure the sheet in place with tape.	_____	_____

Using Specialized Pediatric Immobilization Devices	Yes	No
1. Position a pediatric patient in a Pigg-O-Stat for an AP chest radiograph.	_____	_____
2. Position a pediatric patient on a Velcro strap restraint board.	_____	_____
3. Position a pediatric patient on an Octostop restraint board.	_____	_____

Comments: _____

_____

_____

Evaluator's Signature: _____

Student's Signature: _____

CHAPTER 15 VITAL SIGNS, OXYGEN, CHEST TUBES, AND LINES

Patient Care Laboratory Activities

STUDENT NAME: _____ DATE: _____

LAB 15.1   Monitoring Patient Vital Signs

Objective

- To measure a patient's vital signs of temperature, pulse, respiration, and blood pressure

Equipment

- Thermometer
- Blood pressure kit

Procedures

- On completion of this laboratory activity, the student will be able to perform the following skills:

Temperature: Oral Method	Yes	No
1. Place the oral thermometer under the patient's tongue.	_____	_____
2. Ensure that the thermometer is kept in place until a stable reading is obtained.	_____	_____
3. Read the oral thermometer, and record the reading.	_____	_____

Respiration	Yes	No
1. Measure a patient's respiration by observing the patient's chest or abdomen for a 60-second period.	_____	_____
2. Record the number of respirations per minute.	_____	_____

Pulse	Yes	No
1. Measure a patient's pulse rate at the radial artery near the wrist for a 60-second period.	_____	_____
2. Record the patient's pulse rate per minute.	_____	_____

Blood Pressure	Yes	No
1. Obtain a sphygmomanometer and stethoscope.	_____	_____
2. Place the cuff of the sphygmomanometer on the patient's upper arm midway between the elbow and shoulder.	_____	_____
3. Inflate the cuff above the systolic pressure to stop blood flow to the arm.	_____	_____
4. With the stethoscope placed over the brachial artery in the antecubital fossa of the elbow, slowly release the cuff of the sphygmomanometer.	_____	_____
5. When the first sound of blood flow is heard through the stethoscope, record the systolic pressure reading.	_____	_____
6. When the sound of blood flowing through the arm ceases, record the diastolic pressure reading.	_____	_____

Comments: _____

_____

_____

Evaluator's Signature: _____

Student's Signature: _____

CHAPTER 17 INFECTION CONTROL

Patient Care Laboratory Activities

STUDENT NAME: _____ DATE: _____

LAB 17.1   Proper Hand-Washing Technique

Objective
- To demonstrate proper hand-washing technique

Equipment
- Sink
- Soap
- Toweling

Procedure
- On completion of this laboratory activity, the student will be able to perform the following procedure:

Hand Washing	Yes	No
1. Approach the sink. Consider it to be contaminated. Avoid contact with clothing. Use foot or knee levers when available. If not, use toweling to handle all controls. Adjust water flow to avoid splashing. Adjust water temperature to comfort.	_____	_____
2. Wet hands thoroughly with water, keeping the hands lower than the elbows.	_____	_____
3. Apply soap. Soap should be available in liquid form and can be applied by using foot or knee levers. Soap can also be dispensed from a pump.	_____	_____
4. Use a firm, vigorous, rotary motion, beginning at the wrist and working toward the fingertips. Rub the palms, back of the hands, between the fingers, and under the nails.	_____	_____
5. Rinse and allow water to run down over hands.	_____	_____
6. Repeat the entire process to cleanse from the elbow to the fingertips.	_____	_____
7. Turn off the water. Use toweling on handles if foot or knee levers are not available.	_____	_____
8. Dry from the elbow to the fingertips, never returning to an area.	_____	_____

Comments: _____

_____

_____

Evaluator's Signature: _____

Student's Signature: _____

CHAPTER 17 INFECTION CONTROL

Patient Care Laboratory Activities

STUDENT NAME: _____ DATE: _____

LAB 17.2   Contact Precautions Technique

Objective
- To demonstrate the proper method for performing a radiographic examination on a patient with contact precautions

Equipment
- Cassettes and cassette bags
- Gowns, gloves, caps, masks, goggles
- Portable machine
- Lead aprons

Procedure
- On completion of this laboratory activity, the student will be able to perform the following procedure:

Contact Precautions	Yes	No
1. Determine the correct number of cassettes needed for the examination, and place each cassette into a protective bag.	_____	_____
2. Move the portable machine to the isolated room.	_____	_____
3. Locate the isolation supplies for the room.	_____	_____
4. Remove all ornamentation, including watch, rings, earrings, and other such items, and place them in a pocket.	_____	_____
5. Put on a lead apron.	_____	_____
6. Wash hands as described previously.	_____	_____
7. Put on a clean gown, making sure it is sufficiently long to cover most of the uniform. Pick up the gown from the inside near the armhole openings and gently shake it open. Put one arm in and then the other. First tie the neck strings and then tie the waist strings.	_____	_____
8. Put on a mask, tying it securely, and then a cap. Goggles may also be worn, if available.	_____	_____
9. Put on the gloves. These gloves should be clean but need not be sterile.	_____	_____
10. Direct an assistant to put on a gown, gloves, and cap.	_____	_____
11. Enter the isolated area and explain to the patient who you are and what you are doing.	_____	_____
12. Position the patient and the cassette.	_____	_____
13. Direct the assistant to manipulate the machine and make the exposure.	_____	_____
14. Remove the cassette from behind the patient. Fold back the edge of the protective bag, never touching the inside. Direct the assistant to remove the cassette, never touching the outside. Place the covering into an appropriate container. Instruct the assistant to remove the portable equipment from the room.	_____	_____
15. Untie the waist ties of the gown.	_____	_____
16. Untie the neckties of the gown and pull the gown forward and down from the shoulders. Pull the gown off so that the sleeves are inside out and the front of the gown is folded inward. Avoid touching the front of the gown. Discard into an appropriate container.	_____	_____
17. Remove the gloves. Remove the first glove with the other gloved hand, never touching the inside of the glove. Grasp the top of the glove and pull it inside out. Remove the other glove with the exposed hand, touching the inside only. Discard into an appropriate container.	_____	_____
18. Remove the cap and then the mask, touching the mask's ties or elastic only.	_____	_____
19. Wash hands.	_____	_____
20. Direct the assistant to follow the same protocol. Clean the portable equipment with an antiseptic.	_____	_____
21. Wash hands one last time.	_____	_____

Comments: _____

_____

_____

Evaluator's Signature: _____

Student's Signature: _____

CHAPTER 18 ASEPTIC TECHNIQUES

Patient Care Laboratory Activities

STUDENT NAME: _____ DATE: _____

LAB 18.1   Opening a Sterile Package

Objective
- To demonstrate the proper technique for opening a sterile package

Equipment
- Sterile package and table

Procedures
- On completion of this laboratory activity, the student will be able to perform the following procedures:

Opening a Sterile Package on a Table	Yes	No
1. Place the package on the center of the surface with the top flap of the wrapper set to open away from you.	_____	_____
2. Pinch the first flap on the outside of the wrapper between the thumb and index finger by reaching around (not over) the package. Pull the flap open and lay it flat on the far surface.	_____	_____
3. Use the right hand to open the right flap and the left hand to open the left flap.	_____	_____
4. Grasp the turned-down corner, and pull down the fourth and final flap, being sure not to touch the inner surface of any of the package with an unsterile object such as a sleeve.	_____	_____

Opening a Sterile Package While Holding It	Yes	No
1. Hold the package in one hand, with the top flap opening away from you.	_____	_____
2. Pull the top flap well back, and hold it away from both the contents of the package and the sterile field.	_____	_____
3. Drop the contents gently onto the sterile field from approximately 6 inches above the field and at a slight angle, making sure that the package wrapping does not touch the sterile field at any time.	_____	_____

Comments: _____
_____
_____

Evaluator's Signature: _____

Student's Signature: _____

CHAPTER 18 ASEPTIC TECHNIQUES

Patient Care Laboratory Activities

STUDENT NAME: _____ DATE: _____

LAB 18.2   Sterile Gowning Technique

Objective
- To demonstrate the proper sterile technique for self-gowning and for gowning another person

Equipment
- Surgical gown

Procedures
- On completion of this laboratory activity, the student will be able to perform the following procedures:

Self-Gowning	Yes	No
1. Stand approximately 12 inches from the sterile area, pick up the gown by the folded edges, and lift it directly up from the package. The gown is folded so that the outside faces away.	_____	_____
2. Step back from the table, making sure no objects are near the gown. Holding the gown at the shoulders, allow it to unfold gently. Do not shake the gown.	_____	_____
3. Place the hands inside the armholes, and guide each arm through the sleeves by raising and spreading the arms.	_____	_____
4. Direct an unsterile assistant to stand behind and reach inside the sleeves, grasp the sleeves, and pull them gently to adjust the gown.	_____	_____
5. For the open technique of gloving, the sleeves are pulled over the hands. For the closed technique of gloving, keep the hands and fingers covered by the sterile gown.	_____	_____
6. Direct an assistant to fasten the back and waistband of the gown.	_____	_____

Gowning Another Person	Yes	No
1. After gowning and gloving using sterile technique, pick up the sterile gown by the neck band, hold it at arm's length, and allow it to unfold.	_____	_____
2. Hold the gown by the shoulder seams, with the outside facing the sterile person.	_____	_____
3. Protect the sterile gloves by placing both hands under the back panel of the gown's shoulder.	_____	_____
4. Direct the person being gowned to slip the arms into the sleeves in a downward motion, sliding the gown up to the mid upper arms.	_____	_____
5. A nonsterile circulator pulls the gown up and fastens the back and waistband of the gown.	_____	_____
6. Gently pull the cuff back over the person's hands, being careful that your gloved hands do not touch the bare hands.	_____	_____

Comments: _____

_____

_____

Evaluator's Signature: _____

Student's Signature: _____

CHAPTER 18 ASEPTIC TECHNIQUES

Patient Care Laboratory Activities

STUDENT NAME: _____ DATE: _____

LAB 18.3   Sterile Gloving Technique

Objective
- To demonstrate proper sterile technique for the closed and open methods of self-gloving and for gloving another person

Equipment
- Surgical gloves
- Surgical gown

Procedures
- On completion of this laboratory activity, the student will be able to perform the following procedures:

Self-Gloving: Closed Technique	Yes	No
1. Have an assistant open the glove package so that the right glove is on his or her right side.	____	____
2. After donning a sterile gown with the fingers still inside the cuff of the gown, pick up the glove and lay it palm-down over the cuff of the gown. The fingers of the glove face toward you.	____	____
3. Working through the gown sleeve, grasp the cuff of the glove and bring it over the open cuff of the sleeve.	____	____
4. Unroll the glove cuff so that it covers the sleeve cuff.	____	____
5. Pull the glove on by grasping the glove cuff and advancing the hand into the glove.	____	____
6. Proceed with the opposite hand, using the same technique. Never allow the bare hand to contact the gown cuff edge or outside of glove.	____	____
7. Adjust the fingers until comfortable.	____	____

Self-Gloving: Open Technique	Yes	No
1. Pick up the glove by its inside cuff with one hand. Do not touch the outside surface of the glove or the glove wrapper.	____	____
2. Slide the glove onto the opposite bare hand, leaving the cuff down.	____	____
3. With the gloved (and now sterile) hand, pick up the other glove by reaching under the cuff, being sure to touch only the outside surface of the glove with the sterile gloved hand.	____	____
4. Pull the glove onto the hand without touching the inside surface of the glove, which is actually the outside surface of the folded cuff.	____	____
5. Interlock your hands and remember to keep them at or above waist level.	____	____

Removal of Gloves	Yes	No
1. Grasp the cuff of one glove, pull it inside out, and place it in the gloved hand.	____	____
2. Reach inside the cuff of the gloved hand, pull the glove inside out and over the glove that you are holding, and discard.	____	____
3. Wash and dry your hands.	____	____

Gloving Another Person	Yes	No
1. After gloving using sterile technique, open the sterile package and pick up the right gloves, placing the palm away from the person. Slide the fingers under the glove cuff and spread them so that a wide opening is created. Keep the thumbs under the cuff.	____	____
2. The person thrusts his or her hand into the glove. Be sure to have an extremely good grasp on the cuff because considerable force will be exerted when the hand is pushed down into the tight glove.	____	____
3. Gently release the cuff while rolling it over the wrist.	____	____
4. Proceed with the left glove using the same technique.	____	____

Comments: _____
_____
_____

Evaluator's Signature: _____
Student's Signature: _____

CHAPTER 19 NONASEPTIC TECHNIQUES

Patient Care Laboratory Activities

STUDENT NAME: _____ DATE: _____

LAB 19.1   Assisting Patients with a Urinal and a Bedpan

Objective
- To demonstrate proper technique for assisting a patient with a urinal and a bedpan

Equipment
- Urinal
- Bedpan
- Gloves

Procedures
- On completion of this laboratory activity, the student will be able to: perform the following procedures:

Assisting a Patient with a Urinal	Yes	No
1. Put on clean, disposable gloves, and raise the cover sheet sufficiently to permit adequate visibility while being careful not to expose the patient excessively.	_____	_____
2. Spread the patient's legs, and place the urinal between them. Place the penis into the urinal far enough so that it does not slip out, and hold the urinal in place by the handle until the patient finishes voiding.	_____	_____
3. Remove the urinal, empty it, remove the gloves, and wash hands.	_____	_____

Assisting a Patient with a Bedpan	Yes	No
1. Remove the bedpan cover, and place it at the end of the table.	_____	_____
2. If the patient is able to move, place one hand under the lower back and ask the patient to raise the hips. Place the pan under the hips, being sure the patient is covered with a sheet.	_____	_____
3. Direct the patient to sit up, if possible, so that the head is elevated approximately 60 degrees.	_____	_____
4. When the patient has finished using the bedpan, put on clean, disposable gloves. Direct the patient to lie back. Place one hand under the lumbar area, and instruct the patient to raise up at the hips.	_____	_____
5. Remove the pan, cover it, and empty it in the designated area. Rinse it thoroughly with cold water, and return it to the area where used equipment is placed.	_____	_____
6. Offer the patient a wet paper towel or washcloth to wash hands and a paper towel to dry them. Remove the gloves and wash hands.	_____	_____

Comments: _____

_____

_____

Evaluator's Signature: _____

Student's Signature: _____

CHAPTER 20 MEDICAL EMERGENCIES

Patient Care Laboratory Activities

STUDENT NAME: _____ DATE: _____

LAB 20.1   The Heimlich Maneuver (Abdominal Thrusts)

Objective
- To simulate the Heimlich maneuver on a conscious adult, a pregnant victim, and an infant victim

Equipment
- None

Procedures
- On completion of this laboratory activity, the student will be able to perform the following procedures:

Conscious Adult	Yes	No
1. Assess the victim to determine whether he or she is choking.	_____	_____
2. Stand behind the victim, and wrap both arms around him or her, clutching one fist with the other hand.	_____	_____
3. Place the thumb side of the fist at the midline of the victim's abdomen, above the navel and well below the sternum.	_____	_____
4. Hold the elbows out from the victim, and exert pressure inward and upward.	_____	_____
5. Administer each thrust separately, repeating the procedure quickly 6 to 10 times or until the obstructing object is expelled.	_____	_____

Pregnant Victim	Yes	No
1. Stand behind the pregnant victim, placing both arms under the victim's armpits and around the victim's chest. Place the thumb side of the fist in the center of the sternum and the second hand over the fist.	_____	_____
2. Apply backward thrusts until the obstructing object is expelled.	_____	_____

Infant Victim	Yes	No
1. Hold the infant along your arm, with the head lower than the trunk, and support the infant by holding the jaw.	_____	_____
2. Rest the arm holding the infant on your thigh, and, using the heel of the hand, deliver four back blows between the infant's scapulae.	_____	_____
3. Continue to support the head and neck, and turn the infant over.	_____	_____
4. Place the index finger on the sternum just below the intermammary line. Using two or three fingers, deliver four chest thrusts.	_____	_____
5. Alternately repeat back blows and chest thrusts until the obstructing object is expelled.	_____	_____

Comments: _____

_____

_____

Evaluator's Signature: _____

Student's Signature: _____

CHAPTER 22 PRINCIPLES OF DRUG ADMINISTRATION

Patient Care Laboratory Activities

STUDENT NAME: _____ DATE: _____

LAB 22.1   Filling a Syringe From an Ampule and a Vial

Objective
- To demonstrate proper technique for filling a syringe from an ampule and a vial

Equipment
- Glass ampule
- Vial
- Syringe
- Needle

Procedures
- On completion of this laboratory activity, the student will be able to perform the following procedures:

Filling a Syringe From a Glass Ampule	Yes	No
1. Direct an assistant to flick the top of the neck of the ampule until all the liquid is at the bottom of the container.	_____	_____
2. Direct the assistant to snap off the top of the ampule with a gauze pad.	_____	_____
3. Open a syringe package. Open a needle package, and insert the needle on the end of the syringe without letting the end of the syringe or the end of the needle touch anything but each other.	_____	_____
4. Withdraw the contents of the ampule, being careful not to let the shaft of the needle touch the broken edge of the ampule.	_____	_____
5. After use, dispose of the ampule in an appropriate receptacle and the syringe and needle into an acceptable sharps biohazard container.	_____	_____

Filling a Syringe From a Vial	Yes	No
1. Break the seal, expose the rubber stopper, and wipe the stopper with an alcohol swab.	_____	_____
2. Open a syringe package, and pull back the syringe plunger to pull air into the syringe equal to the amount of drug that will be withdrawn from the vial.	_____	_____
3. Open a needle package, and insert the needle on the end of the syringe without letting the end of the syringe or the end of the needle touch anything but each other.	_____	_____
4. Invert the vial, and, with the dominant hand, insert the needle without letting the tip of the needle touch anything but the rubber stopper of the vial.	_____	_____
5. With the tip of the needle in the fluid, inject air equal to the volume of drug to be removed. Pull back on the plunger until the correct amount of drug has been drawn into the syringe.	_____	_____
6. Remove the needle, and hold the syringe with the needle pointing up while tapping it with a finger to move any air bubble toward the hub, where it can be expelled by gently pushing on the plunger of the syringe.	_____	_____
7. After use, dispose of entire syringe and needle into an acceptable sharps biohazard container.	_____	_____

Comments: _____
_____
_____

Evaluator's Signature: _____
Student's Signature: _____

CHAPTER 22 PRINCIPLES OF DRUG ADMINISTRATION

Patient Care Laboratory Activities

STUDENT NAME: _____ DATE: _____

LAB 22.2 Preparing a Drip Infusion Setup

Objective
- To demonstrate the proper technique for setting up a drip infusion set

Equipment
- Intravenous (IV) pole
- Drip infusion set
- Saline solution bag

Procedure
- On completion of this laboratory activity, the student will be able to perform the following procedure:

Preparing a Drip Infusion Setup	Yes	No
1. Check the expiration date. Remove the administration set from the box, and straighten the tubing while checking for any cracks or holes.	_____	_____
2. Slide the clamp up to the drip chamber, and close it.	_____	_____
3. Place the bag on a hard surface, remove the protective cap from the tubing insertion port on the bag, and wipe it with an alcohol swab.	_____	_____
4. Remove the protective cap from the spike on the drip chamber of the tubing, and insert the spike into the port.	_____	_____
5. Check again to make certain the clamp is closed, hang the bag on the IV pole, and squeeze the drip chamber until it is half full.	_____	_____
6. Prime the IV setup by removing the protective cap from the end of the tubing and holding it over a sink or wastebasket.	_____	_____
7. Taking care to preserve the sterility of the cap and of the end of the tubing, release the clamp and allow the solution to run freely until all air bubbles are cleared from the tubing.	_____	_____
8. Reclamp the tubing to stop the flow, and replace the protective cap over the end of the tubing.	_____	_____

Comments: _____

_____

_____

Evaluator's Signature: _____

Student's Signature: _____

CHAPTER 22 PRINCIPLES OF DRUG ADMINISTRATION

Patient Care Laboratory Activities

STUDENT NAME: _____ DATE: _____

LAB 22.3   Venipuncture and Intravenous Drug Injection

Objective
- To demonstrate the proper technique for venipuncture and IV drug injection

Equipment
- Disposable gloves
- Gauze, tape, and/or adhesive bandage strip
- Butterfly needle or intravenous IV catheter
- Syringe
- Tourniquet
- Venipuncture training arm kit

Procedure
- On completion of this laboratory activity, the student will be able to perform the following procedure:

Venipuncture and Intravenous Drug Injection	Yes	No
1. Wash hands thoroughly.	_____	_____
2. Check two patient identifiers.	_____	_____
3. Explain the procedure to the patient. Ask the patient about any allergies.	_____	_____
4. Assemble all needed supplies, and prepare the drug for administration.	_____	_____
5. Put on disposable gloves.	_____	_____
6. Once an appropriate site for venipuncture has been selected, cleanse it with an alcohol swab, using a circular motion while moving from the center to the outside. Allow the area 30 seconds to dry.	_____	_____
7. Apply a tourniquet above the site, using sufficient tension to impede the flow of blood in the vein. Ask the patient to open and close the fist to fully distend the vein. When the vein has been identified, ask the patient to hold the fist in a clenched position.	_____	_____
8. To stabilize the median cephalic vein, place the thumb on the tissue just above or below the site, and gently pull the skin and vein toward the hand if below and toward the shoulder if above.	_____	_____
9. Hold the needle with the bevel facing upward. Pinch together the wings of the butterfly needle tightly.	_____	_____
10. Insert the needle into the vein at a 15–30-degree angle, and gently advance it into the vein. Blood will flow back into the tubing when the needle is correctly positioned.	_____	_____
11. If the tubing of the butterfly needle has not previously been filled with solution, then allow the blood to flow from the hub before attaching the syringe to ensure that no air bubbles are contained in the system.	_____	_____
12. If using an IV catheter to inject the solution, insert the needle into the vein at a 15–30-degree angle, and gently advance into the vein.	_____	_____
13. Upon blood flashback visualization in the catheter chamber, lower the catheter to be parallel with the skin. Advance the entire catheter unit before threading the flexible plastic portion of the catheter into the vein. Advance the plastic sheath of the catheter into the vein while pulling the needle back away from the sheath and maintaining a taut pressure on the patient's skin. Most catheters have a spring release button to retract the needle. Once the needle is retracted, blood will flow freely.	_____	_____
14. Remove the tourniquet and inject the drug. If using the catheter, you will need to apply a syringe to administer the drug.	_____	_____
15. Unless otherwise instructed, remove the butterfly needle, and apply gentle pressure to the site with a gauze.	_____	_____
16. If using the catheter, remove the plastic sheath that is in the patient's vein and apply gentle pressure with gauze once the catheter is removed.	_____	_____
17. Dispose of the syringe, needle, and other supplies in appropriate receptacles.	_____	_____
18. Record all relevant information in the patient's chart.	_____	_____

Comments: _____

_____

_____

Evaluator's Signature: _____

Student's Signature: _____

CHAPTER 1 INTRODUCTION TO IMAGING AND RADIOLOGIC SCIENCES

1. The term used to describe energy transmitted through matter is:
   a. ionization.
   b. physiology.
   c. radiation.
   d. therapy.
2. Special protection should be taken to prevent excessive exposure to:
   a. energy.
   b. electromagnetic energy.
   c. ionizing radiation.
   d. radio waves.
3. Which of the following specialties uses a nonionizing form of radiation?
   a. nuclear medicine technology
   b. radiation therapy
   c. radiography
   d. sonography
4. The discovery of x-rays occurred in:
   a. 1858.
   b. 1876.
   c. 1895.
   d. 1898.
5. An individual who specializes in using x-rays to create images of the body is known as a:
   a. diagnostic medical sonographer.
   b. nuclear medicine technologist.
   c. radiographer.
   d. radiation therapist
6. An effective treatment of atherosclerosis that uses a special catheter with a balloon tip is termed:
   a. angiography.
   b. angioplasty.
   c. arteriography.
   d. cardiac catheterization.
7. A discipline that visualizes sectional anatomy by the recording of a predetermined plane in the body is:
   a. computed tomography.
   b. cardiovascular interventional technology.
   c. nuclear medicine technology.
   d. radiation therapy.
8. Radiography of the breast is termed:
   a. angiography.
   b. cytotechnology.
   c. histology.
   d. mammography.
9. The study of diseases of muscles and bones is termed:
   a. neurology.
   b. orthopedics.
   c. oncology.
   d. urology.
10. An individual who specializes in carrying out treatments designed to correct or improve the function of a particular body part or system is known as a:
    a. diagnostician.
    b. histologist.
    c. technologist.
    d. therapist.

CHAPTER 2 PROFESSIONAL ORGANIZATIONS

1. Which of the following is a voluntary process through which an agency grants recognition to an individual on demonstration, usually by examination, of specialized professional skills?
   a. accreditation
   b. certification
   c. licensure
   d. registration
2. Which of the following is a listing of individuals holding certification credentials in a particular profession?
   a. accreditation
   b. certification
   c. licensure
   d. registry
3. What organization certifies individuals in radiography?
   a. American Society of Radiologic Technologists
   b. American Registry of Radiologic Technologists
   c. Joint Review Committee on Education in Radiologic Technology
   d. Radiological Society of North America
4. Which of the following organizations represents the interests of radiologic technologists to the public and federal government?
   a. American Registry of Radiologic Technologists
   b. American Society of Radiologic Technologists
   c. International Society of Radiographers and Radiologic Technologists
   d. American Roentgen Ray Society

5. What purpose is served by the *standards* document for a profession?
   a. It sets the legal and ethical standards for a profession.
   b. It determines the minimum standards for an individual to become certified by a registry organization.
   c. It establishes the sponsorship of a joint review committee.
   d. It specifies the requirements for accreditation of an educational program by a joint review committee.

6. Which of the following is the process by which a governmental agency (usually at the state level) grants permission to individuals to practice their profession?
   a. accreditation
   b. certification
   c. licensure
   d. registration

7. Which title is granted to a radiographer after successful completion of the American Registry of Radiologic Technologist's examination in radiography?
   a. radiologic technologist
   b. radiologic technologist, radiographer
   c. registered technologist
   d. registered technologist, radiographer

8. Which of the following organizations is a sponsor of the Joint Review Committee on Education in Radiologic Technology and the American Registry of Radiologic Technologists?
   a. Society of Nuclear Medicine
   b. American Society of Radiologic Technologists
   c. American Healthcare Radiology Administrators
   d. Radiological Society of North America

9. Which of the following is a voluntary peer process through which an agency grants recognition to an institution for a program of study that meets specified criteria?
   a. accreditation
   b. certification
   c. licensure
   d. registration

10. Approximately how many individuals are registered by the American Registry of Radiologic Technologists?
   a. 10,000
   b. 90,000   *not on test*
   c. 250,000
   d. 330,000

CHAPTER 3 EDUCATIONAL SURVIVAL SKILLS

1. Stress is defined as:
   a. a feeling of anxiety and fear.
   b. not having enough time to complete commitments.
   c. a breaking point.
   d. demand on time, energy, and resources with some threat included.

2. Causes of stress include:
   a. individual perception of wants
   b. poor physical health
   c. lack of time management
   d. all of the above

3. The best ways to reduce stress are by:
   a. managing finances better and saving money
   b. controlling time, thinking positively, and buffering stressors
   c. choosing a nonmedical profession and vacationing often
   d. avoiding worry and practicing relaxation

4. When taking a test, always:
   a. cram the night before.
   b. arrive early and review notes just before the test.
   c. answer all questions you know first, then go back and repeat, leaving the most difficult questions for last.
   d. review your test, but do not change answers.

5. In-control language:
   a. is used when driving to class
   b. is positive and expresses choice
   c. identifies where others are wrong
   d. is critical and powerful

6. The biggest thief of time is:
   a. indecision.
   b. worry.
   c. traffic.
   d. mistakes.

7. When managing time, practice self-management, which includes which of the following?
   a. setting your alarm and limiting phone calls and texting
   b. doing only the important tasks
   c. prioritizing, setting limits, and providing for self-care
   d. avoiding worry

8. Good study habits include:
   a. reading out loud and writing down important facts.
   b. planned group activity.
   c. a regular plan for study and review.
   d. all of the above.

9. Stress buffers include:
   a. exercise and good nutrition.
   b. taking a personal day off work.
   c. avoiding studying the night before a test.
   d. avoiding worry.

10. Vitamins and minerals depleted as a result of stress are:
   a. iron, B_{12}, and C.
   b. B complex, C, and magnesium.
   c. magnesium, E, and B complex.
   d. A, E, and C

CHAPTER 4 CRITICAL-THINKING AND PROBLEM-SOLVING STRATEGIES

1. Students in medical professions often learn to apply theories through the review of a real-life situation or scenario. What is this activity called?
   a. code review
   b. case study
   c. role playing
   d. laboratory practice

2. Which of the following is (are) characteristic of professional critical thinking?
   a. sound professional judgment
   b. uncomfortable and challenging decision making

c. quick and inventive response

d. action based on professional knowledge and experience

e. all of the above

3. What is the first step involved in problem solving associated with critical thinking?

a. Identify and clarify the problem.

b. Remove yourself from the situation.

c. Brainstorm all possible solutions.

d. Analyze how the problem affects you personally.

4. The second step involved in problem solving associated with critical thinking is to undergo an objective examination of the problem. What element(s) of this step is (are) reflected below?

a. implications of the problem

b. safety risks and potential liability

c. technical considerations

d. number and type or types of solutions required

e. all of the above

5. What is the primary factor in determining the solution to the problem in critical thinking?

a. the solution that gives the most profit for the health care institution

b. the solution that most closely resembles what the most experienced radiologic science profession in the department would do

c. the solution that results in the least damage to your reputation

d. the solution that provides the best outcome for the patient

6. In what aspect of the education program for a radiologic science professional is the student exposed to real-life experiences that allow him or her to transfer knowledge into action?

a. cognitive

b. classroom

c. laboratory

d. clinical

7. Analyzing personal values and feelings and managing uncomfortable ethical situations are components of what type of critical thinking?

a. affective

b. cognitive

c. psychomotor

d. technical

8. Which of the following describes a situation in which technical critical-thinking skills are required?

a. A patient arrives for a routine procedure and asks questions.

b. A female patient responds that she is pregnant before a procedure.

c. A male patient requests that he be permitted to go to the bathroom before the procedure.

d. A trauma patient has a broken femur, and specialized hip radiographs are required.

9. You are working the 4:00 AM to midnight shift in the emergency room, and as you enter a room to identify your patient for a chest x-ray, you witness a nurse, the head nurse, preparing for an injection. As you peer through the door, you see her brush the needle against the bed sheet and then before you can say anything, she puts the needle into the patient's vein. Identify the problem.

a. Use of a dirty needle is a violation of standard precautions

b. The patient may acquire an infection as a result of the injection

c. The nurse is in a position of authority.

d. All of the above

10. For the scenario in question 9, which of the following would be the most appropriate next step in solving this problem?

a. Take no action; this is not your problem.

b. Ask the patient if he or she saw the needle touch the bed sheet.

c. Bring to the nurse's attention that you saw the needle touch the sheet outside the patient room.

d. Report the nurse to the CEO of the hospital.

CHAPTER 5 INTRODUCTION TO CLINICAL EDUCATION

1. Clinical procedures and activities are performed in what setting?

a. classroom

b. hospital/cancer center

c. laboratory

d. library

2. Cognitive learning includes:

a. attitudes, values, and beliefs.

b. physical actions, neuromuscular manipulations, and coordination.

c. assistance, observation, and performance.

d. knowledge, reason, and judgment.

3. "The observable, successful achievement of performance objectives" defines which of the following?

a. objective

b. competency

c. affective

d. learning outcome

4. A qualified medical imaging and radiologic sciences professional directly supervises a student by:

a. reviewing the request in relation to the student's achievement

b. evaluating the condition of the patient in relation to the student's knowledge

c. being present while the student conducts the treatment/examination

d. reviewing and approving the treatment/examination

e. all of the above

5. A clinical instructor works directly with the students in the clinical setting and provides students with one-on-one instruction and evaluation. Which of the following must a successful clinical instructor possess?

a. knowledge of diagnostic and therapeutic procedures

b. competence in clinical instruction and evaluation techniques

c. patience and willingness to guide students to clinical success

d. all of the above

6. Disciplinary action may be initiated if a student commits which serious infraction?
   a. disclosure of confidential information
   b. falsification of records
   c. cheating
   d. intoxication
   e. all of the above

7. Which of the following may be assessed to determine students' knowledge or comprehension of clinical skills?
   a. communication with staff and patients
   b. manipulation of exposure factors or setting for treatment plan
   c. evaluating the radiographic image or ensuring the appropriate treatment plan
   d. none of the above
   e. all (a-c)

8. Of the following, which is a communication method used to assure an effective handoff of patients from one healthcare worker to another?
   a. HIPAA
   b. TeamSTEPPS
   c. IPE
   d. SBAR

9. In order to perform diagnostic or therapeutic procedures competently students in medical imaging and radiologic sciences programs, must always:
   a. observe a qualified medical imaging and radiologic sciences professional.
   b. develop and refine the appropriate skills and behaviors.
   c. assist the radiologist or radiation oncologist as much as possible.
   d. perform as many diagnostic or therapeutic procedures as possible.
   e. all of the above

10. Which of the following is an approach to teaching students and healthcare workers how to interact and work with each other in the clinical setting?
    a. SBAR
    b. TeamSTEPPS
    c. IPE
    d. HIPAA

not on test

CHAPTER 6 RADIOLOGY ADMINISTRATION

1. The driving and guiding force that outlines the reason for the existence of a hospital is its:
   a. chief executive officer.
   b. medical director.
   c. mission statement.
   d. adherence to The Joint Commission guidelines.

2. The board of directors employs _____, who interacts with the medical staff to ensure coordination and quality of patient care and services.
   a. an insurance agent
   b. a radiology chairman
   c. a vice president of nursing
   d. a president or chief executive officer

3. Forces causing hospitals to reorganize include:
   a. state regulators
   b. economic hardships
   c. total quality management
   d. The Joint Commission

4. When an organization focuses on quality or patient safety, it:
   a. undergoes a cultural revolution.
   b. prohibits employees from participating in groups.
   c. encourages employees to focus on one department to the exclusion of others.
   d. lowers workers' perceptions of patient or physician expectations.

5. The management function that charts a course of action for the future to enable coordinated and consistent fulfillment of goals and objectives is:
   a. coordinating.
   b. planning.
   c. communicating.
   d. setting goals.

6. The management function that involves the development of a structure or framework that identifies how people do their work is:
   a. staffing.
   b. planning.
   c. organizing.
   d. coordinating.

7. The management function that involves getting the right people to do the work and developing their abilities is:
   a. staffing.
   b. organizing.
   c. directing.
   d. describing.

8. Performance standards or guidelines used to measure progress toward the goals of the organizations are defined as:
   a. employee evaluations.
   b. feedback.
   c. controlling.
   d. The Joint Commission guidelines.

9. The internal hospital committee that ensures safe operations for the facility for both patients and employers is the:
   a. safety committee.
   b. certificate of need.
   c. hazardous chemicals group.
   d. radiation safety committee.

10. Besides acquiring a strong knowledge of technical skills, a radiologic technology student should develop:
    a. a broad range of procedural abilities.
    b. referrals of patients from physicians.
    c. skills in magnetic resonance imaging, computed tomography, ultrasonography, and nuclear medicine.
    d. superior skills in interactive relationships.

CHAPTER 7 RADIOGRAPHIC IMAGING

1. The process by which a beam of x-ray photons is reduced as it passes through matter is known as:
   a. density.
   b. attenuation.

c. fog.

d. processing.

2. Computed radiography uses which of the following as its image receptor?

a. photostimulable phosphor plate

b. charge-coupled device

c. radiographic film

d. all of the above

3. The factor that controls the amount of x-radiation produced by the x-ray tube is:

a. milliampere-seconds (mAs)

b. source-to-image distance (SID)

c. object-to-image distance (OID)

d. kilovoltage peak

4. What mAs value would result using the 500 mA setting at 0.25 second?

a. 12.5 mAs

b. 20 mAs

c. 125 mAs

d. 2000 mAs

5. Which of the following image receptor systems does NOT use light during exposure? *not on test*

a. direct capture DR

b. indirect capture DR

c. computed radiography

d. film/screen radiography

6. A radiograph is made using 40 mAs at a 40-inch SID. If the image must be repeated at a 72-inch SID, what mAs value is necessary to maintain the same exposure? *not on test*

a. 12 mAs

b. 13 mAs

c. 120 mAs

d. 130 mAs

7. The 15% rule helps to explain the effect of _____ on exposure. *not on test*

a. grids

b. mAs

c. SID

d. kilovoltage peak

8. Which of the following is NOT a radiographic contrast medium? *not on test*

a. barium compounds

b. air

c. iodine compounds

d. water

9. The most common cause of radiographic unsharpness is:

a. motion

b. detector characteristics

c. increased OID

d. decreased SID

10. What term in digital imaging is used to describe a numeric representation of the quantity of exposure received by a digital image receptor?

a. window level

b. exposure indicator

c. window width

d. exposure latitude

CHAPTER 8 RADIOGRAPHIC AND FLUOROSCOPIC EQUIPMENT

1. The component of the radiographic system that produces radiation is the:

a. collimator.

b. high tension transformer.

c. x-ray tube.

d. goniometer.

2. The selection of radiographic exposure factors such as mAs and kVp is performed at the operator:

a. control console.

b. fluoroscopic tower.

c. image receptor assembly.

d. x-ray tube.

3. The quantity of electrons for x-ray exposure is determined by the mAs. This is calculated by:

a. dividing the milliamperage by the kVp.

b. multiplying the milliamperage by the exposure time.

c. adding the milliamperage and the exposure time.

d. adding the kVp and the exposure time.

4. The primary components of the x-ray tube important to x-ray production are the:

a. the high-voltage cables and tube support mechanism.

b. anode bearings and rotor.

c. diode and triode.

d. anode and cathode.

5. The component that controls the size and shape of the x-ray exposure field is the:

a. x-ray tube housing.

b. collimator assembly.

c. anode.

d. goniometer.

6. True digital image receptors are referred to as: *not on test*

a. flat panel detectors

b. photostimulable phosphor technology (PSP)

c. storage phosphor technology (SPT)

d. analog systems

7. All of the following are typical features of radiographic tables EXCEPT:

a. they have motorized, variable height adjustment.

b. they permit four-way "floating" tabletop mobility.

c. the tabletop materials offer high attenuation to lower patient dose.

d. they have electric locks on tabletop motions.

8. The component that supports and permits the x-ray tube to be moved in different directions is the:

a. tube stand or overhead tube crane assembly.

b. Bucky mechanism and cassette tray.

c. upright image receptor.

d. collimator assembly.

9. In a fluoroscopic system, the surface or face of the fluoroscopic detector is considered: the:

a. lead curtain

b. thin film transistor

c. scatter source

d. primary barrier

10. All of the following are true of fluoroscopy EXCEPT:
    a. the lead protective apron attached to the fluoroscopic carriage is of little value in reducing operator dose.
    b. it permits "real-time" imaging of dynamic patient functions.
    c. modern day fluoroscopy systems record images electronically rather than using cassettes.
    d. dose reduction features such as last image hold (LIH), pulsed fluoroscopy, and electronic shuttering are essential.

CHAPTER 9 BASIC RADIATION PROTECTION AND RADIOBIOLOGY

1. Which of the following is not necessary for x-rays to be produced?
   a. a source of electrons
   b. rapid particle acceleration
   c. a source of protons
   d. instantaneous deceleration

2. For pair production to occur, the energy of the incoming x-ray photon must be at least:
   a. 10 keV.
   b. 1.02 keV.
   c. 10 MeV.
   d. 1.02 MeV.

3. The interaction of x-rays with matter that constitutes the greatest hazard to patients in diagnostic radiography is:
   a. photoelectric interaction.
   b. Compton interaction.
   c. classic coherent scattering.
   d. pair production.

4. The unit used to measure the amount of energy absorbed in any medium is the:
   a. Sievert.
   b. Gray.
   c. Coulombs per kilogram.
   d. Air kerma.

5. The maximum accumulated whole-body dose for a 35-year-old occupational worker is:
   a. 85 mSv.
   b. 5 mSv.
   c. 35 mSv.
   d. 0.5 mSv.

6. According to the law of Bergonie and Tribondeau, the characteristics that determine the sensitivity of a cell to radiation are:
   a. mitotic activity and metabolic function.
   b. metabolic function and cell type.
   c. mitotic activity and structure and function of the cell.
   d. cell type and life span of the cell.

7. The intensity of radiation from a radiographic tube was 35 mR at a distance of 2.5 m from the tube. What would the intensity be at a distance of 4 m from the tube, all other factors remaining the same?
   a. 5.5 mR
   b. 55 mR
   c. 14 mR
   d. 90 mR

8. Which of the following is not a component of an optically stimulated luminescence (OSL) dosimeter?
   a. exposure meter
   b. plastic blister pack
   c. aluminum oxide strip
   d. metal filters

9. What is the annual dose limit for occupational exposure?
   a. 10 mSv
   b. 25 mSv
   c. 50 mSv
   d. 100 mSv

[handwritten: Know this]

10. Lead absorbs x-rays through the process of _____.
    a. classical coherent scattering
    b. the Compton effect
    c. the photoelectric effect *[handwritten: → absorbed dose]*
    d. pair production

CHAPTER 10 HUMAN DIVERSITY

1. Human diversity consists of characteristics associated with:
   a. age.
   b. ethnicity.
   c. gender.
   d. lifestyle.
   e. all of the above.

2. Individuals born between 1981 and 1995 are generally referred to as:
   a. the baby boom generation
   b. generation X
   c. generation Y
   d. the lost generation

3. Over the next three decades, which of the following age groups is expected to be the fastest-growing segment of the population?
   a. 35+
   b. 55+
   c. 65+
   d. 75+
   e. 85+

4. Which one of the following does not relate to a person's ethnicity?
   a. dress
   b. language
   c. religion
   d. race

5. Which of the following is not one of the ways that culturally different individuals have interacted with the US majority culture in the past?
   a. assimilation
   b. biculturalism
   c. multiculturalism
   d. a and b
   e. b and c

6. Government statutes to protect people from discrimination are based on:
   a. ethnicity or race.
   b. disability.

c. age.

d. all of the above.

e. none of the above.

7. Sexual orientation regards an individual's designation as any of the following EXCEPT:

a. asexuality.

b. bisexuality.

c. heterosexuality.

d. homosexuality. .

8. Approximately what percentage of world's population has some type of disability?

a. 5

b. 10

c. 15

d. 20

9. Which of the following is considered the most profound step that the United States has ever undertaken to prevent discrimination toward people with a disability?

a. The *Civil Rights Act* of 1964

b. The *Rehabilitation Act* of 1973

c. The *Americans with Disabilities Act* of 1990

d. The *Human Rights Declaration* of 1999

10. Of the following, which one is not considered an element that may contribute to the ability of an organization to become culturally competent?

a. valuing diversity

b. institutionalizing cultural knowledge

c. possessing the capacity for cultural self-assessment

d. ignoring cultural norms and values

e. developing of adaptations for the delivery of services that reflect an understanding of a multicultural environment

CHAPTER 11 PATIENT INTERACTIONS

1. The highest level of Maslow's hierarchy of needs is:

a. self-actualization.

b. belonging.

c. physiologic.

d. self-esteem.

2. The word ambulatory means that the patient:

a. must be confined to a wheelchair.

b. must be moved by ambulance.

c. can be moved by stretcher.

d. can walk.

3. Which of the following would you not want to discuss with a patient?

a. hobbies

b. medical chart

c. ability to walk

d. weather

4. Questions about the diagnosis of an examination from a patient or visitor are best answered by:

a. explaining that only a radiologist can read radiographs.

b. providing the best diagnosis available.

c. explaining that the results are not available yet.

d. suggesting that the question is inappropriate.

5. Which method is effective in communicating with a patient?

1. professional appearance

2. touch

3. pantomime techniques

a. 1 only

b. 1 and 2 only

c. 2 and 3 only

d. 1, 2, and 3

6. When is touching a patient valuable?

a. for emotional support

b. for emphasis

c. for palpation

d. all of the above

7. Which of the following characterize the development of a toddler (1 to 3 years of age)?

a. understands simple abstractions

b. is unable to understand more than one word for something

c. is unable to take the viewpoint of another

d. all of the above

8. Of the changes that occur in geriatric patients that are especially important when patients are undergoing radiologic examinations, which of the following may produce patient paranoia about potential falls with potential for permanent loss of mobility?

a. osteoporotic loss of bone mass

b. arthritis

c. decreased muscle strength

d. atrophied muscle mass

9. Which of the following is considered to be the first stage of acceptance of dying for a terminally ill patient?

a. anger

b. frustration

c. denial and isolation

d. shock

10. Which of the following permits the patient to begin to work through the various stages that precede dying?

a. suspicious awareness

b. mutual pretense

c. open awareness

d. all of the above

CHAPTER 12 HISTORY TAKING

1. Which of the following is undesirable for conducting a clinical history interview?

a. clarifying terminology

b. asking open-ended questions

c. asking vague questions

d. repeating information

2. Which of the following includes a description of the color, quantity, and consistency of blood or other body substances?

a. localization

b. chronology

c. quality

d. occurrence

3. Which of the following is the determination of a precise area, usually through gentle palpation or careful wording of questions?
   a. localization
   b. chronology
   c. quality
   d. occurrence

4. Which of the following is (are) usually included as part of the chronology of a clinical history?
   a. onset
   b. duration
   c. frequency
   d. all of the above

5. Which of the following includes the tone of voice, the speed of speech, and the position of the speaker's extremities and torso?
   a. nonverbal communication
   b. palpation
   c. quality
   d. facilitation

6. What term describes the primary medical problem as defined by the patient?
   a. chief complaint
   b. palpation
   c. onset
   d. nonverbal communication

7. Which of the following describes an undesirable method of questioning that provides information that may direct the answer toward a suspected symptom or complaint?
   a. facilitation
   b. palpation
   c. nonverbal communication
   d. leading question

8. Which of the following is (are) part of the sacred seven elements of the patient clinical history?
   a. localization
   b. aggravating factors
   c. quality
   d. all of the above

9. Which of the following is (are) desirable method(s) of conducting a clinical history interview?
   a. positive nonverbal communication
   b. defining and specifying terms
   c. subjectiveness
   d. a and b

10. Which term describes gentle touching to determine the precise location of a symptom or complaint?
   a. nonverbal communication
   b. palpation
   c. quality
   d. facilitation

CHAPTER 13 SAFE PATIENT MOVEMENT AND HANDLING TECHNIQUES

1. Which of the following is the foundation on which a body rests?
   a. center of gravity
   b. base of support

   c. orthostatic hypotension
   d. biomechanics

2. What term is used to describe the drop in blood pressure some patients experience when they stand up quickly?
   a. center of gravity
   b. base of support
   c. orthostatic hypotension
   d. a and b

3. Where is the human center of gravity located?
   a. at the center of the diaphragm
   b. within 1 to 2 inches of the umbilicus
   c. midway between the hip joints
   d. at approximately sacral level two

4. Which of the following transfers can be used to move a patient from a wheelchair to an examination table?
   a. pivot
   b. assisted standing
   c. standby assist
   d. all of the above

5. Toward which side should all transfers be initiated?
   a. left
   b. right
   c. patient's weak side
   d. patient's strong side

6. What causes patients to feel lightheaded, queasy, or faint when they stand up quickly from a sitting or supine position?
   a. increased respiration from the effort of standing
   b. decreased blood pressure
   c. increased body temperature
   d. increased pulse rate

7. What term describes the hypothetical point around which all mass appears to be concentrated?
   a. center of gravity
   b. base of support
   c. orthostatic hypotension
   d. a and b

8. If a patient arrives in a wheelchair and on a sling, which type of transfer is indicated?
   a. hydraulic lift
   b. pivot
   c. standby assist
   d. cart to table by means of a moving device

9. How can the base of support be increased?
   a. standing on one toe
   b. standing on one foot
   c. standing with the legs apart
   d. bending the knees with the feet together

10. What is the minimum number of persons to use for a cart-to-table transfer when no moving devices are available?
   a. one
   b. two
   c. three
   d. four

CHAPTER 14 IMMOBILIZATION TECHNIQUES

1. Voluntary motion is under the control of the:
   a. technologist.
   b. patient.
   c. radiologist.
   d. student.
2. The most important communication that occurs in a radiology department takes place between the radiographer and the:
   a. administrator.
   b. patient.
   c. radiologist.
   d. student.
3. A key component to effective communication with a patient is:
   a. establishing rapport
   b. assessing the patient's physical condition
   c. introducing the patient to the radiologist
   d. giving a detailed, technical explanation of the examination
4. What is the most commonly used immobilization device?
   a. sheet restraint
   b. cervical collar
   c. positioning sponge
   d. Velcro straps
5. Which of the following might be used to immobilize a patient for an upright lateral chest radiograph?
   a. sandbags
   b. Velcro straps
   c. head clamps
   d. positioning sponge
6. Which of the following is an example of a spinal trauma immobilization device?
   a. air splint
   b. antishock garment
   c. traction splint
   d. backboard
7. When is removing a cervical collar permissible?
   a. before the initial radiographic examination
   b. after a radiographer makes the exposure
   c. after the physician has reviewed the images and determined it is safe
   d. after a paramedic reads the radiograph and approves removal
8. Which immobilization device is radiopaque?
   a. sponge
   b. cervical collar
   c. sandbag
   d. none of the above
9. The Pigg-O-Stat is an immobilization device used for which pediatric examination?
   a. upper extremity
   b. pelvis
   c. skull
   d. chest
10. One of the greatest fears of a geriatric patient is:
    a. falling
    b. being unable to hear the radiographer
    c. having to lie on a radiolucent pad
    d. getting lost on the way to the radiology department

CHAPTER 15 VITAL SIGNS, OXYGEN, CHEST TUBES, AND LINES

1. Rectal thermometry is believed to most accurately reflect core body temperature measures. Use of which alternative thermometer provides measures that closely correlate to the rectal method?
   a. oral
   b. temporal artery
   c. axillary
   d. tympanic
2. A patient is thought to have suffered cardiac arrest. The _____ peripheral artery may be assessed to verify the effectiveness of chest compressions during cardiopulmonary resuscitation.
   1. Apical
   2. Femoral
   3. Radial
      a. 1, 2
      b. 1, 3
      c. 2, 3
      d. 1, 2, and 3
3. In the healthy adult the normal range for blood pressure is:
   a. systolic less than 95 mm Hg, diastolic less than 60 mm Hg.
   b. systolic less than 60 mm Hg, diastolic greater than 95 mm Hg.
   c. systolic less than 120 mm Hg, diastolic less than 80 mm Hg.
   d. systolic less than 80 mm Hg, diastolic greater than 120 mm Hg.
4. Hypoxia is:
   a. a drug that must be prescribed by a physician.
   b. necessary for cellular repair.
   c. a state describing oxygen-deficient tissue.
   d. necessary for cellular function.
5. Which of the following devices can be classified as a high-flow oxygen delivery device?
   a. air-entrainment mask
   b. nasal cannula
   c. simple mask
   d. nonrebreathing mask
6. Regarding oxygen delivery, all of the following are true EXCEPT:
   a. oxygen dose is ordered in liters per minute or in concentration as a fractional concentration of oxygen.
   b. the maximum dose should always be given to obtain the desired results.
   c. the oxygen flowmeter is green.
   d. the regulator attached to the oxygen tank consists of a flowmeter and pressure manometer.
7. An artificial airway is inserted into a patient's the trachea and connected to a mechanical ventilator. In this circumstance, all of the following are true statements EXCEPT:
   a. the ventilator delivers a minimum set respiratory rate.
   b. the inspiratory volume is preset.
   c. a consistent Fio_2 is delivered.
   d. during chest imaging, the radiographer must fully extend the patient's neck for proper head position.

8. A properly placed endotracheal tube will be radiographically confirmed when the:
   a. distal tip is positioned 1 inch inferior to the tracheal bifurcation.
   b. distal tip is positioned 1 inch superior to the tracheal bifurcation.
   c. distal tip is positioned adjacent to the vocal folds.
   d. cuff is positioned between the vocal folds.

9. Thoracostomy tubes are:
   a. used to monitor pulmonary arterial pressures.
   b. central venous lines used to administer parenteral nutrition.
   c. chest tubes used to drain the intrapleural space.
   d. used to administer oxygen with mechanical ventilators.

10. A patient is admitted to the emergency room and chest images are ordered. The order states the following: Unless sitting up or standing erect, the patient has dyspnea. In this case the patient has which of the following?
   a. tachypnea
   b. bradypnea
   c. apnea
   d. orthopnea

CHAPTER 16 BASIC CARDIAC MONITORING: THE ELECTROCARDIOGRAM

not testing over Ch 16

1. Regarding the electrocardiographic tracing, all of the following are true EXCEPT:
   a. repolarization of atrial muscle cells is represented by the P wave.
   b. the QRS-complex represents depolarization of ventricular muscle cells.
   c. the S portion of the QRS complex represents a return to the baseline (isoelectric point).
   d. the U wave is theorized to represent repolarization of the papillary muscles and Purkinje fibers.

2. When multiplying heart rate times stroke volume, the product is:
   a. systolic pressure
   b. diastolic pressure
   c. cardiac cycle
   d. cardiac output

3. Depending on the cause and severity of an arrhythmia, treatment may include which of the following?
   a. cardiac pacemakers or ICD devices
   b. ablation therapy
   c. cardioversion external shock therapy
   d. all of the above might be useful in treating an arrhythmia

4. Systolic pressures greater than _____ mm Hg generally ensure adequate perfusion of tissues.
   a. 80
   b. 90
   c. 100
   d. 120

5. Rhythmic contraction and relaxation of the chambers of the heart are controlled by principal cell types to include which of the following?
   1. working cardiac cells
   2. specialized neural conductive cells
   3. striated muscle cells
   a. 1, 2
   b. 1, 3
   c. 2, 3
   d. 1, 2, and 3

6. All of the following are true of atrial fibrillation EXCEPT:
   a. it is always fatal.
   b. it is caused by additional ectopic pacemaker firings in the atria that exceed SA node firings.
   c. the atria syncytium quivers instead of fully contracting.
   d. formation of atrial emboli is a potential complication.

7. To ensure a normal sequence for each cardiac cycle, each P wave should be followed by a:
   a. T wave
   b. U wave
   c. QRS complex
   d. PR wave

8. When the resting membrane potential is reversed, _____ occurs and myocardial cells are stimulated to contract.
   a. depolarization
   b. repolarization
   c. cardiac action potential
   d. dysrhythmia

9. All of the following are visible on an ECG tracing EXCEPT:
   a. depolarization of atrial muscle
   b. atrial contraction
   c. depolarization of ventricular muscle
   d. repolarization of ventricular muscle

10. For analysis of an ECG tracing, which of the below indicates regular rhythm?
   1. QRS complexes (RR intervals) are consistent for evaluating ventricular rhythm.
   2. The duration of the QRS complex exceeds 0.20 seconds (five small squares).
   3. Intervals between P waves (PP intervals) are consistent for atrial rhythm.
   a. 1, 2
   b. 1, 3
   c. 2, 3
   d. 1, 2, and 3

CHAPTER 17 INFECTION CONTROL

1. Microorganisms that cause infectious diseases can be classified as:
   a. lytic.
   b. endogenous.
   c. pathogenic.
   d. nosocomial.

2. The best method of preventing the spread of aerosol infections is by:
   a. the patient wearing a mask.
   b. the health care worker wearing a gown.
   c. hand washing.
   d. all of the above.

3. All of the following are types of indirect transmission EXCEPT:
   a. fomite.
   b. vector.
   c. aerosol.
   d. touching.
4. The common cold is an example of an infection by a:
   a. bacterium.
   b. virus.
   c. fungus.
   d. protozoan.
5. The term that best describes the absolute removal of all life forms is:
   a. antisepsis
   b. medical asepsis
   c. disinfection
   d. sterilization
6. A person is bitten by a mosquito and develops an infection. This type of transmission is known as
   a. vector
   b. fomite
   c. nosocomial
   d. iatrogenic
7. A health care worker is accidentally punctured with a contaminated needle. This type of transmission is known as:
   a. vector
   b. fomite
   c. nosocomial
   d. iatrogenic
8. An outpatient develops a staphylococcal infection after a surgical procedure. This type of transmission is known as:
   a. vector
   b. fomite
   c. nosocomial
   d. more than one of the above, but not all
9. An infectious microbe can gain entrance into the human body by:
   a. ingression
   b. penetration
   c. both a and b
   d. neither a nor b
10. Hand washing uses which of the following methods of infection control?
   a. chemical
   b. physical
   c. sterile
   d. a and b

CHAPTER 18 ASEPTIC TECHNIQUES

1. A pacemaker prevents bradycardia by:
   1. sensing the patient's heartbeats.
   2. pacing the heart when it does not contract.
   3. producing electrical impulses.
      a. 1 and 2
      b. 1 and 3
      c. 2 and 3
      d. 1, 2, and 3

2. What type of catheter is the Foley?
   a. retention balloon
   b. straight
   c. coiled
   d. self-cleansing
3. When handling sterile gloves with a nonsterile hand, which of the following is not considered sterile?
   a. outside of the cuff
   b. inside of the cuff
   c. fingertips of the glove
   d. thumb of the glove
4. Outside air is prevented from entering the pleural cavity through the chest tube by the:
   a. collection chamber.
   b. water seal chamber.
   c. suction control chamber.
   d. first compartment.
5. The goal of good sterile technique is to:
   a. protect the health care worker from infection.
   b. remove all infected material.
   c. protect the patient from infection.
   d. remove all viable microorganisms.
6. The first rule of caring for a tracheostomy patient is:
   a. watch for secretions.
   b. establish communication.
   c. contact the nurse in charge of the patient.
   d. attempt to finish the procedure as quickly as possible.
7. The purpose of the surgical hand scrub is to:
   1. remove debris and transient microorganisms from the hands, nails, and forearms.
   2. destroy infected material.
   3. inhibit rapid rebound growth of microorganisms.
      a. 1 and 2
      b. 1 and 3
      c. 2 and 3
      d. 1, 2, and 3
8. All of the following are true in regard to Foley catheters EXCEPT:
   a. this type of catheter is held in place by an inflatable balloon at the end.
   b. this type of closed drainage system catheter is used for a long-tern use and sutured to the skin.
   c. this type of catheter is used primarily to empty the bladder.
   d. this type of catheter can be made of varying materials such as latex or plastic.
9. What parts of a gown are considered sterile?
   1. sleeves
   2. front from the waist up
   3. back from below the waist
      a. 1 and 2
      b. 1 and 3
      c. 2 and 3
      d. 1, 2, and 3
10. Neonatal portable radiography requires the most care to maintain asepsis; which one of the following will best ensure asepsis of the infant?

1. careful attention paid to everything that the radiographer comes in contact with and proper cleaning protocols followed.
2. hand washing after each patient
3. wiping down the machine before each patient
   a. 1 and 2
   b. 1 and 3
   c. 2 and 3
   d. 1, 2, and 3

CHAPTER 19 NONASEPTIC TECHNIQUES

not on test

1. The most common types of nasogastric tubes is:
   a. Levin.
   b. Salem-sump.
   c. Miller-Abbott.
   d. Cantor.
2. How can leakage from a double-lumen tube be prevented?
   a. Clamp with a hemostat.
   b. Clamp with a regular clamping device.
   c. Use a pistonlike syringe.
   d. Leakage is not a problem with a double-lumen tube.
3. Bedpans should be:
   a. rinsed between uses.
   b. sterilized between uses.
   c. disposed of after use.
   d. none of the above.
4. Hypertonic solution is used when:
   a. fluid must be of the same osmolarity as that of the interstitial spaces of the colon.
   b. stool must be softened.
   c. the patient cannot tolerate large amounts of fluid.
   d. infant safety is a primary concern.
5. The normal adult patient should be able to tolerate how much fluid from a cleansing enema?
   a. 200 mL
   b. 500 mL
   c. 1000 mL
   d. 1500 mL
6. What should be done if cramping occurs during a barium enema?
   a. The patient should be told to use deep oral breathing.
   b. The enema should be stopped.
   c. The bag should be raised.
   d. Both a and b should be done.
7. Desirable characteristics of a barium suspension include:
   1. rapid flow.
   2. good mucosal adhesion.
   3. thick layering.
   a. 1 only
   b. 1 and 2
   c. 1 and 3
   d. 1, 2, and 3
8. A postural drop in blood pressure can occur after a barium enema as a result of:
   a. a reaction from the barium
   b. dehydration

c. trapping of barium in the transverse colon
   d. none of the above
9. With a double-barrel colostomy, the proximal stoma delivers_____ and the distal stoma produces _____:
   a. stool/mucus
   b. mucus/stool
   c. mucus/flatus
   d. solids/fluids
10. Approximately what percentage of colostomy patients has recurrences of cancer?
    a. 10%
    b. 20%
    c. 30%
    d. 40%

CHAPTER 20 MEDICAL EMERGENCIES

1. In working with a patient, which of the following would be the first priority for attention?
   a. providing an open airway
   b. splinting a fractured extremity
   c. controlling bleeding
   d. treating shock
2. Which of the following signs or symptoms is typically associated with a deteriorating head injury?
   a. increasing pulse rate
   b. increasing respiratory rate
   c. lethargy
   d. thirst
3. Which of the following actions would help prevent a patient from going into shock?
   a. minimizing pain
   b. providing emotional support
   c. maintaining a normal body temperature
   d. all of the above
4. A patient suffering from hypoglycemia needs which of the following?
   a. rest
   b. insulin
   c. carbohydrates
   d. a and c
5. Where should the heel of the hand be placed when performing chest compressions during cardiopulmonary resuscitation on an adult?

 not on test

   a. near the sternal angle
   b. at the xiphoid process
   c. two fingers above the xiphoid process
   d. anywhere along the length of the sternum
6. *Syncope* is a medical term for which of the following?
   a. dizziness
   b. fainting
   c. hemorrhage
   d. nosebleed
7. Which of the following is typically associated with shock?
   a. decreasing pulse rate
   b. decreasing blood pressure
   c. fever
   d. flushed face

8. The Heimlich maneuver is used in response to which of the following situations?
   a. asthmatic crisis
   b. cardiac arrest
   c. choking
   d. wound dehiscence

9. How long can the brain be deprived of oxygen before cerebral function impairment is likely?
   a. 30 seconds
   b. 60 seconds
   c. 2 to 3 minutes
   d. 4 to 6 minutes

not on test

10. Which of the following actions is appropriate in handling a patient who begins a violent seizure?
    a. Restrain the patient in any way possible.
    b. Ensure an open airway, putting your hands into the victim's mouth if necessary.
    c. Attempt to prevent the patient from injuring himself or herself.
    d. All of the above are true.

CHAPTER 21 PHARMACOLOGY

1. Who is the person licensed to prepare and dispense drugs?
   a. nurse
   b. radiologist
   c. physician
   d. pharmacist

2. The name given to a drug manufactured by a specific company is the
   a. trade (brand) name
   b. chemical name
   c. generic name
   d. nonproprietary name

3. A drug that relieves pain without causing a loss of consciousness is a(an):
   a. sedative
   b. analgesic
   c. anesthetic
   d. hypnotic

4. The following is true of a schedule II drug:
   a. does not have a high potential for drug abuse
   b. has a currently accepted medical use
   c. has a lack of accepted safety for use
   d. will not lead to abuse of the drug or other substances.

not on test

5. What class of drug is Benadryl?
   a. diuretic
   b. antibiotic
   c. anticholinergic
   d. antihistamine

6. In case of emergency, a patient would be treated with the following arrhythmia drug:
   a. Adenosine
   b. Cardiazem
   c. Narcan
   d. both a and b

not on test

7. It is recommended that this medication used for type 2 diabetes be temporarily discontinued before the use of radiographic contrast agents.
   a. Glipizide
   b. Metformin
   c. Pioglitazone
   d. Sitagliptin

8. This agent used to treat anemia may transiently affect magnetic resonance diagnostic imaging studies for up to 3 months after the last dose.
   a. Canagliflozin
   b. Pregabalin
   c. Duloxetine
   d. Ferumoxytol

not on test

9. Which of the following reverses respiratory depression associated with opioids?
   a. Flumazenil
   b. Epinephrine
   c. Naloxone
   d. Atropine

10. Which of the following is classified as a general anesthetic?
    a. Propofol
    b. Xylocaine
    c. Fentanyl
    d. Enoxaparin

CHAPTER 22 PRINCIPLES OF DRUG ADMINISTRATION

1. Which are the appropriate methods to determine the *right* patient before drug administration?
   1. Confirm type of medication
   2. Check patient's identification band
   3. Ask the patient to verify name and/or date of birth
      a. 1 only
      b. 2 and 3
      c. 1 and 2
      d. All of the above

2. What is the appropriate next step, when the incorrect patient is identified?
   a. continue with the procedure
   b. make the correction on the patient's armband
   c. go with the patient to have another armband made with correct patient information
   d. call the ordering physician

3. Volume is measured in:
   1. milliliters.
   2. cubic centimeters.
   3. liters.
      a. 1 only
      b. 2 only
      c. 1 and 3
      d. 1, 2, and 3

not on test

4. If a drug is administered PO, the patient receives the medicine:
   a. subcutaneously.
   b. parenterally.

c. topically.
d. by mouth.

5. This method of drug delivery has a rapid onset because the drug is absorbed directly into the bloodstream.
   a. oral.
   b. topical
   c. sublingual
   d. parenteral

6. All of the following are methods to ensure safe injections EXCEPT:
   a. use of safety needles
   b. injecting a drug without a physician order
   c. following facility protocol
   d. correct patient identification

7 Parenteral drug administration includes all of the following routes except:
   a. Subcutaneous
   b. Sublingual
   c. Intravenous
   d. Intramuscular

8. Which of the following statements expresses the correct relation between lumen diameter and gauge number?
   a. As the diameter increases, the gauge number increases.
   b. As the diameter decreases, the gauge number decreases.
   c. As the diameter decreases, the gauge number increases.
   d. As the diameter increases, the gauge number stays the same.

9. When using an angiocath it is best to:
   a. use a bifurcated vein
   b. use a vein valve
   c. wash hands and use a clean work surface
   d. use a specialist

10. Which vein is best suitable for venipuncture?
    a. femoral vein
    b. popliteal vein
    c. cephalic vein
    d. brachial vein

CHAPTER 23 CONTRAST MEDIA AND INTRODUCTION TO RADIOPHARMACEUTICALS

1. Contrast media are used in radiographic imaging to:
   a. increase the radiographic density of the area of interest.
   b. enhance the subject contrast of the area of interest.
   c. decrease the radiographic density of the area of interest.
   d. lower the subject contrast of the area of interest.

2. Radiographic images that demonstrate few density differences define:
   a. low subject contrast
   b. high subject contrast
   c. low x-ray photon absorption
   d. high x-ray photon absorption

3. A negative contrast agent will:
   a. increase density and is radiopaque.
   b. decrease density and is radiopaque.
   c. decrease density and is radiolucent.
   d. increase density and is radiolucent.

4. A radiopharmaceutical is a:
   a. radioactive contrast agent.
   b. molecular imaging contrast agent.
   c. radiographic contrast agent.
   d. radioactive organ specific pharmaceutical.

5. Contrast media that dissociate into two molecular particles are known as:
   a. ionic agents.
   b. low osmolality agents.
   c. nonionic agents.
   d. oil-based agents.

6. Hydroxyl groups on nonionic water-soluble iodinated contrast media increase:
   a. osmotic effects.
   b. solubility.
   c. blood pressure.
   d. bronchospasm.

7. External contamination of a short-lived diagnostic radioisotope is a problem because it might:
   a. cause major harm to the patient and the caregiver.
   b. be misconstrued as a pathologic condition on an image.
   c. burn a patient.
   d. disable a gamma camera.

8. Which one of the following drugs should be discontinued 48 hours before and 48 hours after administration of water-soluble iodine contrast media?
   a. insulin
   b. glucagons
   c. beta-blockers
   d. metformin

9. What can be done to reduce allergic-like effects for a patient who will receive water-soluble iodine contrast media?
   a. premedicate with steroids and antihistamines
   b. give intravenous fluids
   c. instruct the patient to drink warm salt water before the procedure
   d. give a negative contrast agent with the iodinated medium

10. Which of the following acute reactions to contrast media usually requires no medical treatment?
    a. bronchospasm
    b. laryngeal edema
    c. urticaria
    d. seizures

CHAPTER 24 PROFESSIONAL ETHICS

1. A personal value system can be defined in terms of:
   a. virtues.
   b. values.
   c. ethical principles.
   d. morals.
   e. all of the above.

2. Professional ethics can be best defined as:
   a. reflective decision making.
   b. rules of right living.
   c. the science of rightness and wrongness of human conduct.

d. a common concern for collective self-discipline.

e. rules promulgated by professional societies.

3. Which of the following statements is NOT true?
   a. Ethics apply to specific groups.
   b. Laws apply to political subdivisions.
   c. Morals apply to individuals.
   d. Morals control individuals within a group.
   e. Ethics control a group from within.

4. Which of the following statements is true?
   a. Codes of ethics are usually written by individuals.
   b. Religious writings form the basis for ethical control.
   c. Codes of ethics are a form of legislation.
   d. Conscience controls individual morality.
   e. Laws provide an internal control for society.

5. Which of the following statements is NOT true?
   a. Ethical dilemmas may have competing moral principles.
   b. Ethical dilemmas involve decisions based on human values.
   c. Ethical dilemmas are easily solved by codes of ethics.
   d. Ethical dilemmas can be resolved by problem solving.
   e. Ethical dilemmas invite a wide range of personal opinions.

6. Moral rules are best applied to ethical dilemmas when:
   a. religious beliefs are strongly held.
   b. religious beliefs are not strongly held.
   c. the ethical dilemma is very narrow in scope.
   d. the ethical dilemma is very wide in scope.
   e. all individuals agree to use moral rules.

7. Action to benefit others is defined as:
   a. veracity
   b. fidelity
   c. beneficence
   d. justice
   e. autonomy

8. Which is NOT a step in the problem-solving process?
   a. identifying the problem
   b. developing alternative solutions
   c. selecting the best solution
   d. defending your selection
   e. determining ethical sanctions

9. The strict observance of promises or duties is defined as:
   a. fidelity
   b. justice
   c. autonomy
   d. confidentiality
   e. veracity

10. Generally accepted customs of right living and conduct are:
    a. codes
    b. morals
    c. laws
    d. ethics
    e. rules

CHAPTER 25 HEALTH RECORDS AND HEALTH INFORMATION MANAGEMENT

1. Which of the following is not a function of a hospital health information management department?
   a. coding of diagnoses and operative procedures and diagnosis-related group (DRG) assignment
   b. documenting relevant patient information in the medical record
   c. quality management and performance improvement activities
   d. appropriate release of medical information

2. The prospective payment system is a payment system based on which of the following?
   a. the DRG or the ambulatory patient classification (APC)
   b. the coding system based on the *International Classification of Diseases*, 10th revision, Clinical Modification (ICD-10-CM)
   c. the Current Procedural Terminology (CPT) coding system
   d. the resource-based relative value system (RBRVS)

3. Which of the following is an example of an organization that accredits hospitals and other health care institutions in the United States?
   a. American Hospital Association
   b. American Medical Association
   c. The Joint Commission
   d. American College of Radiology

4. The chief complaint, included in a patient's history, is a statement made by the:
   a. physician.
   b. patient.
   c. admitting officer.
   d. admitting nurse.

5. The Health Insurance Portability and Accountability Act of 1996 (HIPAA) legislation affects radiology and other hospital departments by its focus on:
   a. patient record confidentiality.
   b. facility reimbursement.
   c. quality management and performance improvement.
   d. risk management.

6. Which of the following is not required to be included in a patient's health record?
   a. medical history
   b. radiology reports
   c. incident reports
   d. physical examination report

7. Criteria used in performance improvement activities must be all of the following EXCEPT:
   a. clinically valid.
   b. diagnosis or procedure oriented.
   c. generally acceptable to department staff.
   d. written.

8. Assessment of problems in performance improvement activities must be:
   a. ongoing.
   b. physician directed.
   c. subjective.
   d. objective.

9. In making a correction to an entry in the paper health record, the documenter should:
   a. line out the error, authenticate, and insert correct information.

b. erase the incorrect information, and insert correct information.

c. leave the incorrect entry alone, and add the new correct information.

d. remove the incorrect page from the record, and begin a new page of documentation.

10. The organization (chart order, forms) of a hospital patient record is determined by:

a. the accrediting body's suggested format.

b. Medicare regulations.

c. the American Hospital Association–suggested format

d. the hospital's own preference

CHAPTER 26 MEDICAL LAW

1. If a technologist threatens a patient during the course of a procedure and has an apparent immediate ability to perform the threatened act, which of the following torts may be claimed?

a. assault

b. battery

c. negligence

d. false imprisonment

2. The legal theory of respondeat superior requires that:

a. the employee is responsible for the actions of the employee.

b. each person is responsible for his or her superior.

c. the employer is responsible for the employee's actions.

d. the employee is responsible for the employer's actions.

3. A technologist who has completed a procedure on a patient leaves the area grumbling, "I hate to do AIDS patients because I am afraid of catching the disease." A member of the housekeeping staff hears the technologist and asks who has AIDS. The technologist responds by giving the patient's name and room number. After this incident, housekeeping personnel refuse to clean the room. One person from housekeeping tells the story to members of the housekeeper's church, where the patient is also a member. After learning of the patient's condition, the church asks the patient not to return. What type of complaint might be brought against the technologist?

a. negligence

b. defamation

c. assault

d. false imprisonment

4. The claim of false imprisonment requires the patient to show proof that the technologist restrained his or her freedom without consent. The defenses a technologist may raise include all of the following EXCEPT the:

a. risk that the patient was going to hurt himself or herself.

b. risk that the patient was going to hurt the technologist.

c. life-threatening condition of the patient's health.

d. need for motionless images.

5. In a case in which the legal theory of res ipsa loquitur is being raised, the evidence presented must show all the following elements EXCEPT that the:

a. injury would not have occurred except for negligence.

b. patient contributed to his or her injury

c. defendant was in complete control.

d. patient did not contribute to his or her injury in any way.

6. A consent form has been signed by a patient who will be undergoing an excretory urogram. A witness should sign the form after the patient. Who is the best witness?

a. a member of the patient's family

b. the radiographer performing the procedure

c. a ward clerk who has no relationship with the patient or the procedure

d. the patient's physician

7. Informed consent requires that the patient be given enough information to make an educated decision about his or her health care. The information the patient needs to make this decision includes all of the following EXCEPT:

a. how the procedure will be performed.

b. the benefits of the procedure.

c. the alternatives to the procedure.

d. the cost of the procedure.

8. What complaint may be brought against a technologist if he or she touches a patient in any way without the patient's permission?

a. assault

b. battery

c. false imprisonment

d. harassment

9. A radiographer is performing an abdominal series on a patient from the emergency department. To complete the examination, the patient must be moved from a supine to an upright position using the remote control on the table. During this movement, the patient falls from the table and suffers a fractured hip. A complaint of negligence is brought against both the radiographer and the hospital. The elements that the patient (plaintiff) must prove include all the following EXCEPT:

a. a breach of the duty to the patient.

b. an injury.

c. a direct causal relation between the breach of duty and the injury.

d. that the radiographer acted outside of his or her scope of practice.

10. A patient consents to a procedure in the radiology department, but after it has started, he decides that he does not want the procedure completed. The technologist should:

a. stop immediately.

b. complete the procedure because the patient may not revoke consent once it is given.

c. stop the procedure as soon as it is safe to do so.

d. none of the above should be done.

Note: Page numbers followed by "f" indicate figures and "t" indicate tables "b" indicate boxes.